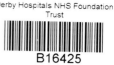
This book is due for return on or before the last date shown below.

# RENAL CELL CARCINOMA

# RENAL CELL CARCINOMA

**Brian I. Rini, MD**
Department of Solid Tumor Oncology and Urology
Cleveland Clinic Taussig Cancer Institute
Cleveland Clinic
Associate Professor of Medicine
Case Western Reserve University
Lerner College of Medicine
Cleveland, Ohio

**Steven C. Campbell, MD, PhD**
Professor of Surgery
Glickman Urological and Kidney Institute
Cleveland Clinic
Cleveland, Ohio

2009
PEOPLE'S MEDICAL PUBLISHING HOUSE
SHELTON, CONNECTICUT

People's Medical Publishing House
2 Enterprise Drive, Suite 509
Shelton, CT 06484
Tel: 203-402-0646
Fax: 203-402-0854
E-mail: info@pmph-usa.com

© 2009 BC Decker Inc

09 10 11 12/PMPH/9 8 7 6 5 4 3 2 1

ISBN 978-1-60795-003-5
Printed in China by People's Medical Publishing House of China
Copy editor/typesetter: diacriTech; Cover designer: Mary McKeon

## Sales and Distribution

*Canada*
McGraw-Hill Ryerson Education
Customer Care
300 Water St
Whitby, Ontario L1N 9B6
Canada
Tel: 1-800-565-5758
Fax: 1-800-463-5885
www.mcgrawhill.ca

*Foreign Rights*
John Scott & Company
International Publisher's Agency
P.O. Box 878
Kimberton, PA 19442
USA
Tel: 610-827-1640
Fax: 610-827-1671

*Japan*
United Publishers Services Limited
1-32-5 Higashi-Shinagawa
Shinagawa-ku, Tokyo 140-0002
Japan
Tel: 03-5479-7251
Fax: 03-5479-7307
Email: kakimoto@ups.co.jp

*United Kingdom, Europe,*
*Middle East, Africa*
McGraw Hill Education
Shoppenhangers Road
Maidenhead
Berkshire, SL6 2QL
England
Tel: 44-0-1628-502500
Fax: 44-0-1628-635895
www.mcgraw-hill.co.uk

*Singapore, Thailand, Philippines,*
*Indonesia, Vietnam, Pacific Rim, Korea*
McGraw-Hill Education
60 Tuas Basin Link
Singapore 638775
Tel: 65-6863-1580
Fax: 65-6862-3354
www.mcgraw-hill.com.sg

*Australia, New Zealand*
Elsevier Australia
Tower 1, 475 Victoria Avenue
Chatswood NSW 2067
Australia
Tel: 0-9422-8553
Fax: 0-9422-8562
www.elsevier.com.au

*Brazil*
Tecmedd Importadora e Distribuidora
de Livros Ltda.
Avenida Maurilio Biagi 2850
City Ribeirao, Rebeirao, Preto SP
Brazil
CEP: 14021-000
Tel: 0800-992236
Fax: 16-3993-9000
Email: tecmedd@tecmedd.com.br

*India, Bangladesh, Pakistan,*
*Sri Lanka, Malaysia*
CBS Publishers
4819/X1 Prahlad Street 24
Ansari Road, Darya, New Delhi-110002
India
Tel: 91-11-23266861/67
Fax: 91-11-23266818
Email:cbspubs@vsnl.com

*People's Republic of China*
PMPH
Bldg 3, 3rd District
Fangqunyuan, Fangzhuang
Beijing 100078
P.R. China
Tel: 8610-67653342
Fax: 8610-67691034
www.pmph.com

# Contents

# Preface

Kidney cancer has been re-energized by novel therapeutics and innovative surgical advances. This clinical atlas of Renal Cell Carcinoma (RCC) contains timely and informative updates about all aspects of the diagnosis and management of RCC. Front and center is the biology of renal cell carcinoma, which has been greatly elucidated over the last few years and has laid the groundwork for discovery of therapeutically-relevant pathways. Both the immunobiology of kidney cancer, which has been of historic interest, as well as new pathways such as those involving vascular endothelial growth factor (VEGF) and mammalian target of rapamycin (mTOR), are extensively detailed. Updates on ever-changing pathologic analysis of RCC are discussed and are of clinical interest. The bulk of the chapters in this Atlas deal with the practical management of the continuum of kidney cancer, ranging from the dilemma of the small renal mass, through locally advanced disease and finally, to the metastatic patient.

Different treatment approaches are discussed within the context of each of these clinical scenarios, and surgical and therapeutic advances are highlighted. In addition, special populations such as patients requiring palliative care, those with brain or bone metastasis and those with inherited renal cell carcinoma are expertly discussed.

We trust that you will find this atlas up-to-date and informative. We wish to express our sincere appreciation to a truly distinguished set of authors for sharing their time, knowledge and skills in producing this volume which, ultimately, attempts to achieve the goal of educating physicians about renal cell carcinoma with the intent of advancing the care of kidney cancer patients.

Brian I. Rini, MD

Steven C. Campbell, MD, PhD
November 2008

# Contributors

KAMRAN AHRAR, MD
Department of Urology
University of Texas
MD Anderson Cancer Center
Houston, Texas

CHIRAG J. AMIN, MD
Indiana Hemophilia and Thrombosis Center
Indianapolis, Indiana

ANDREW J. ARMSTRONG, MD, ScM
Duke Comprehensive Cancer Center
Departments of Medicine & Surgery
Durham, North Carolina

BERTRAND BILLEMONT, MD
Department of Medical Oncology
Cochin Hospital
Paris, France

ARIE BELLDEGRUN, MD, FACS
Department of Urology
University of California, Los Angeles School
    of Medicine
Los Angeles, California

STEVEN C. CAMPBELL, MD, PhD
Department of Urological Oncology
Glickman Urological and Kidney Institute
Cleveland Clinic
Cleveland, Ohio

DANIEL R. CARRIZOSA, MD, MS
Department of Internal Medicine
University of North Carolina at Chapel Hill
Chapel Hill, North Carolina

DAVID Y. T. CHEN, MD
Fox Chase Cancer Center
Temple University School of Medicine
Department of Urology
Philadelphia, Pennsylvania

TONI K. CHOUEIRI, MD
Harvard University
Department of Genitourinary Oncology
Boston, Massachusetts

MELLAR P. DAVIS, MD, FCCP
Harry R. Horowitz Center for Palliative Medicine
Taussig Cancer Center
Cleveland Clinic
Cleveland, Ohio

TIM EISEN, PhD, FRCP
University of Cambridge
Department of Oncology
Cambridge, England

CHRISTOPHER P. EVANS, MD, FACS
Department of Urology
University of California
Davis School of Medicine
Sacramento, California

JAMES H. FINKE, PhD
Department of Immunology
Lerner Research Institute
Cleveland, Ohio

KEITH T. FLAHERTY, MD
Abramson Cancer Center
University of Pennsylvania
Philadelphia, Pennsylvania

KYLE A. FURGE, PhD
Department of Computational Biology
Van Andel Research Institute
Grand Rapids, Michigan

DANIEL J. GEORGE, MD
Departments of Medicine and Surgery
Duke University Medical Center
Durham, North Carolina

PAUL A. GODLEY, MD, PhD, MPP
Department of Medicine
University of North Carolina at Chapel Hill
Chapel Hill, North Carolina

GUILHERME GODOY, MD
Department of Urology
New York University School of Medicine
New York, New York

BRIAN R. HERTS, MD
Department of Radiology
Cleveland Clinic Lerner College of Medicine
Cleveland, Ohio

GARY R. HUDES, MD
Genitourinary Malignancies Program
Department of Medical Oncology
Fox Chase Cancer Center
Philadelphia, Pennsylvania

THOMAS E. HUTSON, DO, PharmD, FACP
Baylor-Sammons Cancer Center
Dallas, Texas

HASSAN IZZEDINE, MD, PhD
Pitie-Salpetriere Hospital
Department of Nephrology
Paris, France

WILLIAM Y. KIM, MD
Department of Hematology/Oncology
Lineberger Comprehensive Cancer Center
Chapel Hill, North Carolina

JENNIFER S. KO, MD
Departments of Hematology and Oncology
Cleveland Clinic
Cleveland, Ohio

VITALY MARGULIS, MD
Department of Urology
The University of Texas
MD Anderson Cancer Center
Houston, Texas

SURENA F. MATIN, MD, FACS
Department of Urology
University of Texas
MD Anderson Cancer Center
Houston, Texas

DAVID F. MCDERMOTT, MD
Department of Medicine
Beth Israel Deaconess Medical Center
Boston, Massachusetts

M. DROR MICHAELSON, MD, PhD
Department of Medicine
Massachusetts General Hospital
Boston, Massachusetts

KATHERINE L. NATHANSON, MD
University of Pennsylvania School of Medicine
Department of Medicine
Philadelphia, Pennsylvania

ERIC C. NELSON, MD
Department of Urology
University of California
Davis School of Medicine
Sacramento, California

ANDREW C. NOVICK, MD
Glickman Urological and Kidney Institute
Cleveland Clinic
Cleveland, Ohio

REBECCA L. O'MALLEY, MD
Department of Urology
New York University
New York, New York

ALLAN PANTUCK, MD, MS, FACS
Department of Urology
University of California, Los Angeles
Los Angeles, California

AHMAD RAHMAN, MB, BS
Royal Marsden Hospital
London, England

W. KIMRYN RATHMELL, MD, PHD
Departments of Hematology & Oncology
Lineberger Comprehensive Cancer Center
University of North Carolina at Chapel Hill
Chapel Hill, North Carolina

BRIAN I. RINI, MD
Department of Solid Tumor Oncology and Urology
Cleveland Clinic Taussig Cancer Institute
Case Western Reserve University
Cleveland, Ohio

OLIVIER RIXE, MD, PHD
National Cancer Institute
Medical Oncology Branch
Bethesda, Maryland

RENEE N. SALAS, BS
Cleveland Clinic Lerner College of Medicine
Case Western University
Cleveland, Ohio

ABRAHAM B. SCHWARZBERG, MD
Department of Medicine
Massachusetts General Hospital
Boston, Massachusetts

BRIAN SHUCH, MD
Department of Urology
University of California, Los Angeles
Los Angeles, California

GURU SONPAVDE, MD
Department of Medicine
Baylor College of Medicine
Houston, Texas

ANDREW J. STEPHENSON, MD, FRCS(C)
Department of Urology
Cleveland Clinic
Cleveland, Ohio

SAMIR S. TANEJA, MD
Department of Urology
New York University School of Medicine
New York, New York

BIN T. TEH, MD, PHD
Department of Cancer Genetics
Van Andel Research Institute
Grand Rapids, Michigan

BIN S. TEH, MD
Department of Radiation Oncology
Methodist Hospital
Houston, Texas

FREDERIC THIBAULT, MD
Pitie-Salpetriere Hospital
Department of Urology
Paris, France

ROBERT G. UZZO, MD, FACS
Department of Surgery
Fox Chase Cancer Center
Philadelphia, Pennsylvania

YU-NING WONG, MD, MSCE
Department of Medical Oncology
Fox Chase Cancer Center
Philadelphia, Pennsylvania

CHRISTOPHER G. WOOD, MD, FACS
Department of Urology
University of Texas MD Anderson Cancer Center
Houston, Texas

MING ZHOU, MD, PHD
Department of Pathology
Cleveland Clinic
Cleveland, Ohio

# Pathology of Renal Cell Carcinomas

**MING ZHOU, MD, PHD**

Different types of tumors have been described in the kidney. Arising from the renal tubular epithelial cells, renal cell carcinoma (RCC) makes up over 90% of the primary tumors in adult kidneys. It comprises a group of heterogenous diseases with divergent clinical, pathologic, and molecular characteristics. Traditionally, RCC has been classified based primarily on histology. Specific genetic alterations in renal tumors have been increasingly elucidated. Hence, 2004 World Health Organization (WHO) classification of renal tumors (Table 1) also included these genetic findings aiming to put forward a pathologic classification scheme that combines both morphologic and molecular features of RCC.[1] Furthermore, the association of several RCC subtypes with specific inherited cancer syndromes was recognized. In this chapter, we review the pathologic and molecular characteristics of different histologic subtypes of RCC, as well as the pathologic prognostic parameters.

## Table 1. 2004 WORLD HEALTH ORGANIZATION CLASSIFICATION OF RENAL CELL NEOPLASMS

Renal cell carcinoma
    Clear cell renal cell carcinoma
    Multilocular clear cell renal cell carcinoma
    Papillary renal cell carcinoma
    Chromophobe renal cell carcinoma
    Carcinoma of the collecting ducts of Bellini
    Renal medullary carcinoma
    Xp11 translocation carcinomas
    Carcinoma associated with neuroblastoma
    Mucinous tubular and spindle cell carcinoma
    Renal cell carcinoma, unclassified
Papillary adenoma/renal cortical adenoma
Oncocytoma

## HISTOLOGIC SUBTYPES OF RCC

### Clear Cell Type

Accounting for 60 to 70% of all RCCs, clear cell type (clear cell RCC) is the most common histologic subtype. It predominantly affects male patients (male:female ratio = 2:1), with a peak incidence in the sixth and seventh decades of life.[2] The majority of clear cell RCC arises sporadically, with < 5% of the cases presenting as part of the inherited cancer syndromes,[3] including von Hippel-Lindau syndrome, tuberous sclerosis (TS), Birt-Hogg-Dube syndrome, and constitutional chromosomal 3 translocation syndrome. As a general rule, familial clear cell RCC presents at a younger age and is more likely to be multifocal and bilateral.

### Pathology

Most clear cell RCC presents as a solitary and well-demarcated mass. Hemorrhage, necrosis, cystic degeneration, and calcification are frequently found, especially in larger tumors. It is characteristically golden yellow due to rich lipid content of the tumor cells (Figure 1A). Multifocal and bilateral tumors occur in < 5% of sporadic cases, but they are more often associated with inherited cancer syndromes.

Microscopically, several architectural patterns, including solid, alveolar, and acinar, and occasionally cystic, tubular, or pseudopapillary, can be found in clear cell RCC, and more than one pattern can be seen in one tumor. The tumor cells have clear cytoplasm due to the loss of cytoplasmic lipid and glycogen during tissue processing and slide preparation (Figure 1B).[4]

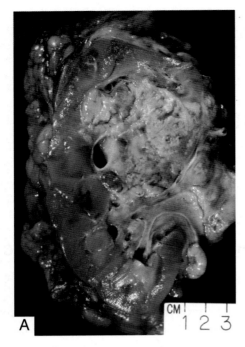

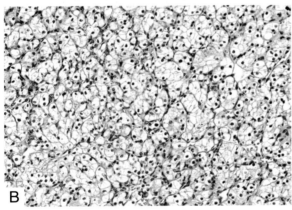

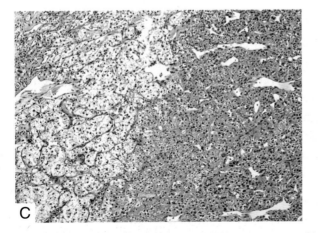

**Figure 1.** Clear cell renal cell carcinoma (RCC) forms a mass with distinctive yellow or light orange color due to rich lipid content in the tumor cells (A). It is composed of compact nests of tumor cells with clear cytoplasm separated by delicate arborizing vasculature (B). High-grade component of a clear cell RCC has more eosinophilic and granular cytoplasm (C), right half of the image.

It contains a regular network of thin-walled blood vessels, a distinct and consistent feature that is diagnostically quite helpful. High-grade clear cell RCC often lose the cytoplasmic clarity and acquires more eosinophilic and granular cytoplasm (Figure 1C). Such tumors were termed *granular cell*–type RCC in the past. Although some RCCs with granular cytoplasm are now classified as clear cell RCC, many are of other histologic subtypes. Therefore, granular cell RCC is not considered a specific subtype. The term is antiquated, and its use is discouraged.

### Genetics

Chromosome 3p alterations are detected in vast majority of sporadic clear cell RCC.[5–7] At least three different regions on 3p are implicated, including 3p25-6, which harbors, among others, von Hippel-Lindau (*VHL*) gene; 3p21-22 (including *RASSF1A* and *DRR1*); and 3p11-12 (*FHIT*). Duplication of 5q22~qter is the second most common cytogenetic finding and may be associated with better prognosis. Other cytogenetic alterations involve chromosomes 6q, 8p, 9, 11q, 14q, 17p, 18q, 19p.[8]

Mutations in *VHL* gene has been found in 22 to 71% of sporadic clear cell RCC[9,10] Inactivation of *VHL* gene by promoter hypermethylation is seen in another 20% of cases. Together, inactivation of *VHL* gene by different mechanisms occurs in > 70% of sporadic clear cell RCC. Therefore, it seems that inactivation of the *VHL* gene plays a critical role in the development of clear cell RCC.

### Multilocular Cystic RCC

Multilocular cystic RCC (MLCRCC) is an uncommon (< 5%) variant of clear cell RCC.[11,12] These tumors form well-circumscribed, encapsulated, and entirely cystic masses (Figure 2A). Microscopically, it is composed of variably sized cysts that are lined with one or several layers of flat or plump clear cells (Figure 2B). No expansile cellular nodules are allowed. The nuclei are almost always of low grade with dense chromatin. If strict diagnostic criteria are applied, MLCRCC has a favorable prognosis. No local or distant metastasis has been documented after complete surgical resection.[11]

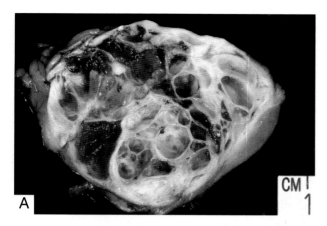

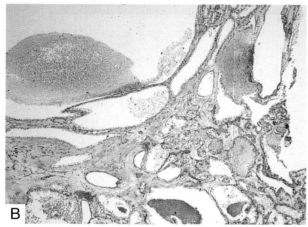

**Figure 2.** Multilocular cystic renal cell carcinoma is well circumscribed with a fibrous capsule in this partial nephrectomy specimen. It consists entirely of cysts of variable sizes (A). The cystic septa are thin without solid component. Microscopically, the cysts are lined with one or several layers of tumor cells with clear cytoplasm and uniformly small, dense, and low-grade nuclei (B).

## Papillary Type

Papillary type RCC (PRCC) accounts for 10 to 15% of RCCs.[2] The gender and age distributions are similar to those of clear cell RCC. However, PRCC has a better prognosis than the latter with a 5-year survival approaching 90% in some series. However, high-grade variants can behave in a highly aggressive manner.

### Pathology

Grossly, PRCC presents as a well-circumscribed mass with a pseudocapsule. Hemorrhage and necrosis are frequently seen, and some tumors appear entirely necrotic and friable (Figure 3A). Bilateral and multifocal tumors are more common in PRCC

than in other subtypes. Microscopically, PRCC has variable proportions of papillae, tubulopapillae, and tubules. The papillae characteristically contain delicate fibrovascular cores expanded with foamy histiocytes (Figure 3B). Necrosis, hemorrhage, hemosiderin deposition in tumor cells, macrophages, stromal cells, and psammomatous calcification are common.

Two types of PRCC are recognized based on the histology.[13] Accounting for about two-thirds of PRCC, type I tumor cells contains papillae that are lined with single layer of tumor cells with scant pale cytoplasm and low-grade nuclei (Figure 3B). In contrast, type II tumor cells have abundant eosinophilic cytoplasm and large pseudostratified nuclei with prominent nucleoli (Figure 3C). Patients with type I PRCC have a better prognosis than those with type II tumor.

### Genetics

Chromosomal gain, including trisomy or tetrasomy 7 and 17, and loss of Y chromosome are the most common cytogenetic changes in PRCC.[5,14] Loss of heterozygosity at 9p13 is associated with shorter survival.[15] Type I and II PRCCs have distinct genetic features, with 7p and 17p gains more commonly seen in type I tumors.[16] Patterns of allelic imbalance also differ between type I and II tumors.[17]

## Chromophobe Type

Chromophobe type RCC (chromophobe RCC) accounts for approximately 5% of RCCs.[2] The prognosis is significantly better than that of clear cell RCC, with mortality < 10%. Most cases are sporadic although rare familial cases are associated with Birt-Hogg-Dube syndrome.[3]

### Pathology

Chromophobe RCC is usually solitary and forms a circumscribed and nonencapsulated mass with homogenous light brown cut surface (Figure 4A). The tumor cells are large and polygonal and have finely reticulated cytoplasm due to numerous

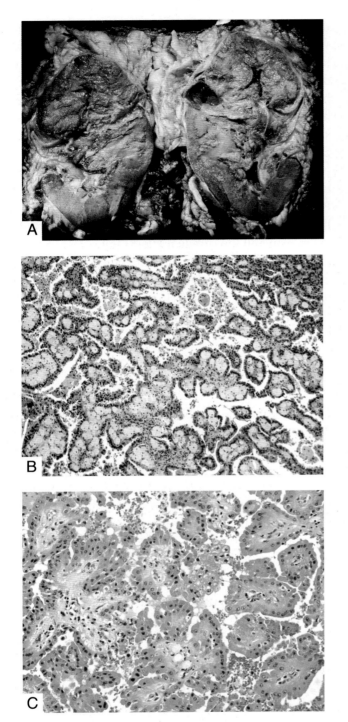

Figure 3. Papillary renal cell carcinoma has a tumor capsule and is entirely necrotic (A). Type I tumors are composed of papillae covered by a single layer of tumor cells with scant cytoplasm. The fibrovascular cores are expanded with foamy histiocytes (B). In contrast, type II tumor cells have abundant eosinophilic cytoplasm and large pseudostratified nuclei with prominent nucleoli (C).

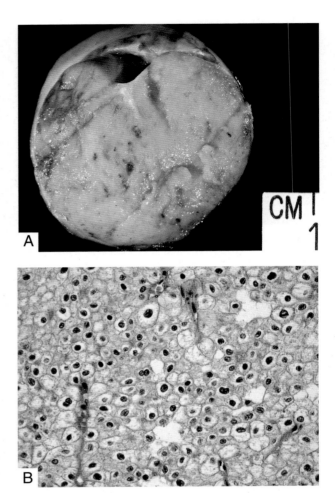

Figure 4. Chromophobe renal cell carcinoma forms a circumscribed nonencapsulated mass with a homogenous light brown cut surface (A). The large and polygonal tumor cells have finely reticulated cytoplasm, prominent cell border, and irregular nuclei with perinuclear clearing (B).

cytoplasmic microvesicles, prominent cell border resembling plant cells, and irregular, often wrinkled, nuclei with perinuclear clearing (Figure 4B).

Chromophobe RCC with these features is referred to as classical type. Not infrequently the tumor comprises predominantly of cells with intensely eosinophilic cytoplasm, hence termed *eosinophilic* variant.[18] However, there is no difference in the clinical characteristics between the two variants, and such distinction is purely for the purpose of pathologic diagnosis. Chromophobe RCC, especially the eosinophilic variant, should be distinguished from renal oncocytoma, a benign renal neoplasm with similar, sometimes overlapping, histology. The distinction can usually be made based on histologic examination, although immunohistochemistry or cytogenetic studies may be required in difficult cases. One such test is Hale's colloidal iron stain that reacts with the mucopolysaccharide content of microvesicles of tumor cells in chromophobe RCC, but not in other neoplasms, including oncocytoma.[19]

## Genetics

Chromophobe RCC harbors extensive chromosomal loss, most commonly involving chromosomes 1, 2, 6, 10, 13, 17, and 21.[8] Occasionally, chromophobe RCC can occur in Birt-Hogg-Dube syndrome, an autosomal dominant disorder characterized by mutations in Birt-Hogg-Dube (*BHD*) gene, *folliculin*, on 17p11.2.[20] However, *BHD* mutations are rarely found in sporadic chromophobe RCC.

## Carcinoma of the Collecting Ducts of Bellini

Carcinoma of the collecting ducts of Bellini (CDC) is a rare (< 1% of renal tumors) and poorly defined entity. Typically, it is centrally located and forms a firm gray mass with infiltrative borders. The highly pleomorphic tumor cells form irregular tubules and/or tubulopapillae that infiltrate in a desmoplastic stroma (Figure 5). Only very limited genetic data are available.[21] The diagnosis of CDC is one of exclusion as CDC may morphologically resemble other poorly differentiated carcinomas such as high-grade RCC or urothelial carcinoma, and these entities should be ruled out before rendering a diagnosis of CDC.

Two recent studies from Japan and Europe reaffirmed that CDC is a highly aggressive disease with grave outcomes.[22,23] It usually presents at advanced stage, with a high rate of distant metastasis at the time of diagnosis. Standard gemcitabine- and carboplatin-based chemotherapy is ineffective for metastatic or recurrent lesions. However, CDC is no more lethal than the stage-matched clear cell RCC, with similar cancer-specific survival in nephrectomized patients.[22]

## Renal Medullary Carcinoma

Renal medullary carcinoma (RMC) is an exceedingly rare and highly aggressive renal tumor of renal medulla, occurring in patients with sickle cell trait; therefore, most patients are of African heritage in the United States, and RMC is referred to as the "seventh sickle cell nephropathy."[24a] The tumor comprises high-grade tumor cells arranged in solid sheets or more commonly in a reticular pattern with microcystic or yolk sac–like areas. The stroma is desmoplastic (Figure 6) and resembles CDC histologically, although the latter typically occurs in older patients without sickle cell trait. RMC also shares similarities with high-grade urothelial carcinoma, given its central location, infiltrative pattern, and high-grade cytology.[24] Most RMCs do

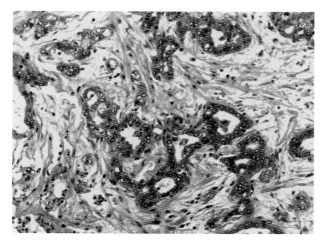

**Figure 5.** Carcinoma of the collecting ducts consists of high-grade tumor cells forming complex and angulated tubules or tubulopapillary structures embedded in a remarkably desmoplastic stroma.

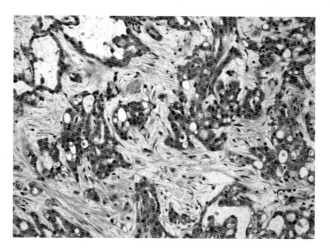

**Figure 6.** Renal medullary carcinoma comprises high-grade tumor cells arranged in irregular nests with microcystic formation. The stroma is desmoplastic.

not respond to chemotherapy or radiation therapy. However, two recent publications reported three adolescent and young adult patients who responded to cisplatin or carboplatin in combination with gemcitabine and paclitaxel.[25,26] The prognosis is dismal, although rare cases of long-term survival have been reported, raising the question whether young patients with sickle cell traits should be surveyed closely in order to facilitate early detection of RMC in these patients.[24]

## Mucinous Tubular and Spindle Cell Carcinoma

In contrast to the male predominance in other RCC subtypes, mucinous tubular and spindle cell carcinoma (MTSCC) predominantly affects female patients, with a male to female ratio of 1:4. It has a wide age range of 17 to 82 years (mean 53 years). On gross examination, the tumor appears as well-circumscribed, homogeneous, tan-white-pinkish lesion, sometimes centered in the renal medulla. As its name implies, microscopically, MTSCC is composed of elongated cords and collapsed tubules with slit-like spaces embedded in a lightly basophilic myxoid background (Figure 7). The tumor cells are usually spherical or oval with scant cytoplasm and low-grade nuclear features.[1,27,28] Tumors with mucin-poor histology and either tubular- or spindle-cell predominance may be mistaken for the solid

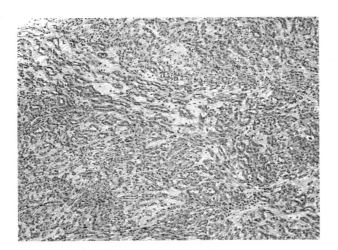

**Figure 7.** Mucinous tubular and spindle cell carcinoma is composed of elongated cords and collapsed tubules with slit-like spaces embedded in a lightly basophilic myxoid background microscopically. The tumor has low-grade nuclear features.

variant of PRCC.[29] Immunohistochemically, it also shares similar staining patterns of AMACR, CK7, and EMA with PRCC.[30] These findings initially raised the possibility that MTSCC and PRCC are related tumors. However, such speculation is not supported by the limited cytogenetic results. A few cases showed multiple numerical chromosome aberrations, but no clear-cut karyotypic aberration pattern is so far discernible.[13] However, the chromosomal gains of 7 and 17 and loss of Y characteristic of PRCC, and 3p alterations typical of clear cell RCC, have not been demonstrated in MTSCC.[31,32] The prognosis seems favorable, with majority of the patients free of disease after surgical resection.

## Renal Carcinoma Associated with Xp11.2 Translocations/*TFE3* Gene Fusions

RCC associated with Xp11.2 translocation/*TFE3* gene fusion (Xp11.2 RCC) is a distinct clinico-pathologic entity defined by the chromosomal translocation involving *TFE3* gene on chromosome Xp11.2 that results in overexpression of the TFE3 protein.[33] The translocation partner genes discovered so far include *PRCC* on 1q21, *ASPL* on 17q26, and *PSL* on 1p34, and *NonO* on Xq12.

Grossly, Xp11.2 RCC resembles clear cell RCC. The morphology varies with different chromosomal translocations; however, the most distinctive histologic feature is clear cell–lined pseudopapillary structures with hyaline nodules and psammomatous calcification frequently present within the fibrovascular cores (Figure 8A). A nested pattern made up of cells with voluminous eosinophilic cytoplasm is commonly seen. The diagnosis can be confirmed by positive nuclear immunostain for TFE3 (Figure 8B).

Xp11.2 typically affects children. Although RCC accounts for < 5% of pediatric renal tumors, Xp11.2 RCC makes up a significant proportion of these cases. The RCC with *ASPL-TFE3* translocation characteristically presents at advanced stage and also with lymph node metastasis but often pursues an indolent clinical course.[34] Recent studies show that Xp11.2 RCC also affects adult patients, with a striking female predominance. Similar to its pediatric counterpart, Xp11.2 RCC presents with

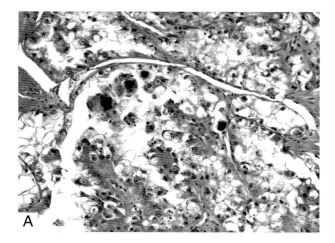

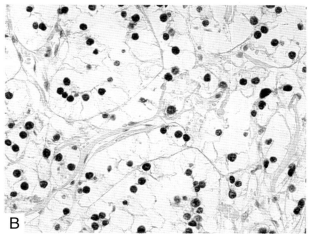

**Figure 8.** ASPL-TFE3 renal cell carcinoma with t(X;17) (p11.2;q25) consists of nested to pseudopapillary structure–lined tumor cells with abundant clear, sometimes eosinophilic, cytoplasm. Psammomatous calcification is also present (A). The tumor cells are positive for nuclear TFE3 protein by immunostain (B).

lymph node metastasis at advanced stage in majority of the cases. Unlike its pediatric counterparts, the adult disease often follows a very aggressive clinical course, with a higher mortality within 2 years of surgery.[35,36]

## Carcinoma Associated with Neuroblastoma

Rarely, RCC occurs in the long-term survivors of neuroblastoma.[37] All affected children were diagnosed with neuroblastoma at 2 years of age or younger, and the majority had advanced-stage neuroblastoma. RCC was diagnosed at age ranging from 5 to 14 years and occurred after a period of 3 to 11.5 years (average 9 years) following the neuroblastoma diagnosis. Although some authors have attributed this association to radiation or chemotherapy prescribed for neuroblastoma, genetic predisposition is also implicated since some patients had neither therapy. Morphologically, many of these tumors are typical clear cell RCC. However, some tumors have solid and papillary architecture with oncocytoid cells. Little is known about the molecular characteristics of these tumors.

## Unclassified Type

Two to 5% of RCCs do not fit into any of the subtypes in the 2004 WHO classification; hence are termed *RCC, unclassified type*. It is important to understand that RCC of unclassified type is a diagnostic category, rather than a true biologic entity. It represents a heterogeneous group of tumors with little in common in terms of clinical, morphologic, or genetic features. As our understanding of RCC increases, this category is destined to diminish and perhaps eventually will disappear.

## Papillary Adenoma

According to WHO definition, papillary adenomas are epithelial neoplasms with papillary or tubular architecture, < 5 mm in size, and with low-grade nuclei. They are the most common renal cell neoplasm, frequently as incidental findings in nephrectomy and autopsy specimens. Its incidence increases with age and also in long-term dialysis patients with acquired renal cystic disease or in scarred kidneys in patients with chronic pyelonephritis or renal vascular disease. Papillary adenomas are benign.

## Pathology

Papillary adenomas appear as small (< 5 mm), well-circumscribed, yellow or white nodules in the renal cortex. They have papillary, tubular, or tubulopapillary architecture similar to PRCC (Figure 9).[38] The cells lining those structures have uniform small nuclei and inconspicuous nucleoli similar to Fuhrman grade 1 or 2 nuclei.

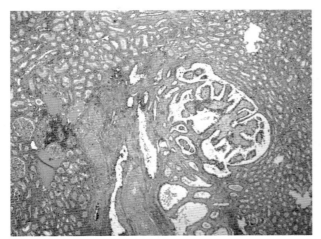

**Figure 9.** Papillary adenoma comprises small collection of papillae that are lined with cells with uniform small nuclei and inconspicuous nucleoli.

## Genetics

The earliest genetic changes observed in papillary adenomas are combined trisomy 7 and 17, and loss of chromosome Y, changes that are also present in PRCC.[39] Additional genetic alterations have been reported as they evolve into PRCC. The cytogenetic findings support the hypothesis that papillary adenoma is the precursor to PRCC.

## Renal Oncocytoma

Renal oncocytoma accounts for approximately 5% of renal cell neoplasms and occurs in a wide age range, with a peak incidence in the seventh decade of life. Most cases are sporadic, although familial cases have been reported in association with Birt-Hogg-Dube syndrome and familial renal oncocytoma syndrome.[3]

## Pathology

Oncocytomas are typically solitary, well-circumscribed, nonencapsulated tumors with homogeneous cut surface and a characteristic dark brown coloration (Figure 10A).[4] A central stellate scar is seen in one-third of the cases and is more common in larger tumors.

Renal oncocytoma is characterized by bright eosinophilic cells arranged in nested, microacinar, or microcystic pattern associated with loose hypocellular and hyalinized stroma (Figure 10B). The tumor cells are round to polygonal and with granular,

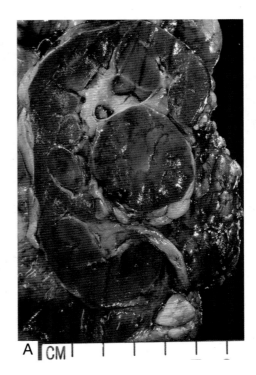

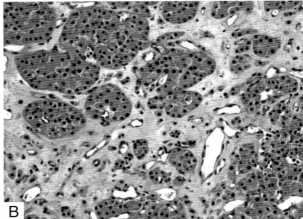

**Figure 10.** Renal oncocytoma forms solitary, well-circumscribed, nonencapsulated mass with homogeneous dark brown cut surface (A). It consists of bright eosinophilic cells nested in a loose stroma. The tumor cells are uniform, round to polygonal, with granular eosinophilic cytoplasm and regular round nuclei (B).

eosinophilic, and mitochondria-rich cytoplasm, and uniform round nuclei with evenly dispersed chromatin. Mitoses are in general absent and should raise the possibility of an RCC if present. Extension of oncocytoma cells into the perinephric fat, or rarely into vascular space, is well documented and does not appear to adversely affect the prognosis.

When multiple oncocytomas are present, along with oncocytic change in renal tubules, microcysts lined with oncocytic cells, and clusters of neoplastic oncocytes among renal tubules, the term oncocytosis is applied.[40] It is often seen in Birt-Hogg-Dube syndrome.[41]

### Genetics

Most oncocytomas are composed of a mixed population of cells with normal and abnormal karyotypes.[42] Some cases demonstrate loss of chromosomes 1 and 14.[43] Occasionally, t(5; 11) is observed.[44]

## RCC IN INHERITED CANCER SYNDROMES

Only < 5% of the cases occur in the setting of inherited cancer syndromes, including von Hippel-Lindau disease (VHLD), hereditary PRCC (HP RCC), hereditary leiomyomatosis/RCC (HLRCC), Birt-Hogg-Dube syndrome, and TS. Each inherited cancer syndrome predisposes patients to distinct subtype(s) of RCC. Renal involvement can range from solitary to bilateral and multifocal. Age of onset is also variable although most cases seem to occur at an earlier age.[3]

VHLD is caused by germ line mutations in *VHL* gene, a tumor-suppressor gene that plays a critical role in hypoxia-inducible signal transduction pathway. Loss of VHL protein leads to the activation of many hypoxia-inducible genes, including genes in angiogenesis (vascular endothelial growth factor), cell growth (platelet-derived growth factor β), and transforming growth factor α), glucose transport (*Glut-1*), acid–base balance (*CA IX*), and red cell production (*erythropoietin*). These factors then activate many intracellular signal transduction pathways, including PI3 kinase-Akt-mTOR and Ras-raf-erk-mek pathways, and contribute to the carcinogenesis of not only VHLD but also sporadic clear cell RCC. Renal lesions in VHLD are always clear cell RCC and tend to be bilateral and multifocal. In resected specimens, hundreds of microscopic tumor foci can be identified. VHLD-related RCC develops early, with a mean age of onset of 37 years compared with 61 years for sporadic clear cell RCC. With improved management of the central nervous system manifestations of the syndrome, RCC is now the leading cause of death. However, patients with VHLD with renal involvement fare better in 10-year survival than their sporadic counterparts.

HPRCC is associated with a germ line mutation in the tyrosine kinase domain of the *c-MET* protooncogene on chromosome 7q31 and develops type I PRCC.[45] Gain-of-function mutations in *c-MET* result in derangement of cellular processes that contribute to carcinogenesis, including angiogenesis, cell motility, proliferation, and morphogenic differentiation. However, sporadic PRCC infrequently has *c-MET* mutations.

HLRCC is an autosomal dominant disease and contains mutations in fumarate hydratase (*FH*) gene on chromosome 17.[46] Patients are at risk for cutaneous and uterine leiomyomas and PRCC of type II histology. The histologic hallmark is the prominent eosinophilic nuclei.[37] RCC in this syndrome can be particularly aggressive.

RCC is also part of the stigmata in Birt-Hogg-Dube syndrome,[47] an autosomal dominant disorder characterized by benign skin tumors (fibrofolliculomas, trichodiscomas of hair follicles and skin tag), renal epithelial neoplasms, and spontaneous pneumothorax. Renal neoplasms are often multifocal and bilateral and present in the forms of hybrid oncocytic tumors, with features of both chromophobe RCC and oncocytoma, chromophobe RCC, oncocytomas, clear cell RCC, and, occasionally, PRCC. *BHD*, the gene implicated in the syndrome, encodes a potential tumor suppressor gene folliculin on 17p11.2. *BHD* mutations are rarely found in sporadic chromophobe RCC or renal oncocytoma.

## HISTOLOGIC PROGNOSTIC FACTORS FOR RCC

Prognosis of RCC patients is influenced by many clinical, pathologic, and molecular factors. The pathologic parameters include histologic subtypes, tumor size, nuclear grade, sarcomatoid differentiation, tumor necrosis, vascular invasion, and status of surgical margins. Many of these parameters, including the tumor size and extent (whether it has spread out of the kidney), vascular and adrenal gland invasion, and lymph node metastasis, have been incorporated into tumor–node–metastasis (TNM) staging for RCC published by American Joint Committee on Cancer.[48] Other parameters have also been shown by many studies to be prognostically relevant and important, and will be discussed below.

## Histologic Subtypes

Many studies have shown differences in survival rates among patients with different subtypes of RCC. Histologic subtypes often correlate with TNM stages and other pathologic parameters. Clear cell RCC usually demonstrates worse pathologic features compared with PRCC and chromophobe RCC, including larger tumor size, higher Fuhrman nuclear grade, pathologic tumor stage, and likelihood to develop distant metastasis. By univariate analysis, most studies found that clear cell RCC fares worse than PRCC and chromophobe RCC. In a study by Cheville and colleagues, the 5- and 10-year cancer-specific survival were 68.9 and 60.3% for clear cell RCC, 90.1 and 81.9% for PRCC, and 88.1 and 83.3% for chromophobe RCC.[2] By multivariate analysis,

however, the histologic subtypes have not been found to be independent predictors of the clinical outcomes. Nevertheless, histologic classification of RCC is still clinically important since different subtypes may exhibit diverse therapeutic response. For example, Upton and colleagues found that 20% of clear cell RCC responded to interleukin 2–based therapy compared with 6% of nonclear cell RCC.[49]

## Fuhrman Nuclear Grading

Fuhrman grading system, the most widely used grading system for RCC, is based on the nuclear size, irregularity of the nuclear membrane, and nucleolar prominence and is categorized into grades 1 to 4 (Figure 11). Most studies have confirmed that Fuhrman nuclear grade is an independent prognostic

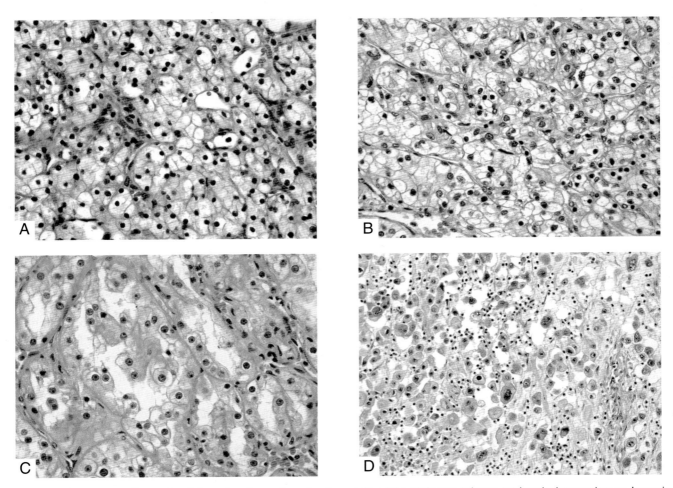

**Figure 11.** Fuhrman grading system is based on the nuclear size, irregularity of the nuclear membrane, and nucleolar prominence. In grade 1 renal cell carcinoma (RCC), nuclei are uniformly small and dense (A). Grade 2 nuclei have smooth open chromatin but inconspicuous nucleoli (B). In grade 3 RCC, nuclei have open chromatin and prominent nucleoli that are visible at low magnification (C). Grade 4 nuclei are markedly pleomorphic, hyperchromatic with single or multiple macronucleoli (D).

predictor for clear cell RCC and RCC, not otherwise specified.[50] Grades 1 and 2 may be grouped together as low grade since the two are not significantly different in prognosis in multivariate analysis.[51] Furthermore, grouping Fuhrman grades into low grade (grades 1 and 2) and high grade (grades 3 and 4) can improve the interobserver agreement and still preserve its prognostic significance.[52]

The prognostic significance of Fuhrman grading for PRCC and chromophobe RCC, however, remains controversial. For PRCC, Fuhrman nuclear grade correlates with clinical outcomes in univariate analysis; however, there is no significant correlation in multivariate analysis. One study demonstrated that only the nucleolar component, but not other components, of the Fuhrman grading system, including nuclear size and shape, was significantly associated with survival in both univariate and multivariate analyses.[53] Only a few studies addressed the prognostic significance of Fuhrman nuclear grade in chromophobe RCC using univariate analysis. A recent study found that Fuhrman grading does not correlate with survival, therefore is not appropriate for chromophobe RCC.[54]

## Sarcomatoid Differentiation

Sarcomatoid differentiation is present in 1 to 6.5% of RCCs and can arise in any subtype of RCC.[55] Therefore, sarcomatoid RCC is not considered a distinct subtype of RCC by current WHO classification; rather, it is thought to represent transformation to a higher grade, more aggressive form of RCC.

RCC with sarcomatoid differentiation is typically associated with other adverse pathologic features, including large tumor size, extension into perinephric fat and vessels, and presence of hemorrhage and necrosis. Sarcomatoid component appears as bulging lobulated areas with white to gray, firm and fibrous cut surface within the RCC (Figure 12A). Histologically, the sarcomatoid component ranges from malignant spindle cells to those resembling leiomyosarcoma, fibrosarcoma, angiosarcoma, rhabdomyosarcoma, and other sarcomas. The coexisting RCC component, including clear cell, papillary, chromophobe RCC, and sometimes, collecting duct RCC, can often be identified and used to classify the RCC with sarcoma-

toid differentiation (Figure 12B). However, such classification may not be possible if the sarcomatoid element entirely overruns the RCC component.

Sarcomatoid differentiation is an adverse prognostic indicator, as RCC with sarcomatoid differentiation often presents as a high-stage and high-grade disease with frequent distant metastasis. Sarcomatoid differentiation in RCC is associated with poor clinical outcome independent of TNM stage, nuclear grade, and tumor size in both univariate and multivariate analyses.[56]

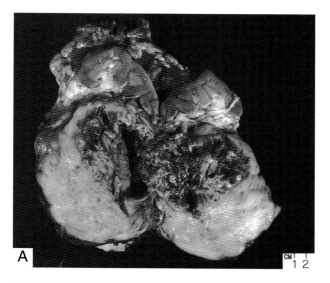

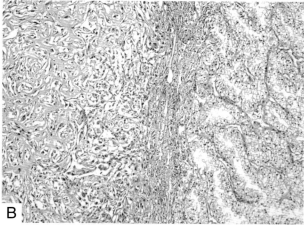

**Figure 12.** Renal cell carcinoma (RCC) with sarcomatoid differentiation. The center of this renal tumor is golden yellow with hemorrhage and necrosis, characteristic of clear cell RCC. The periphery of the tumor, however, is replaced with sarcomatoid component that has myxoid, fleshy cut surface (A). Next to the clear cell RCC component, malignant spindle cells embedded in dense fibrous tissue constitute the sarcomatoid differentiation (B), left half of the image.

## Rhabdoid Differentiation

RCC cells can also assume the so-called rhabdoid morphology with large eccentric nuclei, macronucleoli, and prominent acidophilic globular cytoplasm (Figure 13). Approximately 5% of RCC cases exhibit various amounts of rhabdoid component. The presence of rhabdoid component is also associated with high Fuhrman grade and tumor stage, extrarenal extension, and poor outcomes.[57,58]

## Tumor Necrosis

Tumor necrosis, identified either macroscopically or microscopically, is an adverse pathologic factor and is associated with worse clinical outcomes in both univariate and multivariate analyses. In a Mayo Clinic study, histologic necrosis is associated with twice the risk of death from RCC compared to those without necrosis.[2] Several studies also reported that the presence and extent of histologic necrosis in RCC were independent predictors of survival in localized but not metastatic cases.[59,60] Therefore, two outcome prediction models, SSIGN from Mayo Clinic, and the postoperative outcome nomogram from MSKCC, incorporate tumor necrosis in their models.[61,62] However, tumor necrosis is not prognostically useful for PRCC since it is commonly observed in this tumor type.

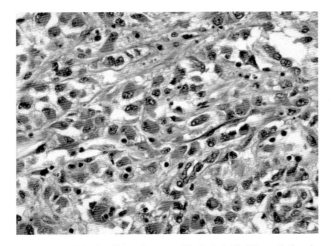

**Figure 13.** Renal cell carcinoma with rhabdoid differentiation has tumor cells with the so-called rhabdoid morphology with large eccentric nuclei, macronucleoli, and prominent acidophilic globular cytoplasm.

## Invasion of Urinary Collecting System

Involvement of the collecting system, including renal calyces, pelvis, and ureter, occurs most frequently in high-stage and high-grade RCC. Uzzo and colleagues found that collecting system invasion did not portend a worse prognosis in high-stage (T3 or higher) tumor, whereas it was an adverse pathologic feature in low-stage RCC.[63] Several studies found that collecting system invasion provides independent prognostic significance, particularly in low-stage (I and II) patients, associated with greater risk of death and shorter recurrence-free survival compared with those without collecting system invasion.[64,65] However, another study did not confirm the independent prognostic value of the involvement of the collecting system, although such a finding was associated with worse prognosis in the univariate analysis.[66]

## Microvascular Invasion

Microvascular invasion, defined as invasion of small vessel, detected only microscopically, is present in 13.6 to 44.6% of RCC and is more common in RCC of higher stage, nuclear grade, and larger size. The current TNM staging does not take into consideration the microscopic vascular invasion; rather, it only recognizes the grossly identifiable involvement of vessels as T3b or T3c. However, microscopic vascular invasion is associated with higher cancer-specific mortality and higher likelihood of disease recurrence independent of other prognostic parameters including tumor grade and size.[67,68]

## Renal Parenchymal Margin Status

Positive renal parenchymal margin in nephron-sparing surgery indicates incomplete resection of RCC and is associated with poor prognosis. However, the width of the margins does not seem to correlate with prognosis as long as the surgical margins are free of tumor.[69–71]

# REFERENCES

1. Eble J, et al. Tumours of the urinary system and male genital organs. Lyon: IAPC Press; 2004.
2. Cheville JC, et al. Comparisons of outcome and prognostic features among histologic subtypes of renal cell carcinoma. Am J Surg Pathol 2003;27:612–24.
3. Cohen D, Zhou M. Molecular genetics of familial renal cell carcinoma syndromes. Clin Lab Med 2005;25:259–77.
4. Murphy W, Grignon D, Perlman E. Tumors of the kidney, bladder, and related urinary structures. Washington, DC: American Registry of Pathology; 2004.
5. Hoglund M, et al. Dissecting karyotypic patterns in renal cell carcinoma: an analysis of the accumulated cytogenetic data. Cancer Genet Cytogenet 2004;153:1–9.
6. Linehan WM, et al. Genetic basis of cancer of the kidney: disease-specific approaches to therapy. Clin Cancer Res, 2004;10(18 Pt 2):6282S–9S.
7. Strefford JC, et al. A combination of molecular cytogenetic analyses reveals complex genetic alterations in conventional renal cell carcinoma. Cancer Genet Cytogenet 2005; 159:1–9.
8. Jones TD, Eble JN, Cheng L. Application of molecular diagnostic techniques to renal epithelial neoplasms. Clin Lab Med, 2005;25:279–303.
9. Banks RE, et al. Genetic and epigenetic analysis of von Hippel-Lindau (VHL) gene alterations and relationship with clinical variables in sporadic renal cancer. Cancer Res 2006; 66:2000–11.
10. Gimenez-Bachs JM, et al. Determination of vhl gene mutations in sporadic renal cell carcinoma. Eur Urol 2005.
11. Suzigan S, et al. Multilocular cystic renal cell carcinoma: a report of 45 cases of a kidney tumor of low malignant potential. Am J Clin Pathol 2006;125:217–22.
12. Nassir A, et al. Multilocular cystic renal cell carcinoma: a series of 12 cases and review of the literature. Urology 2002;60:421–7.
13. Delahunt B, et al. Morphologic typing of papillary renal cell carcinoma: comparison of growth kinetics and patient survival in 66 cases. Hum Pathol 2001;32:590–5.
14. Brunelli M, et al. Gains of chromosomes 7, 17, 12, 16, and 20 and loss of Y occur early in the evolution of papillary renal cell neoplasia: a fluorescent in situ hybridization study. Mod Pathol 2003;16:1053–9.
15. Schraml P, et al. Allelic loss at the D9S171 locus on chromosome 9p13 is associated with progression of papillary renal cell carcinoma. J Pathol 2000;190:457–61.
16. Jiang F, et al. Chromosomal imbalances in papillary renal cell carcinoma: genetic differences between histological subtypes. Am J Pathol 1998;153:1467–73.
17. Sanders ME, et al. Unique patterns of allelic imbalance distinguish type 1 from type 2 sporadic papillary renal cell carcinoma. Am J Pathol 2002;161:997–1005.
18. Thoenes W, et al. Chromophobe cell renal carcinoma and its variants—a report on 32 cases. J Pathol 1988;155:277–87.
19. Tickoo SK, Amin MB, Zarbo RJ. Colloidal iron staining in renal epithelial neoplasms, including chromophobe renal cell carcinoma: emphasis on technique and patterns of staining. Am J Surg Pathol 1998;22:419–24.
20. Vira M, Linehan WM. Expanding the morphological and molecular genetic phenotype of kidney cancer. J Urol 2007;177:10–1.
21. Antonelli A, et al. The collecting duct carcinoma of the kidney: a cytogenetical study. Eur Urol 2003;43:680–5.
22. Karakiewicz PI, et al. Collecting duct renal cell carcinoma: a matched analysis of 41 cases. Eur Urol 2007;52:1140–5.
23. Tokuda N, et al. Collecting duct (Bellini duct) renal cell carcinoma: a nationwide survey in Japan. J Urol 2006;176:40–3; discussion 43.
24. Watanabe, IC, et al. Renal medullary carcinoma: report of seven cases from Brazil. Mod Pathol 2007;20:914–20.
24a. Davis CJ, Jr, et al. Renal Medullary carcinoma. The seventh sickle cell nephropathy. Am J Surg Pathol 1995;19:1–11.
25. Bell MD. Response to paclitaxel, gemcitabine, and cisplatin in renal medullary carcinoma. Pediatr Blood Cancer 2006;228.
26. Strouse JJ, et al. Significant responses to platinum-based chemotherapy in renal medullary carcinoma. Pediatr Blood Cancer 2005;44:407–11.
27. Ferlicot S, et al. Mucinous tubular and spindle cell carcinoma: a report of 15 cases and a review of the literature. Virchows Arch 2005;447:978–83.
28. Kuroda N et al. Review of mucinous tubular and spindle-cell carcinoma of the kidney with a focus on clinical and pathobiological aspects. Histol Histopathol 2005; 20:221–4.
29. Fine SW, et al. Expanding the histologic spectrum of mucinous tubular and spindle cell carcinoma of the kidney. Am J Surg Pathol 2006;30:1554–60.
30. Paner GP, et al. Immunohistochemical analysis of mucinous tubular and spindle cell carcinoma and papillary renal cell carcinoma of the kidney: significant immunophenotypic overlap warrants diagnostic caution. Am J Surg Pathol 2006;30:13–9.
31. Brandal P et al. Genomic aberrations in mucinous tubular and spindle cell renal cell carcinomas. Mod Pathol 2006; 19:186–94.
32. Cossu-Rocca P et al. Renal mucinous tubular and spindle carcinoma lacks the gains of chromosomes 7 and 17 and losses of chromosome Y that are prevalent in papillary renal cell carcinoma. Mod Pathol 2006;19:488–93.
33. Argani P, Ladanyi M. Translocation carcinomas of the kidney. Clin Lab Med 2005;25:363–78.
34. Argani P, et al. Primary renal neoplasms with the ASPL-TFE3 gene fusion of alveolar soft part sarcoma: a distinctive tumor entity previously included among renal cell carcinomas of children and adolescents. Am J Pathol 2001;159:179–92.
35. Argani P, et al. Xp11 translocation renal cell carcinoma in adults: expanded clinical, pathologic, and genetic spectrum. Am J Surg Pathol 2007;31:1149–60.
36. Meyer PN, et al. Xp11.2 translocation renal cell carcinoma with very aggressive course in five adults. Am J Clin Pathol 2007;128:70–9.
37. Merino MJ, et al. The morphologic spectrum of kidney tumors in hereditary leiomyomatosis and renal cell carcinoma (HLRCC) syndrome. Am J Surg Pathol 2007;31:1578–85.
38. Grignon DJ, Eble JN. Papillary and metanephric adenomas of the kidney. Semin Diagn Pathol 1998;15:41–53.

39. Kovacs G, et al. Cytogenetics of papillary renal cell tumors. Genes Chromosomes Cancer 1991;3:249–55.

40. Tickoo SK, et al. Renal oncocytosis: a morphologic study of fourteen cases. Am J Surg Pathol 1999;23:1094–101.

41. Pavlovich CP, et al. Renal tumors in the Birt-Hogg-Dube syndrome. Am J Surg Pathol 2002;26:1542–52.

42. Lindgren V, et al. Cytogenetic analysis of a series of 13 renal oncocytomas. J Urol 2004;171(2 Pt 1):602–4.

43. Presti JC Jr, et al. Comparative genomic hybridization for genetic analysis of renal oncocytomas. Genes Chromosomes Cancer 1996;17:199–204.

44. Sinke RJ et al. Fine mapping of the human renal oncocytoma-associated translocation (5;11)(q35;q13) breakpoint. Cancer Genet Cytogenet 1997;96:95–101.

45. Schmidt L, et al. Germline and somatic mutations in the tyrosine kinase domain of the MET proto-oncogene in papillary renal carcinomas. Nat Genet 1997;16:68–73.

46. Launonen V, et al. Inherited susceptibility to uterine leiomyomas and renal cell cancer. Proc Natl Acad Sci USA 2001;98:3387–92.

47. Murakami T, et al., Identification and characterization of Birt-Hogg-Dube associated renal carcinoma. J Pathol 2007; 211:524–31.

48. Greene F. et al. AJCC cancer staging handbook. 6th ed. New York: Springer; 2002.

49. Upton MP, et al. Histologic predictors of renal cell carcinoma response to interleukin-2-based therapy. J Immunother 2005;28:488–95.

50. Novara G. et al. Grading systems in renal cell carcinoma. J Urol 2007;177:430–6.

51. Rioux-Leclercq N, et al. Prognostic ability of simplified nuclear grading of renal cell carcinoma. Cancer 2007;109:868–74.

52. Lang H, et al. Multicenter determination of optimal interobserver agreement using the Fuhrman grading system for renal cell carcinoma: assessment of 241 patients with > 15-year follow-up. Cancer 2005;103:625–9.

53. Sika-Paotonu D, et al. Nucleolar grade but not Fuhrman grade is applicable to papillary renal cell carcinoma. Am J Surg Pathol 2006;30:1091–6.

54. Delahunt B, et al. Fuhrman grading is not appropriate for chromophobe renal cell carcinoma. Am J Surg Pathol 2007;31:957–60.

55. de Peralta-Venturina M, et al. Sarcomatoid differentiation in renal cell carcinoma: a study of 101 cases. Am J Surg Pathol 2001;25:275–84.

56. Cheville JC, et al. Sarcomatoid renal cell carcinoma: an examination of underlying histologic subtype and an analysis of associations with patient outcome. Am J Surg Pathol 2004;28:435–41.

57. Gokden N, et al. Renal cell carcinoma with rhabdoid features. Am J Surg Pathol 2000;24:1329–38.

58. Leroy X, et al. Renal cell carcinoma with rhabdoid features: an aggressive neoplasm with overexpression of p53. Arch Pathol Lab Med 2007;131:102–6.

59. Lam JS, et al. Clinicopathologic and molecular correlations of necrosis in the primary tumor of patients with renal cell carcinoma. Cancer 2005;103:2517–25.

60. Lee SE, et al. Significance of macroscopic tumor necrosis as a prognostic indicator for renal cell carcinoma. J Urol 2006;176(4 Pt 1):1332–7; discussion 1337–8.

61. Frank I, et al. An outcome prediction model for patients with clear cell renal cell carcinoma treated with radical nephrectomy based on tumor stage, size, grade and necrosis: the SSIGN score. J Urol 2002;168:2395–400.

62. Sorbellini M, et al. A postoperative prognostic nomogram predicting recurrence for patients with conventional clear cell renal cell carcinoma. J Urol 2005;173:48–51.

63. Uzzo RG, et al. Renal cell carcinoma invading the urinary collecting system: implications for staging. J Urol 2002; 167:2392–6.

64. Klatte T, et al. Prognostic relevance of capsular involvement and collecting system invasion in stage I and II renal cell carcinoma. BJU Int 2007;99:821–4.

65. Palapattu GS, et al. Collecting system invasion in renal cell carcinoma: impact on prognosis and future staging strategies. J Urol 2003;170:768–72; discussion 772.

66. Terrone C, et al. Prognostic value of the involvement of the urinary collecting system in renal cell carcinoma. Eur Urol 2004;46:472–6.

67. Antunes AA, et al. Microvascular invasion is an independent prognostic factor in patients with prostate cancer treated with radical prostatectomy. Int Braz J Urol 2006;32: 668–75; discussion 675–7.

68. Madbouly K, et al. Microvascular tumor invasion: prognostic significance in low-stage renal cell carcinoma. Urology 2007;69:670–4.

69. Castilla EA, et al. Prognostic importance of resection margin width after nephron-sparing surgery for renal cell carcinoma. Urology 2002;60:993–7.

70. Sutherland SE, et al. Does the size of the surgical margin in partial nephrectomy for renal cell cancer really matter? J Urol 2002;167:61–4.

71. Timsit MO, et al. Prospective study of safety margins in partial nephrectomy: intraoperative assessment and contribution of frozen section analysis. Urology 2006;67:923–6.

# 2

# Epidemiology and Screening of Renal Cell Carcinoma

DANIEL R. CARRIZOSA, MD, MS

PAUL A. GODLEY, MD, PHD, MPP

In adults, renal cell carcinoma (RCC) accounts for 2% of all new cancer cases worldwide and nearly 80% of all primary malignant kidney tumors.[1] In 2008 over 54,390 new cases of kidney cancer were expected in the United States, and this malignancy accounts for about 13,010 cancer-related deaths each year.[2] A small portion of kidney cancers arise in the renal pelvis and are typically transitional cell carcinomas, whereas more than 85% arise in the renal parenchyma and these are usually adenocarcinomas.[3] Less than 10% of kidney cancers are composed of rarer types including oncocytomas and chromophobe carcinoma.[4,5] The potential etiologic factors for RCC are very diverse. This chapter examines the risk factors for RCC and discusses the current guidelines for screening for this neoplasm.

## DESCRIPTIVE EPIDEMIOLOGY

From 1994 to 2003, incidence rates of kidney cancer have continued to increase in both men and women (Figure 1); in 2003, the age-adjusted incidence rate in men (16.9 per 100,000 cases) was nearly twice that in women (8.9 per 100,000 cases).[6] From 2000 to 2003, in the United States, the mean age at diagnosis for all kidney cancers was 65 years and the mean age at death was 71 years.[7,8] From 1994 to 2003, incidence rates consistently increased with

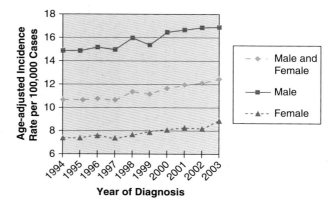

**Figure 1.** Surveillance, Epidemiology, and End Results (SEER) age-adjusted incidence rates by sex for kidney and renal pelvis cancer (all ages, all races SEER 13 registries for 1994 to 2003).

age until a plateau is reached at about age 75 for men and 80 for women (Figure 2).[6] As incidence rates of cancer have increased, mortality has overall reached a plateau of about 4.2 deaths per 100,000 people (Figure 3).[7]

Fortunately, though the incidence of kidney cancer has increased, the number of cancers that present at an advanced stage has decreased. From 1995 to 2002, the number of cancers diagnosed at a localized stage has increased by 12% compared with 1975 to 1979 (Figure 4).[9] This rise in total incidence and particularly that of limited stage disease is in part due to the higher sensitivity and overall increase in abdominal imaging of RCC.[10,11]

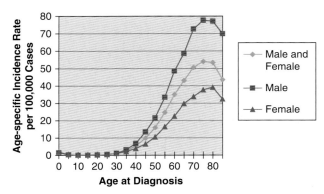

**Figure 2.** Age-specific (crude) Surveillance, Epidemiology, and End Results (SEER) incidence rates by sex for kidney and renal pelvis cancer (all races SEER 13 registries for 1994 to 2003).

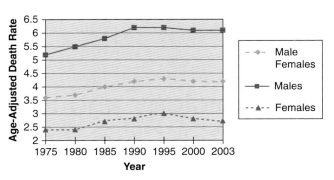

**Figure 3.** Age-adjusted US death rates by year (Surveillance, Epidemiology, and End Results Cancer Statistics Review 1975 to 2003).

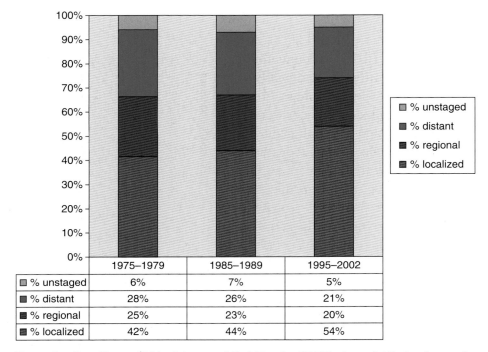

| | 1975–1979 | 1985–1989 | 1995–2002 |
|---|---|---|---|
| ▣ % unstaged | 6% | 7% | 5% |
| ■ % distant | 28% | 26% | 21% |
| ■ % regional | 25% | 23% | 20% |
| ■ % localized | 42% | 44% | 54% |

**Figure 4.** Surveillance, Epidemiology, and End Results (SEER) stage distribution by sex for kidney and renal pelvis cancer (all ages, all races SEER 9 Registries for 1975 to 1979, 1985 to 1989, 1995 to 2002).

Consistent with this relative decrease in advanced disease, overall 5-year survival rates due to kidney cancer have increased by 13.7% from 1975 to 2002 (51.7 vs 65.4%).[9] By 2002, 10-year survival for patients with kidney cancer was 83% for localized disease and a dismal 7% for distant disease.[9] The high discrepancy between survival rates helps spur the argument for generalized screening in the hopes of continuing to decrease the rate of patients diagnosed with distant disease.

## GENERAL POPULATION

### Risk Factors and Risk Markers

As with all cancers, causes and risk factors for RCC are continuously being analyzed. The majority of data are from case–control studies and a few cohort studies. The largest study reported includes 1,732 cases and 2,309 controls from a multicenter, multinational investigation.[12] Because of space constraints, not every article published regarding RCC risk is cited, but certain studies (mainly large-cohort studies) are used to emphasize the major findings in the literature.

## Cigarette Smoking

Cigarette use has been consistently described as a risk for RCC.[13] The use of cigarettes can account for 20 to 30% of RCC in men and 10 to 20% in women.[12,13] In 2005, a meta-analysis showed a relative risk for RCC of 1.54 and 1.22 and a dose-dependent risk in heavy smokers (> 21 cigarettes daily) of 2.03 and 1.58 in male and female smokers, respectively.[14] Cohort studies of US veterans support an increased risk of RCC due to smoking and also a clear dose–response relationship.[15,16] Further support is shown by a significant decrease (between 15 and 30%) in RCC risk after quitting smoking for greater than 15 to 20 years.[14]

## Obesity

Multiple studies have linked obesity to an increased risk of RCC in both men and women.[17–22] Two of these studies showed a similar relative risk increase of 1.07/U of rising body mass index.[20,22] The increase in incidence of obesity in Western culture could account for part of the increased incidence of RCC, and it has been estimated that more than 40% of RCC in the United States and more than 30% of RCC in Europe could be attributed to obesity.[20,23] Multiple mechanisms (lipid peroxidation leading to deoxyribonucleic acid adducts, increased estrogens, increased insulin-like growth factor I, and increased arterionephrosclerosis) have been proposed to potentially link obesity and RCC.[23–26]

## Hypertension and Antihypertensive Medications

Many epidemiologic studies have examined the possible link between hypertension and RCC and have found excess risks ranging from 20% to almost 200%.[27] Unfortunately, it is very difficult to disentangle coincident risks from hypertension alone, the use of antihypertensive medications, and the presence of other related comorbid states. Further complicating

the analysis, early-stage RCCs can induce increased blood pressures.[28] The majority of epidemiologic evidence suggests that it is hypertension and not antihypertensive drugs that influence RCC, but a recent comprehensive review of the literature by Dhote and collegues suggest that there is not enough evidence in the literature to support hypertension as a risk factor—only a risk marker.[27,29] The mechanisms of lipid peroxidation (similar to obesity), increased angiogenic factors, increased growth factors, and subtle damage to the microtubules have all been implicated as increasing RCC risk in patients with hypertension.[24,30–33] Regarding antihypertensive medication, studies are inconsistent about this possible link with RCC. Animal models have shown a link between both loop and thiazide diuretics and kidney tumors in rats.[13] Two cohort studies that observed patients who were admitted and treated with diuretics showed a possible link with RCC, but more recent studies that have carefully controlled for hypertension seem to refute the earlier findings.[34–37] Except diuretics, no other antihypertensive medications have been strongly associated with RCC.[38]

## Occupation

Though some links between RCC and occupation have been reported in the literature, RCC is not generally considered an occupationally associated tumor.[13] Exposure to asbestos, polycyclic aromatic hydrocarbons, solvents, gasoline/petroleum products, metals (eg, cadmium), vinyl chloride, and pesticides have all been associated with RCC, but none have shown consistent risk in epidemiologic studies, possibly due to small sample sizes, recall bias, and short duration of follow-up.[27] Interestingly, gasoline has now been shown not to be a risk factor for RCC, and that the animal models that had shown this link developed RCC due to a unique sex- and species-related compound ($\alpha$2-microglobulin) irrelevant to humans.[39] The only chemical that might show a possible link with RCC is trichloroethylene (TCE) based on three large studies conducted in Germany.[40] Subsequent analysis of the original three studies and newer inquiries have weakened the link between TCE and RCC.[41–43] One study did show a possible mutation in the von Hippel-Lindau (VHL) gene only in patients exposed to TCE; thus, biologic plausibility makes this chemical a possible risk factor.[44]

## Reproductive and Hormonal Factors

There are reports in the literature of the possible link between hormonal status and RCC. One large study from Sweden showed that increased number of births increased the risk of RCC by about 15%.[45] Congruently, prolonged use of oral contraceptives (greater than 10 years) in nonsmoking women showed a moderate decrease in risk of RCC (odds ratio [OR] = 0.4, 95% confidence interval [CI] = 0.1–1.0).[46] After hysterectomy or oophorectomy, population studies also showed an increase in RCC (OR = 2.3, 1.7, 1.8).[47–49] However, other population studies conflict with these observations.[50,51] Potential mechanisms have been studied preclinically and include the growth of renal adenomas and carcinomas in rats exposed to estrogen and the discovery of sex hormone receptors on renal tumors.[52,53]

## Diet

As with many other cancers, diet is considered to be important in RCC, but very little epidemiologic evidence supports a firm link between any specific food and RCC. Many studies have shown some possible links to either greater or lesser risks of RCC, specifically in women.[54] Fruit and vegetable consumption and alcohol intake seem to provide a protective effect in large cohorts of women.[55–57] In particular, a large case–control study based on the Iowa cancer registry noted a decreased risk of RCC (OR = 0.5, 95% CI = 0.2–0.9) associated with three servings of alcohol per week in women compared with no association in men.[58] Other studies had linked increased protein consumption with RCC, but a recent study failed to show this as a risk factor.[59] Overall, evidence is lacking to support diet as a risk factor for RCC.[28]

## Other Risk Factors

In addition to the risk factors mentioned above, several other potential risk factors for RCC have been studied. First, patients with preexisting renal conditions like kidney or ureteral stones have shown little or no increase in RCC.[27,29] Second, the link between kidney malignancies and analgesics has not been clearly shown in the literature except for phenacetin, which has not been on the US market since 1983.[27] In addition to phenacetin, another discontinued carcinogen is thoratrast, an α-particle–emitting radiologic contrast medium. A 40-year Swedish follow-up study showed that thoratrast increased the risk of RCC by 3.4 times (95% CI = 1.4–7.0), but this risk was only statistically significant in men.[60] Finally, patients with a first-degree relative may have a higher incidence of RCC due to an unknown genetic polymorphism.[61,62]

## Screening

The rationale for screening is the early identification of a disease, allowing for more effective treatment. The disease needs to be found prior to the critical point when therapy becomes either less effective or harder to apply.[63] In addition, the disease must cause substantial burden of suffering, and a good screening test must be available that is inexpensive, safe, highly sensitive and specific, and accepted by patients and clinicians.[64] Although the burden of suffering from RCC is sufficient for screening, the testing of asymptomatic individuals for RCC does not yet meet other criteria.

In screening, it is important to remember that RCC is generally only curable when diagnosed as localized and amenable to surgical resection. Multiple studies have shown that there is a survival advantage when it is found early or incidentally. Thompson and Peek showed that 87% of incidentally found tumors were localized versus only 42% of symptomatic tumors, and that 5-year survival was improved with early detection.[65] Another recent study confirmed that incidental detection was also associated with improved survival.[66] Finally, in Iceland, incidental detection of RCC showed a 76% 5-year survival versus 44% in patients with symptomatic tumors.[67]

Though early detection can be beneficial, the major problem with screening the general population is the overall low incidence of RCC. As described previously, RCC accounts for 2% of cancer cases worldwide. A screening test would need to be 100% sensitive and 100% specific to avoid a high number of unnecessary, potentially harmful, and expensive tests.[68] If the test's specificity is even one or two points off 100% in a low-incidence disease, the number of false positives would outnumber true positives by a factor of 10 or more. Because some patients could have benign renal adenomas that can be initially difficult to differentiate from RCC, screening may not be beneficial or cost effective. This is especially true due to the anatomic location of the kidney, making it more difficult to perform biopsy without possible excess morbidity or mortality. Currently, there are no guidelines or medical society endorsements for screening asymptomatic patients for RCC in any country. In the United States, screening asymptomatic patients for bladder cancer or RCC with a urinalysis for microhematuria is also discouraged.[69]

Some authors have argued than on a comparative basis, screening for RCC should still be considered. Turney and colleagues report that the annual death rate in the UK for RCC (0.6%) is similar to those for breast cancer (2.2%) and abdominal aortic aneurysm rupture (0.9%); the latter two disease states have national screening programs in the UK.[70] They postulate that cost-effectiveness could possibly be reached by combining ultrasound screening for RCC with that of abdominal aortic aneurysm. Two other studies also advocate ultrasound screening but found only 192 RCCs in 219,640 patients (0.09%) and 15 RCCs in 6678 patients (0.22%).[71,72] These numbers are consistent with other studies that have looked at confirmed RCC when using ultrasonography (Table 1). Even though ultrasonography is relatively inexpensive, the cost of diagnostic procedures to find this small number of tumors would be astronomical.[73–75]

**Table 1. PUBLISHED STUDIES OF CONFIRMED POSITIVE ULTRASOUND SCREENING TESTS FOR RENAL CELL CARCINOMA**

| Study | No. of Patients | % Confirmed RCC |
|---|---|---|
| Mihara et al.[71] | 219,640 | 0.09 |
| Malaeb et al.[72] | 6,678 | 0.22 |
| Fields et al.[73] | 500 | 0.2 |
| Tsuboi et al.[74] | 60,604 | 0.02 |
| Spouge et al.[75] | 7,925 | 0.3 |

[72]Adapted from Malaeb et al.

Computed tomography (CT) has also been studied in the screening of RCC. Fenton and Weiss reviewed the literature on screening CT.[76] The use of screening CT has increased in the United States, and this study found that the pooled prevalence was 0.21%, similar to the numbers found in ultrasound studies. As CT is considerably more expensive than ultrasonography, this modality has an even lower chance of gaining acceptance for general screening. Of note, the study did conclude that the asymptomatic RCCs found by CT are likely to progress to being symptomatic or clinically relevant, refuting some beliefs that the natural history of RCC found incidentally is different from that of clinically diagnosed cancer.[75]

Given the low incidence of RCC in the general population and the preponderance of data against generalized screening, most authors have recommended focusing our efforts at early detection on well-described target populations, such as patients with end-stage renal failure and possible familial etiologies.

## END-STAGE RENAL DISEASE AND ACQUIRED RENAL CYSTIC DISEASE PATIENTS

### Epidemiology

Over 260,000 individuals have end-stage renal disease in the United States.[77] Studies have shown that the incidence of acquired renal cystic disease is about 7% in patients with chronic renal failure and 22% in patients on maintenance dialysis.[78] Greater than 50 to 80% of patients may be affected after 10 or more years of dialysis.[79,80] Studies have shown a five-fold increase in RCC in patients with acquired renal cystic disease, with the overall incidence increasing linearly with time on maintenance dialysis.[81,82] As in other patients with RCC, dialysis patients who have their cancer found by screening have their risk of death reduced by 35%.[83] Diagnosis of acquired cystic kidney disease can be made by multiple imaging modalities including ultrasonography, CT, or magnetic resonance imaging.[84] Interestingly, some studies suggest that RCC and acquired renal cystic disease might be two separate entities because some patients develop RCC while on maintenance dialysis without any evidence of cystic changes.[85–87]

## Screening

Guidelines for screening patients on maintenance dialysis are controversial. Yearly screening has been suggested for patients who have been on maintenance dialysis for more than 3 years.[79,87–89] Because the incidence is still relatively low, some authors recommend only evaluating patients when they are symptomatic (flank pain or hematuria) or screening young patients who have acquired cystic kidney disease or who may be on maintenance dialysis for a long duration.[84,90] Assuming an incidence of RCC of 0.9 percent per year, Sarasin and collegues calculated a 1.6-year gain in life expectancy with screening, specifically in young dialysis patients with a presumed long life span and few comorbidities.[91] These data likely show that screening may be of little benefit in older patients with frequent comorbidities, a population similar to the majority of US dialysis patients. CT is the imaging modality of choice at most centers for the diagnosis of RCC in kidneys of patients with acquired cystic kidney disease.[92]

## RENAL TRANSPLANT PATIENTS

### Epidemiology/Screening

RCC in transplant patients is a key consideration when both transplanted and native kidneys are entered into the mix. The incidence of transmitted RCC with a transplanted kidney is low, and more commonly, RCC arises from native kidneys.[93,94] The US Renal Data System reports a 3-year cumulative incidence of RCC, in both native and transplanted kidneys, of 2.2%.[95] Data suggest that the inherent immunosuppression in transplant patients does not seem to affect risk of RCC; instead, an inherent defect in the native kidney associated with end-stage renal disease increases risk of RCC.[96] Screening of native kidneys annually or biannually has been advocated by several authors, but the benefits of screening this population has not been demonstrated.[97,98]

## VHL PATIENTS

### Epidemiology/Screening

VHL disease is an autosomal-dominant disease that affects multiple organ systems. In all, 25 to 40% of VHL patients develop RCC, and incidence increases to over 60% if cystic lesions are present in the kidney.[99,100] Before the advent of CT, 13 to 42% of VHL patients died from metastatic RCC.[101] Renal involvement is typically multifocal and bilateral, and tumors have clear-cell histology.[102] Patients at risk of VHL should be offered genetic counseling. VHL testing accuracy is as high as 100% in experienced laboratories.[103] CT of the abdomen and pelvis for both RCC and other anomalies often commences at age 18 and is then performed annually.[104] Other authors recommend starting in the same age range, with CT or ultrasonography performed biannually.[105] Clearly, the incidence of RCC and other abnormalities is high enough to warrant frequent screening, and these patients should also be carefully observed for the other manifestations of this disease.

## OTHER HIGH-RISK STATES

### Epidemiology/Screening

In addition to VHL, other hereditary forms of RCC are known. Hereditary papillary RCC (HPRCC) is a familial syndrome consisting of activating mutations of the MET protooncogene and is reported in several families.[106–109] Because of the small numbers, incidence and screening recommendations are not available, but the disorder appears to have a considerable malignant potential, with the earliest age of presentation of RCC of 18, making frequent and early screening essential.[106] In addition to HPRCC, patients with tuberous sclerosis appear to have an increased risk of RCC.[110,111] Because of the rarity of RCC and of tuberous sclerosis, it is difficult to show a strong association between the two and therefore controversy still exists in the literature.[68] When patients with tuberous sclerosis develop RCC, they have an early age of onset and usually have multifocal disease, suggesting an inherited predisposition.[112]

Despite these associations, a recent meta-analysis failed to demonstrate a clear association between tuberous sclerosis and RCC.[113] Most authors continue to recommend frequent screening with ultrasonography or CT for early detection of RCC and to screen for another common renal occurrence: angiomyolipoma.[114–118]

## SUMMARY

Since 1994, the incidence of kidney cancer continues to rise, in part due to increased frequency and accuracy of abdominal imaging. Cigarette smoking, obesity, and hypertension have been linked to an increased risk of developing RCC. Other risk factors have either a weak or little association with an increased incidence of kidney cancer.

In the general population, no current guidelines recommend screening the asymptomatic patient for RCC. The subpopulations of dialysis patients, transplant patients, and those patients with familial forms of RCC do have recommendations for asymptomatic screening due to their increased risk of developing RCC, although even in these subgroups, screening should be performed selectively, taking into account patient age and comorbidities.

## REFERENCES

1. Parkin CM, Whelan SL, Ferlay J, et al. Cancer incidence in five continents. Lyon, France: International Agency for Research on Cancer, vol. VIII; 2002. IARC Scientific Publications No. 155.
2. Jemel A, Siegal R, Ward E, et al. Cancer statistics, 2008. CA Cancer J Clin 2008;58:71–96.
3. Chow WH, Devesa SS, Warren J, et al. Kidney cancer incidence trends in the United States. JAMA 1999; 281:1628–31.
4. Linehan WM, Lerman MI, Zbar B. Identification of the von Hippel-Lindau (VHL) gene. JAMA 1995;273:564–70.
5. Zbar B, Lerman M. Inherited carcinomas of the kidney. Adv Cancer Res 1998;75:163–201.
6. Surveillance, Epidemiology, and End Results (SEER) Program (www.seer.cancer.gov). SEER*Stat Database: Incidence— SEER 13 Regs Public Use, Nov 2005 Sub (1992–2003), National Cancer Institute, DCCPS, Surveillance Research Program, Cancer Statistics Branch, released April 2006, based on the November 2005 submission.
7. Ries LAG, Harkins D, Krapcho M, et al., editors. SEER Cancer Statistics Review, 1975–2003, National Cancer Institute. Bethesda, MD, http://seer.cancer.gov/csr/1975_2003/, based on November 2005 SEER data submission, posted to the SEER Web site 2006 in Table I-11. http://seer. cancer.gov/csr/1975_2003/results_single/sect_01_ table.11_2pgs.pdf
8. Ries LAG, Harkins D, Krapcho M, et al. editors. SEER Cancer Statistics Review, 1975–2003, National Cancer Institute. Bethesda, MD, http://seer.cancer.gov/csr/1975_ 2003/, based on November 2005 SEER data submission, posted to the SEER Web site 2006 in Table I-13. http://seer.cancer.gov/csr/1975_2003/results_single/sect_0 1_table.13_2pgs.pdf
9. Surveillance, Epidemiology, and End Results (SEER) Program (www.seer.cancer.gov). SEER*Stat Database: Incidence— SEER 17 Regs Public Use, Nov 2005 Sub (1973–2003 varying), National Cancer Institute, DCCPS, Surveillance Research Program, Cancer Statistics Branch, released April 2006, based on the November 2005 submission.
10. Homma Y, Kawabe K, Kitamura T, et al. Increased incidental detection and reduced mortality in renal cancer—recent retrospective analysis at eight institutions. Int J Urol 1995;2:77–80.
11. Jayson M, Sanders H. Increased incidence of serendipitously discovered renal cell carcinoma. Urology 1998;51:203–5.
12. McLaughlin JK, Lindblad P, Mellemgaard A, et al. International renal-cell cancer study. I. Tobacco use. Int J Cancer 1995;60:194–8.
13. McLaughlin JK, Lipworth L. Epidemiologic aspects of renal cell cancer. Semin Oncol 2000;27:115–23.
14. Hunt JD, van der Hel OL, McMillan GP, et al. Renal cell carcinoma in relation to cigarette smoking: meta-analysis of 24 studies. Int J Cancer 2005;114:101–8.
15. McLaughlin JK, Hrubec A, Blot WJ, et al. Smoking and cancer mortality among US veterans: a 26-year follow-up. Int J Cancer 1993;55:32–36.
16. Coughlin SS, Neaton JD, Randall B, et al. Predictors of mortality from kidney cancer in 332,547 men screened for the Multiple Risk Factor Intervention Trial. Cancer 1997;79:2171–7.
17. Wolk A, Gridley G, Niwa S, et al. International renal-cell cancer study. VII. Role of diet. Int J Cancer 1996;65:67–73.
18. Prineas RJ, Folsom AR, Zhang ZM, et al. Nutrition and other risk factors for renal cell carcinoma in postmenopausal women. Epidemiology 1997;8:31–6.
19. Chow WH, Gridley G, Fraumeni JF Jr, Jarvholm B. Obesity, hypertension and risk of kidney cancer in men. N Engl J Med 2000;343:1305–11.
20. Bergstrom A, Hsieh CC, Lindlbad P, et al. Obesity and renal cell cancer—a quantitative review. Br J Cancer 2001;85:984–90.
21. Calle EE, Rodriguez C, Walker-Thurmond K, Thun MJ. Overweight, obesity and mortality from cancer in a prospectively studied cohort of US adults. N Engl J Med 2003;348:1625–38.
22. Bjorge T, Tretli S, Engelend A. Relation of height and body mass index to renal cell carcinoma in two million Norwegian men and women. Am J Epidemiol 2004;160:1168–76.
23. Calle EE, Kaaks, R. Overweight, obesity and cancer: epidemiological evidence and proposed mechanisms. Nat Rev 2004;4:579–91.
24. Gago-Dominguez M, Castelao JE, Yuan JM, et al. Lipid peroxidation: a novel and unifying concept of the etiology of

renal cell carcinoma (United States). Cancer Causes Control 2002;13:287–93.

25. Kasiske BL, O'Donnell MP, Keane WF. The Zucker rat model of obesity, insulin resistance, hyperlipidemia, and renal injury. Hypertension 1992;19:I110–5.

26. Huang Z, Willett WC, Manson JE, et al. Body weight, weight change, and risk for hypertension in women. Ann Intern Med 1998;128:81–8.

27. Chow WH, Devesa SS, Moore, LE. Epidemiology of renal cell carcinoma. In: Nicholas J, Vogelzan N, editors. Comprehensive textbook of genitourinary oncology. 3rd ed. Philadelphia: Lippincott Williams & Wilkins; 2006. p. 669–79.

28. Lipworth L, Tarone RE, McLaughlin JK. The epidemiology of renal cell carcinoma. J Urol 2006;176:2353–8.

29 Dhote R, Thiounn N, Debre B, Vidal-Trecan G. Risk Factors for adult renal cell carcinoma. Urol Clin North Am 2004;31:237–47.

30. Scaglione R, Argano C, Parrinello G, et al. Relationship between transforming growth factor β1 and progression of hypertensive renal disease. J Hum Hypertens 2002; 16:641–45.

31. Shimbukuro T, Ohmoto Y, Naito K. Transforming growth factor-beta1 and renal cell cancer: cell growth, mRNA expression and protein production of cytokines. J Urol 2003;169:1865–9.

32. Johnson RJ, Herrera-Acosta J, Schreiner GF, et al. Subtle acquired renal injury as a mechanism of salt-sensitive hypertension. N Engl J Med 2002;346:913–23.

33. Mazzali M, Jefferson JA, NI A, et al. Microvascular and tubulointerstitial injury associated with chronic hypoxia-induced hypertension. Kidney Int 2003;63:2088–93.

34. Mellemgaard A, Moller H, Olsen JH. Diuretics may increase risk of renal cell carcinoma. Cancer Causes Control 1992;3:309–12.

35. Lindblad P, McLaughlin JK, Rasgon SA, et al. Risk of kidney cancer among patients using analgesics and diuretics: a population-based cohort study. Int J Cancer 1993;55:5–9.

36. McLaughlin JK, Chow WH, Mandel JS, et al. International renal-cell cancer study. VIII. Role of diuretics, other antihypertensive medications and hypertension. Int J Cancer 1995;63:216–21.

37. Yuan JM, Castelao JE, Gago-Dominguez M, et al. Hypertension, obesity and their medications in relation to renal cell carcinoma. Br J Cancer 1998;77:1508–13.

38. Fryzek JP, Poulsen AH, Johnsen SP, et al. A cohort study of antihypertensive treatments and risk of renal cell cancer. Br J Cancer 2005;92:1302–6.

39. McLaughlin JK. Renal cell cancer and exposure to gasoline: a review. Environ Health Perspect 1993;101 Suppl 6:111–4.

40. Bruning T, Pesch B, Wiesenhutter B, et al. Renal cell cancer risk and occupational exposure to trichloroethylene: results of a consecutive case-control study in Arnsberg, Germany. Am J Ind Med 2003;43:274–85.

41. Green LC, Lash TL. Re: renal cell cancer correlated with occupational exposure to trichloroethylene. J Cancer Res Clin Oncol 1999;125:430–2.

42. Cherrie JW, Kromhout H, Semple S. The importance of reliable exposure estimates in deciding whether trichloroethylene can cause kidney cancer. J Cancer Res Clin Oncol 201;127:400–4.

43. McLaughlin JK, Blot WJ. A critical review of epidemiology studies of trichloroethylene and perchloroethylene and risk of renal cell cancer. Int Arch Occup Environ Health 1997;70:222–31.

44. Brauch H, Weirich G, Hornauer MA, et al. Trichloroethylene exposure and specific somatic mutations in patients with renal cell carcinoma. J Natl Cancer Inst 1999;20:123–25.

45. Lambe M, Lindblad P, Wuu J, et al. Pregnancy and risk of renal cell cancer: a population-based study in Sweden. Br J Cancer 2002;86:1425–9.

46. Mellemgaard A, Lindblad P, Schlehofer B, et al. International renal-cell cancer study III. Role of weight, height, physical activity and use of amphetamines. Int J Cancer 1995; 60:350–4.

47. Mellemgaard A, Engholm G, McLaughlin JK, Olsen JH. Risk factors for renal-cell carcinoma in Denmark. III. Role of weight, physical activity and reproductive factors. Int J Cancer 1994;56:66–71.

48. Chow WH, McLaughlin JK, Mandel JS, et al. Reproductive factors and the risk of renal cell cancer among women. Int J Cancer 1995;60:321–4.

49. Gago-Dominguez M, Castelao JE, Yuan JM, et al. Increased risk of renal cell carcinoma subsequent to hysterectomy. Cancer Epidemiol Biomarkers Prev 1999;8:999–1003.

50. Lindblad P, Mellemgaard A, Schelhofer B, et al. International renal-cell cancer study. V. Reproductive factors, gynecologic operations and exogenous hormones. Int J Cancer 1995;61:192–8.

51. Adami H-O, Persson I, Hoover R, et al. Risk of cancer in women receiving hormone replacement therapy. Int J Cancer 1989;44:833–9.

52. Weisz J, Fritz-Wolz G, Clawson GA, et al. Induction of nuclear catechol-O-methytransferase by estrogens in hamster kidney: implications for estrogen-induced renal cancer. Carcinogenesis 1998;19:1307–12.

53. Corte-Vizcaino V, Llombart-Bosch A. Estrogen and progesterone receptors in the diethylstilbestero-induced kidney neoplasms of the Syrian golden hamster: correlation with histopathology and tumoral stages. Carcinogenesis 1993;14:1215–19.

54. Dhote R, Pellicer-Coeuret M, Thiounn N, et al. Risk factors for adult renal cell carcinoma: a systematic review and implications for prevention. BJU Int 2000;86:20–7.

55. Rashidkhani B, Lindblad P, Wolk A. Fruits, vegetables and risk of renal cell carcinoma: a prospective study of Swedish women. Int J Cancer 2005;113:451–5.

56. Adami H-O, McLaughlin JK, Hsing AW, et al. Alcoholism and cancer risk: a population-based cohort study. Cancer Causes Control 1992;3:419–25.

57. Rashidkhani B, Akesson A, Lindblad P, Wolk A. Major dietary patterns and risk of renal cell carcinoma in a prospective cohort of Swedish women. J Nutr 2005; 135:1757–62.

58. Parker AS, Cerhan JR, Lynch CF, et al. Gender, alcohol consumption, and renal cell carcinoma. Am J Epidemiol 2002; 155:455–62.

59. Wolk A, Gridley G, Niwa S, et al. International renal-cell cancer study. VII. Role of diet. Int J Cancer 1996;65:67–73.

60. Nyberg U, Nilsson B, Travis LB, et al. Cancer incidence among Swedish patients exposed to radioactive

thorotrast: a forty-year follow-up survey. Radiat Res 2002;61:2201–9.

61. Schlehofer B, Pommer W, Mellemgaard A, et al. International renal-cell cancer study. VI. The role of medical and family history. Int J Cancer 1996;66:723–26.

62. Gago-Dominguez M, Yuan JM, Castelao JE, et al. Family history and risk of renal cell carcinoma. Cancer Epidemiol Biomarkers Prev 2001;10:10001–4.

63. Hutchison GB. Evaluation of preventive services. J Chronic Dis 1960;11:497–508.

64. Fletcher RH, Fletcher SW, Wagner EH. Clinical epidemiology: the essentials. 3rd ed. Baltimore: Williams & Wilkins; 1996.

65. Thompson IM, Peek M. Improvement in survival of patients with renal cell carcinoma—the role of the seredipitously detected tumor. J Urol 1998;140:487–40.

66. Rodriguez-Rubio FI, Diez-Caballero F, Martin-Marquina A, et al. Incidentally detected renal cell carcinoma. Br J Urol 1996;78:29–32.

67. Gudbjartsson T,.Thoroddsen A, Petursdottir V, et al. Effect of incidental detection for survival of patients with renal cell carcinoma: results of population-based study of 701 patients. Urology 2005;66:1186–91.

68. Cohn EB, Campbell SC. Screening for RCC. In: Bukowski RM, Novick AC, editors. Renal cell carcinoma–molecular biology, immunology, and clinical management. New Jersey: Humana Press;2000. p. 93–110.

69. Guide to Clinical Preventive Services. Recommendations of the US Preventive Services Task Force. Rockville, MD: Agency for Healthcare Research and Quality, June 2006. AHRQ Publication No. 06-0588. http://www.ahrq.gov/clinic/pocketgd06/

70. Turney BW, Reynard JM, Cranston DW. A case for screening for renal cancer. BJU Int 2006;97:220–1.

71. Mihara S, Koruda K, Yoshioka R, Koyama W. Early detection of renal cell carcinoma by ultrasonographic screening—based on the results of 13 years screening in Japan. Ultrasound Med Biol 1999;25:1033–9.

72. Malaeb BS, Martin JD, Littooy FN, et al. The utility of screening renal ultrasonography: identifying renal cell carcinoma in an elderly asymptomatic population. BJU Int 2005;95:977–81.

73. Fields SI, Calvert-Hill MA. Clinical efficacy of screening the entire abdomen during real-time ultrasound examination. J Clin Ultrasound 1985;13:411–3.

74. Tsuboi N, Horiuchi K, Kimura G, et al. Renal masses detected by general health checkup. Int J Urol 2000;7:404–8.

75. Spouge AR, Wilson SR, Wooley B. Abdominal sonography in asymptomatic executives. Prevalence of pathologic findings, potential benefits, and problems. J Ultrasound Med 1996;15:763–7.

76. Fenton JJ, Weiss NS. Screening computed tomography—will it result in overdiagnosis of renal carcinoma. Cancer 2004;100:986–90.

77. Garella S. The cost of dialysis in the USA. Nephrol Dial Transplant 1997;12:10–21.

78. Narasimhan N, Golper T, Wolfson M, et al. Clinical characteristics and diagnostic considerations in acquired renal cystic disease. Kidney Int 1986;30:748–52.

79. Ishikawa I. Acquired cystic disease: mechanisms and manifestations. Semin Nephrol 1991;11:671–84.

80. Ishikawa I, Saito Y, Shikura N, et al. Ten-year prospective study on the development of renal cell carcinoma in dialysis patients. Am J Kidney Dis 1999;34:452–8.

81. Levine E. Acquired cystic kidney disease. Radiol Clin North Am 1996;34:947–64.

82. Hughson M, Buchwald D, Fox M. Renal neoplasia and acquired cystic kidney disease in patients receiving long-term dialysis. Arch Pathol Lab Med 1986;110:592–601.

83. Ishikawa I, Rymon H, Yamada Y, Kakuma T. Renal cell carcinoma detected by screening shows better patient survival than that detected following symptoms in dialysis patients. Ther Apher Dial 2004;8:468–73.

84. Ishikawa I, Ishii H, Shinoda A, et al. Renal cell carcinoma of the native kidney after renal transplantation. A case report and review of the literature. Nephron 1991;58:354–358.

85. Chandhoke PS, Torrence RJ, Clayman RV, Rothstein M. Acquired cystic disease of the kidney: management dilemma. J Urol 1002;147:969–74.

86. Terasawa Y, Suzuki Y, Morita M, et al. Ultrasonic diagnosis of renal cell carcinoma in hemodialysis patients. J Urol 1994;152:846–51.

87. Marple JT, MacDougall M, Chonko AM. Renal cancer complicating acquired cystic kidney disease. J Am Soc Nephrol 1994;4:1951–6.

88. Grantham, JJ. Acquired cystic kidney disease. Kidney Int 1991;40:143–52.

89. MacDougall ML, Welling LW, Wiegmann TB. Prediction of carcinoma in acquired cystic disease as a function of kidney weight. J Am Soc Nephrol 1990;1:828–31.

90. Fick GM, Gabow PA. Hereditary and acquired cystic disease of the kidney. Kidney Int 1994;46:951–64.

91. Sarasin FP, Wong JB, Levey AS, Meyer KB. Screening for acquired cystic kidney disease: a decision analytic perspective. Kidney Int 1995;48:207–19.

92. Cowie A. Renal imaging in patients requiring renal replacement therapy. Semin Dial 2002;15:237–49.

93. Carver BS, Zibari GB, McBride V, et al. The incidence and implications of renal cell carcinoma in cadaveric renal transplants at the time of organ recovery. Transplantation 1999;67:1438–40.

94. Muruve NA, Shoskes DA. Genitourinary malignancies in solid organ transplant recipients. Transplantation 2005;80:709–16.

95. U.S. Renal Data System. USRDS 2003 Annual data report: atlas of end-stage renal disease in the United States, Bethesda, MD: National Institutes of Health, National Institute of Diabetes and Digestive and Kidney Diseases, 2003.

96. Penn I. Primary kidney tumors before and after renal transplantation. Transplantation 1995;59:480–5.

97. Kliem V, Kolditz M, Behrend M, et al. Risk of renal cell carcinoma after kidney transplantation. Clin Transplant 1997;11:255–8.

98. Doublet JD, Peraldi MN, Gattegno B, et al. Renal cell carcinoma of native kidneys: prospective study of 129 renal transplant patients. J Urol 1997;158:42–4.

99. Lonser RR, Glenn GM, Walther M, et al. von Hippel-Lindau disease. Lancet 2003;361:2059–67.

100. Herring JC, Enquist EG, Chernoff A, et al. Parenchymal sparing surgery in patients with hereditary renal cell carcinoma: 10-year experience. J Urol 2001;165:777–81.

101. Walther MM, Choyke PL, Glenn G, et al. Renal cancer in families with hereditary renal cancer: prospective analysis of a tumor size threshold for renal parenchymal sparing surgery. J Urol 1999;161:1475–9.

102. Poston CD, Jaffe GS, Lubensky IA, et al. Characterization of the renal pathology of a familial form of renal cell carcinoma associated with von Hippel-Lindau disease: clinical and molecular genetic implications. J Urol 1995;153:22–6.

103. Stolle C, Glenn G, Zbar B, et al. Improved detection of germline mutations in the von Hippel-Lindau disease tumor suppressor gene. Hum Mutat 1998;12:417–23.

104. Choyke PL, Glenn GM, Walther MM, et al. von Hippel-Lindau disease: genetic, clinical and imaging features. Radiology 1995;194:629–42.

105. Levine E, Collins DL, Horton WA, et al. CT screening of the abdomen in von Hippel-Lindau disease. Am J Roentgenol 1982;139:505–10.

106. Zbar B, Glenn G, Lubensky I, et al. Hereditary papillary renal cell carcinoma: clinical studies in 10 families. J Urol 1995;153:907–12.

107. Schmidt L, Duh FM, Chen F, et al. Germline and somatic mutations in the tyrosine kinase domain of the MET proto-oncogene in papillary renal carcinomas. Nat Genet 1997;16:68–73.

108. Schmidt L, Junker K, Weirich G, et al. Two North American families with hereditary papillary renal carcinoma and identical novel mutations in the MET proto-oncogene. Cancer Res 1998;58:1719–22.

109. Zhuang Z, Park WS, Pack S, et al. Trisomy 7-harbouring non-random duplication of the mutant MET allele in hereditary papillary renal carcinomas. Nat Genet 1998;20:66–9.

110. Sampson JR. The kidney in tuberous sclerosis: manifestations and molecular genetic mechanisms. Nephrol Dial Transplant 1996;11:34–7.

111. Bernstein J, Robbins TO, Kissane JM. The renal lesions of tuberous sclerosis. Semin Diagn Pathol 1986;3:97–105.

112. Washeka R, Hanna M. Malignant renal tumors in tuberous sclerosis. Urology 1991;37:340–3.

113. Tello R, Blickman JG, Buonomo C, Herrin J. Meta analysis of the relationship between tuberous sclerosis complex and renal cell carcinoma. Eur J Radiol 1998;27:131–8.

114. Robertson FM, Cendron M, Klauber GT, Harris BH. Renal cell carcinoma in association with tuberous sclerosis in children. J Pediatr Surg 1996;31:729–30.

115. Bjornsson J, Short MP, Kwiatkowski DJ, Henske EP. Tuberous sclerosis-associated renal cell carcinoma. Clinical, pathological, and genetic features. Am J Pathol 1996;149:1201–8.

116. Aoyama T, Fujikawa K, Yoshimura K, et al. Bilateral renal cell carcinoma in a patient with tuberous sclerosis. Int J Urol 1996;3:150–1.

117. Dickinson M, Ruckle H, Beaghler M, Hadley HR. Renal angiomyolipoma: optimal treatment based on size and symptoms. Clin Nephrol 1998;49:281–6.

118. Lemaitre L, Robert Y, Dubrulle F, et al. Renal angiomyolipoma: growth followed up with CT and/or US. Radiology 1995;197:598–602.

# 3

# Diagnosis and Management of Inherited Renal Cancer

KATHERINE L. NATHANSON, MD
ANDREW J. STEPHENSON, MD

## OVERVIEW OF INHERITED RENAL CANCERS

Inherited renal cancer syndromes are estimated to account for less than 3% of all renal cancers. The identification and elucidation of these syndromes have important implications not only for the management of the families with hereditary renal cancer but for our understanding of the biologic basis of sporadic renal cancer. Familial renal cancer syndromes are divided into two major groups (Tables 1 and 2). We focus on genetic syndromes in which adult-onset renal cancer is one of the major manifestations of disease. These syndromes include von Hippel-Lindau disease (vHL), autosomal dominant inherited susceptibility to clear cell renal cancer, hereditary papillary renal cell carcinoma (HPRCC), hereditary leiomyomatosis and

**Table 1. AUTOSOMAL DOMINANT CANCER-SUSCEPTIBILITY SYNDROMES ASSOCIATED WITH A SIGNIFICANTLY INCREASED RISK OF RENAL CANCER**

| Syndrome | Gene | Chromosome | Type of Renal Cancer | Additional Features |
|---|---|---|---|---|
| von Hippel-Lindau disease | VHL | 3p25–36 | Clear cell | Central nervous-hemangioblastoma (brain, spine, retina); adrenal-pheochromocytoma; ear-endolymphatic sac tumors; pancreas-cysts, neuroendocrine tumors |
| Familial clear cell renal cancer with chromosome 3 translocation | ? | Translocation through chromosome 3 | Clear cell | — |
| Familial clear cell renal cancer | ? | ? | Clear cell | — |
| Hereditary papillary renal cell carcinoma | MET | 7q31 | Type 1 papillary | — |
| Hereditary leiomyomatosis and renal cell carcinoma | FH | 1q42 | Type 2 papillary (large nucleoli surrounded by a clear halo within the nuclei); collecting duct cancer; occasional clear cell | Skin-cutaneous leiomyomas; uterus-leiomyomas, leiomyosarcoma |
| Birt-Hogg-Dube syndrome | FLCN | 17p11.2 | Hybrid oncocytic tumors (oncocytoma/chromophobe); occasional clear cell | Skin-fibrofolliculomas; lung-cysts, pneumothorax |

**Table 2. GENETIC SYNDROMES IN WHICH RENAL CANCER HAS BEEN REPORTED AS AN OCCASIONAL FEATURE**

| Syndrome | Gene | Chromosome | Type of Renal Cancer | Major Disease Features |
|---|---|---|---|---|
| Papillary thyroid cancer–papillary renal cancer | ? | 1p21 | Papillary | — |
| Cowden syndrome | PTEN | 10q23 | Clear cell | Breast, fibrocystic disease, breast cancer; thyroid, multinodular goiter, papillary thyroid cancer; uterus, leiomyomas, endometrial cancer; mucocutaneous, trichilemmomas, papillomatous papules, acral keratosis; central nervous system, macrocephaly, Lhermitte-Duclos |
| Hereditary paraganglioma/pheochromocytoma syndrome | SDHB | 1p36.1–p35 | Clear cell | Paraganglioma; extraadrenal pheochromocytoma; adrenal pheochromocytoma |
| Tuberous sclerosis complex | TSC1 | 9q34 | Angiomyolipoma clear cell | Central nervous system, cortical tubers, subependymal nodules, subependymal astrocytoma; renal, cysts, angiomyolipomas; cardiac, rhabdomyomas; mucocutaneous, angiofibromas, ungal fibromas, hypomelanotic macules, dental pits; lung, lymphangiomyomatosis |
| | TSC2 | 16p13.3 | | |
| Hyperparathyroidism–jaw tumor syndrome | CDC73 | 1q25 | — | Parathyroid adenomas; ossifying fibromas of the jaw; uterine tumors |

renal cell carcinoma (HLRCC), and Birt-Hogg-Dube syndrome (BHD). Each of these inherited diseases is associated with a specific type of renal cancer—clear cell renal cell carcinoma (ccRCC), type 1 papillary cancer, type 2 papillary cancer, and hybrid chromophobe/oncocytoma cancer, respectively. The identification of each of the underlying genes for the inherited forms of renal cancer has significantly increased our understanding of the biology of their sporadic counterparts. Furthermore, our understanding of the disrupted pathways has lead to the development and use of targeted therapeutics in renal cancer.

Each of the hereditary kidney cancer syndromes is associated with varying risks of renal cell carcinoma of specific histologic subtypes and varying extrarenal manifestations. As such, successful management of the patients with the hereditary renal cancer syndromes requires a multidisciplinary team approach that is specific to each syndrome. The management of renal cortical tumors that arise in the setting of hereditary renal cancer syndromes differs substantially from that of sporadic renal tumors because of their earlier age of onset and their tendency for multifocality, bilaterality, and local recurrence in retained kidneys. For patients with vHL and HPRCC, thousands of tumors at different stages of evolution may be observed upon histopathologic evaluation of nephrectomy specimens.[1,2] Given the potential for the development of multiple bilateral tumors over an individual's lifetime, the primary goal in the management of patients with hereditary renal cancer syndromes is preventing the development of distant metastases while preserving renal function and minimizing the number of interventions for the treatment of these lesions.

## AUTOSOMAL DOMINANT CANCER-SUSCEPTIBILITY SYNDROMES ASSOCIATED WITH A SIGNIFICANTLY INCREASED RISK OF RENAL CANCER

### von Hippel-Lindau Disease

#### Genetics of vHL

vHL is an autosomal dominant cancer-susceptibility syndrome in which patients develop hemangioblastomas of the brain, spine, and retina; ccRCC; pancreatic cysts; pancreatic neuroendocrine tumors; endolymphatic sac tumors (ELSTs); and pheochromocytomas. von Hippel first recognized its familial nature[3]; Lindau recognized that the retinal lesions were part of a larger heritable syndrome that affected the central nervous system.[4] In the modern scientific literature, Melmon and Rosen were the first to describe a vHL family in 1964.[5] vHL was the first of the hereditary renal cancer syndromes delineated and was well described prior to gene identification in 1993.[6–9] vHL is prevalent in all ethnic groups and is estimated to occur in 1 in 35,000 people.[10] The penetrance of vHL is estimated at over 90% by age 65. Prior to modern screening techniques, the median age of death was less than 50 years.[11] The mean age of diagnosis is 24.7 years (median 22 years), with patients presenting with clinical symptoms as early as age 5.[12]

After the etiologic gene *VHL* on chromosome 3p25–26 was identified, a strong genotype–phenotype correlation with mutational type predictive of disease was observed (Table 3). Patients with type 1 mutations (in general, truncating mutations) have a decreased penetrance of pheochromocytoma compared with those with type 2 mutations (in general, missense mutations).[12–17] Families with type 2 mutations have either a high (type 2A) or low (type 2B) risk of ccRCC; type 2C families only develop pheochromocytoma.

Genetic testing for mutations in *VHL*, which includes screening for point mutations and large deletions, detects nearly 100% of individuals with vHL.[18] There have been several case reports on mosaicism for a *VHL* mutation identified in parents whose children were diagnosed with vHL.[19,20] The *VHL* gene is a classic tumor suppressor, and loss of the wild-type allele is found in hemangioblastomas, pancreatic neuroendocrine tumors, renal cysts, and ccRCC in patients with vHL.[21–24] Somatic point mutations within and hypermethylation of *VHL* have been identified in 40 to 70% and 5 to 20% of clear cell renal cancers, respectively.[25–29] The most comprehensive study of sporadic ccRCC found somatic biallelic inactivation of *VHL* in 74%.[30] However, somatic mutations found in *VHL* differ from those found in vHL, with missense mutations distributed throughout the gene rather than clustered in the α-domain.[12,30] Thus, the

| vHL Disease Type | Risk of Tumor Types Observed in vHL Families | | | Germline VHL Mutation Types |
| --- | --- | --- | --- | --- |
| | HB | RCC | PHEO | |
| 1 | High | High | Low | Full gene deletions, partial gene deletions, nonsense mutations, and splice acceptor mutations |
| 2A | High | Low | High | Missense mutations (Tyr98His, Tyr112His) |
| 2B | High | High | High | Partial gene deletions, non sense mutations, and mis sense mutations |
| 2C | No | No | High | Missense mutations (Ser80Leu, Val84Leu, Leu188Val) |

Table 3. **RISK OF MAJOR MANIFESTATIONS OF VHL BY MUTATION STATUS**

HB = hemangioblastoma; PHEO = pheochromocytoma; RCC = renal cell cancer; vHL = von Hippel-Lindau disease.

majority of sporadic ccRCC have inactivated *VHL* and thus loss of pVHL function.

The protein from the VHL gene (pVHL) contains two functional domains, the α- and β-domains, which are involved in binding to elongin C and pVHL substrates, respectively.[31–34] pVHL participates in a complex containing elongin C, elongin B, CUL2, and Rbx1, the main function of which is to ubiquinate the alpha regulatory subunits of the hypoxia-inducible factor (HIF) family and target them for degradation.[35] HIF functions as a transcription factor that regulates adaptation to tissue hypoxia.[36–39] pVHL also regulates additional genes, independent of HIF; however, the role of those targets is not as well understood.[40–43]

### Renal Cancer in vHL

Thirty-five percent of patients with vHL are diagnosed with ccRCC, with a mean age at diagnosis of $39.7 \pm 10.7$ years.[12] With the advent of genetic testing, the frequency of renal cancer diagnosis has increased and average age of diagnosis has decreased compared with older series.[11] Renal cysts are observed in over 60% of patients. The wild-type allele of *VHL* is lost consistently in renal cysts, suggesting that the loss is an important initiating event in tumorigenesis.[24] Frameshift and nonsense mutations confer a high penetrance of ccRCC, with risk of 70% at age 50.[12] Full and partial gene deletions confer a lower risk, with risk of ccRCC of 40% at age 50. As discussed above, type 2A missense mutations confer a high risk of ccRCC, whereas other missense mutations, types 2B and 2C, do not appear to be associated with renal cancer.[37] Type 2B mutations impair binding of elongin C to pVHL, and type 2A mutations are within the HIF-binding site (β-domain).[44] Type 2A mutations have been associated with the retention of HIF2α activity and increased growth compared with type 2B mutations.[45,46] These results implicate a biologic difference accounting for the variability risk of renal cancer associated with different types of mutations.

ccRCC is the only type of renal cancer found in patients with vHL. Given the multifocality and bilaterality of renal cell carcinomas in vHL (Figure 1)

and the propensity for the interval development of metachronous tumors, nephron-sparing approaches (partial nephrectomy, thermal ablative therapies, or observation) should be used in the management of these lesions whenever possible. Prior to the institution of familial screening, abdominal computed tomography (CT), and an aggressive surgical approach to ccRCC, tumors were often diagnosed at an advanced stage, necessitating radical nephrectomy. As such, renal manifestations were a major cause of morbidity and mortality; 13 to 42% of patients died from ccRCC and 25 to 33% developed end-stage renal disease.[47–49]

Novick and Streem reported the results of partial nephrectomy in nine patients with vHL between 1981 and 1986.[47] Despite successful partial nephrectomy in all patients, distant metastases developed in two patients, six patients developed local recurrences (three of whom required renal-replacement therapy after treatment), and one patient was continuously disease free over a median follow-up of 7 years. The authors concluded that bilateral nephrectomy and renal transplantation may be a more acceptable alternative to nephron-sparing approaches, conferring the highest probability of cure. Steinbach and colleagues reported a 33% cancer-specific mortality rate at 10 years among 65 patients diagnosed with vHL prior to 1993.[49] Over a short-term follow-up (median 68 months), only 44 patients (32%) retained both kidneys, and 15

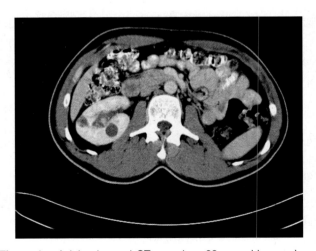

**Figure 1.** Axial enhanced CT scan in a 33-year-old man shows both renal cysts and cystic renal cell carcinoma in the right kidney. A left nephrectomy had been performed previously for ccRCC.

(23%) developed end-stage renal disease requiring transplantation or dialysis.

Goldfarb and colleagues reported the outcome of bilateral nephrectomy and renal transplantation in 32 patients with vHL between 1974 and 1996 in a multicenter study.[50] There was no difference in overall survival, graft survival, or renal function between the patients with vHL and a matched cohort of 32 patients without vHL undergoing renal transplantation. The 5-year survival of the patients with vHL was 65%, and three patients (9%) died of metastatic ccRCC despite bilateral nephrectomy and renal transplantation.

In contemporary series, 85 to 90% of patients with vHL are diagnosed with renal masses less than 6 cm, and only in 11% of patients progression to distant metastases.[51] Given the low reported rate of metastasis among patients with sporadic renal cortical neoplasms less than 3 cm, investigators have adopted a policy of initial observation for ccRCCs less than 3 cm and immediate intervention for lesions greater than 3 cm in patients with vHL.[51] Over a follow-up of 5 years, Walther and colleagues reported no evidence of metastatic disease progression and no requirement for renal transplantation or dialysis in 52 patients with ccRCCs less than 3 cm at diagnosis.[51] In contrast, distant metastases developed in 11 of 44 patients (25%) with lesions greater than 3 cm, including 3 of 27 patients (11%) with lesions between 3 and 6 cm. In a recent update of this series, Duffey and colleagues confirmed the safety of this approach.[52] Over a median follow-up of 41 months, all 108 patients with lesions less than 3 cm remained free of distant metastases and avoided renal transplantation and dialysis: 37 (34%) remained on observation without intervention and 104 (96%) retained both kidneys. For the 71 patients (66%) who required intervention for interval growth of lesions greater than 3 cm, an average of 1.7 procedures per patient were performed, and 97% of these were nephron-sparing procedures (partial nephrectomy or percutaneous ablative procedures). In contrast, for the 63 patients with lesions greater than 3 cm who underwent treatment for renal tumors, a nephron-sparing approach was successfully used in only 68% of instances, and only

34 patients (54%) retained both kidneys at their last follow-up.

## Other Manifestations of vHL

In addition to renal cancer, the most prevalent manifestations of vHL include hemangioblastomas of the retina and central nervous system and pheochromocytomas. Retinal hemangioblastomas have been reported in 37 to 73% of patients.[12,54] The prevalence of cerebellar and spinal hemangioblastomas is reported at 57 and 25%, respectively, with mean ages of diagnosis of 29.9 and 33.3 years.[12,54] Cerebellar hemangioblastomas are more common than spinal hemangioblastomas. The growth pattern of hemangioblastomas is variable and unpredictable; cysts associated with hemangioblastomas cause more acute issues as they enlarge more quickly.[54]

Twenty percent of patients with vHL develop pheochromocytomas, with the mean age of diagnosis of 20 years. Although the risk of pheochromocytoma is highest in patients with missense mutations in surface amino acids ($p =.004$), pheochromocytomas do develop in patients with other mutations, with lower penetrance.[12] The mean age of diagnosis is highest in vHL patients with loss of function mutations in VHL, 27.8 ($\pm$ 9.7 years), compared with those with surface missense mutations, 21.7 ($\pm$ 10.5 years). Individuals as young as 5 years with vHL have been diagnosed with pheochromocytoma.[55] Patients with vHL can develop extraadrenal pheochromocytomas but do not develop paragangliomas of the head and neck.

Other less common manifestations of vHL include ELSTs (11 to 16% of patients), pancreatic cysts (35 to 70% of patients), pancreatic neuroendocrine tumors, and epididymal or broad ligament cystadenoma.[56,57] Pancreatic cysts are extremely common and generally do not need to be treated. Pancreatic neuroendocrine tumors are generally nonsecreting but can cause problems due to obstruction of the biliary tree. ELSTs can cause sensorineural hearing loss and vestibulopathy; unfortunately, these can arise from very small ELSTs, and as such, they need immediate treatment when identified.[57]

## Medical and Surgical Management of vHL

Standard screening recommendations for patients with vHL include (1) annual retinal examination for angiomas starting in infancy, (2) annual biochemical screening for elevated catecholamines and metanephrines starting at age 2, (3) baseline magnetic resonance imaging (MRI) of the craniospinal axis and annual screening starting at age 11, and (4) CT or baseline MRI of the abdomen, annual ultrasound screening of the abdomen from age 8 to 18, and annual CT or MRI screening starting at age 18.[56] Additional screening recommendations can include increased retinal screening to every 6 months from ages 15 to 30 and routine imaging for ELSTs rather than targeted screening based on symptoms of hearing loss and tinnitus.[57,58] Despite the known genotype–phenotype correlations, patients with classic vHL are offered the same standard screening regimen because although the penetrance of different manifestations may vary, they are still at risk. Patients with type 2C vHL (pheochromocytoma only) continue to have the same screening as other patients with vHL but biannually or even every 3 years rather than annually. Patients with bilateral nephrectomies continue to have abdominal imaging for pancreatic cysts, neuroendocrine tumors, and pheochromocytomas.

The mainstay of current therapy for vHL is surgical management of tumors. The technique of partial nephrectomy differs in vHL-related tumors compared with sporadic tumors because of the high probability of recurrent tumors within retained renal units. Given the frequent need for treatment of local recurrences within retained renal units, hilar dissection is minimized and tumors are removed without clamping of the renal vessels wherever possible.[59] Gerota's fascia is preserved and reapproximated at the end of the procedure to facilitate future exploration. vHL tumors are often surrounded by a pseudocapsule, and a technique by which tumors are enucleated without wedge resection by dissecting within this pseudocapsule has been described.[60] Resection of large cysts is attempted, small cysts are unroofed, and the cyst wall is ablated with the argon-beam coagulator. Intraoperative ultrasonography is used as up to 25% of small renal masses may be missed on preoperative imaging.[61] No attempt is made to resect deep intraparenchymal cysts. Management of other intraabdominal manifestations of vHL also can be performed safely at the same setting.[62]

Given that approximately 60% of lesions are less than 3 cm at diagnosis in contemporary vHL series, minimally invasive ablative procedures have been explored as alternatives to observation for these small lesions, but experience with these modalities in patients with vHL is limited at this time.[63,64] Shingleton and Sewell reported the results of percutaneous cryoablation in four patients with vHL with tumors of 2.8 to 5.0 cm.[63] They reported a reduction in tumor size and no enhancement between 2 to 23 months after treatment although two patients required re-treatment. Hwang and colleagues reported the results of percutaneous or laparoscopic radiofrequency ablation (RFA) for 24 tumors in 17 patients with hereditary renal tumors.[62] After 1 year of follow-up, all lesions decreased in size, and only one tumor exhibited enhancement on follow-up CT evaluation. Concerns regarding incomplete tumor destruction using RFA have been reported when treated lesions have been subject to immediate surgical resection.[65,66] In a series of 264 patients with small sporadic renal masses treated with percutaneous RFA ($n = 88$) or laparoscopic cryoablation ($n = 176$), the proportion of patients without evidence of central enhancement on 6-month CT evaluation was 86 and 89%, respectively.[67] However, there was evidence of viable malignancy on routine 6-month biopsy in 35% of RFA-treated lesions (including 25% of lesions without central enhancement) compared with 7% of lesions treated by laparoscopic cryoablation. All lesions without enhancement were biopsy negative. Salvage surgery for ablation-resistant lesions is frequently complicated by extensive perinephric scarring (particularly after cryoablation), and radical nephrectomy is often necessary.[68] On the basis of these results, ablative procedures for patients with vHL must be considered investigational at this time.

Pheochromocytomas in patients with vHL tend to be recurrent, bilateral, and benign.[69] Because of the morbidity associated with bilateral adrenalectomy and steroid-replacement therapy, an approach of observation for lesions less than 3.5 cm that are nonfunctional and asymptomatic has been adopted for patients with vHL. Intervention (either open or laparoscopic partial adrenalectomy) is reserved for lesions greater than 3.5 cm or if there is evidence of catecholamine hypersecretion.[69]

Novel chemotherapeutics, such as Sunitinib (reviewed in other chapters), have been developed that target many of the pathways perturbed in both sporadic renal cancer and vHL. These drugs currently are approved for metastatic sporadic ccRCC and are in clinical trials for use in vHL and, as such, may substantially change the way in which patients with vHL are treated in the near future.

## Autosomal Dominant Familial Clear Cell Renal Cancer

### Familial Clear Cell Renal Cancer

There have been two reports on familial clear cell renal cancer, defined as ≥ two first-degree relatives with ccRCC.[70,71] Unlike classic hereditary renal cancer syndromes, the families had solitary lesions diagnosed at variable ages. Chromosome 3 translocations and mutations in *VHL*, *MET*, and *CUL2* were excluded as causative. No gene has been identified that accounts for familial non-VHL ccRCC as of yet. As these families were described prior to identification of the causative genes for HLRCC and BHD, it is possible that they had one of these syndromes.

### Familial Clear Cell Renal Cancer with Chromosome 3 Translocation

Nine chromosome 3 translocations associated with multifocal renal cancer have been reported.[72–82] A preponderance of patients have bilateral ccRCC. The age of diagnosis varies but is later than in classic hereditary renal cancer syndromes, with the average age of diagnosis ranging from the early forties to late sixties.[73–75,77,79,82,83] Although the earliest reported age of diagnosis is 25, penetrance appears to be incomplete, and not all translocation carriers develop renal cancer.[84] The translocation breakpoints are at different points along both chromosomes; several have been cloned, and no consistent genetic

change has been identified.[78,80,82,85–88] Based on these results, it has been hypothesized that there is increased loss, through nondisjunction, of the derivative chromosome 3 during mitosis.[72,77] With loss of one allele, only one additional event, likely a mutation in or loss of *VHL*, needs to occur to predispose to the development of clear cell renal cancer.

Patients with multifocal, site-specific ccRCC, particularly if they have a positive family history, should be screened with a karyotype if they do not carry a mutation in *VHL*. There are no standard screening recommendations for carriers of a chromosome 3 translocation, and recommendations are based on expert opinion. Carriers of translocations should have abdominal CT or MRI done annually, noting that there are carriers who never develop renal cancer. Given the youngest age of diagnosis at 25, screening should start prior to that age. Observation of ccRCC until they reach 3 cm, as in patients with vHL, is a reasonable approach in this patient population.

## Hereditary Papillary Renal Cell Carcinoma

HPRCC is characterized by multifocal, bilateral, type 1 papillary renal cell carcinomas. Unlike the other hereditary kidney cancer syndromes, there are no extrarenal manifestations of HPRCC, and renal cysts are uncommon.[89,90] The average age of onset of renal tumors is 46.[2] Ornstein and colleagues described 1,000 to 3,000 microscopic papillary tumors within the renal parenchyma of patients with HPRCC.[2] Through linkage studies, the region containing the etiologic gene was narrowed down to 7q31.1–34, and the relevant gene is the Met protooncogene.[91] Subsequent studies have suggested that mutations in the tyrosine kinase domain of *MET* are present in a minority of sporadic type 1 papillary renal cancers.[92,93] No germ line mutations were identified in series of patients with sporadic type 1 papillary renal cancer, suggesting that mutation screening is only necessary for individuals with disease patterns consistent with hereditary disease.[94]

Annual screening with CT or MRI for the type 1 papillary renal cancers is recommended for individuals with HPRCC as this type of renal cancers can be isodense with the surrounding parenchyma and hence missed by ultrasound.[95] In addition, as the tumors are hypovascular, they can be mistaken for renal cysts. The management of renal tumors in patients with HPRCC follows a strategy similar to that used for VHL.[51]

## Hereditary Leiomyomatosis and Renal Cancer

### Genetics of HLRCC

HLRCC is an autosomal syndrome characterized by the development of cutaneous and uterine leiomyomas and renal cancer. An autosomal dominant syndrome with multiple cutaneous and uterine leiomyomas (MCUL) was described in 1973 by Reed and colleagues.[96] In 2001, two families with renal cancer and MUCL were reported by Launonen and colleagues, and they termed this hereditary leiomyomatosis and renal cancer.[97] They also noted the aggressiveness and the distinct histology of the renal cancers in patients with HLRCC.[98] The mutated gene in HLRCC is fumarate hydratase (FH),[99] which encodes the enzyme that converts fumarate to malate in the Krebs cycle. Although individuals with a single mutation in FH develop HLRCC, those with biallelic mutations (homozygous or compound heterozygotes) develop fumarate hydratase deficiency (FHD), in which patients develop fumaric aciduria, progressive encephalopathy, hypotonia, failure to thrive, and seizures.[100–106] Relatives of patients with FHD have been reported to develop cutaneous and uterine leiomyomas and are at risk to develop renal cancer.[99,106]

In a report on 56 HLRCC families seen at the NCI, 52 (93%) were found to have mutations in FH.[107,108] All types of point mutations have been reported in addition to large genomic deletions.[99,107,109] No genotype–phenotype correlations have been reported. Consistent with a postulated role as a tumor suppressor gene, loss of the wild-type allele is observed in cutaneous and uterine leiomyomas, as well as in renal cancer in individuals with FH mutations.[97–99,109,110] Fumarate hydratase enzymatic activity is lower in patients with MCUL and HLRCC and has been proposed as a screening recommendation for family members.[111]

### Renal Cancer in HLRCC

In the series from the National Institutes of Health, 32% of families with MCUL and HLRCC had an individual with renal cancer.[109] In families ascertained on the basis of multiple cutaneous leiomyomas, the frequency of renal cancer is low, at 1 to 2% and 16% in two series.[108,109] However, in families ascertained on the basis of either renal or cutaneous disease, the frequency of renal cancer is much higher, at 62%, suggesting that the predisposition to renal cancer is clustered in families. The standardized incidence ratio (SIR) has been calculated at 6.5 for renal cancer in HLRCC in a study comparing Finnish families with FH mutations and the general population.[110]

The predominant pathologic type of renal cancer associated with HLRCC is type 2 papillary cancer; however, other types of renal cancers are observed, including collecting duct and ccRCC. Patients also can have predominantly cystic lesions, as well as the more common solid tumors.[110] Independent of underlying architecture, cells in the renal cancers associated with HLRCC have large nuclei with inclusion-like orangiophilic or eosinophilic nucleoli surrounded by a clear halo.[112] Renal cancers associated with HLRCC tend to be early onset, high grade, and aggressive. Metastatic renal cancers have been reported in individuals as young as 17.[113] The mean age of diagnosis is 40, substantially less than that of sporadic renal cancer, with 10 of 19 (53%) patients either dead or living with advanced disease with a median follow-up of 34 months.[114] Thus, the natural history of renal cancer in HLRCC is distinct from other hereditary renal cancer syndromes, which tend to exhibit multifocal disease with a relatively benign natural history.

### Other Manifestations of HLRCC

The most frequent nonrenal manifestation of HLRCC is the uterine leiomyomas that develop in 75 to 98% of women.[97,99,107] The leiomyomas tend to be early onset and severe, with 68% diagnosed before the age of 30.[107] Most women have surgical treatment of their leiomyomas, with many having hysterectomies before the age of 30. Uterine leiomyosarcomas have been observed in the European population and in Finland, the SIR being 71.[110] Leiomyosarcomas have not been reported in the North America population, potentially as hysterectomy is more frequent.

Cutaneous leiomyomas are painful, pink-purplish nodules that affect individuals in a disseminated or segmental distribution. Cutaneous leiomyomas are benign tumors that arise from the piloerector apparatus.[108] Not all patients with HLRCC develop the cutaneous lesions, but most families have at least one person with cutaneous disease. Leydig cell tumors also have been reported in patients with HLRCC. Screening of sporadic Leydig cell tumors also identified a second male patient with a germ line mutation, suggesting that patients with Leydig cell tumors should be asked about pertinent family history.[115]

### Medical and Surgical Management of HLRCC

The increased risk of early-onset aggressive renal cancer in HLRCC necessitates screening and quick intervention. Although there are no standard guidelines for renal cancer screening, patients have been diagnosed as young as 17. Thus, screening should start at age 15, with abdominal/pelvic CT or MRI annually. Given the aggressive nature of these lesions, radical nephrectomy at diagnosis regardless of tumor size is the recommended treatment strategy.

## Birt-Hogg-Dube Syndrome

### Genetics of BHD

BHD is an autosomal dominant syndrome characterized by the development of fibrofolliculomas, renal cancer, predominantly hybrid oncocytic tumors, lung cysts, and pneumothoracies.[116,117] The gene for BHD was mapped to 17p12q11.2.[118,119] The gene in which mutations are associated with BHD was identified and named folliculin (*FLCN*).[120] The protein has no homology to previously identified proteins but was found to be conserved across species and expressed in a wide range of normal tissues including the skin, lung, and kidney. The function of the protein remains largely unknown, but recent studies implicate FLCN as acting in the mTOR pathway, potentially as activating Tor2.[121,122]

Mutations in *FLCN* are found in 69 to 85% of BHD families.[123–125] Multiple groups have noted that mutations are most frequently found within a $C_8$ tract in exon 11, as either insertions or deletions.[123,126,127] When the most common mutations, 1733insC and 1733delC, were compared, 1733insC was associated with a higher rate of renal cancers ($p = .03$).[123] More recent studies have suggested an association of mutations in exon 9 with lung cysts and thus pneumothorax ($p = .0002$).[124] *FCLN* was validated as a tumor suppressor gene, and, unusually, the second allele of *FCLN* is most frequently inactivated by point mutation rather than loss.[128] Mutations in *FLCN* are infrequently identified in sporadic renal cancers.[129,130]

### Renal Cancer in BHD

Although renal cancer was not included in the initial descriptions of BHD, an association between renal cancer and BHD was noted in 1993.[131,132] In the largest study of patients with BHD, 20% (38/187) of individuals from 24 families, representing 45% of families in total, had renal cancers.[123] The renal cancers in each patient ranged from a solitary lesion to multifocal bilateral cancers. Occurrence of renal cancer in BHD was predominant in men (27 men and 11 women), and the average age of diagnosis was 48 (range 31 to 71).[123]

A wide range of renal cancers has been observed in patients with BHD, even within the same kidney. The most common type of tumor is an unusual hybrid oncocytic tumor (mixed oncocytoma and chromophobe tumor). Observation of a hybrid oncocytic tumor in any patient should prompt an evaluation for BHD as it is so characteristic of this disease. On the basis of studies of sporadic cancer, it has been suggested that oncocytomas and chromophobe tumors share a common cell of origin and have similar gene expression profiles.[133,134] In a series of 84 tumors from 10 patients with BHD, 67% were hybrid oncocytic tumors, 23% chromophobe tumors, 7% clear cell tumors, and 3% oncocytomas.[135] There can be multiple types of renal cancer within a kidney and multiple cell types within a BHD-associated renal cancer. Small nodules of tumors similar to the large hybrid oncocytic tumors have been observed throughout the kidney, consistent with cancer-susceptibility syndromes in which all cells are predisposed to develop disease.[136] Although the malignant potential of the hybrid tumors has not been entirely elucidated, it appears to be low.[134,135,137] The various studies have not noted features suggestive of metastatic behavior such as the presence of distant metastases, vascular invasion, or tumor necrosis. Unfortunately, the ccRCC that arise in patients with BHD are aggressive and prone to metastasis. The clear cell tumors have been shown to have loss of 3p and/or mutations in *VHL*.[136] BHD accounts for familial oncocytoma in some cases.[132,138] In summary, patients with BHD can develop multifocal, bilateral renal cancers, the vast majority of which are oncocytic hybrid tumors. However, patients are at risk of malignant disease from ccRCC.

### Other Manifestations of BHD

The other major manifestations of BHD are found on the skin and in the lungs. Fibrofolliculomas of the skin appear in the twenties to thirties and are considered characteristic of BHD (Figure 2).[126,139] Patients can have from only a few fibrofolliculomas on their cheeks to extensive involvement of the face, neck, and upper back. Fibrofolliculomas are abnormal growths of the hair follicles, with epithelial

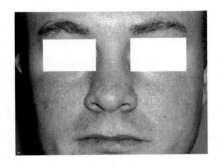

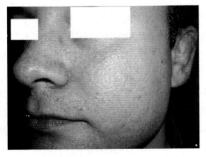

**Figure 2.** Fibrofolliculomas in a patient with BHD.

strands extending into the surrounding stroma. The lesions do not cause any problems for patients beyond cosmetic.

Lung cysts and pneumothoracies also are a component of BHD.[132] The relative risks of pneumothorax has been estimated to be 32 to 50%.[125] Of 198 patients from 89 families, 177 (89%) had lung cysts and 48 (24%) had pneumothoracies.[124] Mutations in *FLCN* also have been found in familial isolated spontaneous pneumothorax and in patients with multiple lung cysts.[143–145] BHD likely is the most common cause of familial pneumothorax.[146]

### Medical and Surgical Management of BHD

Patients do not necessarily have all the three major manifestations of BHD: renal cancer, lung cysts/pneumothorax, or fibrofolliculomas; they can have any combination of findings. This feature of BHD is of particular importance to note when counseling family members of a proband with BHD. All family members need to have genetic testing for mutations in *FLCN*, whether or not they have fibrofolliculomas.

There are no standard screening recommendations or clinical care recommendations for the manifestations of BHD in families with known disease. The risk of renal cancer is the main concern. On the basis of screening recommendations for other hereditary renal cancers, annual screening of the kidneys by CT starting in the early thirties seems reasonable. Because the number and volume of lung cysts are associated with risk of pneumothorax, a baseline chest CT is important. Screening after the initial study depends on the initial findings, with those with multiple cysts requiring annual CT scanning and pulmonary consultation. On the basis of the risk of pneumothorax, patients are advised to avoid scuba diving. A lower threshold for pleurodesis may be warranted in patients with pneumothorax. Intraoperative monitoring of patients is important during surgery as they are at increased risk of pneumothorax.

The treatment of renal masses in patients with BHD follows a strategy similar to that used for VHL; lesions smaller than 3 cm are observed, and those larger than 3 cm are surgically removed immediately.[135]

## GENETIC SYNDROMES IN WHICH RENAL CANCER HAS BEEN REPORTED AS AN OCCASIONAL FEATURE

### Tuberous Sclerosis Complex

Tuberous sclerosis complex (TSC) is an autosomal dominant syndrome, the main features of which are cortical tubers and subependymal nodules, renal angiomyolipomas and cysts, and cardiac rhabdomyomas.[147] TSC is caused by mutations in two genes, *TSC1* and *TSC2*. The phenotype of TSC is quite variable. Patients can be diagnosed with infantile spasms and seizures during their infancy, or this syndrome cannot be detected until their adult years with multiple renal cysts and angiolipomas. Angiomyolipomas cause morbidity based on their risk of hemorrhage and are treated with embolization.[148] There has been some controversy about an association between a risk of renal cancer and TSC.[149–151] Although the overall risk of renal cancer may not be increased, patients with TSC appear to have an earlier age of diagnosis of renal cancer.

### Cowden Syndrome (PTEN Hamartoma Tumor Syndrome)

Cowden syndrome is associated with an increased risk of benign and malignant tumors of the thyroid, breast, and endometrium and is caused by mutations in *PTEN*.[152] Dermatologic manifestations of Cowden syndrome are very common, seen in essentially all patients by their thirties, and include trichilemmomas, papillomatous papules, and acral and plantar keratoses.[153] Clear cell renal cancer has been reported in patients with Cowden syndrome, but the frequency is unknown.[154,155] A study of renal cancers and cell lines has shown that mutations in *PTEN* are present, particularly in late-stage ccRCCs.[156]

### Hereditary Paraganglioma/ Pheochromocytoma Due to Mutations in SDHB

Several hereditary paraganglioma syndromes have been identified due to mutations in three of the genes encoding the proteins of succinate dehydrogenase complex—*SDHB*, *SDHC*, and *SDHD*.[157] Mutations in *SDHB* are associated with malignant paragangliomas and extraadrenal pheochromocytomas.[158] Early-onset clear cell renal cancer also has been reported in association with *SDHB* mutations.[159] However, the prevalence of renal cancer due to *SDHB* mutations is unknown. *SDHB* mutation carriers have abdominal CT or MRI done anually, based on their risk of extraadrenal and adrenal pheochromocytoma, so renal cancer would be identified if present.

### Hyperparathyroidism–Jaw Tumor Syndrome

The main features of hyperparathyroidism–jaw tumor syndrome (HPT-JT), due to mutations in *CDC73* (*HRPT2*), are fibroosseus tumors of the jaw and parathyroid adenomas.[160] Renal cysts, hamartomas, mesoblastic nephromas, late-onset Wilms' tumors, and a single papillary renal cancer have been described in HPT-JT.[161–163]

### Papillary Thyroid Cancer with Associated Papillary Renal Cancer

In a single, large three-generation family, multiple cases of nodular thyroid disease and papillary thyroid cancer were reported.[164] Two of the family members had multifocal papillary renal cancers and one had oncocytomas.

## REFERENCES

1. Walther MM, Lubensky IA, Venzon D, et al. Prevalence of microscopic lesions in grossly normal renal parenchyma from patients with von Hippel-Lindau disease, sporadic renal cell carcinoma and no renal disease: clinical implications. J Urol 1995;154:2010–4; discussion 4–5.
2. Ornstein DK, Lubensky IA, Venzon D, et al. Prevalence of microscopic tumors in normal appearing renal parenchyma of patients with hereditary papillary renal cancer. J Urol 2000;163:431–3.
3. von Hippel E. Uber eine sehr seltene Erkanung der netzhaut. Graefes Arch Clin Exp Opthalmol 1904;59:83–106.
4. Lindau A. Studien ber kleinbirncysten bau: pathogenese und beziehungen zur angiomatosis retinae. Acta Radiol Microbiol Scand 1926;1 Suppl: 1–128.
5. Melmon KL, Rosen SW. Lindau's disease. Review of the literature and study of a large kindred. Am J Med 1964; 36:595–617.

6. Richards FM, Phipps ME, Latif F, et al. Mapping the von Hippel-Lindau disease tumour suppressor gene: identification of germline deletions by pulsed field gel electrophoresis. Hum Mol Genet 1993;2:879–82.

7. Richards FM, Maher ER, Latif F, et al. Detailed genetic mapping of the von Hippel-Lindau disease tumour suppressor gene. J Med Genet 1993;30:104–7.

8. Latif F, Tory K, Gnarra J, et al. Identification of the von Hippel-Lindau disease tumor suppressor gene. Science 1993;260:1317–20.

9. Maher ER, Bentley E, Yates JR, et al. Mapping of the von Hippel-Lindau disease locus to a small region of chromosome 3p by genetic linkage analysis. Genomics 1991;10:957–60.

10. Maher ER, Iselius L, Yates JR, et al. Von Hippel-Lindau disease: a genetic study. J Med Genet 1991;28:443–7.

11. Maher ER, Yates JR, Harries R, et al. Clinical features and natural history of von Hippel-Lindau disease. Q J Med 1990;77:1151–63.

12. Ong KR, Woodward ER, Killick P, et al. Genotype-phenotype correlations in von Hippel-Lindau disease. Hum Mutat 2007;28:143–9.

13. Zbar B, Kishida T, Chen F, et al. Germline mutations in the von Hippel-Lindau disease (VHL) gene in families from North America, Europe, and Japan. Hum Mutat 1996;8:348–57.

14. Hes F, Zewald R, Peeters T, et al. Genotype-phenotype correlations in families with deletions in the von Hippel-Lindau (VHL) gene. Hum Genet 2000;106:425–31.

15. Chen F, Kishida T, Yao M, et al. Germline mutations in the von Hippel-Lindau disease tumor suppressor gene: correlations with phenotype. Hum Mutat 1995;5:66–75.

16. Brauch H, Kishida T, Glavac D, et al. von Hippel-Lindau (VHL) disease with pheochromocytoma in the Black Forest region of Germany: evidence for a founder effect. Hum Genet 1995;95:551–6.

17. Crossey PA, Foster K, Richards FM, et al. Molecular genetic investigations of the mechanism of tumourigenesis in von Hippel-Lindau disease: analysis of allele loss in VHL tumours. Hum Genet 1994;93:53–8.

18. Stolle C, Glenn G, Zbar B, et al. Improved detection of germline mutations in the von Hippel-Lindau disease tumor suppressor gene. Hum Mutat 1998;12:417–23.

19. Murgia A, Martella M, Vinanzi C, et al. Somatic mosaicism in von Hippel-Lindau Disease. Hum Mutat 2000;15:114.

20. Sgambati MT, Stolle C, Choyke PL, et al. Mosaicism in von Hippel-Lindau disease: lessons from kindreds with germline mutations identified in offspring with mosaic parents. Am J Hum Genet 2000;66:84–91.

21. Vortmeyer AO, Lubensky IA, Fogt F, et al. Allelic deletion and mutation of the von Hippel-Lindau (VHL) tumor suppressor gene in pancreatic microcystic adenomas. Am J Pathol 1997

22. Tse JY, Wong JH, Lo KW, et al. Molecular genetic analysis of the von Hippel-Lindau disease tumor suppressor gene in familial and sporadic cerebellar hemangioblastomas. Am J Clin Pathol 1997;107:459–66.

23. Lubensky IA, Gnarra JR, Bertheau P, et al. Allelic deletions of the VHL gene detected in multiple microscopic clear cell renal lesions in von Hippel-Lindau disease patients. Am J Pathol 1996;149:2089–94.

24. Mandriota SJ, Turner KJ, Davies DR, et al. HIF activation identifies early lesions in VHL kidneys: evidence for site-specific tumor suppressor function in the nephron. Cancer Cell 2002;1:459–68.

25. Yao M, Yoshida M, Kishida T, et al. VHL tumor suppressor gene alterations associated with good prognosis in sporadic clear-cell renal carcinoma. J Natl Cancer Inst 2002;94:1569–75.

26. Kondo K, Yao M, Yoshida M, et al. Comprehensive mutational analysis of the VHL gene in sporadic renal cell carcinoma: relationship to clinicopathological parameters. Genes Chromosomes Cancer 2002;34:58–68.

27. Hamano K, Esumi M, Igarashi H, et al. Biallelic inactivation of the von Hippel-Lindau tumor suppressor gene in sporadic renal cell carcinoma. J Urol 2002;167:713–7.

28. Brauch H, Weirich G, Brieger J, et al. VHL alterations in human clear cell renal cell carcinoma: association with advanced tumor stage and a novel hot spot mutation. Cancer Res 2000;60:1942–8.

29. Gallou C, Joly D, Mejean A, et al. Mutations of the VHL gene in sporadic renal cell carcinoma: definition of a risk factor for VHL patients to develop an RCC. Hum Mutat 1999;13:464–75.

30. Banks RE, Tirukonda P, Taylor C, et al. Genetic and epigenetic analysis of von Hippel-Lindau (VHL) gene alterations and relationship with clinical variables in sporadic renal cancer. Cancer Res 2006;66:2000–11.

31. Kibel A, Iliopoulos O, DeCaprio JA, Kaelin WG Jr. Binding of the von Hippel-Lindau tumor suppressor protein to Elongin B and C. Science 1995;269:1444–6.

32. Kishida T, Stackhouse TM, Chen F, et al. Cellular proteins that bind the von Hippel-Lindau disease gene product: mapping of binding domains and the effect of missense mutations. Cancer Res 1995;55:4544–8.

33. Stebbins CE, Kaelin WG Jr, Pavletich NP. Structure of the VHL-ElonginC-ElonginB complex: implications for VHL tumor suppressor function. Science 1999;284:455–61.

34. Ohh M, Takagi Y, Aso T, et al. Synthetic peptides define critical contacts between elongin C, elongin B, and the von Hippel-Lindau protein. J Clin Invest 1999;104:1583–91.

35. Kaelin WG Jr. Molecular basis of the VHL hereditary cancer syndrome. Nat Rev Cancer 2002;2:673–82.

36. Sowter HM, Raval RR, Moore JW, et al. Predominant role of hypoxia-inducible transcription factor (Hif)-1α versus Hif-2α in regulation of the transcriptional response to hypoxia. Cancer Res 2003;63:6130–4.

37. Raval RR, Lau KW, Tran MG, et al. Contrasting properties of hypoxia-inducible factor 1 (HIF-1) and HIF-2 in von Hippel-Lindau-associated renal cell carcinoma. Mol Cell Biol 2005;25:5675–86.

38. Covello KL, Kehler J, Yu H, et al. HIF-2α regulates Oct-4: effects of hypoxia on stem cell function, embryonic development, and tumor growth. Genes Dev 2006;20:557–70.

39. Hu CJ, Iyer S, Sataur A, et al. Differential regulation of the transcriptional activities of hypoxia-inducible factor 1α (HIF-1α) and HIF-2α in stem cells. Mol Cell Biol 2006;26:3514–26.

40. Maina EN, Morris MR, Zatyka M, et al. Identification of novel VHL target genes and relationship to hypoxic response pathways. Oncogene 2005;24:4549–58.

41. Zatyka M, da Silva NF, Clifford SC, et al. Identification of cyclin D1 and other novel targets for the von Hippel-Lindau tumor suppressor gene by expression array analysis

and investigation of cyclin D1 genotype as a modifier in von Hippel-Lindau disease. Cancer Res 2002;62: 3803–11.

42. Wykoff CC, Sotiriou C, Cockman ME, et al. Gene array of VHL mutation and hypoxia shows novel hypoxia-induced genes and that cyclin D1 is a VHL target gene. Br J Cancer 2004;90:1235–43.

43. Jiang Y, Zhang W, Kondo K, et al. Gene expression profiling in a renal cell carcinoma cell line: dissecting VHL and hypoxia-dependent pathways. Mol Cancer Res 2003;1: 453–62.

44. Clifford SC, Cockman ME, Smallwood AC, et al. Contrasting effects on HIF-1α regulation by disease-causing pVHL mutations correlate with patterns of tumourigenesis in von Hippel-Lindau disease. Hum Mol Genet 2001;10: 1029–38.

45. Knauth K, Bex C, Jemth P, Buchberger A. Renal cell carcinoma risk in type 2 von Hippel-Lindau disease correlates with defects in pVHL stability and HIF-1alpha interactions. Oncogene 2006;25:370–7.

46. Li L, Zhang L, Zhang X, et al. Hypoxia-inducible factor linked to differential kidney cancer risk seen with type 2A and type 2B VHL mutations. Mol Cell Biol 2007;27: 5381–92.

47. Novick AC, Streem SB. Long-term followup after nephron sparing surgery for renal cell carcinoma in von Hippel-Lindau disease. J Urol 1992;147:1488–90.

48. Frydenberg M, Malek RS, Zincke H. Conservative renal surgery for renal cell carcinoma in von Hippel-Lindau's disease. J Urol 1993;149:461–4.

49. Steinbach F, Novick AC, Zincke H, et al. Treatment of renal cell carcinoma in von Hippel-Lindau disease: a multicenter study. J Urol 1995;153:1812–6.

50. Goldfarb DA, Neumann HP, Penn I, Novick AC. Results of renal transplantation in patients with renal cell carcinoma and von Hippel-Lindau disease. Transplantation 1997; 64:1726–9.

51. Walther MM, Choyke PL, Glenn G, et al. Renal cancer in families with hereditary renal cancer: prospective analysis of a tumor size threshold for renal parenchymal sparing surgery. J Urol 1999;161:1475–9.

52. Duffey BG, Choyke PL, Glenn G, et al. The relationship between renal tumor size and metastases in patients with von Hippel-Lindau disease. J Urol 2004;172:63–5.

53. Wong WT, Agron E, Coleman HR, et al. Genotype-phenotype correlation in von Hippel-Lindau disease with retinal angiomatosis. Arch Ophthalmol 2007;125:239–45.

54. Wanebo JE, Lonser RR, Glenn GM, Oldfield EH. The natural history of hemangioblastomas of the central nervous system in patients with von Hippel-Lindau disease. J Neurosurg 2003;98:82–94.

55. Bausch B, Borozdin W, Neumann HP. Clinical and genetic characteristics of patients with neurofibromatosis type 1 and pheochromocytoma. N Engl J Med 2006;354:2729–31.

56. Lonser RR, Glenn GM, Walther M, et al. von Hippel-Lindau disease. Lancet 2003;361:2059–67.

57. Butman JA, Kim HJ, Baggenstos M, et al. Mechanisms of morbid hearing loss associated with tumors of the endolymphatic sac in von Hippel-Lindau disease. JAMA 2007;298:41–8.

58. Dollfus H, Massin P, Taupin P, et al. Retinal hemangioblastoma in von Hippel-Lindau disease: a clinical and molecular study. Invest Ophthalmol Vis Sci 2002;43:3067–74.

59. Herring JC, Enquist EG, Chernoff A, et al. Parenchymal sparing surgery in patients with hereditary renal cell carcinoma: 10-year experience. J Urol 2001;165:777–81.

60. Walther MM, Thompson N, Linehan W. Enucleation procedures in patients with multiple hereditary renal tumors. World J Urol 1995;13:248–50.

61. Walther MM, Choyke PL, Hayes W, et al. Evaluation of color Doppler intraoperative ultrasound in parenchymal sparing renal surgery. J Urol 1994;152:1984–7.

62. Hwang JJ, Uchio EM, Pavlovich CP, et al. Surgical management of multi-organ visceral tumors in patients with von Hippel-Lindau disease: a single stage approach. J Urol 2003;169:895–8.

63. Shingleton WB, Sewell PE Jr. Percutaneous renal cryoablation of renal tumors in patients with von Hippel-Lindau disease. J Urol 2002;167:1268–70.

64. Hwang JJ, Walther MM, Pautler SE, et al. Radio frequency ablation of small renal tumors: intermediate results. J Urol 2004;171:1814–8.

65. Rendon RA, Kachura JR, Sweet JM, et al. The uncertainty of radio frequency treatment of renal cell carcinoma: findings at immediate and delayed nephrectomy. J Urol 2002;167:1587–92.

66. Michaels MJ, Rhee HK, Mourtzinos AP, et al. Incomplete renal tumor destruction using radio frequency interstitial ablation. J Urol 2002;168:2406–9; discussion 9–10.

67. Weight CJ, Kaouk J, Hegarty NJ, et al. MRI is inadequate for monitoring renal tumor destruction following radiofrequency ablation. [In preparation]

68. Nguyen CT, Lane BR, Hegarty N, et al. Management of renal cell carcinoma recurrence after prior thermal ablative therapy. [In preparation]

69. Walther MM, Reiter R, Keiser HR, et al. Clinical and genetic characterization of pheochromocytoma in von Hippel-Lindau families: comparison with sporadic pheochromocytoma gives insight into natural history of pheochromocytoma. J Urol 1999;162:659–64.

70. Teh BT, Giraud S, Sari NF, et al. Familial non-VHL non-papillary clear-cell renal cancer. Lancet 1997; 349:848–9.

71. Woodward ER, Clifford SC, Astuti D, et al. Familial clear cell renal cell carcinoma (FCRC): clinical features and mutation analysis of the VHL, MET, and CUL2 candidate genes. J Med Genet 2000;37:348–53.

72. Bonne AC, Bodmer D, Schoenmakers EF, et al. Chromosome 3 translocations and familial renal cell cancer. Curr Mol Med 2004;4:849–54.

73. Melendez B, Rodriguez-Perales S, Martinez-Delgado B, et al. Molecular study of a new family with hereditary renal cell carcinoma and a translocation t(3;8)(p13;q24.1). Hum Genet 2003;112:178–85.

74. Koolen MI, van der Meyden AP, Bodmer D, et al. A familial case of renal cell carcinoma and a t(2;3) chromosome translocation. Kidney Int 1998;53:273–5.

75. van Kessel AG, Wijnhoven H, Bodmer D, et al. Renal cell cancer: chromosome 3 translocations as risk factors. J Natl Cancer Inst 1999;91:1159–60.

76. Kanayama H, Lui WO, Takahashi M, et al. Association of a novel constitutional translocation t(1q;3q) with familial renal cell carcinoma. J Med Genet 2001; 38:165–70.

77. Eleveld MJ, Bodmer D, Merkx G, et al. Molecular analysis of a familial case of renal cell cancer and a t(3;6)(q12;q15). Genes Chromosomes Cancer 2001;31:23–32.

78. Podolski J, Byrski T, Zajaczek S, et al. Characterization of a familial RCC-associated t(2;3)(q33;q21) chromosome translocation. J Hum Genet 2001;46:685–93.

79. Cohen AJ, Li FP, Berg S, et al. Hereditary renal-cell carcinoma associated with a chromosomal translocation. N Engl J Med 1979;301:592–5.

80. Foster RE, Abdulrahman M, Morris MR, et al. Characterization of a 3;6 translocation associated with renal cell carcinoma. Genes Chromosomes Cancer 2007;46:311–7.

81. Subramonian K, Weston PM, Curley P. Multifocal renal cancer associated with renal artery aneurysm and a unique genetic change. Br J Urol 1998;82:761–2.

82. Kovacs G, Brusa P, De Riese W. Tissue-specific expression of a constitutional 3;6 translocation: development of multiple bilateral renal-cell carcinomas. Int J Cancer 1989;43:422–7.

83. Bodmer D, Eleveld M, Ligtenberg M, et al. Cytogenetic and molecular analysis of early stage renal cell carcinomas in a family with a translocation (2;3)(q35;q21). Cancer Genet Cytogenet 2002;134:6–12.

84. Valle L, Cascon A, Melchor L, et al. About the origin and development of hereditary conventional renal cell carcinoma in a four-generation t(3;8)(p14.1;q24.23) family. Eur J Hum Genet 2005;13:570–8.

85. van den Berg A, van der Veen AY, Hulsbeek MM, et al. Defining the position of the breakpoint of the constitutional t(3;6) occurring in a family with renal cell carcinoma. Genes Chromosomes Cancer 1995;12:224–8.

86. Druck T, Kastury K, Hadaczek P, et al. Loss of heterozygosity at the familial RCC t(3;8) locus in most clear cell renal carcinomas. Cancer Res 1995;55:5348–53.

87. Druck T, Podolski J, Byrski T, et al. The DIRC1 gene at chromosome 2q33 spans a familial RCC-associated t(2;3)(q33;q21) chromosome translocation. J Hum Genet 2001;46:583–9.

88. Rodriguez-Perales S, Melendez B, Gribble SM, et al. Cloning of a new familial t(3;8) translocation associated with conventional renal cell carcinoma reveals a 5 kb microdeletion and no gene involved in the rearrangement. Hum Mol Genet 2004;13:983–90.

89. Zbar B, Tory K, Merino M, et al. Hereditary papillary renal cell carcinoma. J Urol 1994;151:561–6.

90. Zbar B, Glenn G, Lubensky I, et al. Hereditary papillary renal cell carcinoma: clinical studies in 10 families. J Urol 1995;153:907–12.

91. Schmidt L, Duh FM, Chen F, et al. Germline and somatic mutations in the tyrosine kinase domain of the MET proto-oncogene in papillary renal carcinomas. Nat Genet 1997;16:68–73.

92. Schmidt L, Junker K, Nakaigawa N, et al. Novel mutations of the MET proto-oncogene in papillary renal carcinomas. Oncogene 1999;18:2343–50.

93. Lubensky IA, Schmidt L, Zhuang Z, et al. Hereditary and sporadic papillary renal carcinomas with c-met mutations share a distinct morphological phenotype. Am J Pathol 1999;155:517–26.

94. Lindor NM, Dechet CB, Greene MH, et al. Papillary renal cell carcinoma: analysis of germline mutations in the MET proto-oncogene in a clinic-based population. Genet Test 2001;5:101–6.

95. Dharmawardana PG, Giubellino A, Bottaro DP. Hereditary papillary renal carcinoma type I. Curr Mol Med 2004;4:855–68.

96. Reed WB, Walker R, Horowitz R. Cutaneous leiomyomata with uterine leiomyomata. Acta Derm Venereol 1973;53:409–16.

97. Launonen V, Vierimaa O, Kiuru M, et al. Inherited susceptibility to uterine leiomyomas and renal cell cancer. Proc Natl Acad Sci U S A 2001;98:3387–92.

98. Kiuru M, Launonen V, Hietala M, et al. Familial cutaneous leiomyomatosis is a two-hit condition associated with renal cell cancer of characteristic histopathology. Am J Pathol 2001;159:825–9.

99. Tomlinson IP, Alam NA, Rowan AJ, et al. Germline mutations in FH predispose to dominantly inherited uterine fibroids, skin leiomyomata and papillary renal cell cancer. Nat Genet 2002;30:406–10.

100. Gellera C, Uziel G, Rimoldi M, et al. Fumarase deficiency is an autosomal recessive encephalopathy affecting both the mitochondrial and the cytosolic enzymes. Neurology 1990;40:495–9.

101. Bourgeron T, Chretien D, Poggi-Bach J, et al. Mutation of the fumarase gene in two siblings with progressive encephalopathy and fumarase deficiency. J Clin Invest 1994;93:2514–8.

102. Coughlin EM, Christensen E, Kunz PL, et al. Molecular analysis and prenatal diagnosis of human fumarase deficiency. Mol Genet Metab 1998;63:254–62.

103. Bonioli E, Di Stefano A, Peri V, et al. Fumarate hydratase deficiency. J Inherit Metab Dis 1998;21:435–6.

104. Zeng WQ, Gao H, Brueton L, et al. Fumarase deficiency caused by homozygous P131R mutation and paternal partial isodisomy of chromosome 1. Am J Med Genet A 2006;140:1004–9.

105. Phillips TM, Gibson JB, Ellison DA. Fumarate hydratase deficiency in monozygotic twins. Pediatr Neurol 2006;35:150–3.

106. Maradin M, Fumic K, Hansikova H, et al. Fumaric aciduria: mild phenotype in a 8-year-old girl with novel mutations. J Inherit Metab Dis 2006;29:683.

107. Wei MH, Toure O, Glenn GM, et al. Novel mutations in FH and expansion of the spectrum of phenotypes expressed in families with hereditary leiomyomatosis and renal cell cancer. J Med Genet 2006;43:18–27.

108. Toro JR, Nickerson ML, Wei MH, et al. Mutations in the fumarate hydratase gene cause hereditary leiomyomatosis and renal cell cancer in families in North America. Am J Hum Genet 2003;73:95–106.

109. Alam NA, Rowan AJ, Wortham NC, et al. Genetic and functional analyses of FH mutations in multiple cutaneous and uterine leiomyomatosis, hereditary leiomyomatosis and renal cancer, and fumarate hydratase deficiency. Hum Mol Genet 2003;12:1241–52.

110. Lehtonen HJ, Kiuru M, Ylisaukko-Oja SK, et al. Increased risk of cancer in patients with fumarate hydratase germline mutation. J Med Genet 2006;43:523–6.

111. Pithukpakorn M, Wei MH, Toure O, et al. Fumarate hydratase enzyme activity in lymphoblastoid cells and fibroblasts of individuals in families with hereditary leiomyomatosis and renal cell cancer. J Med Genet 2006;43:755–62.

112. Merino MJ, Torres-Cabala C, Pinto P, Linehan WM. The morphologic spectrum of kidney tumors in hereditary leiomyomatosis and renal cell carcinoma (HLRCC) syndrome. Am J Surg Pathol 2007;31:1578–85.

113. Refae MA, Wong N, Patenaude F, et al. Hereditary leiomyomatosis and renal cell cancer: an unusual and aggressive form of hereditary renal carcinoma. Nat Clin Pract Oncol 2007;4:256–61.

114. Grubb RL III, Franks ME, Toro J, et al. Hereditary leiomyomatosis and renal cell cancer: a syndrome associated with an aggressive form of inherited renal cancer. J Urol 2007;177:2074–9; discussion 9–80.

115. Carvajal-Carmona LG, Alam NA, Pollard PJ, et al. Adult leydig cell tumors of the testis caused by germline fumarate hydratase mutations. J Clin Endocrinol Metab 2006; 91:3071–5.

116. Hornstein OP, Knickenberg M. Perifollicular fibromatosis cutis with polyps of the colon—a cutaneo-intestinal syndrome sui generis. Arch Dermatol Res 1975;253:161–75.

117. Birt AR, Hogg GR, Dube WJ. Hereditary multiple fibrofolliculomas with trichodiscomas and acrochordons. Arch Dermatol 1977;113:1674–7.

118. Khoo SK, Bradley M, Wong FK, et al. Birt-Hogg-Dube syndrome: mapping of a novel hereditary neoplasia gene to chromosome 17p12-q11.2. Oncogene 2001;20:5239–42.

119. Schmidt LS, Warren MB, Nickerson ML, et al. Birt-Hogg-Dube syndrome, a genodermatosis associated with spontaneous pneumothorax and kidney neoplasia, maps to chromosome 17p11.2. Am J Hum Genet 2001;69:876–82.

120. Nickerson ML, Warren MB, Toro JR, et al. Mutations in a novel gene lead to kidney tumors, lung wall defects, and benign tumors of the hair follicle in patients with the Birt-Hogg-Dube syndrome. Cancer Cell 2002;2:157–64.

121. van Slegtenhorst M, Khabibullin D, Hartman TR, et al. The Birt-Hogg-Dube and tuberous sclerosis complex homologs have opposing roles in amino acid homeostasis in schizosaccharomyces pombe. J Biol Chem 2007; 282:24583–90.

122. Baba M, Hong SB, Sharma N, et al. Folliculin encoded by the BHD gene interacts with a binding protein, FNIP1, and AMPK, and is involved in AMPK and mTOR signaling. Proc Natl Acad Sci U S A 2006;103:15552–7.

123. Schmidt LS, Nickerson ML, Warren MB, et al. Germline BHD-mutation spectrum and phenotype analysis of a large cohort of families with Birt-Hogg-Dube syndrome. Am J Hum Genet 2005;76:1023–33.

124. Toro JR, Pautler SE, Stewart L, et al. Lung cysts, spontaneous pneumothorax, and genetic associations in 89 families with Birt-Hogg-Dube syndrome. Am J Respir Crit Care Med 2007;175:1044–53.

125. Zbar B, Alvord WG, Glenn G, et al. Risk of renal and colonic neoplasms and spontaneous pneumothorax in the Birt-Hogg-Dube syndrome. Cancer Epidemiol Biomarkers Prev 2002;11:393–400.

126. Leter EM, Koopmans AK, Gille JJ, et al. Birt-Hogg-Dube syndrome: clinical and genetic studies of 20 families. J Invest Dermatol 2007.

127. Khoo SK, Giraud S, Kahnoski K, et al. Clinical and genetic studies of Birt-Hogg-Dube syndrome. J Med Genet 2002;39:906–12.

128. Vocke CD, Yang Y, Pavlovich CP, et al. High frequency of somatic frameshift BHD gene mutations in Birt-Hogg-Dube-associated renal tumors. J Natl Cancer Inst 2005;97:931–5.

129. Murakami T, Sano F, Huang Y, et al. Identification and characterization of Birt-Hogg-Dube associated renal carcinoma. J Pathol 2007;211:524–31.

130. Khoo SK, Kahnoski K, Sugimura J, et al. Inactivation of BHD in sporadic renal tumors. Cancer Res 2003;63:4583–7.

131. Roth JS, Rabinowitz AD, Benson M, Grossman ME. Bilateral renal cell carcinoma in the Birt-Hogg-Dube syndrome. J Am Acad Dermatol 1993;29:1055–6.

132. Toro JR, Glenn G, Duray P, et al. Birt-Hogg-Dube syndrome: a novel marker of kidney neoplasia. Arch Dermatol 1999;135:1195–202.

133. Jones J, Otu H, Spentzos D, et al. Gene signatures of progression and metastasis in renal cell cancer. Clin Cancer Res 2005;11:5730–9.

134. Tickoo SK, Reuter VE, Amin MB, et al. Renal oncocytosis: a morphologic study of fourteen cases. Am J Surg Pathol 1999;23:1094–101.

135. Pavlovich CP, Grubb RL III, Hurley K, et al. Evaluation and management of renal tumors in the Birt-Hogg-Dube syndrome. J Urol 2005;173:1482–6.

136. Pavlovich CP, Walther MM, Eyler RA, et al. Renal tumors in the Birt-Hogg-Dube syndrome. Am J Surg Pathol 2002;26:1542–52.

137. Mai KT, Dhamanaskar P, Belanger E, Stinson WA. Hybrid chromophobe renal cell neoplasm. Pathol Res Pract 2005;201:385–9.

138. Weirich G, Glenn G, Junker K, et al. Familial renal oncocytoma: clinicopathological study of 5 families. J Urol 1998;160:335–40.

139. van Steensel MA, Verstraeten VL, Frank J, et al. Novel mutations in the BHD gene and absence of loss of heterozygosity in fibrofolliculomas of Birt-Hogg-Dube patients. J Invest Dermatol 2007;127:588–93.

140. Collins GL, Somach S, Morgan MB. Histomorphologic and immunophenotypic analysis of fibrofolliculomas and trichodiscomas in Birt-Hogg-Dube syndrome and sporadic disease. J Cutan Pathol 2002;29:529–33.

141. De la Torre C, Ocampo C, Doval IG, et al. Acrochordons are not a component of the Birt-Hogg-Dube syndrome: does this syndrome exist? Case reports and review of the literature. Am J Dermatopathol 1999;21:369–74.

142. Schulz T, Hartschuh W. Birt-Hogg-Dube syndrome and Hornstein-Knickenberg syndrome are the same. Different sectioning technique as the cause of different histology. J Cutan Pathol 1999;26:55–61.

143. Gunji Y, Akiyoshi T, Sato T, et al. Mutations of the Birt Hogg Dube gene in patients with multiple lung cysts and recurrent pneumothorax. J Med Genet 2007; 44: 588–93.

144. Graham RB, Nolasco M, Peterlin B, Garcia CK. Nonsense mutations in folliculin presenting as isolated familial spontaneous pneumothorax in adults. Am J Respir Crit Care Med 2005;172:39–44.

145. Painter JN, Tapanainen H, Somer M, et al. A 4-bp deletion in the Birt-Hogg-Dube gene (FLCN) causes dominantly inherited spontaneous pneumothorax. Am J Hum Genet 2005;76:522–7.

146. Chiu HT, Garcia CK. Familial spontaneous pneumothorax. Curr Opin Pulm Med 2006;12:268–72.

147. Crino PB, Nathanson KL, Henske EP. The tuberous sclerosis complex. N Engl J Med 2006;355:1345–56.

148. Ewalt DH, Diamond N, Rees C, et al. Long-term outcome of transcatheter embolization of renal angiomyolipomas due to tuberous sclerosis complex. J Urol 2005;174:1764–6.

149. Tello R, Blickman JG, Buonomo C, Herrin J. Meta analysis of the relationship between tuberous sclerosis complex and renal cell carcinoma. Eur J Radiol 1998;27:131–8.

150. Al-Saleem T, Wessner LL, Scheithauer BW, et al. Malignant tumors of the kidney, brain, and soft tissues in children and young adults with the tuberous sclerosis complex. Cancer 1998;83:2208–16.

151. Lendvay TS, Marshall FF. The tuberous sclerosis complex and its highly variable manifestations. J Urol 2003;169:1635–42.

152. Liaw D, Marsh DJ, Li J, et al. Germline mutations of the PTEN gene in Cowden disease, an inherited breast and thyroid cancer syndrome. Nat Genet 1997;16:64–7.

153. Gustafson S, Zbuk KM, Scacheri C, Eng C. Cowden syndrome. Semin Oncol 2007;34:428–34.

154. Zbuk KM, Eng C. Cancer phenomics: RET and PTEN as illustrative models. Nat Rev Cancer 2007;7:35–45.

155. Lynch ED, Ostermeyer EA, Lee MK, et al. Inherited mutations in PTEN that are associated with breast cancer, Cowden disease, and juvenile polyposis. Am J Hum Genet 1997;61:1254–60.

156. Kondo K, Yao M, Kobayashi K, et al. PTEN/MMAC1/TEP1 mutations in human primary renal-cell carcinomas and renal carcinoma cell lines. Int J Cancer 2001;91:219–24.

157. Nathanson KL, Baysal BE, Drovdic C, et al. Familial paraganglioma-phaeochromocytoma syndromes caused by *SDHB*, *SDHC* and *SDHD* mutations. In: DeLellis RA, Lloyd RV, Heitz PU, Eng C, editors. Pathology & genetics: tumours of endocrine tumours. Lyon, France: IARC Press; 2004. p. 238–42.

158. Timmers HJ, Kozupa A, Eisenhofer G, et al. Clinical presentations, biochemical phenotypes, and genotype-phenotype correlations in patients with succinate dehydrogenase subunit B-associated pheochromocytomas and paragangliomas. J Clin Endocrinol Metab 2007;92:779–86.

159. Vanharanta S, Buchta M, McWhinney SR, et al. Early-onset renal cell carcinoma as a novel extraparaganglial component of SDHB-associated heritable paraganglioma. Am J Hum Genet 2004;74:153–9.

160. Carpten JD, Robbins CM, Villablanca A, et al. HRPT2, encoding parafibromin, is mutated in hyperparathyroidism-jaw tumor syndrome. Nat Genet 2002;32:676–80.

161. Tan MH, Teh BT. Renal neoplasia in the hyperparathyroidism-jaw tumor syndrome. Curr Mol Med 2004;4:895–7.

162. Teh BT, Farnebo F, Kristoffersson U, et al. Autosomal dominant primary hyperparathyroidism and jaw tumor syndrome associated with renal hamartomas and cystic kidney disease: linkage to 1q21-q32 and loss of the wild type allele in renal hamartomas. J Clin Endocrinol Metab 1996;81:4204–11.

163. Teh BT, Farnebo F, Twigg S, et al. Familial isolated hyperparathyroidism maps to the hyperparathyroidism-jaw tumor locus in 1q21-q32 in a subset of families. J Clin Endocrinol Metab 1998;83:2114–20.

164. Malchoff CD, Sarfarazi M, Tendler B, et al. Papillary thyroid carcinoma associated with papillary renal neoplasia: genetic linkage analysis of a distinct heritable tumor syndrome. J Clin Endocrinol Metab 2000;85:1758–64.

# 4

# Genetics of Sporadic Renal Cell Carcinoma

**KYLE A. FURGE, PHD**

**BIN TEAN TEH, MD, PHD**

The spectrum of genetic abnormalities that occur in cancer ranges from single deoxyribonucleic acid (DNA) nucleotide changes that affect the coding of a single amino acid to chromosomal gains and losses that disrupt transcription of hundreds of genes. Likewise, the molecular genetic defects that occur in sporadic adult renal cell carcinoma (RCC) are also as extensive and complex. This chapter gives an overview of the most common genetic abnormalities that occur in the clear cell, papillary, and chromophobe subtypes of RCC. Large chromosomal abnormalities that occur within RCC are discussed first, followed by a discussion on specific molecular defects that affect individual genes. Finally, a summary of the epigenetic effects, manifested by changes in gene expression, is presented within the context of the chromosomal and molecular genetic abnormalities.

## CYTOGENETICS OF RCC

Arguably, the most significant type of genetic disruption that gives rise to sporadic cancers are abnormalities in chromosome number and structure.[1] A wealth of cytogenetic information specific for RCC has been generated based on allelotyping studies, comparative genomic hybridization studies, and fluorescence *in situ* hybridization studies.[2–11] Included in the allelotyping studies are data generated from loss of heterozygosity, restriction fragment length polymorphisms, and microsatellite polymorphism studies. Taken together, these cytogenetic studies have revealed that the common subtypes of RCC have unique and frequently

occurring sets of chromosomal abnormalities.[12] As the cytogenetic defects occurring in RCC have been observed so repeatedly, quantification of these defects can assist in subclassification of the tumor (Table 1). Moreover, the frequent appearance of these cytogenetic abnormalities suggests that important tumor-modifying genes are located within the regions of frequent amplification or deletion.

The most prominent cytogenetic defect present in sporadic RCC is the loss of the p-arm of chromosome 3 in the clear cell subtype.[2,13,14] This abnormality occurs in approximately 70 to 80% of clear cell tumors and only rarely occurs in the other RCC subtypes. The deletion of chromosome 3p has been linked to the presence of a fragile site on chromosome 3; however, this association is not supported in all cytogenetic studies of this region.[14–17] Irrespective of the fragile site association, loss of

## Table 1. OVERVIEW OF CYTOGENETIC ABNORMALITIES IN SPORADIC RCC

| RCC Subtype | Chromosomal Abnormality |
|---|---|
| Clear cell | 3p loss; 5q gain; 14q loss*; 9/9q loss*; 20 gain* |
| Papillary | |
| Type 1 | 7, 12, 16, 17 gain |
| Type 2 | 17q gain; 9/9p loss*; 8q gain* |
| Chromophobe | |
| Typical | 1, 2, 6, 10, 17, 21 loss |
| Eosinophilic | 1, 2, 6, 10, 17, 21 loss (less frequent) |
| Translocation associated | *TFE3/B* translocations |

*Associated with tumor aggressiveness.
RCC = renal cell carcinoma.

chromosome 3 often results from the formation of an unbalanced translocation between the p-arm of chromosome 3 and another chromosome. Pivotal cytogenetic studies of RCC initially identified loss of chromosome 3p by the presence of a translocation between chromosome 3 and chromosome 8.[13] Subsequent studies have revealed that the most common translocation partner of chromosome 3p is the q-arm of chromosome 5. Similar to the chromosome 8 translocation, the formation of the t(3;5) derivative chromosome results in a net loss of one copy of chromosome 3p and a net gain of one copy of chromosome 5q.[7] As such, gain of the q-arm of chromosome 5 is the second most common cytogenetic defect present within clear cell RCC and occurs in approximately 50 to 60% of tumors.[7] Although loss of chromosome 3p and gain of chromosome 5q are common events in clear cell RCC, this subtype is also associated with deletions of chromosomes 6q, 8p, 9p, and 14q. In addition, several chromosomal abnormalities have been associated with more or less aggressive tumor behavior. Deletion of chromosomes 6q, 8p, or 14q is associated with higher stage tumors,[18–20] although loss of chromosome 9p/9 is associated with cancer recurrence and metastatic progression.[7,9] Gains of chromosomes 12 and 20 are associated with poor prognosis in the clear cell subtype.[18] In contrast, retention of the extra copy of chromosome 5q has been linked to overall good prognosis.[7,21] Comparative analysis of primary clear cell tumors with derivative distal metastases suggests that the metastatic lesions have a very high degree of cytogenetic similarity to the primary tumors. However, deletions of chromosome 9, 10, 17, and 18 did occur more frequently in some of the metastatic tumors.[22]

In contrast to clear cell tumors, loss of chromosome 3p and gain of chromosome 5q are rarely found in papillary tumors. Rather, a distinct set of cytogenetic defects have been identified in papillary RCC. It is worth noting that papillary RCC can be divided into two subtypes, type 1 and type 2, based on morphologic and gene expression profiling differences.[23–25] The cytogenetic abnormalities that are found in papillary RCC also support the partitioning of these tumors into two subtypes. Type 1 papillary RCCs are characterized by frequent gains of chromosomes 3q, 7, 12, 16, 17, and 20. Type 2 papillary RCCs share some of these abnormalities, but gains of chromosome 7, 12, and 17p are less frequent and losses of chromosome 9/9p and gains of chromosome 8q are more frequent. Moreover, the amount of cytogenetic variability is also different between type 1 and type 2 tumors. In type 1 papillary RCC, the tumor cells are cytogenetically homogenous, and it is rare to identify cells that contain abnormalities outside of the set of common abnormalities (ie, outside of defects in chromosomes 3q, 7, 12, 16, 17, and 20). In contrast, type 2 tumor cells often contain numerous additional cytogenetic abnormalities. Moreover, the additional abnormalities are a more chaotic assortment of chromosomes and do not seem to follow a particular pattern. As such, the increased cytogenetic complexity found in the type 2 tumor cells may be a reflection of the advanced stage that is typically associated with these tumors. Like clear cell RCC, in papillary RCC, loss of chromosome 9/9p is also associated with the more aggressive tumors.

Papillary RCC is also associated with several structural chromosomal abnormalities. In addition to occurring in young adults, both primary and secondary pediatric renal adenocarinomas[26,27] are associated with a translocation involving the *TFE3* gene located on Xp11.2.[28–30] The *TFE3* gene encodes a protein that is a member of the helix-loop-helix transcription factor family. Other translocations have been described in papillary RCC that involve the *TFEB* transcription factor. *TFEB* is in the same gene family as *TFE3*, and inappropriate expression, either the TFE3 or TFEB fusion protein, is likely involved in tumor development. It is worth noting that tumors containing the Xp11.2 abnormalities were initially described as aggressive tumors displaying papillary and/or alveolar patterns. Xp11.2 translocation carcinomas are now considered a distinct subtype of RCC.

Chromophobe RCCs contain different chromosomal abnormalities compared with either clear cell or papillary RCC. Chromophobe RCCs contain frequent losses of chromosomes 1, 2, 6, 10, and 17. Indeed, chromophobe RCC cells have lost so much genetic material, that these cells are considered to be severely hypoploid. Interestingly, there does not appear to be a significant difference in the cytogenetics between the typical and eosinophilic variants of chromophobe RCC. Related to chromophobe RCC are renal oncocytomas. Renal oncocytomas are benign tumors that are morphologically similar to chromophobe RCCs.[10] Gene expression profiling studies have demonstrated that renal oncocytoma and chromophobe RCC have very similar overall patterns of gene expression.[31,32] However, although renal oncocytoma and chromophobe RCC share gene expression and morphologic characteristics, these tumors differ in the spectrum of cytogenetic abnormalities that they contain.[10] Unlike chromophobe RCC, renal oncocytoma cells are either karyotypically normal or contain a limited number of chromosomal abnormalities including loss of chromosome Y,[33] loss of chromosome 1,[11,33] or translocations involving chromosome 11.[34]

The unique pattern of cytogenetic abnormalities within the RCC subtypes suggests that each of the common abnormalities will have a prominent role in renal tumor development. Therefore, it is critical to develop a robust understanding of how each of these abnormalities contributes to tumorigenesis. In general, however, identification of specific tumor-modifying genes that are located in regions of frequent cytogenetic change is lacking. This may be due, in part, to the lack of high-resolution mapping studies that are required to narrow the cytogenetic interval in which to search for candidate genes. Addressing this issue will require the application of several new technologies that have been developed for generating high-resolution allelotyping and DNA copy number data including hybridizing labeled DNA to complementary DNA,[35] bacterial artificial chromosome,[36] oligonucleotide,[37] or single-nucleotide polymorphism (SNP) arrays.[38] In the coming years, the analysis of these high-resolution data will shed more light on the role of these recurrent cytogenetic abnormalities. Nevertheless, it is worth mentioning that many cytogenetic abnormalities found in RCC involve large intervals of amplification or deletion. As such, it is possible that multiple genes within a region of amplification or deletion contribute to the cancer phenotype. For example, despite numerous mapping attempts, a narrow region of amplification for chromosome 5q has not been identified.[5,39–41]

Therefore, many challenges may still need to be overcome before robust models are developed that describe the contribution of each chromosomal abnormality to tumor development.

## MOLECULAR GENETICS OF RCC

Several hereditary syndromes include a predisposition to develop renal tumors. One method to identify molecular genetic defects that are present in sporadic RCC has been to perform linkage analysis on rare families that have inherited predispositions for these syndromes. Several oncogenes and tumor suppressor genes that are associated with the development of hereditary kidney cancer have also been implicated in sporadic renal cancers. The most prominent example, the *VHL* gene located on 3p25, was identified by positional cloning in families with autosomal dominant von Hippel-Lindau (*VHL*) disease characterized by a high frequency of clear cell RCC, cerebellar hemangioblastoma, pheochromocytoma, and retinal angioma.[42] Inactivating sequence mutations within the *VHL* gene were subsequently identified in sporadic RCC and associated with clear cell renal tumor development.[43–45] The majority of sporadic clear cell RCCs contain somatic sequence mutations in one allele of the *VHL* gene and loss of the other wild-type allele by chromosome 3p deletion. This mutational pattern follows the classic "two-hit" hypothesis,[46] in which inactivating mutations in one allele of the *VHL* gene coupled with the loss of the remaining wild-type *VHL* allele through chromosome 3p deletion lead to inactivation of VHL function. Although the *VHL* gene affects many processes within the cell,[47] the process that has received the greatest attention in RCC relates to the interaction between VHL and the oxygen-responsive transcription factors known as hypoxia-inducible factors (HIFs).[48–51]

HIFs are transcription factors that respond to changes in the level of cellular oxygen.[52] Under normoxic conditions, HIF is expressed at low levels in most cells. Under conditions of limited oxygen (hypoxia), HIF expression is dramatically increased, and this results in the change in gene expression of a number of metabolic and angiogenic target genes including carbonic anhydrase IX (CA9), glucose transporter 1 (SLC2A1), and vascular endothelial growth factor A (VEGF). There are three well-described HIF isoforms, HIF1, HIF2, and HIF3. The HIFs consist of two subunits, HIFα and HIFβ, that dimerize to form the functional transcription factor.[53] As the β-subunits are constitutively expressed, the amount of the HIF heterodimer present in cells is regulated in large part by changes in the amount of the HIFα subunit. Specifically, at high oxygen concentrations, HIFα is rapidly degraded and subsequently low levels of the heterodimer form. In contrast, at lower oxygen levels, the degradation of HIFα is not as efficient, HIFα levels accumulate, and levels of the functional HIF heterodimer rise.[54]

In normoxic cells, HIFα is rapidly targeted for degradation by one or more of three oxygen-sensitive prolyl hydroxylases, EGLN1/PHD2, EGLN2/PHD1, and EGLN3/PHD3.[50,51,55] Using cellular oxygen as a substrate, EGLNs hydroxylate HIFα on either Pro402 or Pro564. The addition of the hydroxyl group enables binding of the VHL protein (Figure 1). VHL is the recognition component of an ubiquitin E3 ligase complex, and VHL binding results in the ubiquitylation and subsequent degradation of HIFα.[56] In clear cell RCC, without VHL to target HIFα for degradation, hydroxylated HIFα levels accumulate. Although hydroxylated, HIFα still binds with

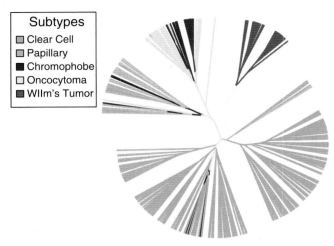

**Figure 2.** Clustering of renal cell carcinomas (RCCs) based on similarities in gene expression. RCCs of several subtypes were organized based on overall similarities in gene expression and displayed as a tree diagram. Gene expression profiles derived from 312 RCC tumors were analyzed. Each tree leaf represents an individual tumor sample and is colored based on the histologic diagnosis. Tumor samples with similar gene expression are found in the same tree branch. Included for comparison are pediatric Wilm's tumors. For some cases, the histologic and gene expression–based classifications disagree. For this analysis, gene expression data were obtained from three independent microarray profiling studies of RCC.[31,32,70] Following data normalization, $log_2$-transformed ratios between tumor expression values and noncancerous tissue expression values were constructed. A total of 7,163 genes were identified as being measured in common between the studies, and 2,654 genes were identified as being well measured (ie, present) in at least 70% of the samples.[31] The samples were then organized using hierarchical clustering (Pearson's correlation and average linkage clustering) and plotted as an unrooted tree dendogram.

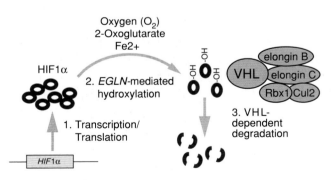

**Figure 1.** Regulation of hypoxia-inducible factors (HIF) levels by protein degradation. A schematic representation of the synthesis and degradation cycle of the HIF1α subunit of the HIF1 transcription factor. Key enzymes in this process are the EGLN/PHD prolyl hydroxylases and the von Hippel-Lindau (VHL) ubiquitin ligase. EGLNs use molecular oxygen as a substrate to add a hydroxyl (–OH) group to HIF1α. VHL then binds to hydroxylated HIF1α and targets it for ubiquitin-mediated degradation. As EGLNs use molecular oxygen as a substrate, the rate of the hydroxylation reaction is influenced by the molecular oxygen concentration inside the cell.

HIFβ to induce transcriptional regulation of metabolic and angiogenesis factors. As cells enter this pseudohypoxic state, the associated change in metabolism and angiogenesis likely contributes to tumor development.

Unlike clear cell RCC, sporadic papillary RCCs have not been associated with *VHL* mutation. In contrast, hereditary papillary RCC syndrome and sporadic type 1 papillary tumors are associated with activating mutations in the MET receptor tyrosine kinase that maps to chromosome 7q31.[57–59] Although sequence mutations in *MET* are observed in a minority of the sporadic cases (15 to 20%), overexpression of the *MET* receptor through amplification of chromosome 7 is commonly observed. As a receptor tyrosine kinase, *MET* possesses a highly glycosylated extracellular ligand binding region, a hydrophobic membrane spanning region, and an intracellular region that contains both a tyrosine kinase domain and a C-terminal multisubstrate binding site.[60,61] Activation of receptor tyrosine kinases usually results from binding a protein growth factor. The growth factor that activates MET is hepatocyte growth factor/scatter factor, referred to as HGF/SF as it was identified independently as both a growth factor for hepatocytes (HGF) and as a fibroblast-derived cell motility factor, scatter factor (SF).[62–64] Since then, HGF/SF-Met signaling has been implicated in a variety of cellular responses including proliferation, motility, and morphogenic differentiation. In both sporadic and hereditary papillary renal carcinoma, missense mutations located in the tyrosine kinase domain of the MET produce a receptor that is active even in the absence of HGF/SF binding. The constitutively active receptor recruits and activates numerous signal transduction proteins including, phosphotidylinositol-3-OH kinase (PI3K), phospholipase C- γ, the GTPases Ras, Rac1/Cdc42, and Rap1, and other signaling molecules. However, a specific mechanism that describes how all, or a subset, of these downstream pathways contribute to papillary tumor growth remains to be developed.

Sporadic type 2 papillary tumors have histologic similarities with hereditary leiomyomatosis and renal cell cancer (HLRCC). The fumarate hydratase (*FH*) gene has been identified as the gene associated with development of HLRCC.[65–67] Fumarate hydratase is one component of the tricarboxylic acid (TCA) cycle, or Krebs cycle, and catalyzes the formation of L-malate from fumarate. In addition to defects in the Krebs cycle, inactivating mutations in the *FH* gene leads to abnormally high levels of fumarate in the cell. Recent work has demonstrated that fumarate binds to and inhibits EGLN/PHD activity.[68,69] The less efficient EGLN/PHD hydroxylation reaction causes HIFα levels to accumulate. Therefore, like inactivation of *VHL* by mutation/chromosome 3p deletion, in hereditary papillary RCC, inactivation of EGLN/PHDs by increased fumarate leads to abnormal upregulation of HIF. Analysis of gene expression data suggests that the *FH* pathway is also deregulated in sporadic type 2 papillary RCCs.[25] Although inactivation of *FH* is described in the computational models, mutations within the *FH* gene, or other genes involved in the TCA cycle, have not been identified. Therefore, the role of the *FH* remains unclear in the sporadic type 2 papillary RCC. Other molecular genetic defects, such as deregulation of the *MYC* gene, may be associated with development of this class of sporadic tumors.[70]

The specific molecular defects that are responsible for the development of chromophobe RCC remain elusive. Patients with Birt-Hogg-Dubé (BHD) syndrome have a propensity to develop renal oncocytoma and chromophobe RCC. This observation strongly suggests that defects in the gene responsible for BHD (a gene commonly referred to as "folliculin," *FLCN*) would be involved in sporadic cases of chromophobe RCC.[71–73] However, sequence mutations in the *FLNC* gene have not been identified in sporadic chromophobe or in other types of renal tumors.[74] Evaluation of rare individuals with multifocal kidney tumors suggests that oncocytic neoplasms morphologically progress from oncocytomas to hybrid tumors with chromophobe carcinoma characteristics.[75] Thus, there is the potential that genetic mechanisms that give rise to renal oncocytoma may also give insight into chromophobe RCC.

Clearly, linkage studies involving hereditary syndromes have yielded significant insight into the development of sporadic RCC. Although the genes identified have given vital clues into the molecular genetic defects present in sporadic RCC, it is likely that these mutations are not the only mutations found in sporadic tumors. Several lines of evidence suggest that additional mutations may be required for sporadic tumor development. As mentioned previously, several large chromosomal aberrations are commonly found in sporadic RCC, suggesting a role for these abnormalities in sporadic tumors. For example, deregulation of other genes that map to chromosome 3p, in addition to *VHL*, may be required for clear cell RCC development. Mice that lack the *VHL* gene form renal cysts, rather than kidney tumors.[76] Although the results in the mouse model system may simply indicate that the model does not faithfully mimic the human disease, this observation may also suggest that additional factors contribute to tumor formation. Mutational events in genes involved in different pathways (such as RASSF1A and CA) have also been implicated in clear cell RCC development and progression.[77] In addition, disruption in Wnt/ β-catenin signaling also gives rise to renal cysts in the mouse.[78] Although the linkage studies give valuable insight into the potential pathways that are deregulated in RCC, additional approaches will be required to identify the specific molecular genetic defects that are present in sporadic RCCs. One approach to identify molecular genetic defects in RCC is the large-scale screening for DNA sequence mutations in sporadic tumors.[79] Although the initial mutational screens in clear cell RCC have not identified frequent mutations in protein kinases, these large-scale sequencing screens hold great promise to identify tumor-modifying genes. An alternative screening method that complements sequencing-based approaches is the application of high-resolution linkage analysis using SNP technology. The clear advantage of this genome-wide linkage analysis is the unbiased examination of thousands to millions of genetic markers. However, the heterogeneity of kidney cancer may present additional challenges. The cytogenetic complexity of RCC suggests that markers of susceptibility in one subtype of RCC may not translate to other types of RCC. As such, each subtype of RCC may have to be examined independently of the other subtypes.

## EPIGENETICS OF SPORADIC RCC

In addition to mutation and cytogenetic screening, comprehensive measurement of gene expression using high-density nucleic acid arrays (ie, gene expression microarrays) has become an important tool for investigating the molecular genetic and epigenetic defects in sporadic RCC. There is now strong evidence that global gene expression profiling can reveal new information in sporadic RCC, including the identification of cytogenetic abnormalities, mechanisms of transformation, and differences in cell lineage/differentiation state. Some of the most straightforward results of the gene expression studies have been the identification of either individual genes or sets of genes that show differences in expression between noncancerous renal tissue and the various subtypes of RCC.[31,32,80–87] Several studies have demonstrated that the gene expression differences between tissue types can involve thousands of genes (Table 2). Therefore, instead of a detailed discussion of the individual genes that are differentially expressed, we will focus on some of the general themes that have emerged from these studies.

One central concept that has emerged is the use of gene expression data to identify tumor cell lineage and/or tumor subtype (Figure 2). This class of gene expression analysis has revealed many potential diagnostic markers for the different subtypes of RCC. Some of these genetic markers include expression of α-methyacyl-CoA racemase for papillary RCC, glutathione S-transferase for clear cell RCC, and more recently the S100A1 gene as a marker to discriminate between renal oncocytoma and chromophobe RCC. Importantly, several other genes such as vimentin, TIMP2, survivin, and adipose differentiation-related have been identified as potential prognostic indicators.[80,88–94] As such, the use of gene expression markers, either single gene markers or multiplexed markers, can complement and extend traditional patient stratification approaches such as tumor–node–metastasis staging, tumor grade, and functional status.[95–98]

In addition to identification of genes that are associated with differences in tumor cell lineage or tumor subtype, genetic markers have also been identified from gene expression data that give insight into the molecular genetic mechanisms of tumor

| Table 2. NUMBER OF DIFFERENTIALLY EXPRESSED GENES BETWEEN TISSUES AND TUMORS* | | | | |
|---|---|---|---|---|
| | Clear Cell | Papillary | Oncocytoma | Chromophobe |
| Noncancerous Kidney | 1,603 | 956 | 1,672 | 1,736 |
| Chromophobe | 1,922 | 1,444 | 776 | — |
| Oncocytoma | 1,845 | 1,335 | — | — |
| Papillary | 1,132 | — | — | — |

*Based on the intersection of three gene expression studies as described in Figure 2.

development and progression. Analysis of gene expression data derived from clear cell RCC revealed an association between *CXCR4* expression, *VHL* inactivation, and poor tumor-specific survival.[99,100] In this case, organ-specific metastasis of RCC to the lung was in part regulated by expression of chemokine receptors in tumor cells (*CXCR4*) and expression of matching a chemokine (*SDF-1*) on the distant organ site. The approach of using gene expression data to quantify the activation or deactivation of specific signal transduction pathways has been shown to be a valid experimental approach in several studies.[101–108] The general design is that sets of genes that are deregulated following overexpression of an oncogene or inactivation of an oncogene are identified from tissue culture experiments.[104,105] The gene expression data derived from a tumor sample is then examined to determine if the same set of genes are also deregulated. A variety of computational approaches, including gene set enrichment analysis,[104,107] singular value decomposition,[105] or parametric statistical tests,[108] can be used to perform this comparison. Using this general experimental approach, several genes associated with insulin-like growth factor 1 (IGF-1) signal transduction were identified as being uniquely expressed in RCC tumor samples versus nondiseased tissues.[109] These data suggest that in addition to VHL inactivation, activation of the IGF-1 pathway may be important for tumor development. Other tumorigenic pathways, such as activation of the transforming growth factor-β pathway in clear cell RCC[110] and of the MYC pathway in type 2 papillary RCC has been identified using similar approaches.[25]

Perhaps a more compelling use of gene expression data is to identify genetic markers that can predict response to treatment. Immunotherapy with interleukin-2 (IL-2) results in a partial response rate of approximately 15% with a smaller percentage (5 to 7%) exhibiting complete remission upon treatment.[111] Although the modest response rate is discouraging, the small percentage of complete responders suggests that identification of specific markers that can predict responsiveness would be highly desirable.[112] Sets of genes have been identified in cell culture models that would predict sensitivity to interferon-α.[113] Other markers that would indicate activation of receptor tyrosine kinases, such

as the VEGF receptor (and sensitivity to sorafenib or sunitinib), or PI3K activation (and sensitivity to temsirolimus or perifosine) have already been identified.[114,115] Although validation of these markers identified from gene expression profiling data is still lacking, the overall experimental approach has high value.

## SUMMARY

We have witnessed tremendous progress in the elucidation of the genetics of sporadic RCC and their clinical implications. However, because of the heterogeneity of the tumors histologically, clinically, and with respect to therapeutic response, further work is warranted to provide even more accurate molecular classification that will benefit the management of patients with RCC. In the coming years, it will become more common to develop detailed genetic portraits of individual tumors. These portraits will include not only cytogenetic and gene expression information, but also much more detailed gene sequence information. Current work is underway to use this molecular data to generate robust diagnostic and prognostic information. In the near future, given the increasing number of drugs approved for RCC treatment, selection of the best treatment for each individual patient will become more important. Incorporation of molecular genetic data can be used to stratify patients into different treatment subgroups. For example, a clear cell tumor with an IL-2–responsive gene expression signature would be evaluated differently compared with a clear cell tumor with activation of the PI3K/AKT pathway due to an activating sequence mutation in the *AKT* gene. In this way, molecular classification could lead to a higher percentage of favorable responses and more effective patient management. Genetic stratification could also be applied iteratively to recurrent disease. Recent studies in lung cancer have shown that one mechanism of resistance to the receptor tyrosine kinase inhibitor gefitinib (Iressa) was the result of upregulation of the *MET* receptor tyrosine kinase.[116] These results suggest that resistance-mediated recurrence (ie, resistance to gefitinib) may cause the tumor to be sensitive to a different class of drugs (ie, sensitive to Met inhibitors). Continued integration, evaluation, and refinement of gene expression and cytogenetic and DNA sequence information will be essential for accurate molecular classification of RCC. Moreover, the design and application of the required infrastructure to accommodate this type of molecular-based stratification will be paramount for its success in the future.

## REFERENCES

1. Duesberg P, et al. Aneuploidy versus gene mutations as cause of cancer. Curr Sci 2001;81:490–500.
2. Zbar B, et al. Loss of alleles of loci on the short arm of chromosome 3 in renal cell carcinoma. Nature 1987;327: 721–4.
3. Kovacs G, et al. Consistent chromosome 3p deletion and loss of heterozygosity in renal cell carcinoma. Proc Natl Acad Sci U S A 1988;85:1571–5.
4. Bugert O, Kovacs G. Molecular differential diagnosis of renal cell carcinomas by microsatellite analysis. Am J Pathol 1996;6:2081–8.
5. Bugert P, Von Knobloch R, Kovacs G. Duplication of two distinct regions on chromosome 5q in non-papillary renal-cell carcinomas. Int J Cancer 1998;76:337–40.
6. Presti JC Jr, et al. Renal cell carcinoma genetic analysis by comparative genomic hybridization and restriction fragment length polymorphism analysis. J Urol 1996; 156:281–5.
7. Gunawan B, et al. Prognostic impacts of cytogenetic findings in clear cell renal cell carcinoma: gain of 5q31-qter predicts a distinct clinical phenotype with favorable prognosis. Cancer Res 2001;61:7731–8.
8. Gunawan B, et al. Cytogenetic and morphologic typing of 58 papillary renal cell carcinomas: evidence for a cytogenetic evolution of type 2 from type 1 tumors. Cancer Res 2003; 63:6200–5.
9. Moch H, et al. Genetic aberrations detected by comparative genomic hybridization are associated with clinical outcome in renal cell carcinoma. Cancer Res 1996;56:27–30.
10. Brunelli M, et al. Eosinophilic and classic chromophobe renal cell carcinomas have similar frequent losses of multiple chromosomes from among chromosomes 1, 2, 6, 10, and 17, and this pattern of genetic abnormality is not present in renal oncocytoma. Mod Pathol 2005;18:161–9.
11. Paner GP, et al. High Incidence of chromosome 1 abnormalities in a series of 27 renal oncocytomas: cytogenetic and fluorescence in situ hybridzation studies. Arch Pathol Lab Med 2006;131:81–5.
12. Kovacs G, et al. The Heidelberg classification of renal cell tumours. J Pathol 1997;183:131–3.
13. Cohen AJ, et al. Hereditary renal-cell carcinoma associated with a chromosomal translocation. N Engl J Med 1979;301:592–5.
14. Kovacs G, Brusa P. Recurrent genomic rearrangements are not at the fragile sites on chromosomes 3 and 5 in human renal cell carcinomas. Hum Genet 1988;80:99–101.
15. Glover TW, et al. Translocation t(3;8)(p14.2;q24.1) in renal cell carcinoma affects expression of the common fragile site at 3p14(FRA3B) in lymphocytes. Cancer Genet Cytogenet 1988;31:69–73.
16. Tajara EH, et al. Loss of common 3p14 fragile site expression in renal cell carcinoma with deletion breakpoint at 3p14. Cancer Genet Cytogenet 1988;31:75–82.
17. Shridhar V, et al. A gene from human chromosomal band 3p21.1 encodes a highly conserved arginine-rich protein and is mutated in renal cell carcinomas. Oncogene 1996;12:1931–9.
18. Elfving P, et al. Prognostic implications of cytogenetic findings in kidney cancer. Br J Urol 1997;80:698–706.
19. Schullerus D, et al. Loss of heterozygosity at chromosomes 8p, 9p, and 14q is associated with stage and grade of nonpapillary renal cell carcinomas. J Pathol 1997;183:151–5.
20. Herbers J, et al. Significance of chromosome arm 14q loss in nonpapillary renal cell carcinomas. Genes Chromosomes Cancer 1997;19:29–35.
21. Nagao K, et al. Allelic loss of 3p25 associated with alterations of 5q22.3 approximately q23.2 may affect the prognosis of conventional renal cell carcinoma. Cancer Genet Cytogenet 2005;160:43–8.
22. Junker K, et al. Genetic alterations in metastatic renal cell carcinoma detected by comparative genomic hybridization: correlation with clinical and histological data. Int J Oncol 2000;17:903–8.
23. Delahunt B, Eble JN. Papillary renal cell carcinoma: a clinicopathologic and immunohistochemical study of 105 tumors. Mod Pathol 1997;10:537–44.
24. Yang XJ, et al. A molecular classification of papillary renal cell carcinoma. Cancer Res 2005;65:5628–37.
25. Furge KA, et al. Identification of deregulated oncogenic pathways in renal cell carcinoma: an integrated oncogenomic approach based on gene expression profiling. Oncogene 2007;26:1346–50.
26. Bruder E, et al. Morphologic and molecular characterization of renal cell carcinoma in children and young adults. Am J Surg Pathol 2004;28:1117–32.
27. Argani P, et al. Translocation carcinomas of the kidney after chemotherapy in childhood. J Clin Oncol 2006;24: 1529–34.
28. Weterman MA, Wilbrink M, Geurts van Kessel A. Fusion of the transcription factor TFE3 gene to a novel gene, PRCC, in t(X;1)(p11;q21)-positive papillary renal cell carcinomas. Proc Natl Acad Sci U S A 1996;93:15294–8.
29. Sidhar SK, et al. The t(X;1)(p11.2;q21.2) translocation in papillary renal cell carcinoma fuses a novel gene PRCC to the TFE3 transcription factor gene. Hum Mol Genet 1996;5:1333–8.
30. Meloni AM, et al. Translocation (X;1) in papillary renal cell carcinoma. A new cytogenetic subtype. Cancer Genet Cytogenet 1993;65:1–6.
31. Takahashi M, et al. Molecular sub-classification of kidney cancer and the discovery of new diagnostic markers. Oncogene 2003;22:6810–6818.
32. Higgins JP, et al. Gene expression patterns in renal cell carcinoma assessed by complementary DNA microarray. Am J Pathol 2003;162:925–32.
33. Brown JA, et al. Fluorescence in situ hybridization analysis of renal oncocytoma reveals frequent loss of chromosomes Y and 1. J Urol 1996;156:31–5.
34. Fuzesi L, et al. Cytogenetic analysis of 11 renal oncocytomas: further evidence of structural rearrangements of 11q13 as a characteristics of chromosomal anomaly. Cancer Genet Cytogenet 1999;107:1–6.

35. Pollack JR, et al. Genome-wide analysis of DNA copy-number changes using cDNA microarrays. Nat Genet 1999;23:41–6.

36. Snijders AM, et al. Assembly of microarrays for genome-wide measurement of DNA copy number. Nat Genet 2001;29:263–4.

37. Barrett MT, et al. Comparative genomic hybridization using oligonucleotide microarrays and total genomic DNA. Proc Natl Acad Sci U S A 2004;101:17765–70.

38. Zhao X, et al. Homozygous deletions and chromosome amplifications in human lung carcinomas revealed by single nucleotide polymorphism array analysis. Cancer Res 2005;65:5561–70.

39. Bugert P, Pesti T, Kovacs G. The tcf17 gene at chromosome 5q is not involved in the development of conventional renal cell carcinoma. Int J Cancer 2000;86:806–10.

40. Bugert P, Kenck C, Kovacs G. A 33 bp minisatellite repeat upstream of the 'mutated in colon cancer' gene at chromosome 5q21. Electrophoresis 1998;19:1362–5.

41. Sultmann H, et al. Gene expression in kidney cancer is associated with cytogenetic abnormalities, metastasis formation, and patient survival. Clin Cancer Res 2005;11:646–55.

42. Latif F, et al. Identification of the von Hippel-Lindau disease tumor suppressor gene. Science 1993;260:1317–20.

43. Iliopoulos O, et al. Tumour suppression by the human von Hippel-Lindau gene product. Nat Med 1995;1:822–6.

44. Chen F, et al. Suppression of growth of renal carcinoma cells by the von Hippel-Lindau tumor suppressor gene. Cancer Res 1995;55:4804–7.

45. Kenck C, et al. Mutation of the VHL gene is associated exclusively with the development of non-papillary renal cell carcinomas. J Pathol 1996;179:157–61.

46. Knudson AG. Mutation and cancer: statistical study of retinoblastoma. Proc Natl Acad Sci U S A 1971;68: 820–3.

47. Maynard MA, Ohh M. von Hippel-Lindau tumor suppressor protein and hypoxia-inducible factor in kidney cancer. Am J Nephrol 2004;24:1–13.

48. Maxwell PH, et al. The tumour suppressor protein VHL targets hypoxia-inducible factors for oxygen-dependent proteolysis. Nature 1999;399:271–5.

49. Ohh M, et al. Ubiquitination of hypoxia-inducible factor requires direct binding to the beta-domain of the von Hippel-Lindau protein. Nat Cell Biol 2000;2:423–7.

50. Ivan M, et al. HIFalpha targeted for VHL-mediated destruction by proline hydroxylation: implications for $O_2$ sensing. Science 2001;292:464–8.

51. Jaakkola P, et al. Targeting of HIF-alpha to the von Hippel-Lindau ubiquitylation complex by $O_2$-regulated prolyl hydroxylation. Science 2001;292:468–72.

52. Schofield CJ, Ratcliffe PJ. Oxygen sensing by HIF hydroxylases. Nat Rev Mol Cell Biol 2004;5:343–54.

53. Wang GL, et al. Hypoxia-inducible factor 1 is a basic-helix-loop-helix-PAS heterodimer regulated by cellular $O_2$ tension. Proc Natl Acad Sci U S A 1995;92:5510–4.

54. Jiang B, et al. Hypoxia-inducible factor 1 levels vary exponentially over a physiological relevant range of $O_2$ tension. Am J Physiol Cell Physiol 1996;271:1172–80.

55. Masson N, et al. Independent function of two destruction domains in hypoxia-inducible factor-alpha chains activated by prolyl hydroxylation. EMBO J 2001;20:5197–206.

56. Kaelin WG. The von Hippel-Lindau protein, HIF hydroxylation, and oxygen sensing. Biochem Biophys Res Commun 2005;338:627–38.

57. Lubensky IA, et al. Hereditary and sporadic papillary renal carcinomas with c-met mutations share a distinct morphological phenotype. Am J Pathol 1999;155:517–26.

58. Schmidt L, et al. Germline and somatic mutations in the tyrosine kinase domain of the MET proto-oncogene in papillary renal carcinomas. Nat Genet 1997;16:68–73.

59. Schmidt L, et al. Novel mutations of the MET proto-oncogene in papillary renal carcinomas. Oncogene 1999;18:2343–50.

60. Cooper CS, et al. Molecular cloning of a new transforming gene from a chemically transformed human cell line. Nature 1984;311:29–33.

61. Park M, et al. Mechanism of met oncogene activation. Cell 1986;45:895–904.

62. Nakamura T, Nawa K, Ichihara A. Partial purification and characterization of hepatocyte growth factor from serum of hepatectomized rats. Biochem Biophys Res Commun 1984;122:1450–9.

63. Stoker M, Perryman M. An epithelial scatter factor released by embryo fibroblasts. J Cell Sci 1985;77:209–23.

64. Bottaro DP, et al. Identification of the hepatocyte growth factor receptor as the c-met proto-oncogene product. Science 1991;251:802–4.

65. Tomlinson IP, et al. Germline mutations in FH predispose to dominantly inherited uterine fibroids, skin leiomyomata and papillary renal cell cancer. Nat Genet 2002;30:406–10.

66. Toro JR, et al. Mutations in the fumarate hydratase gene cause hereditary leiomyomatosis and renal cell cancer in families in North America. Am J Hum Genet 2003;73:95–106.

67. Pollard PJ, et al. Targeted inactivation of fh1 causes proliferative renal cyst development and activation of the hypoxia pathway. Cancer Cell 2007;11:311–9.

68. Isaacs JS, et al. HIF overexpression correlated with biallelic loss of fumarate hydrotase in renal cancer: novel role of fumarate in regulation of HIF stability. Cancer Cell 2005;8:143–53.

69. Pollard PJ, et al. Accumulation of Krebs cycle intermediates and over-expression of HIF1alpha in tumours which result from germline FH and SDH mutations. Hum Mol Genet 2005;14:2231–9.

70. Furge KA, et al. Detection of DNA copy number changes and oncogenic signaling abnormalities from gene expression data reveals MYC activation in high-grade papillary renal cell carcinoma. Cancer Res 2007;67:3171–6.

71. Nickerson ML, et al. Mutations in a novel gene lead to kidney tumors, lung wall defects, and benign tumors of the hair follicle in patients with the Birt-Hogg-Dube syndrome. Cancer Cell 2002;2:157–64.

72. Pavlovich CP, et al. Renal tumors in the Birt-Hogg-Dube syndrome. Am J Surg Pathol 2002;26:1542–52.

73. Schmidt LS, et al. Germline BHD-mutation spectrum and phenotype analysis of a large cohort of families with Birt-Hogg-Dube syndrome. Am J Hum Genet 2005;76: 1023–33.

74. Khoo SK, et al. Inactivation of BHD in sporadic renal tumors. Cancer Res 2003;63:4583–7.

75. Al-Saleem T, et al. The genetics of renal oncocytosis: a possible model for neoplastic progression. Cancer Genet Cytogenet 2004;152:23–8.

76. Rankin EB, Tomaszewski JE, Haase VH. Renal cyst development in mice with conditional inactivation of the von Hippel-Lindau tumor suppressor. Cancer Res 2006;66: 2576–83.

77. Ueki K, et al. Correlation of histology and molecular genetic analysis of 1p, 19q, 10q, TP53, EGFR, CDK4, and CDKN2A in 91 astrocytic and oligodendroglial tumors. Clin Cancer Res 2002;8:196–201.

78. Qian CN, et al. Cystic renal neoplasia following conditional inactivation of apc in mouse renal tubular epithelium. J Biol Chem 2005;280:3938–45.

79. Greenman C, et al. Patterns of somatic mutation in human cancer genomes. Nature 2007;446:153–8.

80. Takahashi M, et al. Gene expression profiling of clear cell renal cell carcinoma: gene identification and prognostic classification. Proc Natl Acad Sci USA 2001;98:9754–9.

81. Gieseg MA, et al. Expression profiling of human renal carcinomas with functional taxonomic analysis. BMC Bioinformatics 2002;3:26.

82. Boer JM, et al. Identification and classification of differentially expressed genes in renal cell carcinoma by expression profiling on a global human 31,500-element cDNA array. Genome Res 2001;11:1861–70.

83. Jones J, et al. Gene signatures of progression and metastasis in renal cell cancer. Clin Cancer Res 2005;11:5730–9.

84. Liou LS, et al. Microarray gene expression profiling and analysis in renal cell carcinoma. BMC Urol 2004;4:9.

85. Yamazaki K, et al. Overexpression of KIT in chromophobe renal cell carcinoma. Oncogene 2003;22:847–52.

86. Skubitz KM, Skubitz AP. Differential gene expression in renal-cell cancer. J Lab Clin Med 2002;140:52–64.

87. Skubitz KM, et al. Differential gene expression identifies subgroups of renal cell carcinoma. J Lab Clin Med 2006; 147:250–67.

88. Moch H, et al. High-throughput tissue microarray analysis to evaluate genes uncovered by cDNA microarray screening in renal cell carcinoma. Am J Pathol 1999;154:981–6.

89. Li G, et al. S100A1: a powerful marker to differentiate chromophobe renal cell carcinoma from renal oncocytoma. Histopathology 2007;50:642–7.

90. Lin F, et al. Expression of S-100 protein in renal cell neoplasms. Hum Pathol 2006;37:462–70.

91. Rocca PC, et al. Diagnostic utility of S100A1 expression in renal cell neoplasms: an immunohistochemical and quantitative RT-PCR study. Mod Pathol 2007;20:722–8.

92. Yao M, et al. Expression of adipose differentiation-related protein: a predictor of cancer-specific survival in clear cell renal carcinoma. Clin Cancer Res 2007;13:152–60.

93. Kosari F, et al. Clear cell renal cell carcinoma: gene expression analyses identify a potential signature for tumor aggressiveness. Clin Cancer Res 2005;11:5128–39.

94. Zhao H, et al. Gene expression profiling predicts survival in conventional renal cell carcinoma. PLoS Med 2006;3:e13.

95. Tsui KH, et al. Prognostic indicators for renal cell carcinoma: a multivariate analysis of 643 patients using the revised 1997 TNM staging criteria. J Urol 2000;163:1090-5; quiz 1295.

96. Gettman MT, et al. Pathologic staging of renal cell carcinoma: significance of tumor classification with the 1997 TNM staging system. Cancer 2001;91:354–61.

97. Han KR, et al. Validation of an integrated staging system toward improved prognostication of patients with localized renal cell carcinoma in an international population. J Urol 2003;170(6 Pt 1):2221–4.

98. Zisman A, et al. Improved prognostication of renal cell carcinoma using an integrated staging system. J Clin Oncol 2001;19:1649–57.

99. Staller P, et al. Chemokine receptor CXCR4 downregulated by von Hippel-Lindau tumour suppressor pVHL. Nature 2003;425:307–11.

100. Yao M, et al. Gene expression analysis of renal carcinoma: adipose differentiation-related protein as a potential diagnostic and prognostic biomarker for clear-cell renal carcinoma. J Pathol 2005;205:377–87.

101. Desai KV, et al. Initiating oncogenic event determines gene-expression patterns of human breast cancer models. Proc Natl Acad Sci U S A 2002;99:6967–72.

102. Ferrando AA, et al. Gene expression signatures define novel oncogenic pathways in T cell acute lymphoblastic leukemia. Cancer Cell 2002;1:75–87.

103. Huang E, et al. Gene expression phenotypic models that predict the activity of oncogenic pathways. Nat Genet 2003;34:226–30.

104. Sweet-Cordero A, et al. An oncogenic KRAS2 expression signature identified by cross-species gene-expression analysis. Nat Genet 2005;37:48–55.

105. Bild AH, et al. Oncogenic pathway signatures in human cancers as a guide to targeted therapies. Nature 2005; 439:353–7.

106. Chi JT, et al. Gene expression programs in response to hypoxia: cell type specificity and prognostic significance in human cancers. PLoS Med 2006;3:e47.

107. Subramanian A, et al. Gene set enrichment analysis: a knowledge-based approach for interpreting genome-wide expression profiles. Proc Natl Acad Sci U S A 2005; 102:15545–50.

108. Kim S, Volsky DJ. PAGE: parametric analysis of gene set enrichment. BMC Bioinformatics 2005;6:144.

109. Riss J, et al. Cancers as wounds that do not heal: differences and similarities between renal regeneration/repair and renal cell carcinoma. Cancer Res 2006;66:7216–24.

110. Copland JA, et al. Genomic profiling identifies alterations in TGFbeta signaling through loss of TGFbeta receptor expression in human renal cell carcinogenesis and progression. Oncogene 2003;22:8053–62.

111. Minasian LM, et al. Interferon alfa-2a in advanced renal cell carcinoma: treatment results and survival in 159 patients with long-term follow-up. J Clin Oncol 1993; 11:1368–75.

112. Atkins MB, Regan M, McDermott D. Update on the role of interleukin 2 and other cytokines in the treatment of patients with stage IV renal carcinoma. Clin Cancer Res 2004;10(18 Pt 2):6342S–6S.

113. Shimazui T, et al. Prediction of in vitro response to interferon-alpha in renal cell carcinoma cell lines. Cancer Sci 2007;98:529–34.

114. Tiwari G, et al. Gene expression profiling in prostate cancer cells with Akt activation reveals Fra-1 as an Akt-inducible gene. Mol Cancer Res 2003;1:475–84.

115. Gerritsen ME, et al. Using gene expression profiling to identify the molecular basis of the synergistic actions of hepatocyte growth factor and vascular endothelial growth factor in human endothelial cells. Br J Pharmacol 2003;140: 595–610.

116. Engelman JA, et al. MET amplification leads to gefitinib resistance in lung cancer by activating ERBB3 signaling. Science 2007;316:1039–43.

5

# Imaging Techniques in Renal Cell Carcinoma

**BRIAN R. HERTS, MD**

## CROSS-SECTIONAL IMAGING TECHNIQUES AND THE APPEARANCE OF RENAL CELL CARCINOMA

Cross-sectional imaging plays a critical role in the diagnosis and characterization of renal masses. Cross-sectional imaging is used to detect and characterize renal masses, stage renal cell carcinoma (RCC), and plan surgery. Renal masses are almost ubiquitous on computed tomography (CT), magnetic resonance (MR), and ultrasonography (US) because benign renal cysts are so common. The difficulty comes when trying to distinguish between a malignant neoplasm and another etiology, such as a benign cyst, neoplasm, vascular lesion, congenital anomaly, or normal variant. Fortunately, because there is a wealth of experience with renal imaging, there is ample data to support the use of cross-sectional imaging as a diagnostic tool for distinguishing between clinically significant and insignificant renal lesions. Clinical signs and symptoms are relegated to a supplementary role in the diagnosis of RCC because most renal lesions are asymptomatic and because cross-sectional imaging has proven to have a high sensitivity and specificity for renal malignancies.

### Computed Tomography

State-of-the-art CT is the gold standard for the detection and characterization of renal masses. CT of the kidneys always includes thin slices, preferably no thicker that 3 mm slice width, reconstructed from submillimeter collimated slices, and imaging before and after intravenous (IV) contrast. The kidneys are optimally scanned during peak concentration of contrast by the tubules; this facilitates differentiation between normal renal parenchyma, which concentrates contrast, and abnormal tissue, which does not have functioning nephrons. This time period after IV contrast is the nephrographic phase (NP) and typically occurs 90 to 120 seconds after the initiation of the IV contrast bolus.

A three-phase CT scan is considered the optimal technique for detecting and characterizing renal masses, as well as for staging RCC (Figure 1). This includes an unenhanced scan, a vascular or corticomedullary phase (CMP) scan, and an NP scan. Several studies have shown that the NP is the most sensitive for the detection of renal tumors, and more renal lesions can be seen when a combination of unenhanced, CMP, and NP scans is used.[1–6]

The CMP occurs shortly after peak arterial enhancement (typically 35 to 40 seconds after the contrast bolus is initiated) and is useful for assessing the renal vasculature and vascular renal lesions.[3,4,7] The enhancement seen on the CMP can also be useful for characterizing lesions.[1] However, when used alone, the CMP can result in lesions being missed and false-positive diagnosis of medullary lesions.[8]

Advantages of CT are high spatial resolution, rapid scan times, easy access, and user familiarity. Limitations to CT include the use of ionizing radiation and risk of contrast nephropathy in patients with renal insufficiency. Technical difficulties can also occur in patients with metallic hardware in the upper lumbar spine that can cause image artifacts at the level of the kidneys.

## MR Imaging

MR is also used to characterize and stage RCC and is used to further characterize indeterminate lesions at CT; MR is more contrast sensitive and tissue sensitive than CT. MR is the test of choice in patients with mild

to moderate renal insufficiency. At standard clinical doses, MR contrast (gadolinium–DTPA) does not appear to have any nephrotoxic effects in patients with mild kidney disease, but at high doses in dialysis patients, there are rare reports of nephrotoxicity and a severe systemic fibrosis.[9,10] As MR evolves, the spatial resolution may match and even surpass that of CT. Until then, and because of the relatively less frequent use of MR in abdominal imaging, CT will remain the gold standard.

Similar to CT, MR imaging must be performed before and after contrast. T2-weighted imaging, in-phase and out-of-phase imaging, and imaging with and without fat saturation are performed without contrast to characterize cystic and fatty lesions (Figure 2). T1-weighted imaging, usually with a fat-saturation breath-hold sequence, is performed before and after contrast during several time points; we scan at 0, 45, 90, and 120 seconds after contrast, using both axial and coronal planes.[11,12] The lack of ionizing radiation allows the more liberal use of scanning after contrast.

Advantages of MR include lack of ionizing radiation and superior tissue characterization. MR is highly sensitive for renal tumors, approaching 100%, and has advantages over CT for the characterization

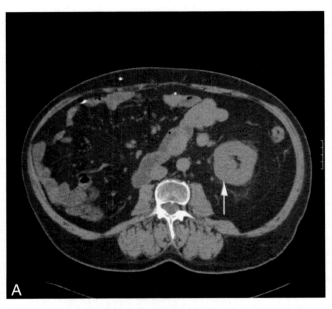

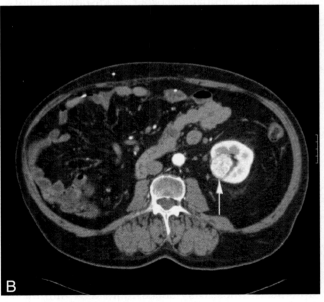

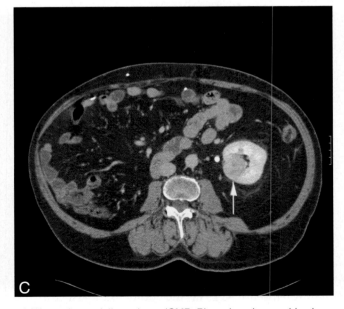

**Figure 1.** Renal cell carcinoma computed tomography (CT). Unenhanced (A), corticomedullary phase (CMP; B), and nephrographic phase (NP; C) axial CT scans show an approximately 2.5-cm, left lower pole, enhancing solid renal neoplasm (arrows). Three scan phase techniques are considered state of the art for the detection and characterization of renal cell carcinoma (RCC). Renal masses are often isodense to normal renal parenchyma on the unenhanced CT (A). On the CMP CT (B), hypervascular masses such as this enhance similar to the renal cortex but on the NP (C), masses are hypodense to normal renal parenchyma because tumors lack functioning nephrons and do not concentrate the contrast that has been filtered into the urine.

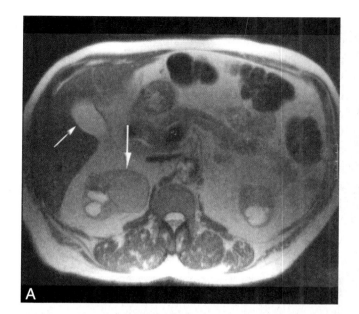

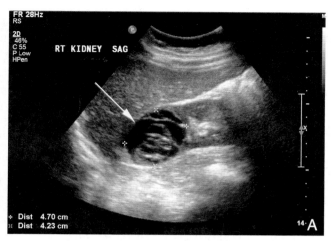

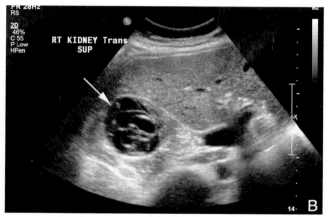

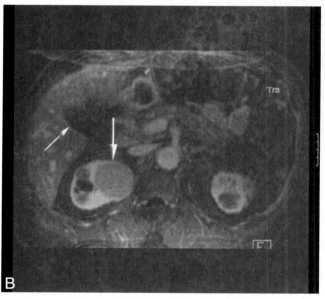

**Figure 2.** Magnetic resonance (MR) techniques. T2 axial (A) and contrast-enhanced T1 volume-interpolated breath-hold sequence subtraction (B) images. The fluid in the gallbladder (thin arrow) is bright on T2-weighted image (A) and dark on T1-weighted image (B). A solid renal cell carcinoma (thick arrow) will enhance after contrast (B) and typically has intermediate signal on T2-weighted images.

**Figure 3.** Cystic renal cell carcinoma (RCC) on ultrasonography (US). Longitudinal (A) and axial (B) sonographic images. Both anechoic and solid components are seen on this US, demonstrating a complex cystic renal mass (arrow) that was RCC at pathology.

of subcentimeter cysts. The sensitivity and specificity of CT and MR for the detection of RCC are nearly equivalent, ranging between 80 and 100%.[13-16]

One limitation of MR is its inability to specify enhancement criteria following contrast in order to distinguish between cystic lesions and hypovascular solid masses. A 15% increase in signal intensity has been advocated as a threshold to determine enhancement in renal tumors.[17] However, signal intensity in MR is based on a relative scale, not on absolute density, as is the Hounsfield unit (HU) scale.[18] Therefore, an image subtraction between pre- and postcontrast MR exams can be used to eliminate the subjectivity of determining enhancement after contrast on MR.[19] A minor limitation of MR is difficulty in detecting calcium in renal lesions because calcium appears as a signal void.

## Ultrasonography

RCC can be hypoechoic, isoechoic, or hyperechoic on US. In general, renal tumors that are large, contour deforming, or partially cystic can be detected sonographically (Figure 3). US is ideal for distinguishing between cystic and solid renal masses.[20] However, US is not the best test for the detection and characterization of most renal tumors for several reasons.

First, small renal tumors are often isoechoic and therefore can only be detected if there is a distortion of the renal contour. Second, the detection of fat within a lesion to identify angiomyolipoma (AML) is less specific with US than with other cross-sectional imaging. Third, US is more user dependent and patient dependent in that body habitus can play a significant role in the sonographic depiction of the kidneys. As a result, the sensitivity and specificity of renal US for detection of renal masses are lower than those of either CT or MR.[18,19] The advantages of renal US include the noninvasive nature of the exam without the use of contrast agents or radiation.

US is performed with a 3- to 6-MHz transducer, and images are obtained through each kidney in both the axial and longitudinal planes. Tissue harmonic imaging can be used to increase the sensitivity of US for renal masses. Cysts will appear as round or oval anechoic structures with a thin or imperceptible wall. Solid and complex cystic masses will either deform the renal contour or be distinguished from the normal renal parenchyma by a difference in echogenicity. The sensitivity of US for the detection of RCC is also dependent on the size of the lesion.[21] The sensitivity may improve with IV contrast agents for US: in one study, sensitivity increased to 97% compared with 70% for gray scale US.[22] US contrast agents are available for use with Doppler US systems but are not in general use in the United States.

The importance of contrast use for the CT and MR detection and staging of RCC cannot be understated. However, a full discussion of the different types of contrast agents used for CT and MR and their limitations and potential complications is beyond the scope of the chapter.

## Imaging Appearance of RCC

Primary neoplasms of renal epithelial origin can be classified as follows: clear cell, granular cell, sarcomatoid adenocarcinoma, chromophobe, papillary, collecting duct, medullary, mixed cell types or as adenocarcinoma not specified, oncocytoma, small cell carcinoma, juxtaglomerular tumor, or carcinoid.[23-25]

Clear cell RCC (CCRCC) is the most common cell type and accounts for 70 to 80% of all RCC.

Clear cell carcinomas are typically hypervascular on CT, with enhancement more avid than that displayed by other subtypes (Figure 4).[26] A hypervascular pattern is present in nearly 50% of clear cell carcinomas compared with 15% of papillary and 4% of chromophobe subtypes.[26,27] Some CCRCC are cystic. There is a large body of literature devoted to distinguishing between benign cystic renal disease and cystic RCC with several indeterminate lesion characteristics. We use the Bosniak criteria to stratify risk of malignancy based on appearance.[28-30] Those cystic masses with clearly solid enhancing elements at CT or

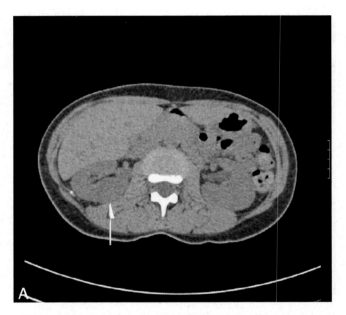

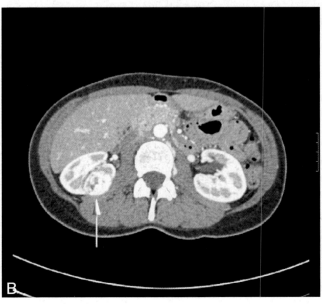

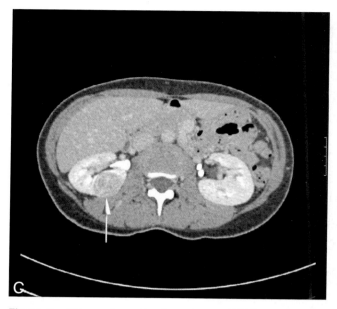

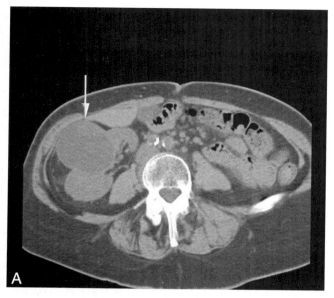

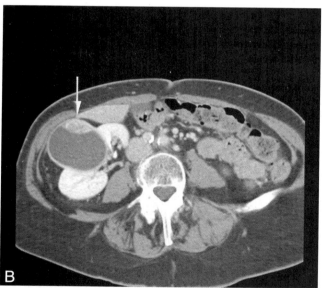

**Figure 4.** Clear cell renal cell carcinoma (RCC) on computed tomography (CT) Unenhanced (A), corticomedullary phase (CMP; B), and nephrographic phase (NP; C)—clear cell RCC (CCRCC), the most common subtype, occurs in approximately 70% of patients. CCRCC (arrow) enhances avidly with intravenous contrast, which is more pronounced on the CMP (B) than on the NP (C).

**Figure 5.** Cystic renal cell carcinoma (RCC) on computed tomography (CT). Noncontrast (A) and nephrographic (B) phase images show a thick-walled cystic mass with a discrete, enhancing nodule along the anterior wall (arrow). RCC can appear as solid, complex cystic or infiltrating masses. Cystic renal masses that contain clearly solid, enhancing elements are Bosniak IV complex cystic lesions and almost always RCC.

MR are usually cystic RCC (Bosniak IV) (Figure 5). On MR, CCRCC is isointense on T1WI and isointense to hyperintense on T2WI (Figure 6).[31] Clear cell carcinomas more commonly invade the renal collecting system.[32] Cystic degeneration is also more common in the clear cell subtype than in the other subtypes (Figure 7). This is true regardless of tumor size. The chromophobe subtype shows homogeneous enhancement in nearly 75% of cases, significantly more than 45 and 65% of clear cell and papillary subtypes, respectively. Calcification occurs equally: in 21 to 25% of clear cell, papillary, and chromophobe subtypes.

Papillary RCC (PRCC) accounts for approximately 10% of RCC and has a better prognosis than CCRCC.[33–35] PRCC can be bilateral and multiple.[35] On CT, PRCC is typically a hypovascular solid mass (Figure 8).[27,36] PRCC rarely invades the collecting system.[32] On MR, PRCC can be hemorrhagic, leading to heterogeneous and increased signal intensity on T1WI and decreased signal intensity on T2WI (Figure 9).[31,35] There are no sonographic features specific for PRCC.

The chromophobe subtype accounts for only a small percentage of RCC and is typically hypovascular on CT, similar to PRCC (Figure 10).[34,37] Collecting or Bellini duct carcinomas are uncommon, accounting for only 1 to 2% of all RCC. Collecting duct RCC (CDRCC) are of medullary origin and typically infiltrate within kidney.[38–42] Metastases occur in approximately one-third of patients

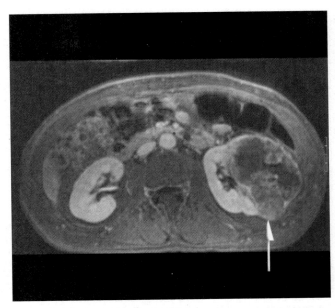

**Figure 6.**   Clear cell renal cell carcinoma on magnetic resonance (MR). Axial subtraction MR volume-interpolated breath-hold image shows a centrally necrotic left renal mass (arrow), a clear cell carcinoma.

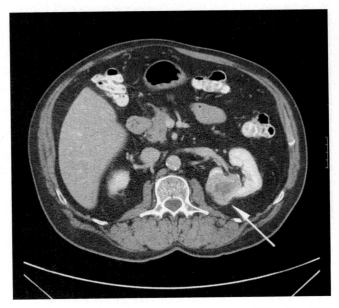

**Figure 7.**   Centrally necrotic renal cell carcinoma (RCC). This RCC (arrow) has mixed enhancement pattern with a low-attenuation region centrally, which shows no enhancement; this represents tumor necrosis at pathology.

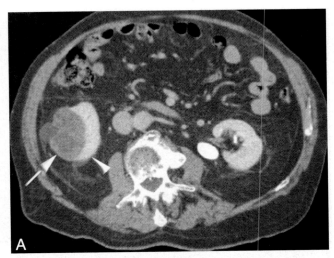

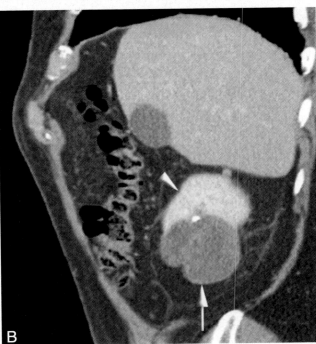

**Figure 8.**   Papillary renal cell carcinoma on computed tomography (CT) Axial (A) and sagittal (B) images demonstrate a hypovascular mass (arrow). Note the large difference in density between the mass and the normal parenchyma (arrowhead) on this nephrographic phase scan. Most papillary renal cell carcinoma are hypovascular on CT and angiography.

with CDRCC and are more common at presentation than with other RCC cell types. Bone metastases from CDRCC are osteoblastic, in contrast to metastases from CCRCC, which are osteolytic.[15] CDRCC tumors are hypovascular on CT and angiography.[36] The differential diagnosis of CDRCC includes high-grade transitional cell carcinoma, squamous cell carcinoma of the renal pelvis, and non-Hodgkin's lymphoma (NHL) (Figure 11).[38,42]

Sarcomatoid RCC is highly aggressive. It typically has an infiltrating appearance on imaging and is usually symptomatic at presentation.[43] Renal sarcoma and sarcomatoid RCC should be considered when there is an extensively infiltrating tumor with extension into the perinephric space and adjacent organs (Figure 12). The differential diagnosis, similar to that for CDRCC, includes TCC and NHL.[44]

Medullary carcinoma, although usually considered a distinct entity, may be an aggressive form of CDRCC that occurs in younger patients. Medullary renal carcinoma has been associated with sickle cell trait but not with sickle cell disease.

Juxtaglomerular tumors are exceedingly uncommon, and few specific imaging details are available.

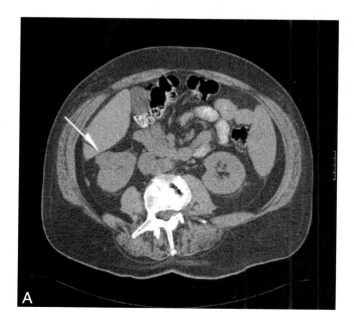

**Figure 9.** Papillary renal cell carcinoma (PRCC) on magnetic resonance (MR). PRCC (arrow), seen here in the upper pole of the right kidney anteriorly, is frequently hyperintense to the normal renal parenchyma in T1-weighted MR imaging.

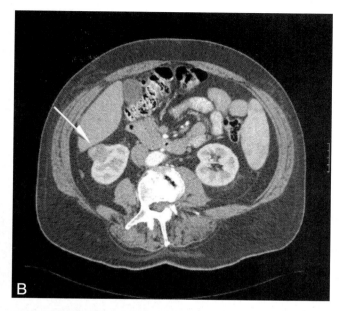

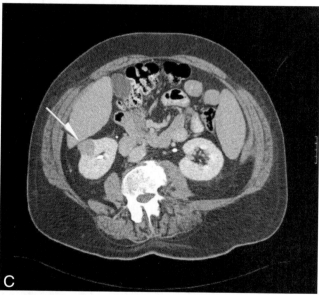

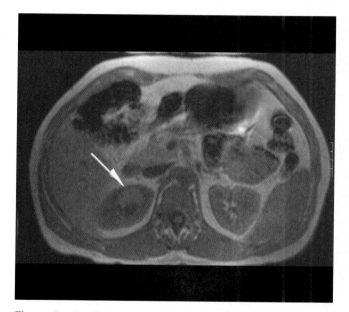

**Figure 10.** Chromophobe renal cell carcinoma (RCC). Chromophobe RCC are hypovascular tumors (arrow) on unenhanced (A), corticomedullary phase (B), and nephrographic phase (C) CT scans, a pattern similar to papillary RCC. Chromophobe RCC rarely have necrosis or hemorrhage and carry a better prognosis than CCRCC. Histologically, they exhibit polyhedral tumor cells with abundant pale cytoplasm and a solid pattern of growth.

Juxtaglomerular tumors are often associated with hypertension and hypokalemia due to the production of renin or renin analogues that activate the renin–angiotensin system.[23] This contrasts with the majority of RCC that are now asymptomatic and discovered incidentally.

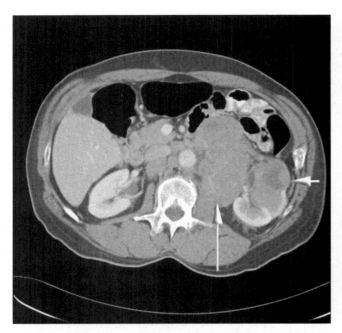

**Figure 11.** Renal non-Hodgkin's lymphoma (NHL). This patient has large bulky retroperitoneal lymphadenopathy (long arrow), out of proportion to the size of the mass (short arrow). This patient has NHL.

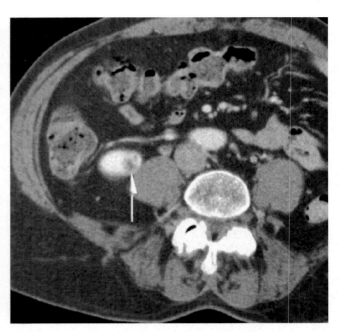

**Figure 13.** Oncocytoma. This small right lower pole tumor is an oncocytoma (arrow). There are no computed tomographic, ultrasonagraphic, or magnetic resonance features specific for oncocytoma, although histologic features have been described that may allow for the diagnosis of oncocytoma on percutaneous biopsy of larger lesions.

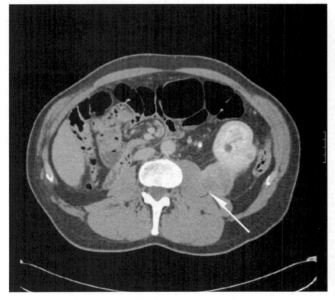

**Figure 12.** Sarcomatoid renal cell carcinoma (RCC). This exophytic sarcomatoid RCC invades into the left iliopsoas muscle complex (arrow). Sarcomatoid tumors are more aggressive and have a worse prognosis than the more common clear cell carcinomas.

## Benign Renal Tumors

Benign primary renal tumors include oncocytoma and AML (Figures 13 and 14). Oncocytoma is hypervascular, similar to clear cell carcinoma. CT cannot reliably distinguish between most RCC and

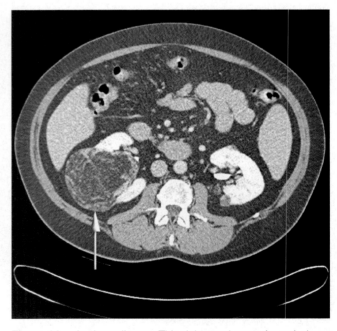

**Figure 14.** Angiomyolipoma. This right renal mass (arrow) shows mixed fat and soft tissue density. Macroscopic fat is diagnostic of an angiomyolipoma, with rare exceptions.

oncocytoma.[45] The histopathologic features of oncocytoma that allow differentiation from RCC on biopsy have recently been described.[46,47] However, it is still difficult to distinguish between

RCC and oncocytoma on percutaneous core needle biopsy. Most AML are able to be characterized by gross fat on CT identified by HU density measurements less than 0 and on MR by fat-suppression techniques. There are a small percentage of AML with minimal fat expression macroscopically. Although these are easy to diagnose at pathology, these AML with minimal fat can be difficult to distinguish from small solid RCC on imaging.

## STAGING OF RCC BY CT AND MR

### Staging with CT and MR

The revised tumor–node–metastasis (TNM) staging criteria more accurately delineate differences in survival rates between Stage I and Stage II disease.[48] Overall, the accuracy of CT and MR for staging is high, between 87 and 100%.[49–54] The major limitation is identifying T3 tumors: those tumors that have spread beyond the renal capsule without direct invasion of adjacent structures. The difference between T1 and T3 or T2 and T3 tumors theoretically has serious prognostic implications, but understaging by CT may not affect the overall prognosis: there was no difference in the 5-year survival rate between patients with clinical stage T1 disease and pathologic stage T1 disease when compared with patients with clinical stage T1 disease and pathologic stage T3 disease.[55] US is not generally used to stage RCC.

### Tumor Size

Tumor size in the TNM staging system is based on the largest dimension at pathology, but clinical staging is based on size at imaging. In general, there is good correlation between CT size and pathological size, but there are some discrepancies.[53,54] Clear cell tumors are typically smaller at pathology than at CT; this may be due to the vascular nature of CCRCC as there is no blood volume within the mass at pathology.[56]

For expected low-stage disease with small primary tumors, a normal chest radiograph will likely suffice for pulmonary staging; for larger

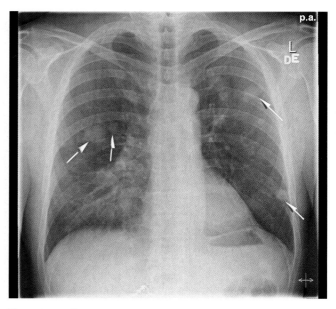

**Figure 15.** Pulmonary metastases on chest radiograph. Multiple round soft tissue masses (arrows) can be seen in this patient with stage IV renal cell carcinoma.

tumors and patients with extensive regional disease or pulmonary symptoms, chest CT is indicated (Figure 15).[57] Pelvic CT is not indicated for the initial staging evaluation of RCC.[58,59]

### Lymphadenopathy

Both CT and MR are highly sensitive for lymphadenopathy (based on 1-cm short-axis diameter), at 89 to 100%.[48,51,52] The appearance of lymph node metastases often mimics that of the primary tumor; for example, lymph node metastases from CCRCC are frequently hypervascular.

At the time of presentation, it is rare that RCC involves the adrenal gland; this is true even more so today with early detection and asymptomatic presentation.[60] Adrenal gland involvement ranges from less than 1% to up to 8% in advanced disease.[61] CT has a high negative predictive value for adrenal involvement, between 94 and 100%.[62,63] Positive predictive value of CT for adrenal involvement is low, less than 30% in some reports (Figures 16 and 17).[62,63] MR is highly sensitive for adrenal involvement and characterizing small adrenal lesions that are commonly lipid-rich adrenal adenomas (Figure 18).

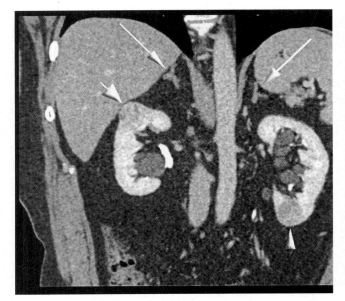

**Figure 16.** Normal adrenal gland on computed tomography. Coronal reformation demonstrating the normal appearance of the adrenal glands (long arrows) in this patient with a right upper pole renal tumor (short arrow). Direct invasion into the ipsilateral adrenal gland is uncommon, even with upper pole tumors. This patient has bilateral tumors with a left lower pole mass (arrowhead).

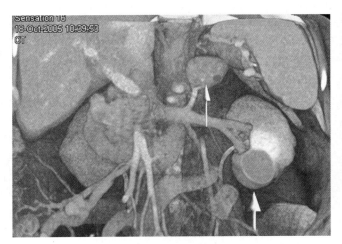

**Figure 17.** Renal cell carcinoma (RCC) and adrenal mass on a three-dimensional volume-rendered computed tomography (CT). This patient has both a lower pole left renal mass (thick arrow) and an adrenal mass (thin arrow). CT has a high specificity for adrenal disease; however, most adrenal masses are usually benign, even in patients with RCC.

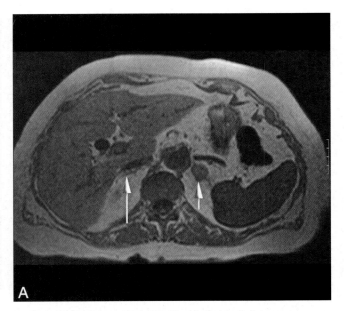

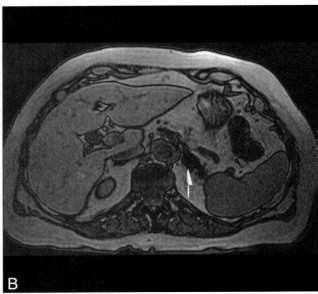

**Figure 18.** Magnetic resonance normal adrenal gland and adrenal adenoma. T1-weighted in-phase (A) and out-of-phase (B) images showing a normal right adrenal gland (long arrow) and a left adrenal adenoma (short arrow). The adrenal adenoma, because of high intracellular lipid content, drops in signal intensity between the in-phase (A) and out-of-phase (B) images as signals from lipid and water cancel.

## Renal Vein and Inferior Vena Cava Tumor

The detection of renal vein invasion or tumor thrombus and its cephalad extent into the inferior venacava (IVC) is critical for proper staging and for surgical planning in patients with RCC (Figures 19–22).[64,65] Briefly, level I tumor thrombus extends only within the renal vein, or into the renal vein and IVC within 2 cm of the renal vein ostia, level II extends within the IVC more than 2 cm from the renal vein ostia but not into the intrahepatic IVC, level III extends into the intrahepatic IVC but not above the hepatic veins, and level IV extends above the hepatic veins including into the

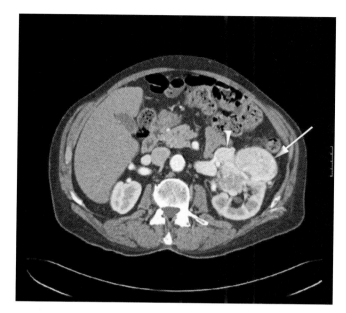

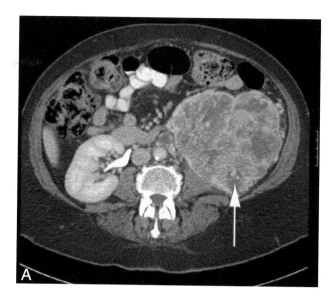

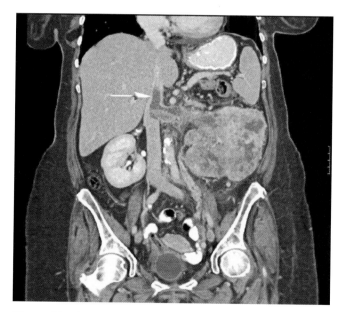

**Figure 19.** Level 1 renal vein tumor thrombus. Level 1 renal vein tumor (arrowhead) from renal cell carcinoma (arrow) either remains within the renal vein, as in this case, or extends into the inferior venacava no more than 2 cm from the renal vein ostium.

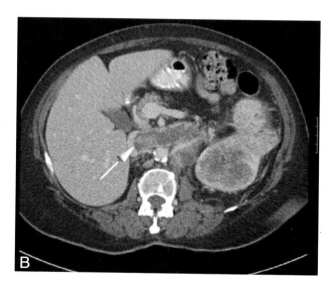

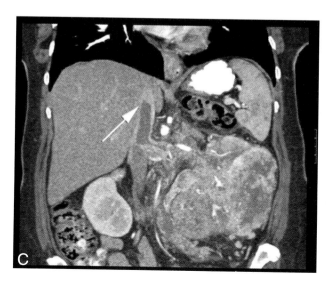

**Figure 20.** Level 2 renal vein tumor thrombus. The tumor and thrombus (arrow) extend more than 2 cm from the renal vein ostia but not within the intrahepatic inferior venacava.

right atrium.[64–66] MR and CT are both highly sensitive for renal vein involvement, with sensitivity and specificity of 85 to 100%.[67] Other methods for imaging tumor thrombus in the IVC and right atrium include transesophageal sonography and angiography.[67–71]

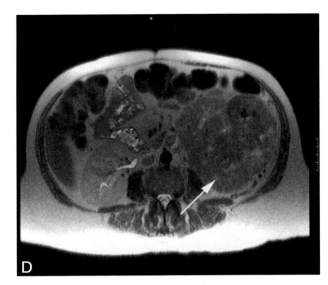

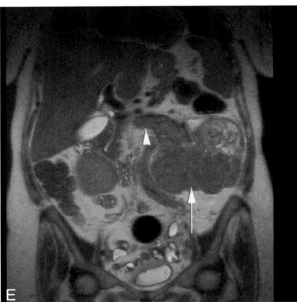

**Figure 21.** Level 3 renal vein tumor thrombus. Axial computed tomography (*CT;* A) showing the heterogeneous nature of the enhancement pattern of the tumor (arrow), axial CT image (B) with left renal vein tumor thrombus (arrow), and coronal reconstruction (C) showing level 3 tumor thrombus (arrow) into the intrahepatic inferior venacava below the hepatic veins. Axial (D) and coronal (E) T2-weighted magnetic resonance image demonstrating the mass (arrow) and vein thrombus (arrowhead).

## Metastatic Disease

Lymph nodes, lung, brain, and bone are the most common sites of metastatic disease from RCC (Figures 23–28). Other sites of metastatic disease include soft tissues, musculature, and pancreas.[72–73] Although rare, peritoneal carcinomatosis has also been reported.[74] As many as 30% of patients with RCC have metastasis at presentation.[75]

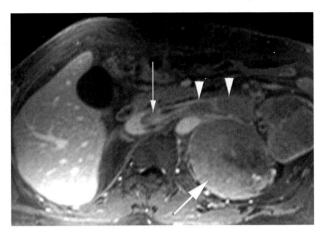

**Figure 22.** Magnetic resonance (MR) of renal vein tumor thrombus. A large renal cell carcinoma (thick arrow) replaces most of the left kidney, and tumor thrombus in the left renal vein (arrowheads) extends into the inferior venacava (thin arrow). MR is slightly more sensitive than computed tomography for renal vein tumor thrombus.

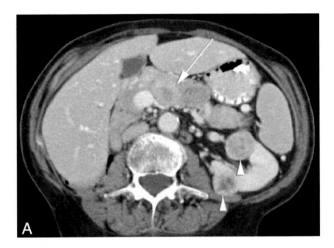

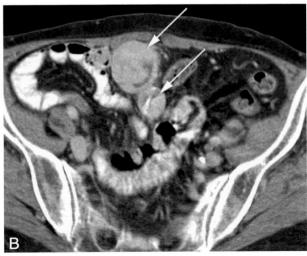

**Figure 23.** Metastatic disease from renal cell carcinoma (RCC). A 65-year-old male, status-post right nephrectomy for RCC. This patient has metastatic disease with (A) two left renal masses (arrowheads), a pancreatic mass (arrow), and (B) mesenteric masses (arrows).

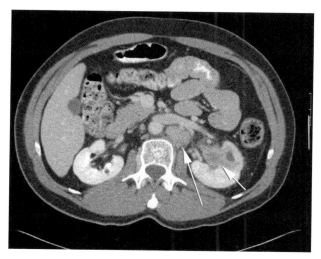

**Figure 24.** Infiltrating renal cell carcinoma with regional lymphadenopathy. Centrally located infiltrating renal tumors (short arrow) include clear cell and medullary renal cell carcinoma, transitional cell carcinoma, and lymphoma. A pathologically enlarged lymph node (long arrow) makes this a stage IIIB tumor.

## SURGICAL PLANNING

Nephron-sparing surgery (NSS) is now a highly regarded treatment option for patients with RCC and, in many instances, is preferred to radical nephrectomy.[76,77] Open extirpative NSS has proven to be a safe and effective therapy for renal neoplasms in patients with a tumor in a unilateral kidney, bilateral renal tumors, or renal insufficiency. This success has expanded the use of NSS to include small renal neoplasms.[78] Laparoscopic partial nephrectomy and ablative therapies, including laparoscopic and percutaneous cryoablation and radiofrequency ablation, are all now being used with success in selective circumstances.[79]

The goal of NSS is to maximally preserve renal function while still achieving the optimal cure or control of RCC. NSS procedures require that the surgeon have a complete understanding of the position of the tumor with respect to the normal parenchymal and vascular anatomy (Figures 29 and 30).

Three-dimensional software image processing using thin slice images from multidetector helical CT acquisitions or state-of-the-art MR sequences can provide anatomic definition to facilitate surgical decision making when considering NSS. Information that was not previously considered when interpreting CT and MR a decade ago is now routinely

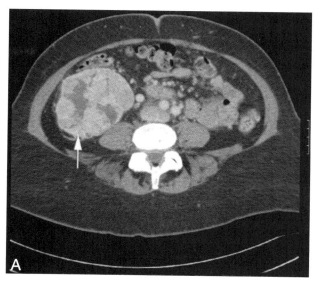

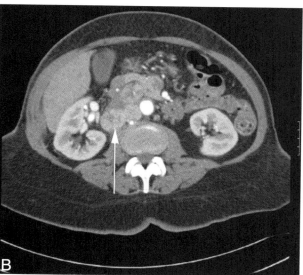

**Figure 25.** Renal cell carcinoma with lymphadenopathy. Axial computed tomography (CT) images show a (A) large right renal mass (arrow) and (B) retroperitoneal lymphadenopathy (arrow). The CT appearance of metastatic lymphadenopathy often mirrors that of the primary tumor.

available, such as the arterial and venous anatomy, the tumor position, and depth of extension into the parenchyma or into the central renal sinus. The proximity of the tumor to the vascular structures and the pelvocalyceal system, and the number and course of the arteries, veins, and ureters can also be delineated by CT and MR (Figures 31–35).[80–82] Accurate surgical planning information helps to minimize postoperative complications such as urinary leak or renal infarct and, again, helps to maximize preserved renal function.

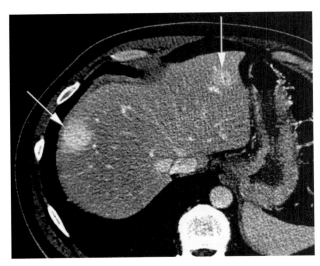

**Figure 26.** Hepatic metastatic disease from renal cell carcinoma (RCC). Two hypervascular lesions from metastatic RCC (arrows) are seen in the liver; the liver attenuation is lower than normal from fatty infiltration.

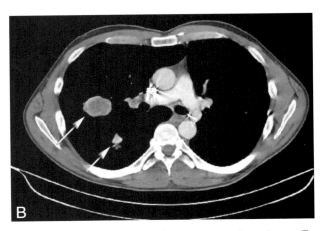

**Figure 28.** Pulmonary metastasis from renal cell carcinoma. Two pulmonary metastases are seen in the right lower lobe (arrows) on (A) wide (lung) and (B) soft-tissue windows. Multiple pulmonary masses are common in patients with late-stage disease.

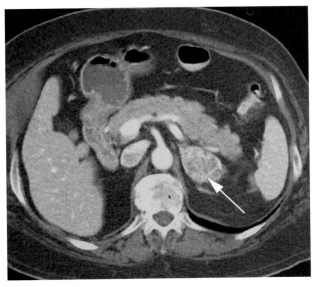

**Figure 27.** Adrenal metastasis from renal cell carcinoma. Axial computed tomography image shows a heterogeneously enhancing left adrenal metastasis (arrow). Adrenal metastases are uncommon at presentation but often resemble the primary tumor.

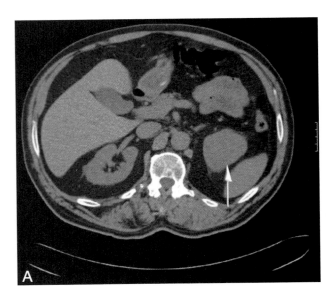

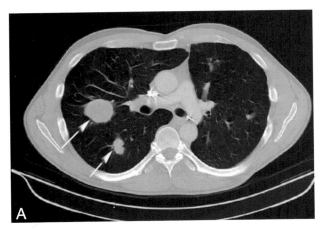

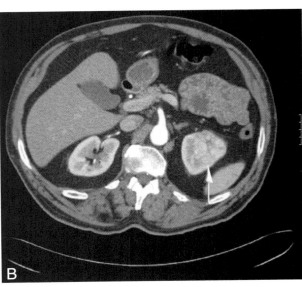

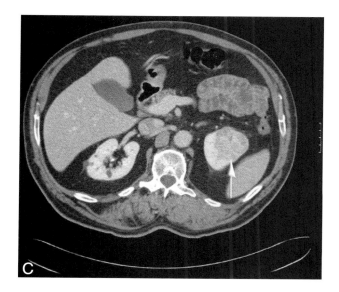

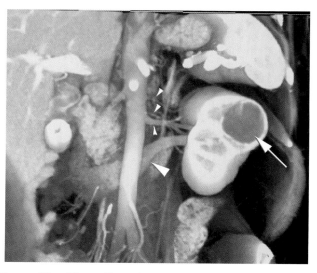

**Figure 30.** Three-dimensional volume-rendered computed tomography of tumor position. Volume-rendered image showing a cystic renal cell carcinoma in the anterior midkidney (arrow). Three left renal arteries (small arrowheads) and a retroaortic left renal vein (large arrowhead) are identified. Renal venous anomalies are common, and retroaortic left renal veins (arrowhead) occur in 5 to 10% of patients. Although venous anomalies do not directly affect outcome, it is important for the surgeon to be aware of these variants in order to control the renal blood supply during surgery.

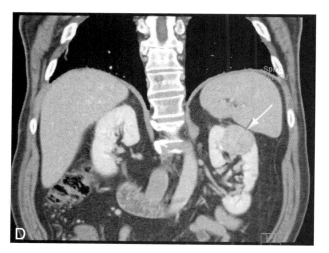

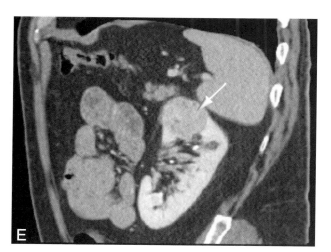

**Figure 29.** Multiplanar reconstructions for surgical planning. Unenhanced (A), corticomedullary phase (B), and nephrographic phase (C) axial images can be used to characterize this lesion (arrow) as a solid enhancing mass. The addition of (D) coronal and (E) sagittal images reconstructed from thin slice (0.75 or 1.0 mm) axial images localizes the tumor (arrow) to the apical, anterolateral portion of the kidney for the urologist.

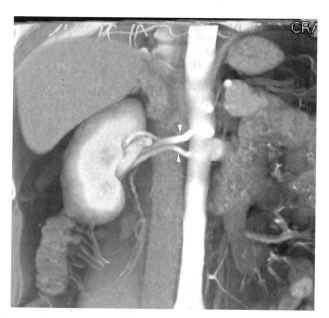

**Figure 31.** Three-dimensional volume-rendered computed tomography showing multiple renal arteries. Two right renal arteries (arrowheads) arise from the aorta approximately 1 cm apart from each other. The arteries are roughly the same size.

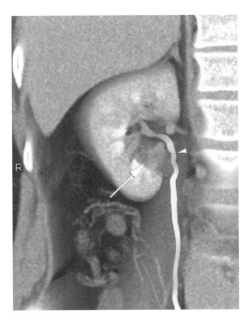

**Figure 32.**    Hilar renal cell carcinoma. This hilar tumor (arrow) demonstrates mass effect on the proximal ureter (arrowhead); there was no invasion of the ureter at surgery.

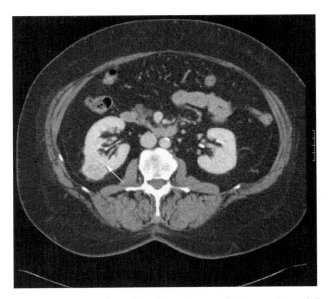

**Figure 33.**    Exophytic peripheral renal mass. This mass is partially exophytic, and the most intrarenal margin (arrow) does not extend to the central sinus fat.

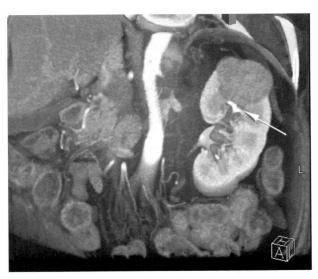

**Figure 34.**    Three-dimensional volume rendering of renal tumor displacing the renal collecting system. The left upper pole tumor can be seen abutting and distorting the upper pole calices (arrow).

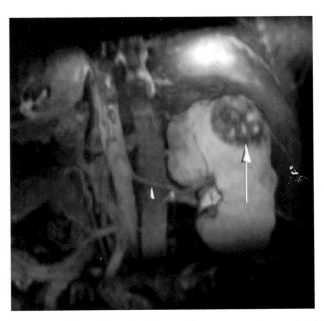

**Figure 35.**    Three-dimensional magnetic resonance image of right renal mass. Three-dimensional volume-rendered image from a posterior projection shows a complex mass in the posterior upper pole of the right kidney (arrow). The retrocaval course of the single right renal artery is also seen (arrowhead).

## SUMMARY

Most RCC are now found incidentally, as part of an exam performed for other abdominal complaints. CT and MR are critical in the diagnosis, evaluation, and management of patients with RCC. Some imaging features suggest histologic subtypes. Imaging is highly accurate for staging.

## REFERENCES

1.  Kopka L, Fischer U, Zoeller G, et al. Dual-phase helical CT of the kidney: value of thecorticomedullary and nephrographic phase for evaluation of renal lesions and preoperative staging of renal cell carcinoma. AJR Am J Roentgenol 1997;169:1573–8.
2.  Kauczor HU, Schwickert HC, Schweden F, et al. Bolus-enhanced renal spiral CT: techniques, diagnostic value and drawbacks. Eur J Radiol 1994;18:153–7.

3. Garant M, Bonaldi VM, Taourel P, et al. Enhancement patterns of renal masses during multiphase helical CT acquisitions. Abdom Imaging 1998;23:431–6.

4. Cohan RH, Sherman LS, Korobkin M, et al. Renal masses: assessment of corticomedullary-phase and nephrographic-phase CT scans. Radiology 1995;196:445–51.

5. Birnbaum BA, Jacobs JE, Ramchandani P. Multiphasic renal CT: comparison of renal mass enhancement during the corticomedullary and nephrographic phases. Radiology 1996;200:753–8.

6. Szolar DH, Kammerhuber F, Altziebler S, et al. Multiphasic helical CT of the kidney: increased conspicuity for detection and characterization of small (< 3-cm) renal masses. Radiology 1997;202:211–7.

7. Herts BR, Coll DM, Lieber ML, et al. Triphasic helical CT of the kidneys: contribution of vascular phase scanning in patients before urologic surgery. AJR Am J Roentgenol1999;1273–7.

8. Herts BR, Einstein DM, Paushter DM. Spiral CT of the abdomen: artifacts and potential pitfalls. AJR Am J Roentgenol 1993;161:1185–90.

9. Rofsky NM, Weinreb JC, Bosniak MA, et al. Renal lesion characterization with gadolinium-enhanced MR imaging: efficacy and safety in patients with renal insufficiency. Radiology 1991;180:85–9.

10. Broome DR, Girguis MS, Baron PW, et al. Gadodiamide-associated nephrogenic systemic fibrosis: why radiologists should be concerned. AJR Am J Roentgenol 2007;188:1–7.

11. Kramer LA. Magnetic resonance imaging of renal masses. World J Urol 1998;16:22–8.

12. Narumi Y, Hricak H, Presti JC Jr, et al. MR imaging of renal cell carcinoma. Abdom Imaging 1997;22:216–25.

13. Walter C, Kruessell M, Gindele A, et al. Imaging of renal lesions: evaluation of fast MRI and helical CT. Br J Radiol 2003;76:696–703.

14. Semelka RC, Shoenut JP, Magro CM, et al. Renal cancer staging: comparison of contrast-enhanced CT and gadolinium-enhanced fat-suppressed spin-echo and gradient-echo MR imaging. J Magn Reson Imaging 1993;3:597–602.

15. Hallscheidt PJ, Bock M, Riedasch G, et al. Diagnostic accuracy of staging renal cell carcinoma using multidetector-row computed tomography and magnetic resonance imaging. J Comput Assist Tomogr 2004;28:333–9.

16. Pretorius ES, Wickstrom L, Siegelman ES. MR imaging of renal neoplasms. Magn Reson Imaging Clin N Am 2000;8:813–36.

17. Hecht EM, Israel GM, Krinsky GA, et al. Renal masses: quantitative analysis of enhancement with signal intensity measurements versus qualitative analysis of enhancement with image subtraction for diagnosing malignancy at MR imaging. Radiology 2004;232:373–8.

18. Ho VB, Allen SF, Hood MN, et al. Renal masses: quantitative assessment of enhancement with dynamic MR imaging. Radiology 2002;224:695–700.

19. Ho VB, Choyke PL. MR evaluation of solid renal masses. Magn Reson Imaging Clin N Am 2004;12:413–27.

20. Helenon O, Correas JM, Balleyquier C, et al. Ultrasound of renal tumors. Eur Radiol 2001;11:1890–901.

21. Tosaka A, Ohya K, Yamada K, et al. Incidence and properties of renal masses and asymptomatic renal cell carcinoma detected by abdominal ultrasonography. J Urol 1990; 144:1097–9.

22. Park BK, Kim SH, Choi HJ. Characterization of renal cell carcinoma using agent detection imaging: comparison with gray-scale ultrasound. Korean J Radiol 2005;6:173–8.

23. Weiss LM, Gelb AB, Medeiros LJ. Adult renal epithelial neoplasms. Am J Clin Pathol 1995;103:624–35.

24. Bostwick DG, Eble JN. Diagnosis and classification of renal cell carcinoma. Urol Clin North Am 1999;26:627–35.

25. Zisman A, Chao DH, Pantuck AJ, et al. Unclassified renal cell carcinoma: clinical features and prognostic impact of a new histological subtype. J Urol 2002;168:950–5.

26. Jinzaki M, Tanimoto A, Mukai M, et al. Double-phase helical CT of small renal parenchymal neoplasms: correlation with pathological findings and tumor angiogenesis. J Comput Assist Tomogr 2000;24:835–42.

27. Herts BR, Coll DM, Novick AC, et al. Enhancement characteristics of papillary renal neoplasms revealed on triphasic helical CT of the kidneys. AJR Am J Roentgenol 2002;178:367–72.

28. Bosniak MA. The current radiological approach to renal cysts. Radiology 1986;158:1–10.

29. Bosniak MA. Difficulties in classifying cystic lesions of the kidney. Urol Radiol 1991;13:91–3.

30. Israel GM, Hindman N, Bosniak MA. Evaluation of cystic renal masses: comparison of CT and MR using the Bosniak classification system. Radiology 2004;231:365–71.

31. Shinmoto H, Yuasa Y, Tanimoto A, et al. Small renal cell carcinoma: MRI with pathological correlation. J Magn Reson Imaging 1998;8:690–4.

32. Uzzo RG, Cherullo EE, Myles J, et al. Renal cell carcinoma invading the urinary collecting system: implications for staging. J Urol 2002;167:2392–6.

33. Delahunt B, Eble JN. Papillary renal cell carcinoma: a clinopathologic and immunohistochemical study of 105 cases. Mod Pathol 1997;10:537–44.

34. Lager DJ, Huston BJ, Timmerman TG, Bonsib SM. Papillary renal tumors. Cancer 1995;76:669.

35. Onishi T, Ohishi Y, Goto H, et al. Papillary renal cell carcinoma: clinicopathological characteristics and evaluation of prognosis in 42 patients. BJU Int 1999; 83:937–43.

36. Ruppert-Kohlmayr AJ, Uggowitzer M, Meissnitzer T, et al. Differentiation of renal clear cell carcinoma and renal papillary carcinoma using quantitative CT enhancement parameters. AJR Am J Roentgenol 2004;183:1387–91.

37. Megumi Y, Nishimura K. Chromophobe renal cell carcinoma. Urol Int 1998;61:172–4.

38. Srigley JR, Eble JN. Collecting duct carcinoma of kidney. Semin Diagn Pathol 1998;15:54–67.

39. Fukuya T, Honda H, Goto K, et al. Computed tomographic findings of Bellini duct carcinoma of the kidney. J Comput Assist Tomogr 1996;20:399–403.

40. Gurocak S, Sozens, Akyurek N, et al. Cortically located collecting duct carcinoma. Urology 2005;65:1226.

41. Pickhardt PJ, Siegel CL, McLarney JK. Collecting duct carcinoma of the kidney: are imaging findings suggestive of the diagnosis? AJR Am J Roentgenol 2001;176:627–33.

42. Pickhardt PJ. Collecting duct carcinoma arising in a solitary kidney: imaging findings. Clin Imaging 1999; 23:115–8.

43. Mian BM, Bhadkamkar NJ, Slaton JW, et al. Prognostic factors and survival of patients with sarcomatoid renal cell carcinoma. Urology 2002;167:65–70.

44. Staelens L, Van Poppel H, Vanuytsel L, et al. Sarcomatoid renal cell carcinoma: case report and review of the literature. Acta Urol Belg 1997;65:39–42.

45. Davidson AJ, Hayes WJ, Hartman DS, et al. Renal oncocytoma and carcinoma: failure of differentiation with CT. Radiology 1993;186:693–6.

46. Wiatrowska BA, Zakowski MF. Fine-needle aspiration biopsy of chromophobe renal cell carcinoma and oncocytoma: comparison of cytomorphologic features. Cancer 1999;87:161–7.

47. Liu J, Fanning CV. Can renal oncocytomas be distinguished from renal cell carcinoma on fine-needle aspiration specimens? A study of conventional smears in conjunction with ancillary studies. Cancer 2001;93:390–7.

48. Javidan J, Strciker HJ, Tamboli P, et al. Prognostic significance of the 1997 TNM classification of renal cell carcinoma. J Urol 2000;162:1277–81.

49. Dinney CP, Awad SA, Gajewski J, et al. Analysis of imaging modalities, staging systems, and prognostic indicators for renal cell carcinoma. Urology 1992;39:122–9.

50. Constantinides C, Recker F, Bruehlmann W, et al. Accuracy of magnetic resonance imaging compared to computerized tomography and selective renal angiography in preoperatively staging renal cell carcinoma. Urol Int 1991;47:181–5.

51. Bechtold RE, Zagoria RJ. Imaging approach to staging of renal cell carcinoma. Urol Clin North Am 1997;24:507–22.

52. Johnson CD, Dunnick NR, Cohan RH, et al. Renal adenocarcinoma: CT staging of 100 tumors. AJR Am J Roentgenol 1987;148:59–63.

53. Cronan JJ, Zeman RK, Rosenfeld AT. Comparison of computerized tomography, ultrasound and angiography in staging renal cell carcinoma. J Urol 1982;127:712–4.

54. Prati GF, Saggin P, Boschiero L, et al. Small renal-cell carcinomas: clinical and imaging features. Urol Int 1993;51:19–22.

55. Roberts WW, Bhayani J, Allaf ME, et al. Pathological stage does not alter the prognosis for renal lesions determined to be stage T1 by computerized tomography. Urology 2005; 173:713–5.

56. Herr HW, Lee CT, Sharma S, et al. Radiographic versus pathologic size of renal tumors: implications for partial nephrectomy. Urology 2001;58:157–60.

57. Lim DJ, Carter F. Computerized tomography in the preoperative staging for pulmonary metastases in patients with renal cell carcinoma. J Urol 1993;150:1112–4.

58. Khaitan A, Gupta NP, Hemal AK, et al. Is there a need for pelvic CT scan in cases of renal cell carcinoma? Int Urol Nephrol 2002;33:13–5.

59. Fielding JR, Aliabadi N, Renshaw AA, et al. Staging of 119 patients with renal cell carcinoma: the yield and cost-effectiveness of pelvic CT. AJR Am J Roentgenol 1999; 172:1721–3.

60. Tsui KH, Shvarts O, Smith RB, et al. Renal cell carcinoma: prognostic significance of incidentally detected tumors. J Urol 2000;163:426–30.

61. Tsui KH, Shvarts O, Barbaric Z, et al. Is adrenalectomy a necessary component of radical nephrectomy? UCLA experience with 511 radical nephrectomies. J Urol 2000; 163:437–41.

62. Sawai Y, Kinochi T, Mano M, et al. Ipsilateral adrenal involvement from renal cell carcinoma: retrospective study of the predictive value of computed tomography. Urology 2002; 59:28–31.

63. Gill IS, McClennan BL, Kerbi K, et al. Adrenal involvement from renal cell carcinoma: predictive value of computerized tomography. J Urol 1994;154:1082–5.

64. Hatcher PA, Anderson EE, Paulson DF, et al. Surgical management and prognosis of renal cell carcinoma invading the vena cava. J Urol 1991;145:20–24.

65. Oto A, Herts BR, Remer EM, Novick AC. Inferior vena cava tumor thrombus in renal cell carcinoma: staging by MR imaging and impact on surgical treatment. AJR Am J Roentgenol 1998;171:1619–24.

66. Gupta NP, Ansari MD, Khaitan A, et al. Impact of imaging and thrombus level in management of renal cell carcinoma extending to veins. Urol Int 2004;72:129–34.

67. Glazer A, Novick AC. Preoperative transesophageal echocardiography for assessment of venal caval tumor thrombi: a comparative study with venacavography and magnetic resonance imaging. Urology 1997; 49:32–4.

68. Lawrentschuk N, Gani J, Riordan R, et al. Multidetector computed tomography vs. magnetic resonance imaging for defining the upper limit of tumour thrombus in renal cell carcinoma: a study and review. BJU Int 2005; 96:291–5.

69. Kallman DA, King BF, Hattery RR, et al. Renal vein and inferior vena cava tumor thrombus in renal cell carcinoma: CT, US, MRI and venacavography. J Comput Assist Tomogr 1992;16:240–7.

70. Goldfarb DA, Novick AC, Lorig R, et al. Magnetic resonance imaging for assessment of vena cava tumor thrombi: a comparative study with venacavography and computerized tomography scanning. J Urol 1990;144:1100–3.

71. Hockley NM, Foster RS, Bihrle R, et al. Use of magnetic resonance imaging to determine surgical approach to renal cell carcinoma with vena caval extension. Urology 1990; 36:55–60.

72. Ng CS, Loyer EM, Iyer RB, et al. Metastases to the pancreas from renal cell carcinoma: findings on three-phase contrast-enhanced helical CT. AJR Am J Roentgenol 1999; 172:1555–9.

73. Ghavamian R, Klein KA, Stephens DH, et al. Renal cell carcinoma metastatic to the pancreas: clinical and radiographic features. Mayo Clin Proc 2000; 75:581–5.

74. Tartar VM, Heiken JP, McClennan BL. Renal cell carcinoma presenting with diffuse peritoneal metastases: CT findings. J Comput Assist Tomogr 1991;15:450–3.

75. Motzer RJ, Bander NH, Nanus DM. Medical progress: renal cell carcinoma. N Engl J Med 1996;335:865.

76. Novick AC. Current surgical approaches, nephron-sparing surgery, and the role of surgery in the integrated immunologic approach to renal-cell carcinoma. Semin Oncol 1995;22:29–33.

77. Novick AC. Nephron-sparing surgery for renal cell carcinoma. Annu Rev Med 2002;53:393–407.

78. Butler BP, Novick AC, Miller DP, et al. Management of small unilateral renal cell carcinomas: radical versus nephron-sparing surgery. Urology 1995;45:34–40; discussion 40–1.

79. Wood BJ, Ramkaransingh JR, Fojo T, et al. Percutaneous tumor ablation with radiofrequency. Cancer 2002;94:443–51.

80. Coll DM, Uzzo RG, Herts BR, et al. 3-dimensional volume rendered computerized tomography for preoperative evaluation and intraoperative treatment of patients undergoing nephron sparing surgery. J Urol 1999; 161:1097–102.

81. Coll DM, Herts BR, Davros WJ, et al. Preoperative use of 3D volume rendering to demonstrate renal tumors and renal anatomy. Radiographics 2000;20:431–8.

82. Wunderlich H, Reichelt O, Schubert R, et al. Preoperative simulation of partial nephrectomy with three-dimensional computed tomography. BJU Int 2000;86:777–81.

# Management of Small Renal Masses

## Active Surveillance of Sporadic Renal Masses

DAVID Y.T. CHEN, MD
YU-NING WONG, MD, MSCE
ROBERT G. UZZO, MD, FACS

The treatment of renal cell carcinoma (RCC) continues to evolve. A major impetus for this evolution has been the increasing incidence of asymptomatic small renal masses (SRMs) found during evaluation of unrelated abdominal complaints. This has led to a more than two-fold increase in the age-adjusted incidence of localized RCC from 1975 to 1995.[1,2] Physicians are now often evaluating asymptomatic patients with presumptively malignant renal masses whose natural history has not been well defined.

Surgical excision remains the gold standard management of RCC.[3–5] However, some patients may be poor surgical candidates due to their age and/or significant comorbid conditions. In these patients, the risks associated with treatment may be greater than the risk of disease progression during active surveillance. Moreover, longevity in the elderly may be affected more by existing medical problems than impacted by an incidentally detected RCC. Despite this, there remains a strong bias to treat all SRMs because the long-term outcome of untreated localized RCC remains unknown and systemic therapies for metastatic RCC (mRCC) have limited efficacy.

Although the outcomes of *treated* RCC have been well established for both localized and mRCC,[6–7] the behavior of *untreated* renal lesions has only recently been examined. Initial results suggest that many SRMs do not demonstrate uniformly aggressive or malignant behavior. Here we review the data on the epidemiology and pathology of the SRM. We then examine the role of renal mass biopsy; discuss indications and outcomes for active surveillance and more recent information regarding growth kinetics, rates, and predictors of cancer progression during active surveillance; and competing causes of death. Last, we describe delayed management strategies and the existing data comparing excision, ablation, and surveillance of the SRM.

## EPIDEMIOLOGY AND PATHOLOGY OF THE SRM

The rising incidence of kidney cancer over the past three decades is primarily due to an increase in the number of SRMs.[1,2,8] Despite the lead-time and length-time biases associated with earlier RCC detection, cancer-specific death rates have not changed

This publication was supported in part by grant #P30 CA006927. Additional funds were provided by Fox Chase Cancer Center via institutional support of the Kidney Cancer Keystone Program.

appreciably.[1,2,8] Hollingsworth and colleagues[8] have noted that despite a rise in RCC incidence and an associated increase in SRM treatment, an unexpected upward trend in kidney cancer-specific and overall mortality rates has occurred. This treatment disconnect of generally earlier RCC detection with increased numbers of patients treated yet paradoxically higher kidney cancer–specific death rates suggests that incidentally detected SRMs may not all be life limiting or clinically meaningful, and a proportion might be unnecessarily treated. These observations raise several important questions, including whether some kidney cancers are intrinsically indolent and do not require treatment, and if so, can these cases be recognized and unneeded intervention avoided.

Clinicians have historically regarded all enhancing renal masses as RCC until proven otherwise. This assumes that all SRMs are equally malignant and require prompt intervention. Unfortunately, this practice results in unnecessary intervention for nearly 20% of individuals in whom a benign lesion is found. Frank and colleagues[9] recognized the relationship between tumor size and frequency of RCC. In their review of 2,935 solid renal tumors, malignant pathology was identified in 87.2% of all cases. The likelihood of a renal lesion being benign was related to its size at presentation (6.3% for tumors $\geq 7$ cm, 21% for tumors 2 to 4 cm, and 30% of tumors < 2 cm.) In their series, the odds for finding cancer increased by 17%, with each 1-cm increase in tumor diameter.[9]

The likelihood of an SRM being benign has also been correlated to age and gender. Renal masses in young women (< 45 years) are more often benign (36 to 41%), whereas only 10 to 20% are benign in similarly aged men.[10,11] For renal masses $\leq 7$ cm, the relative risk (RR) of identifying a benign lesion is 1.8 times more likely in women than in men.[12] More recent data in patients with a $\leq$ 7-cm renal mass also suggest the chance of benign pathology is higher not only in younger women but also in older men (> 75 years).[13]

Even though the majority of SRM may be confirmed as RCC, initial data from the active surveillance literature suggest a heterogeneous biologic behavior. In general, most are indolent lesions that lack a highly aggressive or malignant phenotype.[14] This finding is consistent with a recent analysis of a cohort of clinical T1 tumors, where less than 30% of RCC showed pathologic grade or stage suggestive of potentially aggressive behavior.[13]

## BIOPSY OF THE SRM

Enhancing renal lesions are generally not biopsied, with the diagnosis of RCC confirmed only after surgery. In comparison with other solid malignancies, renal mass biopsy has not been used because of concerns regarding its accuracy and reliability, its risks, and its expected negligible impact on management. Because most enhancing renal masses are RCC, urologists have erred on the side of possible overtreatment for nonmalignant lesions. At present, even the current 2007 National Comprehensive Cancer Network Clinical Practice Guidelines for Kidney Cancer considers renal mass biopsy a nonessential option in the workup of RCC.[15] The main hesitation for routine renal mass biopsy relates to its historic rate of failure and the possibility of an indeterminate or false-negative diagnosis. There is a wide range in the reported accuracy of biopsy outcomes (Table 1). Variability in results has been attributed to differences in mass size and location, the type of imaging used for targeting, the number of biopsies obtained, and the manner of pathologic assessment. In a recent review, renal mass biopsy was found to be accurate in approximately 87% of tumors examined (range 40 to 100%), inadequate in roughly 7% (range 0 to 22%), indeterminate in 8% (range 0 to 36%), false negative in 4% (range 0 to 24%), and false positive in 1% (range 0 to 3%).[16]

The risks of biopsy include hemorrhage, pneumothorax, pseudoaneurysm formation, renal parenchymal injury/kidney loss, and the possibility of tumor seeding. Although with greater tissue sampling, the potential of these complications may increase, the rate of complications from contemporary renal biopsy is low (< 5%),[16] with kidney loss exceedingly rare and mortality not reported.[17,18] Hemorrhage is the most frequent adverse event, with subclinical bleeding commonly identified if routine postbiopsy imaging is performed.[19] However, hemorrhage requiring blood transfusion is infrequent. Although biopsy using smaller

| Table 1.  RESULTS OF MAJOR BIOPSY SERIES (1974–2000) | | | | | | | |
|---|---|---|---|---|---|---|---|
| Reference | Year | No. | No. Inadequate Biopsy (%) | No. Indeterminate Path (%) | No. False Negative (%) | No. False Positive (%) | Accuracy of Diagnosis* (%) |
| Kristensen | 1974 | 34 | 1 (3%) | 4 (12%) | 1 (3%) | 0 (0%) | 28/33 (85%) |
| Karp | 1979 | 23 | 5 (22%) | 1 (6%) | 1 (6%) | 0 (0%) | 16/18 (89%) |
| Murphy | 1984 | 56 | 6 (11%) | 7 (14%) | 1 (2%) | 1 (2%) | 41/50 (82%) |
| Juul | 1985 | 301 | 16 (5%) | 0 (0%) | 25 (9%) | 0 (0%) | 260/285 (91%) |
| Orell | 1985 | 83 | 7 (8%) | 0 (0%) | 0 (0%) | 1 (3%) | 75/76 (99%) |
| Nadel | 1986 | 30 | 0 (0%) | 0 (0%) | 1 (3%) | 0 (0%) | 29/30 (97%) |
| Pilotti | 1988 | 132 | 8 (6%) | 0 (0%) | 0 (0%) | 1 (1%) | 123/124 (99%) |
| Leiman | 1990 | 120 | 26 (22%) | 0 (0%) | 0 (0%) | 2 (2%) | 92/94 (98%) |
| Haubek | 1991 | 169 | 8 (5%) | 0 (0%) | 17 (11%) | 4 (3%) | 137/161 (87%) |
| Cristallani | 1991 | 79 | 7 (9%) | 0 (0%) | 4 (6%) | 1 (1%) | 67/72 (93%) |
| Mondal | 1992 | 92 | 0 (0%) | 4 (4%) | 0 (0%) | 2 (2%) | 86/92 (93%) |
| Niceforo | 1993 | 23 | 0 (0%) | 0 (0%) | 3 (13%) | 0 (0%) | 20/23 (87%) |
| Kelley | 1996 | 43 | 1 (2%) | 6 (14%) | 0 (0%) | 1 (2%) | 35/42 (83%) |
| Campbell | 1997 | 25 | 0 (0%) | 9 (36%) | 6 (24%) | 0 (0%) | 10/25 (40%) |
| Truong | 1999 | 108 | 17 (16%) | 11 (12%) | 1 (1%) | 0 (0%) | 79/91 (87%) |
| Wood | 1999 | 79 | 5 (6%) | 0 (0%) | 0 (0%) | 0 (0%) | 74/74 (100%) |
| Richter | 2000 | 517 | 21 (4%) | 103 (20%) | 6 (1%) | 1 (0%) | 386/496 (78%) |
| Brierly | 2000 | 49 | 8 (16%) | 7 (14%) | 7 (14%) | 1 (2%) | 26/41 (63%) |
| Lechevalier | 2000 | 73 | 15 (21%) | 2 (3%) | 0 (0%) | 0 (0%) | 56/58 (97%) |
| *Total* | | *2036* | *151 (7%)* | *154 (8%)* | *73 (4%)* | *15 (1%)* | *1640/1885 (87%)* |

[16]Adapted From Lane.

*Accuracy of diagnosis = true diagnosis of total biopsies having adequate tissue for assessment.

(> 18-gauge) needles is thought to carry a lower risk of complications, no studies have compared outcomes with different-size needles. Because insufficient tissue yield or indeterminate findings are more likely when using smaller needles for primarily cytologic assessment,[20,21] more recent studies recommend use of the 18-gauge, spring-loaded, automatic biopsy guns and show equally low complication rates obtaining core biopsies through an introducer needle in a coaxial fashion.[17,18] The risk of pneumothorax relates to the location of needle passage, with a posterior and intercostal approach to access the upper pole carrying the greatest risk (14 to 29%) for pleural injury[22]; clinically significant pneumothorax is uncommon. Pseudoaneurysm formation is also rare, typically asymptomatic and therefore likely underdiagnosed.[23,24] When indicated, treatment of pseudoaneurysm is often successful via endovascular angioembolization.[25]

Although tumor seeding via the needle tract has always been a concern, the risk is no greater for RCC than for other malignancies (< 0.01%); with only eight cases identified in the literature, and none since 1994.[16]

Several points have been recommended to optimize renal mass biopsy:

- The mass should be sampled from at least two areas, avoiding obvious necrotic regions. Additional passes show similar risks of complication as a single biopsy attempt.[26]
- Automatic core biopsy needles of 18-gauge allow more reliable tissue retrieval with equal risk as smaller gauge needles.[17,20,21]
- Needle guidance by ultrasound, computed tomography, or magnetic resonance imaging is equally effective. No single modality is universally superior for targeting.[21,27]

- Predominantly cystic lesions have a higher chance of sampling error, tumor spillage, and/or seeding, and biopsy is less advisable.[28]
- Infiltrative lesions that are atypical for RCC and may represent an upper tract urothelial cancer, or sarcoma may have a higher risk for needle tract seeding.

Modern renal mass biopsy results show improved diagnostic accuracy, with sensitivity and accuracy > 95%, (Table 2), and can also provide prognostic information such as RCC subtype and Fuhrman grade. Improved accuracy has occurred in part from the application of newer immunohisto-chemical and molecular methods of tissue analy-sis.[29-32] Therefore, refinements in biopsy technique and tissue assessment are likely to further improve the accuracy of renal mass biopsy in the future.

Renal mass biopsy is currently indicated for select clinical scenarios such as suspected renal metastasis, renal lymphoma, or renal abscess. Additionally, patients with mRCC that is surgically unresectable or patients who are poor operative candidates for cytoreductive nephrectomy may ben-efit from pathologic information obtained by biopsy. The identification of RCC variant type and other molecular features may guide modern targeted sys-temic treatments and provide important prognostic information.[33,34]

## INDICATIONS FOR SURVEILLANCE OF THE SRM

It is helpful to consider indications for surveillance of the SRM as absolute, relative, or elective. An *absolute* indication describes patients in whom surgery is contraindicated due to severe medical comorbidities as treatment that is anticipated to carry excessive risk is not acceptable to most patients or physicians. In the reported active surveil-lance literature, "significant" comorbidity appears to be the primary indication in 36 to 66% of patients.[35,36] Medical comorbidities and competing health risks are major concerns when considering a patient for intervention. Unfortunately, these com-peting health risks may be difficult to measure and are often poorly quantified. For patients with chronic significant disease states that are unlikely to improve, the indication for observation may appear absolute, but given our ability to manage highly complex medical conditions, patients with a true absolute indication for observation are rare.

*Relative* indications for active surveillance include the presence of concomitant but less severe disease states.[37] These conditions include incurable but treatable illnesses such as renal, pulmonary, or cardiac disease, or other concurrent malignancy. The degree of medical comorbidity in patients can be challenging to quantify, and it is often helpful to

### Table 2. RESULTS OF MODERN RENAL MASS BIOPSY (2001 TO PRESENT)

| Reference | Year | No. | No. Inadequate Biopsy (%) | No. Indeterminate Path (%) | No. False Negative (%) | No. False Positive (%) | Accuracy of Diagnosis* (%) |
|-----------|------|-----|----------------------------|-----------------------------|-------------------------|-------------------------|-----------------------------|
| Johnson | 2001 | 44 | 8 (18%) | 0 (0%) | 0 (0%) | 0 (0%) | 36/36 (100%) |
| Hara | 2001 | 33 | 0 (0%) | 0 (0%) | 0 (0%) | 0 (0%) | 33/33 (100%) |
| Caoili | 2002 | 26 | 0 (0%) | 0 (0%) | 0 (0%) | 0 (0%) | 26/26 (100%) |
| Neuzillet | 2004 | 88 | 3 (3%) | 5 (6%) | 0 (0%) | 0 (0%) | 80/85 (94%) |
| Eshed | 2004 | 23 | 1 (4%) | 0 (0%) | 1 (4%) | 0 (0%) | 21/22 (95%) |
| Volpe | 2006 | 49 | 4 (8%) | 0 (0%) | 0 (0%) | 0 (0%) | 45/45 (100%) |
| Barocas | 2006 | 77 | 3 (4%) | 4 (5%) | 0 (0%) | 0 (0%) | 70/74 (95%) |
| Maturan | 2007 | 152 | 0 (0%) | 6 (4%) | 0 (0%) | 0 (0%) | 146/156 (96%) |
| Beland | 2007 | 58 | 3 (5%) | 3 (5%) | 1 (1.7%) | 0 (0%) | 51/55 (93%) |
| *Total* | | 550 | 22 (4%) | 18 (3%) | 2 (0%) | 0 (0%) | 508/532 (95%) |

[16]Adapted From Lane.

*Accuracy of diagnosis = true diagnosis of total biopsies having adequate tissue for assessment.

solicit other medical opinions regarding the severity of these competing risks. Too often the decision to treat an SRM becomes a function of "can we intervene" instead of "should we intervene."

Last, some patients despite having low operative risks may choose to pursue observation out of personal preference. In these *elective* circumstances, the treating physician is obligated to inform the patient of the limited data on the natural history of untreated SRM, the uncertainty in estimating future tumor growth, and the potential for disease progression from untreated RCC. No matter what the indication is for observation, it must be understood that the patient and physician both accept a degree of risk due to the heterogeneous and unpredictable behavior of RCC. In all cases, the primary goal is to balance the risks of treatment and risks of surveillance.

## THE SURVEILLANCE LITERATURE

Initial reports on surveillance were first published in 1995. In total, the outcomes are described for fewer than 400 tumors from 11 documented single-institutional series.[14,35,36,38–47] The majority of these cases were recently reviewed in a meta-analysis that noted similar results between series.[14]

Most untreated SRMs show a slow consistent growth rate, with a mean increase in diameter of 0.35 cm/yr (range 0.1 to 0.7 cm/yr). The incidence of subsequent metastases during surveillance has been a rare event ($\leq 1\%$).[14] With a mean follow-up of nearly 3 years, most patients showed tumor growth, but also avoided treatment and remained without symptoms or evidence of cancer progression. Ultimately, nearly half of the observed masses proceeded with treatment, usually because of interval tumor growth or patient or physician anxiety. In these cases, RCC was confirmed in 92% (range 80 to 100%) of those undergoing delayed management[14,46,47] (Table 3). The high incidence of RCC in this series of initially observed small tumors may be due in part to selection bias. Nonetheless, clear cell RCC was the most common variant (91%), with the remainder papillary RCC. Nuclear-grade data were

| | | | Table 3. PATHOLOGY OF RENAL LESIONS INITIALLY MANAGED BY OBSERVATION | | | | | |
|---|---|---|---|---|---|---|---|
| Author | No. lesions | Mean Lesion Size (cm) | Pathology Available (%) | Benign (%) | RCC (%) | Grade* | Histology |
| Fujimoto[45] | 6 | 2.47 | 6 (100%) | 0 | 6 (100%) | G2 = 5 | Clear cell = 5 |
| Bosniak[41,42] | 40 | 1.73 | 26 (65%) | 4 (15%) | 22 (85%) | G1 = 18, G2 = 4 | NA |
| Oda[44] | 16 | 2.0 | 16 (100%) | 0 | 16 (100%) | G1 = 6, G2 = 9, G3 = 1 | NA |
| Kassouf[39] | 26 | 3.27 | 4 (15%) | 0 | 4 (100%) | NA | Clear cell = 3, Papillary = 1 |
| Volpe[40] | 32 | 2.48 | 9 (28%) | 1 (11%) | 8 (89%) | G2 = 4, G3 = 2, G4 = 2 | Clear cell = 8 |
| Wehle[38] | 29 | 1.83 | 5 (17%) | 1 (20%) | 4 (80%) | NA | NA |
| Kato[43] | 18 | 1.98 | 18 (100%) | 0 | 18 (100%) | G1 = 7, G2 = 8, G3 = 3 | Clear cell = 15, Papillary = 3 |
| Lamb[36]* | 36 | 7.2 | 24 (67%) | 1 (4%) | 23 (96%) | G1 = 3, G3 = 1 | Clear cell = 18, Papillary = 1 |
| Sowery[35] | 22 | 4.08 | 2 (9%) | 0 | 2 (100%) | NA | NA |
| Kunkle[47] | 106 | 2.6 | 42 (40%) | 5 (12%) | 37 (88%) | NA | Clear cell = 24, Papillary = 12, Coll. duct = 1 |
| Kouba[46] | 46 | 2.92 | 14 (30%) | 2 (14%) | 12 (86%) | G1 = 1, G2 = 8, G3 = 2, G4 = 0 | NA |
| Total | 377 | 2.99 | 166 (44%) | 14 (8%) | 152 (92%) | | |

*Pathology presented for Lamb[36] represents pathologic assessment of percutaneous biopsies.

| Table 4. MEAN GROWTH RATES OF CLINICALLY LOCALIZED ENHANCING RENAL LESIONS | | | | | | | |
|---|---|---|---|---|---|---|---|
| Author | Year | N | Average Size on Presentation (cm) | Size Range (cm) | Duration of Follow-up (average months) | Growth Rate Average | Growth Rate Range (cm/yr) |
| Oda[44] | 2001 | 16 | 2.0* | 1.0–4.5 | 25* | 0.54* cm/yr | 0.1–1.35 |
| Kato[43] | 2004 | 18 | 1.98 | 0.8–3.4 | 27 | 0.42 cm/yr | 0.08–1.60 |
| Volpe[40] | 2004 | 32 | 2.48 | 0.9–3.9 | 35 | 0.1 cm/yr | NA |
| Kassouf[39] | 2004 | 26 | 3.27 | 0.9–10.0 | 32 | 0.09 cm/yr | 0–1.2 |
| Bosniak[41,42] | 1995 | 40 | 1.73 | 0.2–3.5 | 39 | 0.36 cm/yr | 0–1.1 |
| Wehle[38] | 2004 | 29 | 1.83 | 0.4–3.5 | 32 | 0.12 cm/yr | NA |
| Lamb[36] | 2004 | 36 | 7.2 | 3.5–20.0 | 28 | 0.39 cm/yr | 0–1.76 |
| Sowery[35] | 2004 | 22 | 4.08 | 2.0–8.8 | 26 | 0.86 cm/yr | NA |
| Fujimoto[45] | 1995 | 6 | 2.47 | 1.8–3.4 | 29 | 0.47 cm/yr | 0.05–0.73 |
| Kunkle[47] | 2007 | 106 | 2.6 | 1.0–12.0 | 29 | 0.19 cm/yr | −1.4–1.60 |
| Kouba[46] | 2007 | 46 | 2.93 | 0.7–6.6 | 36 | 0.35 | 0–5.3 |

N = number of lesions observed in each series.

*median values.

reported in 74% of cases, with most tumors (88%) being of low Fuhrman grade (grades 1 to 2). Only a small percentage of tumors would be considered pathologically aggressive based on pathologic grade and stage.[13]

Although these studies have a relatively short follow-up period, they indicate that SRMs are not equally malignant. Even though tumor growth kinetics may suggest the need for treatment, similar growth rates have been shown for oncocytomas.[14] Conversely, these studies also suggest that as many as 30% of SRMs show a net zero growth during a period of active surveillance[47] and might be candidates for long-term observation (Table 4).

## PREDICTORS OF INTERVAL TUMOR GROWTH

In considering active surveillance of an incidental renal mass, identification of clinical or pathologic predictors of future behavior, such as rapid tumor growth or metastatic spread, is essential. Specifically, rapid tumor growth is believed to indicate an aggressive malignancy. Multiple parameters have been investigated as additional predictors of tumor aggressiveness, including patient demographics, tumor-related symptoms, imaging characteristics, and pathologic and molecular markers in tissue from patients who have had renal mass biopsy.

Patient age is suggested to correlate with aggressiveness. Kouba and colleagues[46] reported a faster mean growth rate in patients 60 years old or younger in a series of 43 patients and noted a significant inverse correlation between average age and growth rate on meta-analysis of several series. However, in our own cohort of 109 patients, patient age did not correlate with or predict tumor growth.[48]

Symptoms may signify a worse tumor behavior. Sowery and Siemens[35] noted that symptomatic tumors had a higher volumetric growth (45.03 cc/yr) compared with asymptomatic lesions (16.12 cc/yr). Unfortunately, initial tumor size was not examined, and the difference in growth rates was not otherwise significant. Recently, Kouba and colleagues[46] found a significantly higher growth rate in symptomatic than in asymptomatic patients, with initial tumor size and mean patient age similar in both groups.

Initial tumor size and degree of cystic components have been examined as radiographic features that might predict tumor growth. In multiple studies, tumor size at presentation does not correlate with growth rate.[14,35,38,41,42,46,47] Even in the series by Lamb and colleagues,[36] where the mean presenting tumor size was large (7.2 cm), the mean growth rate

(0.39 cm/yr) was similar to that seen for markedly smaller renal masses.[14] Comparison of solid versus predominantly cystic lesions also shows similar growth rates, even though a better prognosis is associated with cystic RCC.[35,40,49–52]

Tumor nuclear grade has been investigated as a predictor of growth; however, the association between grade and growth kinetics is inconsistent.[43,44] Additionally, although histologic subtypes of RCC have been implied to have intrinsically better or worse clinical behaviors,[9] the relationship between RCC histology and growth rate has not been examined, despite the reported correlation between disease progression and tumor histology.[53,54]

Several authors have explored the relationship between cellular and molecular markers and tumor growth rate. AgNORs and PCNA are reported to be inversely and significantly related to tumor doubling time in localized tumors,[45] Other parameters, such as Ki-67 immunostaining, tissue microvessel density, or apoptosis as measured by TUNEL assay, have not shown correlation with tumor growth.[43,55] Although these areas of study remain investigational, identification of cellular and molecular markers correlating with tumor growth rate gives the potential for predicting tumor behavior in the future from analysis of tissue from renal mass biopsy.

## PROGRESSION TO METASTATIC DISEASE

The greatest risk of observation of a localized renal mass is development of metastases. It likely rarely occurs, with a ~1% rate of metastatic disease progression documented during active surveillance.[14] Only three cases have been described, and two were associated with significant tumor growth and onset of hematuria; clinical information was not detailed for the third.[14,35,36] Several factors may contribute to and bias the low reported rate of progression in these series, including a relatively short follow-up period; the uncommon use of biopsy, likely allowing inclusion of benign lesions; a small initial tumor size; treatment of enlarging masses, selecting out potentially more aggressive tumors; and selection bias due to their retrospective nature. However, with few cases reported, it is difficult to accurately estimate the rate at which sporadic localized RCC progresses to metastatic disease while under active surveillance.

The risk of progression for sporadic RCC has been compared to the rate reported with familial RCC in von Hippel-Lindau (VHL) disease. Patients with VHL develop multifocal RCC of a more aggressive phenotype than sporadic RCC.[56] For VHL-associated RCC, the risk of metastasis has been correlated with tumor size. Metastatic disease was not seen with a tumor ≤ 3 cm, whereas metastases were recognized in 27.4% of patients when a primary tumor exceeded 3 cm. The likelihood of developing metastatic cancer for VHL-associated RCC positively correlates with increasing tumor size.[57] These findings might serve as potential guidelines and could be cautiously extrapolated to SRMs under surveillance.

## DELAYED MANAGEMENT AND COMPETING CAUSES OF DEATH

To minimize overtreatment of clinically insignificant renal tumors, active surveillance with selective delayed intervention of tumors that reach a defined threshold or endpoint might be appropriate for many SRMs.[58] A similar approach has been proposed for men having low-risk prostate cancer.[59] With RCC, there are several obstacles to applying delayed management: (1) the perception that RCC has an inherently aggressive biological behavior, (2) the inability to predict future tumor growth or behavior, (3) the concern for progression from localized to metastatic disease during observation, (4) historically poorly effective therapy for advanced RCC, and (5) immediate definitive treatment of localized RCC usually results in few and minor impacts on quality of life and long-term function.

Nevertheless, as the natural history of the SRM is increasingly shown to be relatively slow and indolent, the option of delayed management may be reasonable. In an initial report on delayed management in 14 masses treated in a delayed fashion, no patient was upstaged or had died of disease.[46] In a larger study of 87 SRMs managed in a delayed fashion (median delay of 14 months, range 6 to 97) delayed management did not limit or alter ultimate treatment, and only 6% of patients were pathologically upstaged. The majority (84%) of tumors proved to be RCC, of which only 26% demonstrated high-risk pathologic features. The 3-year estimated cancer recurrence–free survival following delayed treatment was 99%; no systemic recurrences, no metastatic progression, and no cancer-related deaths occurred prior to or following intervention.[58]

Delayed management may serve not only to identify potentially more aggressive tumors but also to select out appropriate patients with substantial competing risks of death. This strategy may potentially avert unnecessary interventions for as many as 85% of SRMs. For example, if nearly 20% of all SRM are benign,[9] 30% of SRMs (of which over 80% are RCC) exhibit zero growth over a median of 29 months,[47] and about 23% of SRM < 7 cm are potentially aggressive,[13] we can estimate that only between 10 to 15% of SRMs will demonstrate growth and have a significant biologic potential for metastases in the short to intermediate term. In recognizing the competing causes of noncancer death in patients of various ages, it is plausible that in the elderly, an even smaller fraction of individuals are at significant risk of death from RCC during a specified period of active surveillance. For example, for patients aged 75 to 84 years the 5-year cumulative noncancer death rate is roughly 20% (Table 5). Although recognizing that these data have inherent limitations and biases, a period of active surveillance followed by selective delayed intervention appears to be a reasonable strategy, especially in the elderly and infirmed. A significant shortcoming of this model is that it fails to take into account other motivations for immediate intervention, including social, cultural, legal, and economic concerns.

## EXCISE, ABLATE, OR OBSERVE THE SRM?

Paralleling the increase in early detection and stage migration of RCC has been the development of tissue ablative therapies that afford less invasive and less morbid treatment, shorter hospital stays, and quicker recovery. These newer therapies have come into favor with physicians, patients, and even insurers. Conceptually, they offer an alternative treatment option for the incidental SRM, balancing the benefits of doing "something" against the uncertainty of

doing "nothing." Unfortunately, they have not yet convincingly demonstrated that they alter the inherent natural biology of an SRM. In an effort to address this question, we have recently completed a meta-analysis of the world's literature reporting outcomes of SRM treatment. We analyzed 99 studies involving over 6400 localized renal lesions managed by excision, ablation, or observation between 1980 and 2006. Only studies that examined the treatment of clinically localized sporadic renal masses with information pertaining to disease recurrence and progression were included. Patient age, tumor size, duration of follow-up, available tumor pathologic data, and oncologic outcomes were evaluated. In comparing partial nephrectomy to ablation and observation, significant differences in mean age ($p < .001$), tumor size ($p < .001$), and length of follow-up ($P < .001$) were detected. The incidence of unknown/indeterminate pathology ($p = .003$) was significant for cryoablation (19%), radiofrequency ablation (43%), and observation (54%). Compared with excision by partial nephrectomy, significantly increased local recurrence rates were calculated for cryoablation (relative risk = 7.45) and radiofrequency ablation (RR = 18.23). However, no significant differences were seen in the incidence of progression to metastatic disease when comparing outcomes of excision, ablation, or surveillance.[60]

### Table 5. US POPULATION COMPETING CAUSES OF NONCANCER DEATH BY PATIENT AGE AT 1 AND 5 YEARS

| Age | Overall Survival | Cumulative Noncancer Deaths |
|---|---|---|
| Age 45 to 54 | | |
| 1 year | 99.6% | 0.3% |
| 5 year | 97.9% | 1.5% |
| Age 55 to 64 | | |
| 1 year | 99.1% | 0.6% |
| 5 year | 95.4% | 2.9% |
| Age 65 to 74 | | |
| 1 year | 97.7% | 1.5% |
| 5 year | 89.2% | 7.1% |
| Age 75 to 84 | | |
| 1 year | 94.5% | 4.2% |
| 5 year | 75.5% | 18.7% |
| Age 85+ | | |
| 1 year | 85.4% | 12.9% |
| 5 year | 45.4% | 48.2% |

These data emphasize important points when evaluating the literature regarding the management of an SRM. Specifically, they suggest that not all SRMs are biologically lethal, and we are most likely overtreating a number of these lesions. Moreover, they underscore that the currently used endpoint to assess recurrence following ablation (ie, enhancement on cross-sectional imaging) is imperfect and may not accurately measure the effectiveness of therapy or the long-term survival risks. Therefore, we are likely overestimating the benefit of these modalities and must be aware of these limitations and biases when assessing our own experiences and the published reports of others, particularly when using these data to counsel patients and recommend intervention.

## CONCLUSIONS

The natural history of incidental SRMs is actively being defined. Contrary to traditional belief, the intrinsic degree of malignant behavior and aggressiveness in renal tumors is variable, and although the majority of asymptomatic tumors demonstrate a slow incremental size increase, up to one-third show zero net growth in the short to medium term.[47] The rate of development of symptoms or progression to metastatic disease in untreated patients appears low. Early surveillance data suggest that a proportion of small renal tumors can be safely followed and carries a low risk of morbidity or metastatic spread. Moreover, treatment might be reasonably deferred except for cases demonstrating more rapid growth or onset of symptoms. Delayed intervention for SRMs in initial retrospective studies suggests it to be nearly as effective as immediate treatment, without compromise of treatment options or change in outcomes. However, as there are no recognized and accurate predictors of rapid tumor growth or disease progression, active surveillance should be considered with caution and only following careful review of expected benefits and inherent risks. As the current clinical and radiographic assessment of a renal mass is unable to predict tumor growth or risk of metastasis, the discovery, development, and validation of tumor markers to improve upon pretreatment prognosis is imperative. Renal mass biopsy may be of greater utility and more commonly performed in the future to provide more accurate expectations regarding tumor behavior.

## REFERENCES

1. Chow WH, Devesa SS, Warren JL, Fraumeni JF Jr. Rising incidence of renal cell cancer in the United States. JAMA 1999;281:1628–31.
2. Hock LM, Lynch J, Balaji KC. Increasing incidence of all stages of kidney cancer in the last 2 decades in the United States: an analysis of surveillance, epidemiology and end results program data. J Urol 2002;167:57–60.
3. Butler BP, Novick AC, Miller DP, et al. Management of small unilateral renal cell carcinomas: radical versus nephron-sparing surgery. Urology 1995;45:34–40.
4. Lerner SE, Hawkins CA, Blute ML, et al. Disease outcome in patients with low stage renal cell carcinoma treated with nephron sparing or radical surgery. J Urol 1996; 155:1868–73.
5. Fergany AF, Hafez KS, Novick AC. Long-term results of nephron sparing surgery for localized renal cell carcinoma: 10-year follow-up. J Urol 2000;163:442–5.
6. Bukowski RM. Natural history and therapy of metastatic renal cell carcinoma: the role of interleukin-2. Cancer 1997;80:1198–220.
7. Uzzo RG, Novick AC. Nephron sparing surgery for renal tumors: indications, techniques and outcomes. J Urol 2001;166:6–18.
8. Hollingsworth JM, Miller DC, Daignault S, Hollenbeck BK. Rising incidence of small renal masses: a need to reassess treatment effect. J Natl Cancer Inst 2006;98:1331–4.
9. Frank I, Blute ML, Cheville JC, et al. Solid renal tumors: an analysis of pathological features related to tumor size. J Urol 2003;170:2217–20.
10. Eggener SE, Rebenstein JN, Smith ND, et al. Renal tumors in young adults. J Urol 2004;171:106–10.
11. Siemer S, Hack M, Lehmann J, et al. Outcome of renal tumors in young adults. J Urol 2006;175:1240–3.
12. Snyder ME, Bach A, Kattan MW, et al. Incidence of benign lesions for clinically localized renal masses smaller than 7 cm in radiological diameter: influence of sex. J Urol 2006;176:2391–5.
13. Lane BR, Babineau D, Kattan MW, et al. A preoperative prognostic nomogram for solid enhancing renal tumors 7 cm or less amenable to partial nephrectomy. J Urol 2007;178:429–34.
14. Chawla SN, Crispen PL, Hanlon AL, et al. The natural history of observed enhancing renal masses: meta-analysis and review of the world literature. J Urol 2006; 175:425–31.
15. NCCN Clinical practice guidelines for kidney cancer. 2007.
16. Lane BR, Samplaski MK, Herts BR, et al. Renal mass biopsy: a renaissance? J Urol 2007 (In press).
17. Wood BJ, Khan MA, McGovern F, et al. Imaging guided biopsy of renal masses: indications, accuracy and impact on clinical management. J Urol 1999;161:1470–4.

18. Nadel L, Baumgartner BR, Bernardino ME. Percutaneous renal biopsies: accuracy, safety, and indications. Urol Radiol 1986;8:67–71.

19. Ralls PW, Barakos JA, Kaptein EM, et al. Renal biopsy-related hemorrhage: frequency and comparison of CT and sonography. J Comput Assist Tomogr 1987;11:1031–4.

20. Johnson PT, Nazarian LN, Feld RI, et al. Sonographically guided renal mass biopsy: indications and efficacy. J Ultrasound Med 2001;20:749–53.

21. Rybicki FJ, Shu KM, Cibas ES, et al. Percutaneous biopsy of renal masses: sensitivity and negative predictive value statified by clinical setting and size of masses. AJR Am J Roentgenol 2003;180:1281–7.

22. Hopper KD, Yakes WF. The posterior intercostal approach for percutaneous renal procedures: risk of puncturing the lung, spleen, and liver as determined by CT. AJR Am J Roentgenol 1990;154:115–7.

23. Schmid T, Sandbichler P, Ausserwinkler M, et al. Vascular lesions after percutaneous biopsies of renal allografts. Transpl Int 1989;2:56–8.

24. Matsell DG, Jones DP, Boulden TF, et al. Arteriovenous fistula after biopsy of renal transplant kidney: diagnosis and treatment. Pediatr Nephrol 1992;6:562–4.

25. Nakatani T, Uchida J, Han YS, et al. Renal allograft arteriovenous fistula and large pseudoaneurysm. Clin Transplant 2003;17:9–12.

26. Neuzillet Y, Lechevallier E, Andre M, et al. Accuracy and clinical role of fine needle percutaneous biopsy with computerized tomography guidance of small (less than 4.0 cm) renal masses. J Urol 2004;171:1802–5.

27. Herts BR. Imaging guided biopsies of renal masses. Curr Opin Urol 2000;10:105–9.

28. Israel GM, Bosniak MA. An update of the Bosniak renal cyst classification system. Urology 2005;66:484–8.

29. Beland MD, Mayo-Smith WW, Dupuy DE, et al. Diagnostic yield of 59 consecutive imaging-guided biopsies of solid renal masses: should we biopsy all that are indeterminate? AJR Am J Roentgenol 2007;188:792–7.

30. Zhou M, Roma A, Magi-Galluzzi C. The usefulness of immunohistochemical markers in the differential diagnosis of renal neoplasms. Clin Lab Med 2005;25:247–57.

31. Avery AK, Beckstead J, Renshaw AA, Corless CL. Use of antibodies to RCC and CD10 in the differential diagnosis of renal neoplasms. Am J Surg Pathol 2000; 24:203–10.

32. Barocas DA, Mathew S, Delpizzo JJ, et al. Renal cell carcinoma sub-typing by histopathology and fluorescence in situ hybridization on a needle-biopsy specimen. BJU Int 2007;99:290–5.

33. Upton MP, Parker RA, Youmans A, et al. Histologic predictors of renal cell carcinoma response to interleukin-2 based therapy. J Immunother 2005;28:488–95.

34. David KA, Milowsky MI, Nanus DM. Chemotherapy for non-clear cell renal cell carcinoma. Clin Genitourin Cancer 2006;4:263–8.

35. Sowery RD, Siemens DR. Growth characteristics of renal cortical tumors in patients managed by watchful waiting. Can J Urol 2004;11:2407–10.

36. Lamb GW, Bromwich EJ, Vasey P, et al. Management of renal masses in patients medically unsuitable for nephrectomy—natural history, complications, and outcome. Urology 2004;64:909–13.

37. Mydlo JH, Gerstein M. Patients with urologic cancer and other nonurologic malignancies: analysis of a sample and review of the literature. Urology 2001;58:864–9.

38. Wehle MJ, Thiel DD, Petrou SP, et al. Conservative management of incidental contrast-enhancing renal masses as safe alternative to invasive therapy. Urology 2004;64:49–52.

39. Kassouf W, Aprikian AG, Laplante M, Tanguay S. Natural history of renal masses followed expectantly [discussion 113]. J Urol 2004;171:111–3.

40. Volpe A, Panzarella T, Rendon RA, et al. The natural history of incidentally detected small renal masses. Cancer 2004;100:738–45.

41. Bosniak MA, Birnbaum BA, Krinsky GA, Waisman J. Small renal parenchymal neoplasms: further observations on growth. Radiology 1995;197:589–97.

42. Bosniak MA. Observation of small incidentally detected renal masses. Semin Urol Oncol 1995;13:267–72.

43. Kato M, Suzuki T, Suzuki Y, et al. Natural history of small renal cell carcinoma: evaluation of growth rate, histological grade, cell proliferation and apoptosis. J Urol 2004;172:863–6.

44. Oda T, Miyao N, Takahashi A, et al. Growth rates of primary and metastatic lesions of renal cell carcinoma. Int J Urol 2001;8:473–7.

45. Fujimoto N, Sugita A, Terasawa Y, Kato M. Observations on the growth rate of renal cell carcinoma. Int J Urol 1995;2:71–6.

46. Kouba E, Smith A, McRackan D, et al. Watchful waiting for solid renal masses: insight into the natural history and results of delayed intervention. J Urol 2007;177:466–70.

47. Kunkle DA, Crispen PL, Chen DY, et al. Enhancing renal masses with zero net growth during active surveillance. J Urol 2007;177:849–53.

48. Crispen PL, Wong YN, Greenberg RE, et al. Predicting growth of solid renal masses under active surveillance. Urol Oncol 2007 (In press).

49. Corica FA, Iczkowski KA, Cheng L, et al. Cystic renal cell carcinoma is cured by resection: a study of 24 cases with long-term followup. J Urol 1999;161:408–11.

50. Han KR, Janzen NK, McWhorter VC, et al. Cystic renal cell carcinoma: biology and clinical behavior. Urol Oncol 2004;22:410–4.

51. Nassir A, Jollimore J, Gupta R, et al. Multilocular cystic renal cell carcinoma: a series of 12 cases and review of the literature. Urology 2002;60:421–7.

52. Koga S, Nishikido M, Hayashi T, et al. Outcome of surgery in cystic renal cell carcinoma. Urology 2000;56:67–70.

53. Gudbjartsson T, Hardarson S, Petursdottir V, et al. Histological subtyping and nuclear grading of renal cell carcinoma and their implications for survival: a retrospective nationwide study of 629 patients. Eur Urol 2005;48:593–600.

54. Lau WK, Cheville JC, Blute ML, et al. Prognostic features of pathologic stage T1 renal cell carcinoma after radical nephrectomy. Urology 2002;59:532–7.

55. Oda T, Takahashi A, Miyao N, et al. Cell proliferation, apoptosis, angiogenesis and growth rate of incidentally found renal cell carcinoma. Int J Urol 2003;10:13–8.

56. Grubb RL 3rd, Choyke PL, Pinto PA, et al. Management of von Hippel-Lindau-associated kidney cancer. Nat Clin Pract Urol 2005;2:248–55.

57. Duffey BG, Choyke PL, Glenn G, et al. The relationship between renal tumor size and metastases in patients with von Hippel-Lindau disease. J Urol 2004;172:63–5.

58. Crispen PL, Viterbo R, Fox EB, et al. Delayed intervention of small sporadic renal masses undergoing active surveillance. Cancer 2007. (In press).

59. Klotz L. Active surveillance with selective delayed intervention for favorable risk prostate cancer. Urol Oncol 2006;24:46–50.

60. Kunkle DA, Egleston BL, Uzzo RG. Excise, ablate or observe: The small renal mass dilemma—a meta-analysis and review. J Urol 2007 (In press).

# MANAGEMENT OF SMALL RENAL MASSES

## Energy-Ablative Therapy for Small Renal Masses

**SURENA F. MATIN, MD, FACS**
**KAMRAN AHRAR, MD**

Advances in preoperative staging and modern surgical techniques have led to the increasing popularity of nephron-sparing surgery for small renal tumors. Initial data have shown that partial nephrectomy is as effective as radical nephrectomy for treating tumors less than 4 cm in size.[1] This finding provided the impetus for the use of nephron-sparing surgery for selected tumors 4 to 7 cm in size.[2] Minimally invasive forms of nephron-sparing surgery have gained popularity in the treatment of small, asymptomatic tumors, particularly for elderly patients and patients with multifocal or familial renal cell carcinomas (RCCs). In this climate, nephron-sparing surgery has been integrated with probe-based energy-ablative technologies (using laparoscopic and percutaneous approaches) and this

regimen has rapidly been incorporated into the armamentarium of treatment options for renal tumors.

The application of new technology into clinical care generally involves a transition of that technology from one stage of acceptance to another, that is, the transition from the experimental stage to the developmental stage and, finally, to its recognition as a standard treatment (Figure 1). Current data thus far support the application of cryoablation and radiofrequency ablation (RFA) technology in carefully selected, well-informed patients. In this chapter, we describe the treatment options used for renal tumors and we refer to them according to their current status as an experimental, developmental, or standard treatment option.

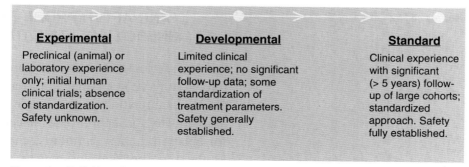

| Experimental | Developmental | Standard |
|---|---|---|
| Preclinical (animal) or laboratory experience only; initial human clinical trials; absence of standardization. Safety unknown. | Limited clinical experience; no significant follow-up data; some standardization of treatment parameters. Safety generally established. | Clinical experience with significant (> 5 years) follow-up of large cohorts; standardized approach. Safety fully established. |

**Figure 1.** Definition of standard, developmental, and experimental terminologies as used in this chapter. Reproduced with permission from Copyright Matin SF2007.

## INDICATIONS FOR PROBE-BASED ENERGY-ABLATIVE THERAPY

### Patient Selection Criteria

About 80% of enhancing renal tumors removed at surgery prove to be RCC.[3] Surgical resection remains the gold standard treatment for patients with RCCs who are eligible for surgery.[4] For some patients, however, surgery is not the ideal treatment option. For example, the majority of incidentally detected renal tumors are encountered in elderly patients with multiple medical comorbidities who may thus be suboptimal candidates for surgical intervention. Some patients have limited renal reserve, owing to renal disease, previous infections, previous surgeries, nephrosclerosis, or vascular disease, which would render surgery for the renal mass a risky option with the threat of hemodialysis. Similar renal functional considerations may also apply to some patients with genetic syndromes such as von Hippel-Lindau disease, who may have extensive multifocal disease. Table 1 summarizes patient selection criteria for probe-ablative therapy. One must consider not only patient and renal function–related factors but also tumor characteristics as well.

### Tumor Selection Criteria

When selecting patients for probe-based energy-ablative therapy, careful attention should be given

### Table 1. FACTORS CONSIDERED IN SELECTING PROBE-ABLATIVE THERAPY OF A SMALL RENAL MASS

Patient factors
  Age (physiologic rather than chronologic)
  Performance status
  Comorbidities
  Critical need for anticoagulation
  Coexistent or recently treated malignancy (other than RCC)
  Acceptance of imperative need for radiographic
    follow-up regimen

Renal factors
  Overall renal function
  Contralateral kidney function
  Previous ipsilateral renal surgery

Tumor factors
  Number of tumors
  Size of tumor
  Symptoms
  Tumor depth (central versus noncentral)
  Tumor location (posterior, anterior, lateral)
  Cystic tumor (contraindicated)

to several tumor-related factors, primarily tumor size. Currently available probe-ablative technology allows for complete eradication of most tumors less than 4 cm in size.[5] Larger tumors may also be treated, if other options are inappropriate because of imperative patient factors, but multiple sessions and repeat ablations may be required, and with the expectation of a lower success rate. Ablative therapy can also be used to provide symptomatic relief, as has been shown in patients with poor renal function suffering from tumor-related hematuria for whom embolization is not an option.[6]

Another consideration is tumor location. Exophytic tumors yield the best chance of success. When tumors extend to the central portion of the kidney (central or mixed tumors), there is a lower chance of treatment success.[5] Ablative therapy has also been used to treat recurrent tumors in the nephrectomy bed when the location is favorable.[7] Tumors located in the posterior or lateral aspect of the kidney are ideally suited for a percutaneous approach; however, positional maneuvering of the patient and the use of various techniques to separate adjacent vital structures are other options, such as creation of an intentional pneumothorax to access upper pole tumors, mechanical separation from bowel using instillation of fluid or gas, or the use of balloon catheters for more anterior tumors.[8–11] However, a laparoscopic approach is probably most ideal for anterior and anteromedial tumors. Cystic tumors are not ideally suited to probe-based energy-ablative approaches because tumor puncture has to be performed before ablation, which poses a risk of tumor seeding.

## EVALUATION BEFORE, DURING, AND AFTER PROBE-BASED ENERGY-ABLATIVE THERAPY

Preablation imaging with renal protocol computed tomography (CT) or magnetic resonance imaging (MRI) examination is the single most important prerequisite for appropriate selection of patients for ablation therapy. Similarly, characteristics such as the size, consistency, pattern of enhancement, location, and proximity to the ureter, bowel, and other vulnerable organs, determine the feasibility of ablative therapy and help to determine whether a percutaneous or laparoscopic approach should be used. The pretreatment discussion includes the risks and benefits of ablation, standard proven therapies, and the need for continued rigorous imaging follow-up after ablation. The preablation laboratory evaluation typically includes complete blood count, serum creatinine level, and prothrombin time tests. Some investigators advocate a preablation biopsy for all patients, whereas others recommend a separately scheduled biopsy only for lesions suspected to not be of primary renal tumors. For patients with a suspected metastasis to the kidney or a lymphoma, a separately scheduled percutaneous biopsy can often prevent unnecessary therapy.[12] As well, recent studies indicate that 27 to 37% of patients referred for percutaneous ablation of renal tumors have benign disease.[13,14] These same studies, however, show a nondiagnostic rate of 12 to 26%.[13,14] Although there is no consensus about the use of separately scheduled percutaneous biopsy in advance of ablation, we recommend obtaining core biopsy samples at the time of ablation for all tumors because subtyping and grading of RCCs have important prognostic implications.[15] In addition, cancer-specific survival (CSS) data cannot be reported accurately without pathologic confirmation of malignancy.

Imaging analysis is an integral part of both pre, intra, and postoperative ablation therapy (Table 2). During laparoscopy, ultrasonography (US) is used to localize and characterize the tumor, guide placement of the probe (RFA electrode or cryo probe), and monitor the iceball formation during cryoablation[16]; however, US is limited in its ability to monitor the extent of RFA.[17] During RFA, gas microbubbles are generated within the ablation zone and are released into the surrounding tissues. These echogenic bubbles often degrade the quality of ultrasound images and preclude its use for repositioning the RFA electrode when creating overlapping areas of ablation.

The use of US, CT, and MRI has been described in association with percutaneous approaches.[18–20] US provides real-time imaging that facilitates tumor targeting and placement of the applicator(s). Similar to its use during laparoscopic procedures, the iceball formation can be monitored by US, although the iceball creates intense acoustic shadowing and precludes assessment of the deep margin of the ablation zone. In most published reports of percutaneous ablation of renal tumors, CT has been used to guide placement of the applicator(s). In this capacity, CT can localize the tumor and other vulnerable organs in the vicinity of the tumor. Using CT guidance, positional or mechanical maneuvers may be used to

| Table 2. MODALITIES USED FOR IMAGING OF LAPAROSCOPIC OR PERCUTANEOUS RFA/CRYOABLATION OF RENAL TUMORS | | | | |
|---|---|---|---|---|
| **Laparoscopic** | | | | |
| Imaging | Preprocedure | Intraprocedure | | Postprocedure |
| | | Targeting | Monitoring | |
| Ultrasound | No | Yes | Yes* | No |
| CT | Yes | No | No | Yes |
| MRI | Yes | No | No | Yes |
| **Percutaneous** | | | | |
| Imaging | Preprocedure | Intraprocedure | | Postprocedure |
| | | Targeting | Monitoring | |
| Ultrasound | No | Yes | No | No |
| CT | Yes | Yes | Yes* | Yes |
| MRI | Yes | Yes | Yes | Yes |

*US is useful for monitoring the iceball during cryoablation, but not for RFA.

*With immediate procedural contrast study.

separate the tumor from neighboring vulnerable structures, facilitating a safe ablation.[8–11]

During CT-guided cryotherapy, the iceball appears as a well-defined area of low density.[21] Unfortunately, noncontrast CT is limited in monitoring the extent of ablation during RFA procedures. Changes in CT density without iodinated contrast are not predictable and are not characteristic of a successful ablation. However, once the planned ablation is completed, contrast-enhanced CT can be performed allowing the operator to assess the extent of ablation. If one or more of the margins appear inadequate, the electrode can be reinserted into the residual tumor for additional treatment. Delayed CT images may be used to confirm patency of the ureter and the absence of hemorrhage in the renal collecting system.

Interventional MRI suites are not yet widely available, but the exquisite soft-tissue differentiation and multiplanar imaging capabilities of MRI have been exploited at a few centers for ablation of renal tumors.[20,22] During MRI-guided cryotherapy, the iceball can be visualized as an area of decreased T2-signal intensity.[22] Similarly, changes in the signal intensity of the ablation zone are sufficiently characteristic to indicate successful RFA of renal tumors and the presence of any residual unablated tumor.[20]

With all energy-ablation therapies, a regimented postoperative follow-up imaging schedule is required to determine the effectiveness of treatment. This is because neither pathology nor long-term data are available to confirm cure. It is critical that patients understand this issue up-front and adhere to a systematic follow-up regimen after ablation. Patients who are unwilling or unable to accept the follow-up regimen should be considered poor candidates for these approaches. On the basis of a recent multi-institutional study, it is felt that a minimum of three studies be performed in the first year—at months 1, 3 or 6, and month 12 after treatment—and then semiannually or annually thereafter.[23] Follow-up studies should consist of renal protocol CT or MRI examinations, and the results should be carefully reviewed and compared with earlier results. Any new enhancement or enlargement of the ablation zone should be viewed as residual unablated tumor or recurrent disease.[24] The absence of shrinkage, even in the setting of no enhancement, is usually a trigger for percutaneous biopsy to ensure absence of residual or recurrent disease. However, most institutions do not routinely perform percutaneous biopsy after ablation.[23] A caveat with the use of only imaging to define success is data suggesting that lack of enhancement may not be the single best surrogate for confirming oncologic efficacy. Gill and colleagues[25] reported two positive needle biopsies after cryoablation when MRI suggested no enhancement. Generally, enhancement is more clearly defined and more reliably obtained with CT scan than with MRI; hence, although it is possible that these findings are due to observer sensitivity, they suggest that using enhancement on imaging as the sole surrogate for determining treatment success may need to be reconsidered.

## PROBE-BASED ENERGY-ABLATIVE THERAPIES

Nearly every known form of energy has been used or investigated in the treatment of small renal masses (Table 3). At present, however, cryoablation and RFA are the most widely used. These technologies can be applied either percutaneously or laparoscopically. The different technical approaches are discussed in a separate section, but it will be impossible to completely differentiate the topics because of the uniqueness of each combination.

Injury to the collecting system is to be expected with either form of energy or type of approach, even with tumors that do not come in contact with the collecting system, because the treatment margin has to include a margin of normal tissue. It is expected that for adequate therapy, with some of the deeper infiltrating tumors, the collecting system will be treated. The two primary concerns in these cases are the development of urinary fistula and the potentially reduced efficacy of the treatment. Studies show that treatment of the collecting system by RFA or cryoablation does not lead to any permanent injury, so long as the collecting system itself is not punctured, because it appears to heal by secondary intent.[26–29] Treatment of lesions close to the collecting system, however, may be associated with a lower efficacy because of a thermal sink from the collecting system and segmental renal vessels as well as the

| Table 3. FORMS OF ENERGY USED FOR THE TREATMENT OF SOLID TUMORS | | | | |
|---|---|---|---|---|
| Classification | Name | Energy/Technology | Result | Effect of energy on tissue |
| Probe-ablative (invasive) | Cryoablation | Cold temperature | Iceball | Mechanical and cellular tissue disruption, denaturation, apoptosis |
| | Radiofrequency | Electrical radiofrequency | Heat, dessication | Protein denaturation |
| | Interstitial laser coagulation | Light | Heat, dessication | Protein denaturation |
| | Microwave thermotherapy | Microwave | Heat, dessication | Protein denaturation |
| | Photodynamic therapy | Light, photobiologic reaction | Singlet oxygen | Oxidative damage, apoptosis |
| Noninvasive | High-intensity focused ultrasound | Sound waves | Heat, cavitation | Protein denaturation, mechanical tissue disruption |
| | Radiation | Gamma and beta particles | Ionizing radiation | Ionization, free radicals, DNA damage, increased membrane permeability |

risk of hematuria with clot obstruction, a phenomenon seen with both cryoablation and RFA.[30,31]

## Cryoablation: Mechanism of Cell Death, Current Technologies, and Results

Cell death from cryoablation occurs because of rapid cooling crystallizing extracellular water and the shift of super cooled intracellular water into the hyperosmotic extracellular space, causing membrane and organelle damage.[32] Intracellular formation of ice crystals subsequently occurs at −40°C and is the main mechanism of cell death during cryoablation.[32,33] During thawing, smaller crystals fuse to form larger ones at temperatures ranging from −25° to −20°C, causing mechanical cell damage.[32,33] A slow thawing rate, therefore, leads to greater destruction because of recrystallization.

Two factors influence cell death: the minimum temperature reached and the rate of cooling. Temperatures between −19° and 0°C result in only 80% cell death.[34,35] Many consider the critical nadir temperature for complete cell death to occur at −20° to −40°C,[33–36] and possibly as low as −60° to −84°C.[37,38] Because the edge of the iceball corresponds to 0°C, it is critical to create an iceball that goes beyond tumor borders by at least 5 to 10 mm to reach the critical nadir value.[34] With respect to the rate of cooling, in-vitro data have shown that a slow cooling rate of 5°C/min requires a nadir temperature of −40°C, whereas if the cooling rate

is increased to 25°C/min, only a −19°C nadir is required for complete cell death.[36] The rate of cooling is generally a concern at the periphery, where cooling is much slower.[33,34] On the basis of this collective data, the concepts of a rapid freeze, slow thaw, and double freeze-thaw cycle have become standard protocols in clinical practice.

Laparoscopic cryoablation was one of the first energy-ablation technologies to be explored for the treatment of small renal masses. The systematic clinical use of laparoscopic cryoablation was explored primarily by one center, using rigorous selection criteria, follow-up imaging and biopsies, with promising initial results.[16] Overall published success rates of cryoablation range from 84.3 to 100%[21,22,25,39–46] (Table 4). Success in most of these cases has been shown by nonenhancement on CT or MRI, but in some cases postoperative biopsies have also identified viable cancer cells.[25,43] In one study with a mean follow-up of 15 months, two of seven patients (29%) with biopsy-proven RCC had recurrent cancer on postcryoablation biopsy.[43] Gill and colleagues[47] have subsequently reported one of the longest follow-up studies of laparoscopic cryoablation, with a CSS rate of 98% in patients with a unilateral sporadic renal tumor and at least 3 years of follow-up. Davol and colleagues[40] reported the results of both open and laparoscopic cryoablation in 48 patients with 3-year radiographic follow-up, showing a 84.3% CSS after one cryoablation, but up to 96.8% after repeated intervention.

## Table 4. RESULTS OF RFA AND CRYOABLATION OF RENAL TUMORS

| First Author, Year | No. Tumors | No. Patients | Size, cm Mean | Size, cm Range | Follow-up, months Mean | Follow-up, months Range | Success Rates |
|---|---|---|---|---|---|---|---|
| **Cryoablation** | | | | | | | |
| Schwartz, 2006 | 85 | 84 | 2.6 | 1.2–4.7 | 10 (in 55 patients) | 3–36 | 83/85 (97.6%); open cryo in 11 patients and unknown approach in 4 |
| Lawatsch, 2005 | 81 | 59 | 2.5 | 1.0–5.0 | 26.8 | NR–61.1 | 57/59 (96.6%) |
| Gill, 2006 | 60 | 56 | 2.3 | 1.0–5.0 | 36 | At least 36 for all patients | 54/56 (96.4%; 2 with positive biopsies); 98% CSS for those with sporadic unilateral renal tumor |
| Davol, 2006 | 51 | 48 | 2.6 | 1.1–4.6 | 36* | 36–110 | 27/32 (84.3% CSS) after one cryoablation, 31/32 (96.8%) after repeat cryo; open cryo in 24 patients |
| Cestari, 2004 | 37 | 37 | 2.6 | 1.0–6.0 | 20.5 | 1–36 | 36/37 (97.3%) |
| Gupta, 2006 | 27 | 20 | 2.5 | 1.0–4.6 | 5.9 (in 12 patients) | 1–10 | 15/16 (93.8%); CT-guided cryoablation |
| Silverman, 2005 | 26 | 23 | 2.6 | 1.0–4.6 | 14 | 4–30 | 24/26 (92.3%); MRI-guided percutaneous cryo |
| Shingleton, 2001 | 22 | 20 | 3.0 | 1.8–7.0 | 9.1 | 3–14 | 19/20 (95%) after 1 treatment, 100% after retreatment; MRI-guided percutaneous cryo |
| Lee, 2003 | 20 | 20 | 2.5 | 1.4–4.0 | 14.2 | 1.4–4.5 | 17/20 (85%) without enhancement |
| O'Malley, 2006 | 15 | 15 | 2.7 | NR | 11.9 | NR | 15/15 (100%) |
| Nadler, 2003 | 15 | 15 | 2.15 | 1.2–3.2 | 15.1 | 4.9–27 | 13/15 (87.7%, 2 with positive biopsies); all exophytic lesions |
| Hruby, 2005 | 11 | 11 | 1.9 | 0.9–2.7 | 11.3 | NR | 11/11 (100%); hilar tumors only |
| **Radiofrequency ablation** | | | | | | | |
| Gervais, 2005 | 100 | 85 | 3.2 | 1.1–8.9 | 27 | 3.5–72 | 3 cm: 52/52 (100%); 3.1–5 cm: 36/39 (92%); > 5 cm: 2/8 (25%) |
| Farrell, 2003 | 35 | 20 | 1.7 | 0.9–3.6 | 9 | 1–13 | 35/35 (100%) |
| Su, 2003 | 35 | 29 | 2.2 | 1–4 | 9 | 1–23 | 33/35 (94%) |
| Mayo-Smith, 2003 | 32 | 32 | 2.6 | 1–5 | 9 | 1–36 | 31/32 (97%) |
| Ahrar, 2005 | 28 | 27 | 3.5 | 1.5–6.5 | 10 | 1–33 | 23/24 (96%) |
| Clark, 2006 | 26 | 22 | 2.2 | 1–4 | 11.2 | 1–31 | 26/26 (100%) |
| Pavlovich, 2002 | 24 | 21 | 2.4 | 1.5–3 | NR | NR | 19/24 (79%) |
| Zagoria, 2004 | 24 | 22 | 3.5 | 1–7 | 7 | 1–35 | 3 cm: 11/11 (100%); > 3cm: 9/13 (69%) |
| Veltri, 2004 | 18 | 13 | 2.5 | 1.5–7.5 | 14 | 3–34 | 3.5 cm: 16/17 (94%); > 3.5 cm, embolized first |
| Mahnken, 2004 | 15 | 14 | 3 | 1–4.5 | 13.9 | NR | 15/15 (100%) Pre-RFA embolization in 6 tumors > 3 cm |
| Ogan, 2002 | 13 | 12 | 2.4 | 1.4–3.6 | 4.9 | 1–13 | 12/13 (92%) |
| Roy-Choudhury, 2003 | 11 | 8 | 3 | 1.5–5.5 | 17 | 10–26 | 9/11 (82%) |
| Lewin, 2004 | 10 | 10 | 2.3 | 1–3.6 | 25 | NR | 10/10 (100%) |
| De Baere, 2002 | 5 | 5 | 3.3 | 3–4 | NR | 6–18 | 5/5 (100%) |

Adapted from Expert Review in Anticancer Therapy, 6 (12):1735–1744, 2006, with permission of Future Drugs Ltd.

CSS = cancer-specific survival; MRI = magnetic resonance imaging; NR = not reported; US = ultrasound.

*Radiographic follow-up. Clinical follow-up was 64 months.

Overall, cryoablation is well tolerated. The most common complication reported is hemorrhage, usually because of fracture of the cryolesion. Pancreatic injury, ureteral injury, clot obstruction, and conversion to open surgery or nephrectomy have also been reported.[30,40,42,46,48]

Small cryoprobes (17 gauge) have recently become available and may facilitate percutaneous and laparoscopic approaches because of their smaller diameter. In fact, several groups have recently reported their early experience with MRI- and CT-guided percutaneous ablation of renal tumors using small cryoprobes.[21,22,49,50] However, the iceball size, which is 2 cm or less, is too small for a single probe to treat a renal tumor—an iceball of about 3 cm would be desired in this setting. Thus, multiple probes must be placed as an array to treat the entire tumor with a margin and must be geometrically centered.[49] Adding to the complexity of whether a single probe is used or multiple ones, is the angulation needed for access to mid- and upper-pole tumors because of interference from the rib cage. Percutaneously, access between the ribs can be accomplished. However, this is risky laparoscopically. Thus, the probes have to be placed in an angulated fashion, which punctures the tumor off the geometric center. The presence of multiple probes can also raise the risk of iceball fracture, which is facilitated by movement of the kidney. Despite these limitations, the initial results reported using new smaller probes are promising but require additional validation.[51]

Because of the recently published 3-year follow-up data and the standardized approach, laparoscopic cryoablation is now considered somewhat more than a developmental technique and, in fact, could be considered a standard technique in experienced hands for judiciously selected patients. At present, the majority of experience with *percutaneous* thermal ablation of renal tumors involves the use of RFA, but percutaneous cryoablation is being investigated at some centers.[21,49,52]

## RFA: Mechanism of Cell Death, Current Technologies, and Results

RFA-induced cell death results from thermal energy created by an alternating electrical current (frequency range, 480–500 kHz) deposited into the tumor via an electrode. The resulting ionic agitation within the tissue creates frictional heating in the immediate vicinity of the electrode, resulting in ablation of a finite volume of tissue.[53] As with cryoablation, the ablation zone should encompass the tumor and a margin of normal tissue. The size and shape of the ablation zone will vary depending on the amount of energy needed, the type of electrode used, the duration of the ablation, and tissue characteristics.[54,55] One advantage of RFA is the ability to perform multiple overlapping ablations with a single electrode allowing the treatment of irregularly shaped, noncircular tumors.

There are currently three monopolar RFA devices capable of delivering up to 250 W of power that are available for use in the United States: the Cool Tip device (Tyco Healthcare, Valleylab, Boulder, CO, USA), the LeVeen needle electrode device (Boston Scientific, Natick, MA, USA), and the RITA device (RITA Medical Systems, Fremont, CA, USA). Monopolar RFA devices consist of three components: a generator, an applicator (electrode), and dispersive electrodes (grounding pads). The energy delivery of each generator is modulated by an internal feedback mechanism monitoring the impedance in the ablated tissue (Valleylab and Boston Scientific generators) or the target temperature in the tumor (RITA generator). All three devices have been used in clinical practice and appear to be equally effective.

The feasibility of RFA for the treatment of renal tumors was established in 1997 in three patients who underwent the procedure before surgical resection.[56] RFA resulted in extensive localized necrosis of the tumor with no damage to adjacent structures. The first case report of successful percutaneous RFA of a renal tumor was published in 1999.[57] Since then, several case series of percutaneous RFA have been published and have reported good success rates determined by imaging studies[5,18–20,58–67] (Table 4). In a study of 85 patients with 100 renal tumors that ranged in size from 1.1 to 8.9 cm in diameter, complete necrosis was achieved in 90% of the cases.[5] Tumor size and noncentral location were found to be independent predictors of complete necrosis after a single ablation session. Complete ablation was achieved in all tumors 3 cm or smaller and 92% of tumors between 3 and 5 cm, but in only 25% of tumors larger than 5 cm. Other studies show a recurrence-free survival rate of 95 to 100% from 2 to 4 years.[68,69] In a study with the longest follow-up available, 15 of 16 (94%) patients with biopsy-proven RCC treated with curative intent were successfully treated at 5 years.[69]

In general, RFA is well tolerated. Perinephric hemorrhage after percutaneous RFA is almost always self-limiting. In a series of 85 patients who underwent renal RFA, only 2 (2.3%) required blood transfusion.[5] In our own experience, RFA of renal tumors in more than 100 patients resulted in two cases (2%) of persistent bleeding: one patient required blood transfusion and the other required blood transfusion and embolization. Hematuria is most likely during RFA of central tumors. Although usually self-limiting, ureteral stent placement may be required to relieve urinary obstruction.[18] RFA of tumors in close proximity to the ureteropelvic junction or the ureter can lead to strictures.[5,70] Other potential complications, such as urine leak and tract seeding, are extremely rare.[5,61] Renal function is preserved when the treatment is carefully applied.[71] RFA is considered to be beyond the developmental stage of clinical acceptance because of the published data, but because of lingering concerns regarding its application (see "RFA versus Cryoablation," below), it is not yet considered a standard therapy. It is, however, a reasonable alternative for carefully selected patients.

## Access Techniques

From a purely anatomic perspective, tumors that are posteriorly or laterally located are accessed percutaneously, whereas lesions that are anterior or in close approximation to the ureter, bowel, or other critical structures are accessed laparoscopically. From a practical standpoint, however, the approach taken often depends on available experience, personnel, and technology. In centers or communities that do not have an involved interventional radiologist, all procedures will be performed laparoscopically, whereas those without an involved urologist will perform most procedures percutaneously. With respect to cost, the percutaneous approach has been shown to have an advantage over laparoscopy, but

this is generally not a consideration for most centers choosing one technology over another.[72,73]

The percutaneous approach is performed by some interventional radiologists under local anesthetic and heavy sedation, whereas others, including our institution, use general anesthesia to minimize patient discomfort, patient movement and to control respiration to minimize renal excursion and optimize targeting. Some surgeons consider the laparoscopic approach to be superior to the percutaneous approach because it adds the ability to visually monitor therapy; however, we are not aware of any direct data supporting this opinion. The use of laparoscopic US (LUS) is critical during laparoscopic procedures because it allows for the accurate positioning of the treatment probe, particularly in the deep portion of the tumor where a margin of treated normal tissue is usually desired; otherwise, the utility of LUS during RFA has limited value because of imaging artifacts that render the LUS image of little value. The advantage of the percutaneous approach is that it is minimally invasive, it is repeatable over time, and is associated with less destruction of tissue planes. A limitation of the laparoscopic approach is that tissue planes are violated, making secondary surgery more difficult because of scarring. With cryoablation, LUS can be used throughout the treatment to monitor progression of the iceball in the intrarenal portions. This ability to monitor the treatment in real-time represents the single greatest advantage of cryoablation over all other technologies discussed in this chapter and represents an important limitation—indeed a potential Achilles' heel—for all other energy-based technologies.

## RFA versus Cryoablation

Comparisons between RFA and cryoablation are inevitable, yet, as we describe below, a direct evaluation using current data is difficult because of inherent differences in how these technologies have been applied, developed, and reported in retrospective studies.

Several early ablate-and-resect studies of RFA were initially performed and have suggested that this technique achieves incomplete ablation.[74,75] These studies were limited in their findings, however, because of several technical factors. First, investigators used less-powerful, and thus less-effective, generators. Newer generators deliver at least 200 to 250 W of energy—double or more the energy provided by older generators. Second, percutaneous ultrasound was used solely for guidance in some procedures, which is inferior to MRI or CT guidance. Third, only a single ablation was performed, whereas an advantage of RFA is the ability to perform multiple overlapping ablations until satisfactory results are achieved. The fourth factor involves the pathologic evaluation. Simple hematoxylin and eosin (H&E) staining was used as a test of viability, but in the acute period it does not accurately reflect tissue necrosis or cells destined to undergo apoptosis.[76] H&E staining soon after ablation is an unreliable measure of viability because it shows preserved parenchymal architecture with little cellular inflammation, poorly defined cytoplasmic borders, decreased eosinophilia, and viable-appearing nuclei.[77,78] Several investigators have instead advocated the use of NADH histochemical staining as a test of viability.[77,79] In two small series, pathologic evaluation of resected tumors shortly after ablation suggested the presence of viable tumor.[74,75] In another study, 10 tumors were ablated shortly before resection.[79] H&E and NADH staining of pathology specimen showed complete ablation in 8 of 10 tumors. At the present time, pathologic evaluation of resected specimens after ablation has not been standardized and remains a subject of investigation.

No systematic ablate-and-resect studies have been performed with cryoablation. Cryoablation was initially championed largely by a single institution, using technology from a single manufacturer in a systematic and entirely laparoscopic application. With strict patient selection criteria, rigorous technical application, and regimented follow-up, excellent results followed.[16,25] In comparison, RFA, probably because of its ease of percutaneous application, was applied by multiple centers, without uniform patient/tumor criteria, using different manufacturers and diverse form of follow-up regimens. Because percutaneous therapy can be easily repeated, the initial treatments were probably not sufficiently aggressive, knowing that some centers follow the strategy of repeating percutaneous therapy as necessary over time, which is not a traditional surgical mentality.[5] With a laparoscopic approach, however, a maximal therapeutic effect must be achieved at that setting because repeat operation is not a feasible option.

Attempted comparisons between cryoablation and RFA have produced misleading findings. In a recent evaluation of these two techniques at a single center, cryoablation appeared to produce better results.[80] A closer look at the study, however, showed that patients undergoing RFA were six times more likely to have centrally located tumors and twice as likely to have a solitary kidney. Patients undergoing RFA, therefore, had adverse factors and were preselected for inferior results in this uncontrolled, retrospective study. In a recent multi-institutional study evaluating the timing of residual or recurrent disease after ablative therapy to determine effective follow-up imaging regimens, Matin and colleagues[23] described a failure rate of 3.9% in patients undergoing cryoablation versus 13.4% in those undergoing RFA. However, most of the failures in percutaneous RFA occurred because of a conservative treatment strategy that favored retreatment rather than aggressive initial therapy.

Because of the absence of well-performed prospective studies, or at the least well-controlled retrospective studies, it would seem reasonable to conclude based on current available data that small, exophytic tumors can likely be treated efficaciously with either cryoablation or RFA. Any further statements regarding the superiority of one energy treatment over another require controlled prospective studies, with uniform patient selection and treatment application and with defined objective endpoints.

## Other Invasive Energy-Ablative Technologies

### Interstitial Laser Ablation or Thermotherapy

Laser light causes tissue destruction by heat. The amount of destruction depends on the power used and the length of treatment, whereas the penetration of light depends on the laser wavelength and tissue pigmentation. The initial report of this technology, published by de Jode and colleagues[81] in 1999, documented its use in three patients. A larger series, reported by the same group in 2002, described its use in nine high-risk patients who had undergone ablation with an neodymium-yittrium-argon laser under MRI guidance.[81,82] After nearly 17 months of follow-up, the lesions did not appear to have shrunk and enhancing tumor volume was decreased by a mean of only 45%.[83] Gettman and colleagues[84] described the use of laser ablation with and without hilar occlusion in an animal model. Viability staining showed the presence of viable cells in the treated zone.

There are many unknowns about the use of laser ablation in the treatment of renal tumors. Ideal wavelengths, power outputs, type of laser, duration of treatment, and size and type of fiber are parameters that have not been systematically studied. This is an experimental technology requiring additional information before it can be applied to patient care.

### Photodynamic Therapy

Whereas in heat-based laser treatment, thermal energy is used primarily for tissue ablation, photodynamic therapy (PDT) relies on a photochemical reaction that generates free radicals causing tissue injury via two interacting components: drug and light. The drug is an intravenously delivered photosensitizer. Laser light of a specific wavelength directed at the tumor activates the photosensitizer at a specific time interval after drug administration. This generates reactive oxygen species, primarily singlet oxygen, that causes mitochondrial, cellular, and microvascular damage.[85,86] The first-generation porphyrin-based photosensitizers had significant light absorption at 640 nm, this wavelength does not penetrate tissues well because of absorption by endogenous porphyrins. Other limitations include a long half-life and significant, prolonged skin phototoxicity.[87,88] Since this initial development, a variety of other photosensitizers have become available. To our knowledge, there is currently one published study evaluating PDT for treatment of renal tumors consisting of preclinical studies in an animal model using a novel vascular-targeted PDT.[89] This is still an experimental technology requiring further preclinical work before any clinical application.

### Microwave Thermotherapy

Microwaves are electromagnetic energy in the range of 30 to 30,000 MHz. Tissue absorbs the microwave energy, resulting in heat. For medical purposes, microwaves are applied by a probe puncture, similar to RFA, cryoablation, and laser therapies. Microwave thermotherapy was first described in 1998 for the clinical setting.[90–92] Since then, various reports, all from Japanese institutions, have described small cohorts of patients being treated with this technology, primarily as an adjunct to laparoscopic partial nephrectomy.[91,93–96] These limited data suggest that microwave thermotherapy has a coagulative effect and can result in reproducible necrosis. However, multiple parameters, including amount and timing of energy, probe configuration, and treatment monitoring remain unanswered. The role of microwaves as monotherapy with curative attempt for RCC is unknown; thus, in this regard, this technology is considered experimental.

## NONINVASIVE ENERGY-ABLATIVE THERAPIES

The ultimate promise of energy-ablative technology is the evolution to noninvasive therapy. Given the absence of a molecular marker for RCC and the uncertainty of diagnosis when excision is not performed, these novel technologies require greater understanding of the biology of RCC than is currently available. Thus, in addition to technical limitations, all the following described technologies require continued careful experimental evaluation.

### High-Intensity Focused Ultrasound

High-intensity focused ultrasound (HIFU) is delivered in the 1-MHz range. The use of HIFU was first described in the treatment of neoplastic tissue in 1975 and in the treatment of kidney tumors in 1991.[97,98] Similar to stone lithotripsy, ultrasonic frequencies are focused by reflectors at a specified distance and onto a single point. The focused ultrasound beam causes tissue destruction by coagulative necrosis at the focal zone and by mechanical tissue disruption.[99,100] The individual ellipsoid

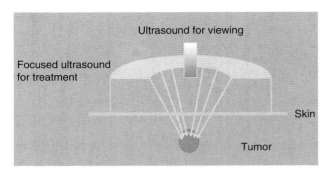

**Figure 2.** Schematic showing the concept of high-intensity focused ultrasound. Reproduced with permission from Copyright Matin SF2007.

lesions are quite small, ranging from 1 to 5 cm × 0.5 to 5 cm in size, and it takes about 4 seconds to generate each lesion, and many of these have to be generated. The kidney moves with respirations, limiting treatment-zone targeting and, because of bone and air (bowel) interference, also limiting access to the lesion. The side effects of this approach are generally low, with skin burns occurring in about 5% of patients and fever in up to 20% of patients.[101–104] General anesthesia is required for treatment. The HIFU unit allows for real-time imaging during treatment (Figure 2). Two units are currently available, one each from Storz Medical (Tuttlingen, Germany) and Chongqing HAIFU (Chongqing, China). Clinical experience with this technology is still quite limited. Most results show incomplete tumor destruction. Complete destruction has been reported in only up to 21% of cases, which is clearly not up to par with current standards.[101–105] Currently, this technology is deemed experimental.

### Radiation Therapy with CyberKnife

Radiation therapy plays a role in the palliative treatment of bony metastases from RCC as well as in the treatment of brain and spinal tumors.[106] Limitations on the application of radiation to the primary renal lesion include a relative radioresistance of RCC, the potential damage to surrounding bowel, and renal movement, which can make targeting difficult. Development of a unit that enables tracking of a mobile organ, such as the kidney, and delivery through multiple windows could avoid these limitations and potentially deliver lethally high doses to a small renal mass without damaging surrounding organs. The CyberKnife (Accuray,

Sunnyvale, CA, USA) is such a unit. CyberKnife is a frameless stereotactic radiation unit mounted on a robotic arm. Ponsky and colleagues[107] investigated the utility of this technology for treatment of renal tissue in a large animal model. Histologic evaluation has shown relative sparing of surrounding normal tissue with discrete necrosis in the area of treatment and a sharp demarcation from surrounding normal renal tissue. Because of these promising initial findings, a phase 1 clinical trial consisting of treatment followed by surgical resection is currently underway for this experimental therapy.

### CONCLUSIONS

RFA and cryoablation represent the two most mature and well-developed energy-ablative technologies for treatment of renal tumors. Either can be applied laparoscopically or percutaneously. The current available literature consists of limited data that does not convincingly prove the superiority of one approach over another. Instead, individual physician preferences, experience, personal comfort with a technology and technique, and institutional biases for a particular technology have been the key drivers. RFA and cryoablation are reasonable alternative options for well-informed patients who are at high-risk for standard surgical approaches. Noninvasive therapies are still experimental and require additional development before their incorporation into clinical care.

### REFERENCES

1. Lam JS, Belldegrun AS, Pantuck AJ. Long-term outcomes of the surgical management of renal cell carcinoma. World J Urol 2006.
2. Patard JJ, Shvarts O, Lam JS, et al. Safety and efficacy of partial nephrectomy for all T1 tumors based on an international multicenter experience. J Urol 2004;171:2181–5.
3. Wehle MJ, Thiel DD, Petrou SP, et al. Conservative management of incidental contrast-enhancing renal masses as safe alternative to invasive therapy. Urology 2004; 64:49–52.
4. Novick AC, Anderson CM, Campbell MF. Ranal Tumors. In: Campbell MF, editor. Campbell's Urology. Vol 8. Philadelphia: Saunders; 2002. p. 2672–731.
5. Gervais DA, McGovern FJ, Arellano RS, et al. Radiofrequency ablation of renal cell carcinoma: part 1, Indications, results, and role in patient management over a 6-year period and ablation of 100 tumors. AJR Am J Roentgenol 2005;185:64–71.

6. Wood BJ, Grippo J, Pavlovich CP. Percutaneous radio frequency ablation for hematuria. J Urol 2001;166:2303–4.

7. McLaughlin CA, Chen MY, Torti FM, et al. Radiofrequency ablation of isolated local recurrence of renal cell carcinoma after radical nephrectomy. AJR Am J Roentgenol 2003;181:93–4.

8. Ahrar K, Matin S, Wallace MJ, et al. Percutaneous transthoracic radiofrequency ablation of renal tumors using an iatrogenic pneumothorax. AJR Am J Roentgenol 2005;185:86–8.

9. Farrell MA, Charboneau JW, Callstrom MR, et al. Paranephric water instillation: a technique to prevent bowel injury during percutaneous renal radiofrequency ablation. AJR Am J Roentgenol 2003;181:1315–7.

10. Kariya S, Tanigawa N, Kojima H, et al. Radiofrequency ablation combined with CO2 injection for treatment of retroperitoneal tumor: protecting surrounding organs against thermal injury. AJR Am J Roentgenol 2005; 185:890–3.

11. Yamakado K, Nakatsuka A, Akeboshi M, Takeda K. Percutaneous radiofrequency ablation of liver neoplasms adjacent to the gastrointestinal tract after balloon catheter interposition. J Vasc Interv Radiol 2003;14:1183–6.

12. Bosniak MA, Birnbaum BA, Krinsky GA, Waisman J. Small renal parenchymal neoplasms: further observations on growth. Radiology 1995;197:589–97.

13. Beland MD, Mayo-Smith WW, Dupuy DE, et al. Diagnostic yield of 58 consecutive imaging-guided biopsies of solid renal masses: should we biopsy all that are indeterminate? AJR Am J Roentgenol 2007;188:792–7.

14. Tuncali K, vanSonnenberg E, Shankar S, et al. Evaluation of patients referred for percutaneous ablation of renal tumors: importance of a preprocedural diagnosis. AJR Am J Roentgenol 2004;183:575–82.

15. Mejean A, Oudard S, Thiounn N. Prognostic factors of renal cell carcinoma. J Urol 2003;169:821–7.

16. Gill IS, Novick AC, Meraney AM, et al. Laparoscopic renal cryoablation in 32 patients. Urology 2000;56:748–53.

17. Leyendecker JR, Dodd GD 3rd, Halff GA, et al. Sonographically observed echogenic response during intraoperative radiofrequency ablation of cirrhotic livers: pathologic correlation. AJR Am J Roentgenol 2002;178:1147–51.

18. Ahrar K, Matin S, Wood CG, et al. Percutaneous radiofrequency ablation of renal tumors: technique, complications, and outcomes. J Vasc Interv Radiol 2005;16:679–88.

19. Farrell MA, Charboneau WJ, DiMarco DS, et al. Imaging-guided radiofrequency ablation of solid renal tumors. AJR Am J Roentgenol 2003;180:1509–13.

20. Lewin JS, Nour SG, Connell CF, et al. Phase II clinical trial of interactive MR imaging-guided interstitial radiofrequency thermal ablation of primary kidney tumors: initial experience. Radiology 2004;232:835–45.

21. Gupta A, Allaf ME, Kavoussi LR, et al. Computerized tomography guided percutaneous renal cryoablation with the patient under conscious sedation: initial clinical experience. J Urol 2006;175:447–52;discussion 452–3.

22. Silverman SG, Tuncali K, vanSonnenberg E, et al. Renal tumors: MR imaging-guided percutaneous cryotherapy – initial experience in 23 patients. Radiology 2005;236:716–24.

23. Matin SF, Ahrar K, Cadeddu JA, et al. Residual and recurrent disease following renal energy ablative therapy: a multi-institutional study. J Urol 2006;176:1973–7.

24. Gervais DA, Arellano RS, McGovern FJ, et al. Radiofrequency ablation of renal cell carcinoma: part 2, Lessons learned with ablation of 100 tumors. AJR Am J Roentgenol 2005;185:72–80.

25. Gill IS, Remer EM, Hasan WA, et al. Renal cryoablation: outcome at 3 years. J Urol 2005;173:1903–7.

26. Sung GT, Gill IS, Hsu TH, et al. Effect of intentional cryo-injury to the renal collecting system. J Urol 2003; 170:619–22.

27. Shingleton WB, Farabaugh P, Hughson M, Sewell P. Effects of cryoablation on short-term development of urinary fistulas in the porcine kidney. J Endourol 2003; 17:37–40.

28. Janzen NK, Perry KT, Han KR, et al. The effects of intentional cryoablation and radio frequency ablation of renal tissue involving the collecting system in a porcine model. J Urol 2005;173:1368–74.

29. Warlick CA, Lima GC, Allaf ME, et al. Clinical sequelae of radiographic iceball involvement of collecting system during computed tomography-guided percutaneous renal tumor cryoablation. Urology 2006;67:918–22.

30. Lane BR, Moinzadeh A, Kaouk JH. Acute obstructive renal failure after laparoscopic cryoablation of multiple renal tumors in a solitary kidney. Urology 2005;????:65.

31. Jacobsohn KM, Ahrar K, Wood CG, Matin SF. Is radiofrequency ablation safe for solitary kidneys? Urology 2007 [in press].

32. Gage AA, Baust J. Mechanisms of tissue injury in cryosurgery. Cryobiology 1998;37:171–86.

33. Baust J, Gage AA, Ma H, Zhang CM. Minimally invasive cryosurgery—technological advances. Cryobiology 1997;34:373–84.

34. Campbell SC, Krishnamurthi V, Chow G, et al. Renal cryosurgery: experimental evaluation of treatment parameters. Urology 1998;52:29–33.

35. Chosy SG, Nakada SY, Lee FT Jr, Warner TF. Monitoring renal cryosurgery: predictors of tissue necrosis in swine. J Urol 1998;159:1370–4.

36. Tatsutani K, Rubinsky B, Onik G, Dahiya R. Effect of thermal variables on frozen human primary prostatic adenocarcinoma cells. Urology 1996;48:441–7.

37. Staren ED, Sabel MS, Gianakakis LM, et al. Cryosurgery of breast cancer. Arch Surg 1997;132:28–33.

38. Seifert JK, Zhao J, Ahkter J, et al. Cryoablation of human colorectal cancer in vivo in a nude mouse xenograft model. Cryobiology 1998;37:30–7.

39. Cestari A, Guazzoni G, dell'Acqua V, et al. Laparoscopic cryoablation of solid renal masses: intermediate term followup. J Urol 2004;172:1267–70.

40. Davol PE, Fulmer BR, Rukstalis DB. Long-term results of cryoablation for renal cancer and complex renal masses. Urology 2006;68:2–6.

41. Hruby G, Reisiger K, Venkatesh R, et al. Comparison of laparoscopic partial nephrectomy and laparoscopic cryoablation for renal hilar tumors. Urology 2006;67:50–4.

42. Lee DI, McGinnis DE, Feld R, Strup SE. Retroperitoneal laparoscopic cryoablation of small renal tumors: intermediate results. Urology 2003;61:83–8.

43. Nadler RB, Kim SC, Rubenstein JN, et al. Laparoscopic renal cryosurgery: the Northwestern experience. J Urol 2003;170:1121–5.

44. O'Malley RL, Berger AD, Kanofsky JA, et al. A matched-cohort comparison of laparoscopic cryoablation and laparoscopic partial nephrectomy for treating renal masses. BJU Int 2007;99:395–8.

45. Rukstalis DB, Khorsandi M, Garcia FU, et al. Clinical experience with open renal cryoablation. Urology 2001;57:34–9.

46. Schwartz BF, Rewcastle JC, Powell T, et al. Cryoablation of small peripheral renal masses: a retrospective analysis. Urology 2006;68:14–8.

47. Gill IS, Remer EM, Hasan WA, et al. Renal cryoablation: outcome at 3 years. J Urol 2005;173:1903–7.

48. Lawatsch EJ, Langenstroer P, Byrd GF, et al. Intermediate results of laparoscopic cryoablation in 59 patients at the Medical College of Wisconsin. J Urol 2006;175:1225–9.

49. Littrup PJ, Ahmed A, Aoun HD, et al. CT-guided percutaneous cryotherapy of renal masses. J Vasc Interv Radiol 2007;18:383–92.

50. Shingleton WB, Sewell PE Jr. Percutaneous renal tumor cryoablation with magnetic resonance imaging guidance. J Urol 2001;165:773–6.

51. Bachmann A, Sulser T, Jayet C, et al. Retroperitoneoscopy-assisted cryoablation of renal tumors using multiple 1.5 mm ultrathin cryoprobes: a preliminary report. Eur Urol 2005;47:474–9.

52. Allaf ME, Varkarakis IM, Bhayani SB, et al. Pain control requirements for percutaneous ablation of renal tumors: cryoablation versus radiofrequency ablation—initial observations. Radiology 2005;237:366–70.

53. Nahum Goldberg S, Dupuy DE. Image-guided radiofrequency tumor ablation: challenges and opportunities—part I. J Vasc Interv Radiol 2001;12:1021–32.

54. Goldberg SN, Gazelle GS, Dawson SL, et al. Tissue ablation with radiofrequency: effect of probe size, gauge, duration, and temperature on lesion volume. Acad Radiol 1995;2:399–404.

55. Goldberg SN, Hahn PF, Tanabe KK, et al. Percutaneous radiofrequency tissue ablation: does perfusion-mediated tissue cooling limit coagulation necrosis? J Vasc Interv Radiol 1998;9:101–11.

56. Zlotta AR, Wildschutz T, Raviv G, et al. Radiofrequency interstitial tumor ablation (RITA) is a possible new modality for treatment of renal cancer: ex vivo and in vivo experience. J Endourol 1997;11:251–8.

57. McGovern FJ, Wood BJ, Goldberg SN, Mueller PR. Radio frequency ablation of renal cell carcinoma via image guided needle electrodes. J Urol 1999;161:599–600.

58. Clark TW, Malkowicz B, Stavropoulos SW, et al. Radiofrequency ablation of small renal cell carcinomas using multi-tined expandable electrodes: preliminary experience. J Vasc Interv Radiol 2006;17:513–9.

59. de Baere T, Kuoch V, Smayra T, et al. Radio frequency ablation of renal cell carcinoma: preliminary clinical experience. J Urol 2002;167:1961–4.

60. Mahnken AH, Rohde D, Brkovic D, et al. Percutaneous radiofrequency ablation of renal cell carcinoma: preliminary results. Acta Radiol 2005;46:208–14.

61. Mayo-Smith WW, Dupuy DE, Parikh PM, et al. Imaging-guided percutaneous radiofrequency ablation of solid renal masses: techniques and outcomes of 38 treatment sessions in 32 consecutive patients. AJR Am J Roentgenol 2003;180:1503–8.

62. Ogan K, Jacomides L, Dolmatch BL, et al. Percutaneous radiofrequency ablation of renal tumors: technique, limitations, and morbidity. Urology 2002;60:954–8.

63. Pavlovich CP, Walther MM, Choyke PL, et al. Percutaneous radio frequency ablation of small renal tumors:initial results. J Urol 2002;167:10–5.

64. Roy-Choudhury SH, Cast JE, Cooksey G, et al. Early experience with percutaneous radiofrequency ablation of small solid renal masses. AJR Am J Roentgenol 2003;180:1055–61.

65. Su LM, Jarrett TW, Chan DY, et al. Percutaneous computed tomography-guided radiofrequency ablation of renal masses in high surgical risk patients: preliminary results. Urology 2003;61:26–33.

66. Veltri A, De Fazio G, Malfitana V, et al. Percutaneous US-guided RF thermal ablation for malignant renal tumors: preliminary results in 13 patients. Eur Radiol 2004;14:2303–10.

67. Zagoria RJ, Hawkins AD, Clark PE, et al. Percutaneous CT-guided radiofrequency ablation of renal neoplasms: factors influencing success. AJR Am J Roentgenol 2004;183:201–7.

68. Varkarakis IM, Allaf ME, Inagaki T, et al. Percutaneous radio frequency ablation of renal masses: results at a 2-year mean followup. J Urol 2005;174:456–60;discussion 460.

69. McDougal WS, Gervais DA, McGovern FJ, Mueller PR. Long-term followup of patients with renal cell carcinoma treated with radio frequency ablation with curative intent. J Urol 2005;174:61–3.

70. Johnson DB, Saboorian MH, Duchene DA, et al. Nephrectomy after radiofrequency ablation-induced ureteropelvic junction obstruction: potential complication and long-term assessment of ablation adequacy. Urology 2003;62:351–2.

71. Johnson DB, Taylor GD, Lotan Y, et al. The effects of radio frequency ablation on renal function and blood pressure. J Urol 2003;170:2234–6.

72. Lotan Y, Cadeddu JA. A cost comparison of nephron-sparing surgical techniques for renal tumour. BJU Int 2005;95:1039–42.

73. Link RE, Permpongkosol S, Gupta A, et al. Cost analysis of open, laparoscopic, and percutaneous treatment options for nephron-sparing surgery. J Endourol 2006;20:782–9.

74. Michaels MJ, Rhee HK, Mourtzinos AP, et al. Incomplete renal tumor destruction using radio frequency interstitial ablation. J Urol 2002;168:2406–9;discussion 2409–10.

75. Rendon RA, Kachura JR, Sweet JM, et al. The uncertainty of radio frequency treatment of renal cell carcinoma: findings at immediate and delayed nephrectomy. J Urol 2002;167:1587–92.

76. Marcovich R, Aldana JP, Morgenstern N, et al. Optimal lesion assessment following acute radio frequency ablation of porcine kidney: cellular viability or histopathology? J Urol 2003;170:1370–4.

77. Corwin TS, Lindberg G, Traxer O, et al. Laparoscopic radiofrequency thermal ablation of renal tissue with and without hilar occlusion. J Urol 2001;166:281–4.

78. Margulis V, Matsumoto ED, Lindberg G, et al. Acute histologic effects of temperature-based radiofrequency ablation on renal tumor pathologic interpretation. Urology 2004;64:660–3.

79. Matlaga BR, Zagoria RJ, Woodruff RD, et al. Phase II trial of radio frequency ablation of renal cancer: evaluation of the kill zone. J Urol 2002;168:2401–5.

80. Hegarty NJ, Gill IS, Desai MM, et al. Probe-ablative nephron-sparing surgery: cryoablation versus radiofrequency ablation. Urology 2006;68:7–13.

81. de Jode MG, Vale JA, Gedroyc WM. MR-guided laser thermoablation of inoperable renal tumors in an open-configuration interventional MR scanner: preliminary clinical experience in three cases. J Magn Reson Imaging 1999;10:545–9.

82. Dick EA, Joarder R, De Jode MG, et al. Magnetic resonance imaging-guided laser thermal ablation of renal tumours. BJU Int 2002;90:814–22.

83. Dick EA, Wragg P, Joarder R, et al. Feasibility of abdomino-pelvic T1-weighted real-time thermal mapping of laser ablation. J Magn Reson Imaging 2003;17:197–205.

84. Gettman MT, Lotan Y, Lindberg G, et al. Laparoscopic interstitial laser coagulation of renal tissue with and without hilar occlusion in the porcine model. J Endourol 2002;16:565–70.

85. Agostinis P, Buytaert E, Breyssens H, Hendrickx N. Regulatory pathways in photodynamic therapy induced apoptosis. Photochem Photobiol Sci 2004;3:721–729.

86. Nieminen AL. Apoptosis and necrosis in health and disease: role of mitochondria. Int Rev Cytol 2003;224:29–55.

87. Brandis A, Mazor O, Neumark E, et al. Novel water-soluble bacteriochlorophyll derivatives for vascular-targeted photodynamic therapy:synthesis, solubility, phototoxicity and the effect of serum proteins. Photochem Photobiol 2005;81:983–993.

88. Mazor O, Brandis A, Plaks V, et al. WST11, A novel water-soluble bacteriochlorophyll derivative;cellular uptake, pharmacokinetics, biodistribution and vascular-targeted photodynamic activity using melanoma tumors as a model. Photochem Photobiol 2005;81:342–51.

89. Matin SF, Tinkey PT, Borne AT, et al. Pilot Trial of Vascular Targeted Photodynamic Therapy for Renal Tissue. J Urol 2008;180:338–342.

90. Kigure T, Harada T, Yuri Y, et al. Experimental study of microwave coagulation of a VX-2 carcinoma implanted in rabbit kidney. Int J Urol 1994;1:23–7.

91. Naito S, Nakashima M, Kimoto Y, et al. Application of microwave tissue coagulator in partial nephrectomy for renal cell carcinoma. J Urol 1998;159:960–2.

92. Muraki J, Cord J, Addonizio JC, et al. Application of microwave tissue coagulation in partial nephrectomy. Urology 1991;37:282–7.

93. Itoh K, Suzuki Y, Miuru M, et al. Posterior retroperitoneoscopic partial nephrectomy using microwave tissue coagulator for small renal tumors. J Endourol 2002;16:367–71.

94. Murota T, Kawakita M, Oguchi N, et al. Retroperitoneoscopic partial nephrectomy using microwave coagulation for small renal tumors. Eur Urol 2002;41:540–5.

95. Terai A, Ito N, Yoshimura K, et al. Laparoscopic partial nephrectomy using microwave tissue coagulator for small renal tumors: usefulness and complications. Eur Urol 2004;45:744–8.

96. Yoshimura K, Okubo K, Ichioka K, et al. Laparoscopic partial nephrectomy with a microwave tissue coagulator for small renal tumor. J Urol 2001;165:1893–6.

97. Vallancien G, Chartier-Kastler E, Chopin D, et al. Focussed extracorporeal pyrotherapy: experimental results. Eur Urol 1991;20:211–9.

98. Longo FW, Longo WE, Tomashefsky P, et al. Interaction of ultrasound with neoplastic tissue. Local effect on subcutaneously implanted Furth-Columbia rat Wilms' tumor. Urology 1975;6:631–4.

99. Rewcastle JC. High Intensity Focused Ultrasound for Prostate Cancer: A Review of the Scientific Foundation, Technology and Clinical Outcomes. Technology in Cancer Research and Treatment 5; 2006.

100. Marberger M, Schatzl G, Cranston D, Kennedy JE. Extracorporeal ablation of renal tumours with high-intensity focused ultrasound. BJU Int 2005;2:52–5.

101. Illing RO, Kennedy JE, Wu F, et al. The safety and feasibility of extracorporeal high-intensity focused ultrasound (HIFU) for the treatment of liver and kidney tumours in a Western population. Br J Cancer 2005;93:890–5.

102. Hacker A, Dinter D, Michel MS, Alken P. High-intensity focused ultrasound as a treatment option in renal cell carcinoma. Expert Rev Anticancer Ther 2005;5:1053–9.

103. Wu F, Wang ZB, Chen WZ, et al. Preliminary experience using high intensity focused ultrasound for the treatment of patients with advanced stage renal malignancy. J Urol 2003;170:2237–40.

104. Kohrmann KU, Michel MS, Gaa J, et al. High intensity focused ultrasound as noninvasive therapy for multilocal renal cell carcinoma: case study and review of the literature. J Urol 2002;167:2397–403.

105. Visioli AG, Rivens IH, ter Haar GR, et al. Preliminary results of a phase I dose escalation clinical trial using focused ultrasound in the treatment of localised tumours. Eur J Ultrasound 1999;9:11–8.

106. Goyal LK, Suh JH, Reddy CA, Barnett GH. The role of whole brain radiotherapy and stereotactic radiosurgery on brain metastases from renal cell carcinoma. Int J Radiat Oncol Biol Phys 2000;47:1007–12.

107. Ponsky LE, Crownover RL, Rosen MJ, et al. Initial evaluation of Cyberknife technology for extracorporeal renal tissue ablation. Urology 2003;61:498–501

# MANAGEMENT OF SMALL RENAL MASSES

## Partial Nephrectomy

### ANDREW C. NOVICK, MD

Renal cortical tumors account for about 3% of all solid neoplasms, with an incidence similar to that of all forms of leukemia combined.[1] The incidence of renal cell carcinoma (RCC) has risen by 2.3 to 4.3% each year during the last three decades, resulting in an estimated 38,890 new diagnoses and 12,840 deaths in 2006 in the United States alone.[1,2] RCC most commonly presents as a unilateral, sporadic tumor, but multifocal sporadic tumors can be present in between 3 and 25% of patients,[3–5] and an additional 1 to 2% of RCC can be attributed to known familial syndromes, such as von Hippel Lindau (VHL) disease.[6]

Wells first described the technique of partial nephrectomy for excision of a renal tumor in 1884, and Czerny was the first to treat a renal malignancy using partial nephrectomy in 1897. Excessive postoperative morbidity limited its application until the 1950s when Vermooten suggested that encapsulated, peripheral renal neoplasms could be removed with only a margin of normal parenchyma around the tumor. Robson and colleagues challenged the oncologic safety of this approach by reporting in 1969 that early ligation of the renal vasculature, removal of the perinephric fat, and excision of all regional lymph nodes reduced the risk of hematologic spread.[7] Robson's radical nephrectomy (RN), which involved excision of the affected kidney outside of its investing (Gerota's) fascia along with the perinephric fat and ipsilateral adrenal gland, was the

standard treatment for RCC for more than 50 years. RN is still the best treatment for larger tumors, which are more likely to invade the perinephric fat, adrenal gland, or other neighboring organs, and is the standard against which all the other treatments for RCC must be judged.

Although RCC used to be referred to as the *internist's* tumor, it may now be more appropriate to refer to it as the *radiologist's* tumor because more than 60% of renal tumors are detected incidentally on abdominal imaging obtained for various reasons. The small renal mass is, therefore, becoming an increasingly common clinical scenario, with a wide range of options for management. Incidentally detected tumors are often small, unlikely to metastasize, and amenable to treatment with partial nephrectomy.[8,9] Recent findings suggest that this approach is greatly underutilized in the United States because only 9.6% of patients with surgically treated renal tumors in a large nationwide hospital database underwent partial nephrectomy.[10]

## CURRENT INDICATIONS FOR PARTIAL NEPHRECTOMY

The increasing detection of small renal masses, advances in CT and MR imaging of the kidney, improved surgical technique and methods to prevent ischemic renal injury, better postoperative management including renal replacement therapy, and long-term cancer-free survival data, have stimulated the expanded usage of partial nephrectomy. Time has shown that open partial nephrectomy (OPN) can be performed safely, with low morbidity and high patient satisfaction, and provides outstanding oncologic and renal functional outcomes at 10 years and longer.[11–14]

Absolute indications for partial nephrectomy include conditions that would render the patient dialysis-dependent upon complete resection of tumor-bearing kidneys, that is, bilateral tumors or tumor in a solitary functioning kidney. Relative indications for partial nephrectomy include the presence of any condition that poses a current or future risk to renal function, such as calculus disease, renal artery stenosis, chronic pyelonephritis, ureteral reflux, or systemic diseases such as diabetes or hypertension. Elective partial nephrectomy is defined as treatment of a single, small (≤ 4 cm), clinically localized RCC in a patient with a normal contralateral kidney. Several reports have shown that partial nephrectomy provides equivalent oncologic and superior renal functional results to RN for these patients.[15–18]

The results of NSS have historically been reported to be less satisfactory in patients with larger (≥ 4 cm) or multiple localized RCCs, and RN has been the treatment of choice in such cases when the opposite kidney is normal.[19] However, recent data have suggested that partial nephrectomy can be performed safely for a single tumor up to 7 cm, and that elective partial nephrectomy may be a reasonable option for any patient with a clinical T1 tumor.[20–22] In one study, cancer-specific mortality occurred in 6.2 and 9.0% of patients with pT1b tumors treated with OPN ($n = 65$) or RN ($n = 576$), respectively.[21] In two other reports, Kaplan–Meier estimates of distant metastasis-free survival were 92 to 94% and 83% following OPN ($n = 91$ and 33) or RN ($n = 841$ and 66) at 5 years, respectively.[20,23] In a fourth report, only 4 of 69 (5.8%) patients undergoing OPN for a pT1b tumor developed distant metastases over a median follow-up interval of 5.8 years[22] In each of these studies, a survival advantage was observed with OPN; the most likely explanation for these findings is the bias inherent in selecting tumors amenable to partial nephrectomy. Expanding the indications for elective partial

nephrectomy to include 4 to 7 cm tumors, therefore, remains somewhat controversial because of the increased likelihood of micrometastases, multicentricity, and perioperative morbidity in patients with larger tumors.

The importance of elective partial nephrectomy is related to functional and quality of life advantages associated with preservation of renal tissue, even in the presence of a normal contralateral kidney. Studies from our center and others have reported that several quality of life parameters are enhanced with preservation of more functioning renal parenchyma.[24] Patients with reduced renal function are prone to develop hyperfiltration renal injury and renal insufficiency.[25] The risk of this problem is directly related to the amount of remaining renal tissue and it is a problem that develops over an extended period of several years. Histopathologically, focal segmental glomerular sclerosis is the hallmark of this lesion on renal biopsy. The clinical harbinger of this problem is proteinuria, which, when present, indicates the need for angiotensin-converting enzyme inhibitor therapy to mitigate progressive loss of renal function.[26]

Several studies have now shown that patients with RCC, who undergo an elective RN, are at increased risk of developing long-term loss of renal function, compared with those treated with partial nephrectomy.[18,27,28] In a recent study by Huang and colleagues, the renal functional outcomes of radical versus partial nephrectomy were reviewed in 662 patients with a single, small (≤ 4 cm) renal tumor, a normal serum creatinine level, and two apparently health kidneys. Interestingly, estimated glomerular filtration rate (EGFR) determinations indicated that 26% of these patients had preexisting renal dysfunction (EGFR < 60 mL/min/1.73 m$^2$). Three years following surgery, the probability of freedom from renal insufficiency (EGFR < 45 mL/min/1.73 m$^2$) was 95% in the partial nephrectomy group and only 64% in the RN group ($p < 0.001$).[28] Although no patient in this study has thus far required dialysis, other large population-based studies have documented that chronic kidney disease is significantly associated with increased risks of hospitalization, cardiovascular morbid events, and death.[29] These data highlight that, unlike live donor nephrectomy patients, patients with RCC have co-morbid problems that can impact long-term renal function; nephron-sparing surgery can mitigate adverse sequelae associated with chronic kidney disease in this setting.

## EVALUATION BEFORE PARTIAL NEPHRECTOMY

Complete evaluation of patients with suspected RCC must include a complete history and physical examination, urinalysis or urine dipstick to screen for hematuria and proteinuria, and laboratory evaluation, including complete blood count, complete metabolic panel, and coagulation factors. Radiographic evaluation, including chest radiograph and abdominal CT or MR imaging, can rule out locally advanced or metastatic disease and aid in surgical planning. Three-dimensional reconstruction of CT or MR images is routinely performed by radiologists at our Urological Institute before partial nephrectomy to accurately delineate the vascular anatomy and relation of the tumor to normal parenchyma. This 2 to 4 minute videotape is reviewed immediately before surgery; hence, the surgeon can anticipate the subtleties of the anatomy.

## OPN

### Operative Technique

It is almost always possible to perform OPN for suspected malignancy in situ by using an operative approach that optimizes exposure of the kidney and renal vasculature. At Cleveland Clinic, we generally perform an extraperitoneal flank incision through the bed of the eleventh or twelfth rib, and use a thoracoabdominal incision for very large, upper pole tumors. After the kidney is fully mobilized, the surgeon has excellent exposure of the peripheral renal vessels and can excise the tumor at skin level. The surgical exposure using an anterior subcostal transperitoneal incision is sub-optimal. Tumor excision can be performed using polar (apical or basilar) segmental excision, wedge resection, or transverse resection. Each technique requires adherence to the basic principles of early vascular control, avoidance of ischemic renal damage, complete tumor excision with free margins and a small surrounding rim of grossly normal parenchyma, precise closure of the collecting system, careful hemostasis, and closure or coverage of the renal defect with adjacent fat, fascia, peritoneum, or Oxycel. Although obtaining a negative surgical margin around the tumor is imperative, the width of this parenchymal margin does not affect the likelihood of recurrence.[30] Intraoperative ultrasound can be used to delineate tumor extension and is especially useful for completely intraparenchymal tumors. Animal models have shown that ischemic intervals longer than 30 minutes are associated with greater renal damage. In clinical practice, the use of hypothermia can reduce the surgical ischemic insult and allow the ischemic interval to be extended safely. In experienced hands, hypothermia has proven unnecessary because most OPN can be readily accomplished with warm ischemic intervals less than 20 to 30 minutes.

### Clinical Outcomes

OPN is the gold standard for nephron-sparing therapy because it is the technique with which the largest experience has been obtained and regarding which the longest follow-up data are available. Several groups have reported oncologic results following OPN for RCC at 5 or more years of follow-up.[11–18,31] A total of 84 (6.3%) distant and 43 (3.2%) local recurrences were detected when considering only the 1,336 patients in the largest series from each institution (Table 1). Oncologic outcomes for the subset of patients undergoing elective OPN are particularly outstanding, with cancer-specific survival rates at 10 years that range from 94.5 to 97%.[12,14] Fergany and colleagues provided data regarding 10-year outcomes in 107 patients who underwent OPN, many of whom had adverse clinical and pathologic features.[12] Preoperative renal insufficiency was present in 39% of patients and NSS was imperative in 90%.[12] Recurrence was more common in patients with systemic symptoms, larger tumors, and advanced pathologic tumor state; cancer-specific survival for the entire cohort was 88% at 5 years and 73% at 10 years.[12]

| | Reference | Number of Patients | Mean Tumor Size (cm) | Follow-up (months) | Survival | | Recurrence | |
|---|---|---|---|---|---|---|---|---|
| | | | | | Overall | Cancer-specific | Distant | Local |
| 5-year outcomes | Steinbach et al, 1995[31] | 110 | 3.3 | 51 | 94% | 98% | 3 (2.7%) | 3 (2.7%) |
| | Lerner et al, 1996[15] | 185 | 4.1 | 44 | 77% | 89% | 32 (17%) | 11 (5.9%) |
| | D'Armiento et al, 1997[16] | 19 | 3.3 | 70 | 95% | 95% | 1 (5%) | 0 (0%) |
| | Barbalias et al, 1999[39] | 41 | 3.5 | 59 | NA | 98% | 1 (2.5%) | 3 (7.3%) |
| | Belldegrun et al, 1999[40] | 146 | 3.6 | 57 | 86% | 93% | 8 (5.5%) | 4 (2.7%) |
| | Hafez et al, 1999[19] | 485 | 2.7 | 47 | 81% | 92% | 28 (5.8%) | 16 (3.2% |
| | Lee et al, 2000[17] | 79 | 2.5 | 40 | 86% | 96% | 3 (3.8%) | 0 (0%) |
| | Lau et al, 2000[18] | 164 | 3.3 | 41 | 91% | 98% | 3 (1.8%) | 5 (3.0%) |
| 10-year outcomes | Herr, 1999[11] | 70 | 3.0 | 120 | 93% | 97% | 2 (2.8%) | 1 (1.4%) |
| | Fergany et al, 2000[12] | 107 | 4.7 | 105 | 45% | 73% | 30 (28%) | 11 (10%) |
| | Fergany et al, 2006[13] | 400 | 4.2 | 44 | 77% | 82% | 69 (17%) | 38 (9.5%) |
| | Pahernik et al, 2006[14] | 381 | 3 | 81 | 69% | 97% | 11 (2.9%) | 9 (2.3%) |
| | **Summary (5-year data)** | **>1300** | **2.5 to 4.7** | **40 to 120** | **77 to 95%** | **89 to 98%** | **2 to 17%** | **0 to 10%** |

Table 1. ONCOLOGIC OUTCOMES OF OPEN PARTIAL NEPHRECTOMY

The most challenging patient candidates for partial nephrectomy are those with cancer in a solitary kidney because the risk of losing renal function is greatest in this setting. I recently reported a personal series of 400 patients who underwent OPN for localized RCC in a solitary kidney between 1980 and 2002.[13] Long-term preservation of renal function was achieved in 95% of these patients, and the 10-year cancer-specific survival rate was 82%. These data lend further support to the efficacy of OPN for RCC even in technically challenging and high-risk patients.

## Laparoscopic Partial Nephrectomy (LPN)

### Technique

LPN attempts to duplicate the surgical principles of OPN while offering the advantages of minimally invasive surgery, that is, decreased postoperative pain, shorter convalencence, and superior cosmesis. Because LPN was first reported in 1993, more than 1,500 patients have now undergone LPN worldwide. At our institution, LPN typically involves transient en bloc renal vascular control, tumor excision with cold scissors, sutured reconstruction of the pelvicaliceal system, and sutured hemostatic suture repair of the renal parenchymal defect over surgical bolsters, performed through either a transperitoneal or retroperitoneal approach.[32] Currently available laparoscopic instrumentation has enabled more reliable control of the renal hilum, without which progress during LPN can be greatly impaired, and the introduction of tissue sealants have resulted in decreased postoperative bleeding complications.[33] Even with such advances, LPN is a technique that demands significant laparoscopic surgical experience and expertise. Techniques to enable cold ischemia during LPN have not been widely embraced; LPN, therefore, requires the surgeon to complete a significant amount of intracorporeal suturing within the time constraints of a safe interval of warm ischemia.

Selection of cases appropriate for LPN should be made carefully considering the individual tumor, patient, and surgeon. In each surgical series, LPN has initially been performed for small (≤ 4 cm), peripheral tumors. With increasing experience, the indications for LPN have been expanded at certain centers to include patients with a centrally located tumor, larger tumor (> 4 cm), tumor abutting the renal hilum, or tumor in a solitary-functioning kidney.[34,35] Nevertheless, increasing depth of invasion, increasing size, proximity to the renal hilum, posterior location, and anomalous renal anatomy makes LPN more challenging. In patients with multiple tumors, impaired renal function, or tumor in a solitary kidney, OPN should be strongly considered because a longer period of warm ischemia in these high-risk patients may lead to greater renal ischemic injury.

| Table 2. ONCOLOGIC OUTCOMES OF LAPAROSCOPIC PARTIAL NEPHRECTOMY | | | | | | |
|---|---|---|---|---|---|---|
| Reference | Number of Patients | Number with RCC | Mean Tumor Size (cm) | Mean Follow-up (months) | Recurrence | Major Complications |
| Lane et al, 2007[36] | 56 | 39 | 2.9 | 68 | 1 local | 8 (14%) |
| Allaf et al, 2004[41] | 48 | 48 | 2.4 | 38 | 2 local | 11%* |
| Abukora et al, 2005[42] | 78 | 65 | 2.3 | 24 | 0 | 15 (19%) |
| Seifman et al, 2004[43] | 40 | 29 | 2.3 | 24 | 0 | 6 (15%) |
| Jeschke et al, 2001[44] | 51 | 38 | 2 | 34 | 0 | 5 (10%) |

*Reported percentage for first 223 cases in Line et al. J Urol 2205;173:1690–4.[45]

## Outcomes

The oncologic outcomes of LPN have been reported by several groups to be excellent at between 1- and 3-year follow-ups (Table 2). Outcomes 5 years after LPN have recently become available in a relatively small number of patients. Of the 56 patients followed at least 5 years after LPN, overall survival was 86% and RCC was present in 39 patients.[36] In these 39 patients, cancer-specific survival is 100% at 5 years, zero have distant metastases, and 1 (2.6%) has developed a de novo local recurrence.[35] In this series, no patient with normal baseline creatinine undergoing elective LPN developed renal insufficiency.[36] Clearly, while the published oncologic and renal functional outcomes of LPN are impressive, analysis of data from a greater number of patients with longer follow-up will be needed to clarify the oncologic efficacy of this approach in comparison with OPN and RN.

## COMPARISON OF OPEN (OPN) AND LPN

In a recent multicenter study, data regarding 1,800 consecutive OPN or LPN operations were collected prospectively or retrospectively in tumor registries at three large referral centers.[37] These centers include Cleveland Clinic, Mayo Clinic, and Johns Hopkins University. Inclusion criteria for this study comprised patients with a single, localized, and suspected sporadic RCC ($\leq$ 7 cm in size), who were treated with LPN or OPN between January 1998 and September 2005. The primary focus of the study was on perioperative parameters and early renal functional outcomes with the two techniques.

OPN was performed in 1,029 patients, and LPN was performed in 771 patients. Patients undergoing

OPN were a higher risk group as defined by a greater percentage presenting symptomatically with reduced performance status, impaired renal function, and tumor in a solitary kidney ($p < 0.0001$). More tumors in the OPN group were > 4 cm and centrally located ($p < 0.0001$), and more proved to be malignant (84 vs 72%, $p = 0.0003$).

On the basis of multivariable analysis, LPN was associated with shorter operative time (201 vs 266 minutes, $p < 0.0001$) and shorter hospital stay (3.3 vs 5.8 days, $p < 0.0001$). However, LPN was also associated with longer warm ischemia time (WIT) (31 vs 20 minutes, $p < 0.0001$) and more postoperative renal/urologic complications (9.2 vs 5.0%, $p = 0.0006$), particularly postoperative hemorrhage (4.7 vs 1.6%, $p = 0.0001$). More patients in the LPN group required a subsequent procedure compared with the OPN group (6.9 vs 3.5%, $p < 0.0001$). The odds of a postoperative renal/urologic complication, hemorrhage, or a subsequent procedure were 2.14, 3.52, and 3.05 times higher after LPN compared with OPN, respectively.

Renal functional outcomes were similar 3 months after LPN and OPN, with 97 and 99% of renal units retaining function. Loss of function in the operated kidney occurred in 16 patients from the LPN group (2.1%) and four patients from the OPN group (0.4%), which was not statistically significant. Three-year cancer-specific survival for patients with a single pT1N0M0 RCC was 99.3 and 99.2% after LPN and OPN, respectively; however, the median follow-up interval was only 1.4 years for patients in the LPN group.

In another recent study from the Cleveland Clinic,[38] we compared the postoperative and renal functional outcomes of patients undergoing OPN or LPN for tumor in a solitary-functioning kidney.

Between 1999 and 2006, 169 OPN and 30 LPN were performed for $\leq 7$ cm tumor in a solitary-functioning kidney. Data were collected in an IRB-approved registry; median follow-up was 2 years. Pre and postoperative glomerular filtration rates (GFR) were estimated by abbreviated MDRD equation. Postoperative dialysis was required acutely after one OPN (0.6%) and three LPN (10%, $p = 0.01$), and dialysis-dependent end-stage renal failure within 1 year occurred after one OPN (0.6%) and two LPN (6.6%, $p = 0.06$). In multivariate analysis, WIT was 9-minute longer ($p = 0.0001$) and the chance of postoperative complication was 2.54-fold higher ($p < 0.05$) with LPN. Longer WIT (> 20 minutes) and preoperative GFR were associated with poorer postoperative GFR in multivariate analysis.

The results of these studies suggest that LPN can achieve early renal functional outcome comparable with OPN when applied to select patients with a single renal tumor $\leq 7$ cm in size. LPN offers the advantages of shorter operative time, reduced hospital stay, and more rapid convalescence. However, LPN is associated with longer intraoperative ischemia time, more postoperative renal/urologic complications (particularly hemorrhage), and more frequent need for a subsequent procedure. OPN remains the preferred approach for more complicated renal tumors such as those that are larger, hilar/intrarenal in location, multicentric, and located within a solitary kidney.

## CONCLUSIONS

The incidence of small renal masses continues to rise worldwide. With the acceptance of elective partial nephrectomy for tumors > 4 cm and potentially for those < 7cm, the percentage of tumors that will be treated with this approach will continue to grow. OPN has become the standard-of-care for tumors amenable to local excision, with established 10-year oncologic and renal functional outcomes. LPN is now being offered at many centers, and 5-year outcomes are available in small subsets of treated patients. Urologists must be knowledgeable about the indications, limitations, and outcomes with each approach so that they can help patients to select the one that best fits the individual tumor, patient, and surgeon.

## REFERENCES

1. Jemal A, Siegel R, Ward E, et al. Cancer statistics, 2006. CA Cancer J Clin 2006;56:106–30.
2. Chow WH, Devesa SS, Warren JL, Fraumeni JF Jr. Rising incidence of renal cell cancer in the United States. JAMA 1999;281:1628–31.
3. Dimarco DS, Lohse CM, Zincke H, et al. Long-term survival of patients with unilateral sporadic multifocal renal cell carcinoma according to histologic subtype compared with patients with solitary tumors after radical nephrectomy. Urology 2004;64:462–7.
4. Lang H, Lindner V, Martin M, et al. Prognostic value of multifocality on progression and survival in localized renal cell carcinoma. Eur Urol 2004;45:749–53.
5. Richstone L, Scherr DS, Reuter VR, et al. Multifocal renal cortical tumors: frequency, associated clinicopathological features and impact on survival. J Urol 2004;171(2 Pt 1):615–20.
6. Cohen HT, McGovern FJ. Renal-cell carcinoma. N Engl J Med 2005;353:2477–90.
7. Robson CJ, Chruchill BM, Anderson W. The results of radical nephrectomy for renal cell carcinoma. J Urol 1969;101:297–301.
8. Frank I, Blute ML, Cheville JC, et al. Solid renal tumors: an analysis of pathological features related to tumor size. J Urol 2003;170(6 Pt 1):2217–20.
9. Patard JJ, Dorey FJ, Cindolo L, et al. Symptoms as well as tumor size provide prognostic information on patients with localized renal tumors. J Urol 2004;172(6, Part 1 of 2):2167–71.
10. Hollenbeck BK, Taub DA, Miller DC, et al. National utilization trends of partial nephrectomy for renal cell carcinoma: a case of underutilization? Urology 2006;67:254–9.
11. Herr HW. Partial nephrectomy for unilateral renal carcinoma and a normal contralateral kidney: 10-year follow-up. J Urol 1999;161:33–4;discussion 34–5.
12. Fergany AF, Hafez KS, Novick AC. Long-term results of nephron sparing surgery for localized renal cell carcinoma: 10-year follow-up. J Urol 2000;163:442–5.
13. Fergany AF, Saad IR, Woo L, Novick AC. Open partial nephrectomy for tumor in a solitary kidney: experience with 400 cases. J Urol 2006 discussion 1633;175:1630–3.
14. Pahernik S, Roos F, Hampel C, et al. Nephron sparing surgery for renal cell carcinoma with normal contralateral kidney: 25 years of experience. J Urol 2006;175:2027–31.
15. Lerner SE, Hawkins CA, Blute ML, et al. Disease outcome in patients with low stage renal cell carcinoma treated with nephron-sparing or radical surgery. J Urol 1996;155:1868–73.
16. D'Armiento M, Damiano R, Feleppa B, et al. Elective conservative surgery for renal carcinoma versus radical nephrectomy: a prospective study. Br J Urol 1997;79:15–9.
17. Lee CT, Katz J, Shi W, et al. Surgical management of renal tumors 4 cm or less in a contemporary cohort. J Urol 2000;163:730–6.
18. Lau WK, Blute ML, Weaver AL, et al. Matched comparison of radical nephrectomy vs. nephron-sparing surgery in patients with unilateral renal cell carcinoma and a normal contralateral kidney. Mayo Clin Proc 2000;75:236–1242.

19. Hafez KS, Fergany AF, Novick AC. Nephron sparing surgery for localized renal cell carcinoma: impact of tumor size on patient survival, tumor recurrence and TNM staging. J Urol 1999;162:1930–3.

20. Leibovich BC, Blute ML, Cheville JC, et al. Nephron sparing surgery for appropriately selected renal cell carcinoma between 4 and 7 cm results in outcome similar to radical nephrectomy. J Urol 2004;171:1066–70.

21. Patard JJ, Shvarts O, Lam JS, et al. Safety and efficacy of partial nephrectomy for all T1 tumors based on an international multicenter experience. J Urol 2004;171(6 Pt 1): 2181–5, quiz 2435.

22. Becker F, Siemer S, Hack M, et al. Excellent long-term cancer control with elective nephron-sparing surgery for selected renal cell carcinomas measuring more than 4 cm. Eur Urol 2006;49:1058–63;discussion 1063–4.

23. Mitchell RE, Gilbert SM, Murphy AM, et al. Partial nephrectomy and radical nephrectomy offer similar cancer outcomes in renal cortical tumors 4 cm or larger. Urology 2006;67:260–4.

24. Clark P, Schover L, Uzzo R, et al. Quality of life and psychological adaptation following surgical treatment for localized renal cell carcinoma: impact of the amount of remaining renal tissue. Urol 2001;57:252.

25. Novick AC, Gephardt G, Guz B, et al. Long-term follow- up after partial removal of a solitary kidney. NEJM 1991;11058–1062.

26. Novick AC, Schreiber MJ. The effect of angiotensin-converting-enzyme inhibition on nephropathy in patients with a remnant kidney. Urol 1995;46:785.

27. McKienan J, Simmons R, Katz J, Russo P. Natural history of chronic renal insufficiency after partial and radical nephrectomy. Urol 2002;59:816–20.

28. Huang WC, Levey AS, Serio AM, et al. Chronic kidney disease after nephrectomy in patients with renal cortical tumors: a retrospective cohort study. Lancet Oncol 2006; 7:735–40.

29. Go AS, Chertow GM, Fan D, et al. Chronic kidney disease and the risks of death, cardiovascular events, and hospitalization. NEJM 2004:351:1296–305.

30. Castilla EA, Liou LS, Abrahams NA, et al. Prognostic importance of resection margin width after nephron-sparing surgery for renal cell carcinoma. Urology 2002; 60:993–7.

31. Steinbach F, Stockle M, Hohenfellner R. Clinical experience with nephron-sparing surgery in the presence of a normal contralateral kidney. Semin Urol Oncol 1995;13:288–91.

32. Gill IS, Desai MM, Kaouk JH, et al. Laparoscopic partial nephrectomy for renal tumor: duplicating open surgical techniques. J Urol 2002;167(2 Pt 1):469–7;discussion 475–6.

33. Gill IS, Ramani AP, Spaliviero M, et al. Improved hemostasis during laparoscopic partial nephrectomy using gelatin matrix thrombin sealant. Urology 2005;65:463–6.

34. Frank I, Colombo JR Jr, Rubinstein M, et al. Laparoscopic partial nephrectomy for centrally located renal tumors. J Urol 2006;175(3 Pt 1):849–52.

35. Gill IS, Colombo JR Jr, Frank I, et al. Laparoscopic partial nephrectomy for hilar tumors. J Urol 2005;174:850–3; discussion 853–4.

36. Lane BR, Gill IS. Five year outcomes of laparoscopic partial nephrectomy. J Urol 2007;177:70–4.

37. Gill I, Kavoussi L, Lane B, et al. Comparison of 1800 laparoscopic and open partial nephrectomies for single renal tumors. J Urology [in press].

38. Lane B, Novick AC, Babineau D, et al. Comparison of laparoscopic and open partial nephrectomy for tumor in solitary kidney. J Urology [in press].

39. Barbalias GA, Liatsikos EN, Tsintavis A, Nikiforidis G. Adenocarcinoma of the kidney: nephron-sparing surgical approach vs radical nephrectomy. J Surg Oncol 1999;72:156–61.

40. Belldegrun A, Tsui KH, deKernion JB, Smith RB. Efficacy of nephron-sparing surgery for renal cell carcinoma: analysis based on the new 1997 tumor-node-metastasis staging system. J Clin Oncol 1999;17:2868–75.

41. Allaf ME, Bhayani SB, Rogers C, et al. Laparoscopic partial nephrectomy: evaluation of long-term oncological outcome. J Urol 2004;172:871–3.

42. Abukora F, Nambirajan T, Albqami N, et al. Laparoscopic nephron sparing surgery: evolution in a decade. Eur Urol 2005;47:488–93;discussion 493.

43. Seifman BD, Hollenbeck BK, Wolf JS Jr. Laparoscopic nephron-sparing surgery for a renal mass: 1-year minimum follow-up. J Endourol 2004;18:783–6.

44. Jeschke K, Peschel R, Wakonig J, et al. Laparoscopic nephron-sparing surgery for renal tumors. Urology 2001;58:688–92.

45. Link RE, Bhayani SB, Allaf ME, et al. Exploring the learning curve, pathological outcomes and perioperative morbidity of laparoscopic partial nephrectomy performed for renal mass. J Urol 2005;173:1690–4.

# 7

# Prognostic Factors in Localized Renal Cell Carcinoma

**BRIAN SHUCH, MD**
**ALLAN PANTUCK, MD, MS, FACS**
**ARIE BELLDEGRUN, MD, FACS**

A variety of clinical and pathologic factors are known to be prognostic markers of tumor progression and influence cancer-specific survival in renal cell carcinoma (RCC). Traditional prognostic factors such as tumor size, grade, and histological features are associated with RCC behavior. Clinical presentation and baseline laboratory studies also play a role in determining outcome. Advancements in molecular biology and genetics have provided insight into the genetic alterations and molecular pathways involved in renal cell carcinogenesis. Many of these molecular changes appear to influence prognosis. Besides providing better understanding of the disease, knowledge of the molecular changes may lead to the development of new therapeutic modalities.

In this chapter, the current prognostic factors important to localized RCC will be summarized, and attention will be given to new markers that may be important to future prognostic models and therapeutic modalities.

## ANATOMICAL FACTORS

### T Stage

Tumor staging provides a common language to stratify patient's disease according to the size of the primary tumor and the degree of distant spread.

Staging is important to renal cell carcinoma, as it helps treatment planning, is useful to estimate prognosis, and serves as the primary basis for clinical trial planning (Figure 1). The American Joint Committee on Cancer (AJCC) determines staging in renal cell carcinoma by the tumor node metastasis (TNM) classification system. The combination of TMN variables is used to stratify patients into four separate tumor stages (I–IV).

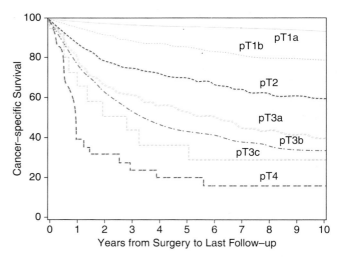

**Figure 1.** Cancer-specific survival based on the 2002 American Joint Committee on Cancer primary tumor classification from 2,746 patients with renal cell carcinoma. Adapted from Frank I et al.[3]

## T1a versus T1b

The lowest T stage encompasses organ-confined tumors less than 7 cm in size. However, even with organ-confined tumors, tumor size appears to be an important prognostic factor. The current concept of distinguishing T1 tumors by size came from analysis of which tumors are amenable to a partial nephrectomy. Several studies demonstrated tumors larger than 4 cm had worse outcome than smaller tumors.[1,2] These findings led to the revision of T1 tumors in the 2002 AJCC TMN system into two subdivisions, T1a (≤ 4 cm) and T1b (> 4 cm). The T1 criteria previously had been reserved for tumors 7.0 cm or less in the 1997 AJCC TMN classification and tumors 2.5 cm or less in the 1987 version. Regardless of the type of therapy, the 5-year cancer-specific survival rates based on the 2002 AJCC TMN system is excellent with T1a and T1b tumors demonstrating survival of 97% and 87%, respectively.[3]

The optimal size cutoff for T1 and T2 tumors is still debated by different centers though there is a uniform agreement that the current 7-cm cutoff is too high. Several groups have reported improved stratification with values anywhere from 4.5 to 5.5 cm, depending on the institution.[4–6] In many of these studies, the survival of patients above the cutoff was similar to T2 patients, therefore, it may be better to simply lower the T1/T2 cutoff rather than to continue a T1a/T1b subclassification.

## T2

The TMN classification system for T2 tumors was changed in 1997 to include tumors greater than 7.0 cm. The T2 tumors demonstrate worse outcome compared with T1 tumors with a 5-year cancer-specific survival of 71%.[7] Similar to what was seen subdividing by size in T1 tumors, Frank and colleagues[8] further improved upon the prognostic accuracy demonstrating T2 tumors larger than 10 cm behave more aggressively than those of 7.0 to 10.0 cm. The 5-year cancer-specific survival for tumors larger than 10.0 cm is 64.1 versus 77.1% for those 7.0 to 10.0 cm. Lam and colleagues[9] determined that tumor size cutoff of 13 cm could also discriniate outcome. For patients with T2 tumors of 13 cm or greater, the 5-year disease-specific survival was

77% compared with 82% for tumors less than 13 cm in size.[9] Both studies suggest creating T2a and T2b subclasses to reflect these findings.

## T3: Tumor Extension and Adrenal Involvement

The 5-year cancer-specific survival for T3 tumors has been shown to be 37 to 53%.[3,7] This broad category includes various clinical situations that involve regional tumor extension.

T3a classification includes tumors that have adrenal involvement or extend into the perinephric fat but not beyond Gerota's fascia. The 5-year cancer-specific mortality for T3a tumors is 36 to 44%.[3,10] Recent data question the prognostic accuracy of including adrenal involvement into the T3a tumor classification. Han and colleagues[10] reported a 12.5 month median survival of patients with direct adrenal extension compared to 36 months for patients with perinephric fat and no adrenal involvement.[10] Tumors with adrenal involvement from direct extension appear to have similar outcome to patients with T4 disease.[10–12] No study has directly evaluated the prognostic significance of ipsilateral adrenal involvement due to direct invasion compared to those that have spread hematogenously.

### Perinephric Fat Involvement

T3a tumors with perirenal fat involvement may have an improved outcome compared to their counterparts with adrenal extension; however, the mortality of this group is significantly worse than those with T2 disease. The presence of fat involvement appears to almost double the risk of death from RCC.[13] In analyzing patients with T3b disease with renal vein (RV) involvement, Leibovich[13] demonstrated that patients with concomitant perinephric fat invasion have worse prognosis. This prompted the recommendation of altering the T3b category to incorporate perinephric fat involvement in the setting of simultaneous venous involvement.

### Venous Involvement

Renal tumors commonly invade into the renal vein and lead to more extensive tumor thrombus in 4 to

9% of newly diagnosed patients with RCC.[14,15] Whether the extent, as opposed to the presence, of tumor thrombus affects overall survival has been a controversial topic. Currently, the 2002 TMN system distinguishes T3b (RV involvement and inferior vena cava [IVC] involvement below diaphragm) from T3c (IVC involvement above diaphragm). Kim and colleagues[14] evaluated 226 patients who underwent radical nephrectomy and RV or IVC tumor thrombectomy to determine how the level of tumor thrombus impacted prognosis.[14] For localized tumors, the 3-year cancer-specific survival with tumor thrombus in the RV, IVC below the diaphragm, and IVC above the diaphragm was 76, 63, and 23%, respectively. On multivariate analysis, patients with RV and IVC involvement below the diaphragm had similar cancer-specific survival. Moinzadeh and Blute both published data that demonstrated that tumor thrombus contained within the RV has improved survival versus all levels of IVC involvement.[15,16]

Moinzadeh and Blute both proposed different classifications than the current T3b and T3c definitions. Consensus has not been reached on which of the current classification systems are most useful at stratifying patients. Larger cohorts of patients will need to be analyzed to determine a more accurate subclassification system to be incorporated into the next AJCC TMN revision.

## Lymph Node Involvement

Performing a regional lymphadenectomy during a nephrectomy can accurately stage localized disease. The risk of lymph node metastasis is dependent on the extent of the disease. For small, localized tumors, the risk of lymph metastasis is small, ranging from 2 to 9%. In the setting of metastatic disease, the presence of lymph node metastasis can approach 50%.[17] The presence of lymph node status has a significant impact on overall outcome with a 5-year disease-specific survival of 11 to 35%.[18–20]

The most recent edition of the TMN classification system distinguished nodal involvement based on the number of lymph nodes involved (pN0 = 0, pN1 = 1, pN2 = 2 or more involved nodes). This system classifies nodal status after a formal lymphadenectomy of eight lymph nodes or more as analysis of a limited number of nodes can lead to understaging. Whether patients with pN1 and pN2 disease have a statistical difference in overall survival is uncertain. If pN2 disease demonstrates worse survival, it will be important to assess the method of lymph node dissection as surgeons may perform a more extensive lymphadenectomy in the setting of more advanced disease.[21]

Terrone and colleagues[22] analyzed patients undergoing open radical nephrectomy and lymph node dissection and determined the five-year disease-specific survival with and without pN+ disease was 18% versus 74.4%.[22] Analysis of patients with positive lymph nodes demonstrated that a cutoff of four positive nodes might impact survival rather than the current system. The concept of lymph node density was also analyzed in this subset. A lymph node density of less than 60% doubled the risk of death and was an independent predictor of survival.[22]

Canfield and colleagues[23] at the M.D. Anderson Cancer Center recently presented data that supports the current subclassification system. In their analysis of 40 patients who underwent nephrectomy for M0N+ disease, 12 and 28 patients had N1 and N2 diseases. The patients with N2 disease had a significantly decreased rate of disease-free recurrence and overall survival (Figure 2).[23]

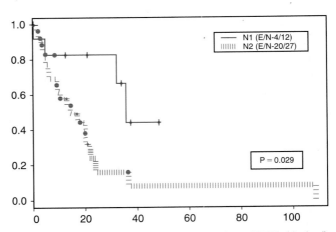

**Figure 2.** Overall survival on M0N1 (solid) vs M0N2 (dashed). Patients with N1 disease have improved survival compared to patients with N2 disease. Adapted from Canfield SE et al.[23]

## TUMOR HISTOLOGY

The histological examination of renal neoplasms was the only adjunct to anatomical information for most of the past century. The cellular classification of subtypes has evolved over that past two decades. Although some older designations have fallen out of favor, other histologic findings have been further characterized and are now believed independent predictors of outcome. The RCC is now best understood as a blanket term to describe all malignant epithelial neoplasms arising from the renal parenchyma. The current classification system was established by the International Union Against Cancer and the AJCC and divides subtypes by histologic appearance and cellular origin.[24]

Whether different histologic variants of RCC display different clinical behaviors remain unclear. The Mayo Clinic demonstrated a 5-year cancer-specific survival of 68.9% for clear cell RCC, 87.4% for papillary RCC, and 86.9% for chromophobe RCC. Clear cell RCC had a worse outcome when controlling for TMN stage and Fuhrman grade, whereas no difference in outcome was noted between papillary and chromophobe RCC.[25] More recent studies have questioned these findings. Patard and colleagues[26] published the results from a large international multicenter study that demonstrated histologic subtype was not an independent predictor of survival (Figure 3).

Papillary RCC has recently been divided into two types (I and II) based on its histologic appearance. Delahunt and colleagues[27] have demonstrated that type II is an independent predictor of poor outcome.

Two additional subtypes arise from the collecting duct rather than the convoluted tubule. Collecting duct carcinoma is a rare variant with very poor outcome.[28] Renal medullary carcinoma, a subgroup of collecting duct carcinoma, is found most frequently in black men with sickle cell trait or disease and also has a poor prognosis.

## TUMOR GRADE

The Fuhrman grading system is the most commonly used grading system for RCC. This system stratifies tumors based on nuclear morphology, including

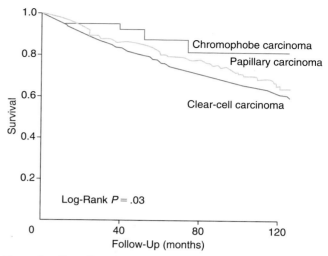

**Figure 3.** Overall survival in 3,056 patients with localized renal cell carcinoma according to histologic sub-type. Controlling for other independent predictors of outcome, histologic sub-type does not appear to be an independent predictor of outcome. Adapted from Patard JJ et al.[26]

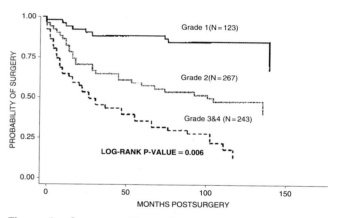

**Figure 4.** Cancer-specific survival based on Fuhrman grade demonstrates worse outcome for high-grade tumors. Adapted from Tsui KH et al.[7]

nuclear and nucleolar size, shape, and content.[29] The Fuhrman nuclear grade correlates with tumor stage, size, metastases, lymph node involvement, renal vein involvement, and perirenal fat involvement.[30]

The role of grade in prognosis has been extensively studied. Tsui and colleagues confirmed the prognostic role of tumor grade in outcome. Fuhrman grade and TMN stage proved to be the most important prognostic factors. The 5-year cancer-specific survival rates for grades 1, 2, and grade 3 or grade 4 are 89, 65, and 46.1%, respectively (Figure 4).[7] Stratifying the groups by stage, low-grade tumors have improved survival compared to high-grade tumors.

Several additional studies have demonstrated that each Fuhrman grade demonstrates an increased risk of disease-specific survival.[31,32] However, each subgroup stratified by Fuhrman grade may not be an independent predictor of survival. Recently, Gudbjartsson and colleagues[32] demonstrated that controlling for other prognostic factors, only Fuhrman grade 4 demonstrated a worse outcome than grades 1 to 3. Similar findings increase the concern over a four-tiered classification system. Lang and colleagues[33] recently recommended collapsing the grading system into a two-tier system.

## TUMOR NECROSIS

Tumor necrosis is a histologic feature believed to be associated with tumor aggressiveness, resulting from rapid tumor enlargement with outgrowth of blood supply. The presence of tumor necrosis is associated with variables such as TMN stage, tumor size, and Fuhrman grade.[34] Its histological presence is an independent predictor of poor outcome in clear cell but not in papillary RCC.[35] Lam and colleagues[34] analyzed the presence of tumor necrosis in both localized and metastatic tumors and determined that its presence is an independent predictor of survival only for localized RCC. Frank and colleagues[36] demonstrated a strong association with risk of death (4.5 times) in clear cell carcinoma and incorporated this finding into an outcome prediction model (SSIGN).

## MICROVASCULAR INVASION

Microvascular invasion is defined as the presence of neoplastic cells in tumor microvessels. The presence of microvascular invasion is known to influence disease recurrence in other genitourinary malignancies such as prostate cancer.[37] As tumor cells are directly accessible to the vasculature, hematologic shedding may allow distant metastasis. The incidence of microvascular invasion in RCC has been estimated to be 25 to 28%.[38,39] It was previously believed that microvascular invasion did not play a prognostic role in RCC; however, recent data suggest otherwise.

Van Poppel and colleagues[38] analyzed a cohort of 180 patients who undergone nephrectomy for localized RCC and demonstrated that microvascular invasion was the most important independent prognostic factor in disease-free survival.[38] Recently, Goncalves [39] confirmed microvascular invasion is an independent predictor of both recurrence and cancer-specific survival and is associated with poor prognostic features, such as tumor size, perirenal fat invasion, Fuhrman grade, lymph node involvement, and sarcomatoid features. Microvascular invasion has been incorporated into a new prognostic nomogram.[40]

## PRESENCE OF SARCOMATOID FEATURES

Farrow and colleagues[41] published the first report of sarcomatoid RCC in 1968 describing it as a unique RCC variant, which contained highly pleomorphic spindle cells. Sarcomatoid features are now considered a high grade form of RCC that may be present in association with any histological subtype, rather than a distinct histologic subtype.[42] Sarcomatoid features are found in less than 5% of RCC.[43] Frequently, these tumors are locally advanced and have metastases at diagnosis.[43] Cangiano and colleagues[43] demonstrated one and two year overall survival was 48 and 34%, respectively. Moch and colleagues[35] demonstrated that sarcomatoid characteristics were an independent predictor of poor outcome for clear cell and papillary RCC, however, it may have a greater prognostic value in papillary subtypes.

The percentage of tumor with sarcomatoid features may influence prognosis, with tumors displaying greater than 5% having worse prognosis.[44] However, several studies have failed to demonstrate a benefit in stratifying the tumor by percentage of sarcomatoid involvement.[43,45]

### Collecting System Involvement

The overall incidence of collecting system involvement is 14%; however, for localized T1 and T2 tumors, this is an infrequent occurrence (3%).[46] Tumors with collecting system involvement have more frequent hematuria, higher T classification, higher Fuhrman grade, positive lymph nodes, and metastatic disease.[47] Uzzo[46] demonstrated that for T1 and T2 tumors only, collecting system involvement was associated with poor prognosis. Palapattu and colleagues[48] confirmed this finding, and also demonstrated that T3 collecting system invasion was associated with a worse survival. A recent study by Terrone and colleagues[47] questioned the impact of collecting system involvement on prognosis. Collecting system invasion did not appear to be an independent predictor of outcome.

## LABORATORY ANALYSIS

### Erythrocyte Sedimentation Rate

The ESR is elevated in 83% of patients with metastatic RCC.[49] Sengupta and colleagues[50] analyzed preoperative values in patients with localized and metastatic disease. Elevated ESR was found to be an independent risk factor for death due to clear cell RCC. More data are needed to evaluate whether ESR is an independent risk factor for localized tumors only.

### C-reactive Protein

C-reactive protein is a nonspecific protein marker of inflammation if elevated after cytoreductive nephrectomy is a marker of poor outcome.[51] For patients with localized RCC, elevated C-reactive protein may also be a marker of poor outcome. Komai and colleagues[52] recently published a cohort of patients with clinically localized disease. Elevated CRP was an independent predictor of poor outcome and more than doubled the risk of recurrence and disease-free survival.[52]

### Thrombocytosis

The presence of thrombocytosis (platelets > 400,000/mm³) is an independent predictor of poor outcome in patients with metastatic RCC.[53] For localized RCC, thrombocytosis may also indicate a more aggressive disease. Gogus and colleagues[54] discovered that thrombocytosis increased with T stage and its presence had a worse disease-specific survival. Bensalah and colleagues[55] found thrombocytosis was associated with larger tumor size, worse the Eastern Cooperative Oncology Group performance scale (ECOG-PS), T stage, Fuhrman grade, lymph node invasion, and distant metastasis. For patients with localized disease, thrombocytosis was strong predictor of worse cancer-specific survival.[55]

Whether thrombocytosis is directly responsible for worse prognostic features or the end result of tumor-mediated inflammatory mechanisms is unclear. Platelet-derived growth factor (PDGF) is an important mechanism in the hypoxia cascade. It is possible that increased production of PDGF could promote tumor growth and lead to a more aggressive phenotype.

## CLINICAL FACTORS

### Incidental Versus Symptomatic Tumors

The widespread use of computed tomography and magnetic resonance imaging scans has greatly altered the presentation of RCC. In 1971, only 7% of tumors were discovered incidentally.[56] Most contemporary series demonstrate that between 40 to 60% of renal tumors are discovered prior to the development of symptoms.[57–59] With more tumors being detected incidentally, RCC has experienced an expected stage migration to smaller and more frequently organ-confined tumors. Tsui and colleagues[7] reported incidental tumors are of smaller size and have lower stage and grade. Thompson and colleagues[59] demonstrated that 87% of incidentally discovered tumors are clinical stage I.

Tumors that present incidentally may represent more indolent disease and have been shown to influence disease-specific survival. The overall 5-year disease-specific survival of incidental tumors is 60 to 92% compared to 40 to 69% for symptomatic tumors.[7, 57–59] Whether the mode of presentation is an independent predictor of outcome is debated in the literature. Several studies have demonstrated no difference in survival when controlling for stage.[36] In contrast to these findings, both Lee and Ficarra published data that demonstrated that mode of presentation was a strong and independent predictor of outcome (Figure 5).[57,58] On the basis of these findings, both the groups recommended inclusion of mode of presentation into future prognostic nomograms.

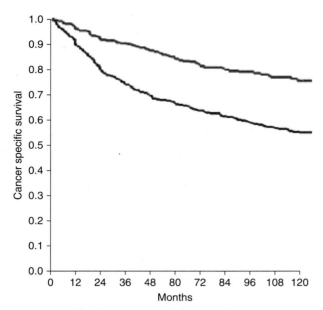

**Figure 5.** Cancer-specific survival for incidental (red) versus symptomatic (blue) localized renal cell carcinoma. While incidental tumors demonstrate improved outcome, there is still a debate whether mode of detection is an independent predictor of outcome. Adapted from Ficarra VT et al[58].

## Performance Status

The ECOG-PS is a scale used to assess the impact of disease on a patient's overall health with higher scores signifying worse status. The Karnofsky scale is a similar system used to stratify patients. The ECOG-PS is an independent prognostic factor of survival in patients with metastatic RCC.[60] As such, clinical trials have incorporated low ECOG-PS score into the inclusion criteria for interleukin-2 based therapy.[61]

The value of ECOG-PS in localized RCC is uncertain. Tsui and colleagues[7] evaluated the role of ECOG-PS in all stages of RCC and found that worse performance status was an independent predictor of poor outcome (Figure 6). Frank and colleagues[36] reviewed patients with all stages of RCC. In their analysis, they evaluated the role of ECOG-PS and another clinical performance scale, the Charlson score. Although they found a significant association with risk of death, neither method proved to be an independent predictor of cancer-specific survival.

## Cachexia-related Symptoms

Kim and colleagues examined patients with localized and metastatic RCC and identified a collection of symptoms termed cachexia-related findings. Presence of these features includes: (1) hypoalbuminemia, (2) weight loss, (3) anorexia, and (4) malaise. These features were independent predictors of a poor prognosis.[62] For localized disease, cachexia is presumably related to the paraneoplastic effects of the primary tumor. Kim and colleagues later analyzed a cohort of 250 patients with localized T1 tumors. The overall incidence of cachexia-related findings was 14.8%.[63] The presence of cachexia-related findings in the setting of localized disease was an independent predictor of worse progression-free survival and disease-specific survival.

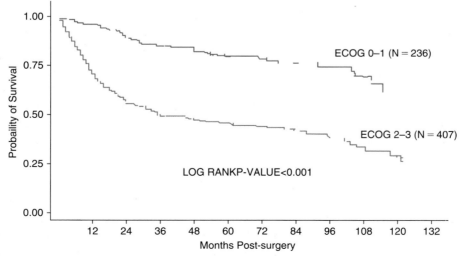

**Figure 6.** Cancer-specific survival for Eastern Cooperative Oncology Group performance scale demonstrates that patients with worse performance status have decreased survival. Adapted from Tsui KH et al[7].

## COMPREHENSIVE INTEGRATED PREDICTION MODELS

Counseling a patient regarding RCC can be challenging due to the complex interaction of multiple factors that influence disease recurrence and survival. Several models have been designed to integrate the anatomic, histologic, and clinical prognostic factors into outcome models. In addition, these prognostic models can identify those at greatest risk of recurrence for selection into adjuvant trials.

### Kattan Nomogram

Recent models have focused on patients with localized disease undergoing radical nephrectomy for RCC. The Kattan nomogram was established to predict the probability of tumor recurrence within five years after surgery. Clinical information including TMN stage, histology, tumor size, and the presence of symptoms for patients with clinically localized RCC were modeled into a nomogram and statistically validated.[64] In a recent study, the nomogram did not accurately predict DFS.[65] A new version of nomogram proposed by Sorbellini and colleagues[40] included tumor size, T classification, symptoms, grade, necrosis, and vascular invasion. The nomogram demonstrated better predictive accuracy, and the authors believed it was an improvement in their previous prognostic model.[40]

### SSIGN score

The Mayo Clinic established a combined outcome model for both localized and metastatic clear cell RCC. In this cohort, TNM stage, tumor size of 5 cm or greater, nuclear grade, and histologic tumor necrosis were all found to be independent predictors of poor survival.[36] These characteristics were assigned a score and incorporated into a scoring algorithm, the SSIGN score. Decreased survival was shown to correlate with increased SSIGN score.

### UCLA Integrated Staging System (UISS)

UCLA designed a prognostic system, the UISS, to predict survival in all histologic subtypes in both localized and metastatic RCC. The UISS contained low-risk, intermediate-risk, and high-risk groups

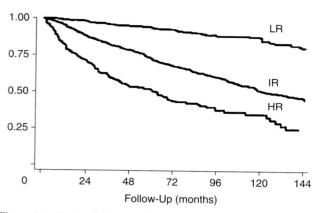

**Figure 7.** Kaplan–Meier survival estimates for 3,119 patients with localized renal cell carcinoma according to the UISS. Adapted from Patard JJ et al.[69]

based on TNM stage, Fuhrman grade, and ECOG-PS (Table 1).[66–68] The UISS was later validated in a large, multicenter, international study consisting of 4,202 patients.[69] For localized RCC, the five-year survival rate for low-risk, intermediate-risk, and high-risk patients was 92, 67, and 44%, respectively (Figure 7).

### Model Validation

A recent multicenter retrospective study attempted to externally validate each prognostic model in patients with localized RCC previously treated with nephrectomy. The patients were assessed with various models including the initial Kattan nomogram, the Yaycioglu model, the Cindolo model, and the UISS.[70] This study validated the ability of each of the models to distinguish groups with different outcome. The postoperative models (the Kattan nomogram and the UISS) appeared to better predict outcome compared with preoperative models (Yaycioglu and Cindolo models). For patients with localized RCC, both the Kattan nomogram and the UISS worked well, and the authors concluded "both models are most likely the same on practical grounds".[70]

## MOLECULAR MARKERS

Tissue and gene-array based technology allows the simultaneous characterization of thousands of genes and proteins in RCC. There are several molecular markers of importance in RCC prognosis, including hypoxia-inducible factors, cell-cycle regulators, mediators of cellular proliferation, cellular adhesion

**Table 1. ASSIGNMENT OF N0M0 PATIENTS POSTNEPHRECTOMY INTO RISK GROUPS ACCORDING TO AJCC T STAGE, FUHRMAN GRADE, AND ECOG PERFORMANCE SCALE**

| T Stage | 1 | | | 2 | 3 | | | | 4 |
|---|---|---|---|---|---|---|---|---|---|
| Grade | 1–2 | 3–4 | | ↓ | 1 | | > 1 | | ↓ |
| ECOG-PS | 0  ≥ 1 | 0  ≥ 1 | | | 0  ≥ 1 | | 0  ≥ 1 | | ↓ |
| Risk | Low | | | Intermediate | | | | | high |

Adapted from Zisman A et al.[67]

AJCC = American Joint Committee on Cancer; ECOG-PS = Eastern Cooperative Oncology Group performance scale.

molecules, and a wide variety of other molecules. We will briefly review several known prognostic markers for localized RCC.

## Hypoxia Inducible Pathway

Hypoxia inducible factors (HIFs) regulate the production of genes such as vascular endothelial growth factor (*VEGF*), *PDGF*, carbonic anhydrase IX (*CAIX*), and transforming growth factor alpha (*TGF-A*).[71,72] Its role in determining prognosis was recently examined in both metastatic and localized tumors.[73] HIF1a is differentially expressed between histological subtypes with clear cell displaying greater expression than either papillary or chromophobe RCC. For clear cell RCC, decreased HIF1a expression was an independent predictor of poor survival.

## Carbonic Anhydrase IX

CA IX is a member of the carbonic anhydrase family that regulates intracellular and extracellular pH during periods of hypoxia. Bui and colleagues[74] reported that 94% of clear cell RCC tumor samples stained positive for CA IX. Low CA IX staining was found to be an independent prognostic indicator of poor survival in patients with metastatic RCC. For patients with advanced nodal disease, decreased expression of CAIX can also predict worse survival; however, survival was not influenced in patients with localized disease.[74,75]

## VHL Status

A function of the VHL protein is to mark HIF1a and HIF2a for proteosomal degradation and to down regulate the hypoxia-induced pathway. The *VHL* gene was identified as the gene associated with von Hippel Lindau disease and sporadic clear cell RCC.[76,77]

Yao and colleagues[78] explored the prognostic capability of *VHL* alterations. The *VHL* alterations were determined to be independent predictors of improved progression-free survival and disease-specific survival for patients with Stage I-III RCC.[78] Parker and colleagues re-examined the association of VHL with prognosis. Immunohistochemistry, was performed on tumor specimens from patients with clear cell RCC. The VHL expression was not associated with any known prognostic factor including tumor size, stage, grade, lymph node involvement, and the presence of metastasis. VHL expression did not alter cancer-specific survival; however, when adjusting for SSIGN score and age, T1 and T2 tumors with no VHL expression were associated with a decreased risk of death (hazard ratio = 0.4). Why the loss of a tumor suppressor gene would lead to improved outcome for localized tumors is unclear at this time. It is possible that tumors that develop in the absence of VHL alterations do so in the setting of nontraditional molecular pathways that convey worse prognosis and outcome.

## REGULATORS OF CELL CYCLE AND APOPTOSIS

### TP53

*TP53* is a tumor suppressor gene, which has been coined the "guardian of the genome." The product of this gene plays a vital role in regulating the cell cycle and inducing apoptosis when DNA damage occurs.[79] Mutant forms of *TP53* have extended half-lives leading to accumulation and detection by immunohistochemical staining.[80] *TP53* expression is found in 16 to 57% of renal tumors and varies with histologic type.[80–82] Shvarts and colleagues[82] examined the prognostic role of *TP53* overexpression in localized RCC. *TP53* staining was found in 57.5% of tumors, and its expression correlated with tumor grade and was an independent predictor of recurrence. The prognostic potential of *TP53* was confirmed by Kim and colleagues[83] who incorporated it into a combined molecular and clinical prognostic model.

### p21

*p21* is an important tumor suppressor gene that plays an important role in cell-cycle control. *p21* is able to induce cell-cycle arrest by inhibiting the cyclin/cyclin-dependent kinases 2 regulation of the G1-S cell-cycle checkpoint.[84] In addition, *p21* has an important role in activation of the apoptotic pathway, and it expression is regulated by the tumor suppressor gene *TP53*.[85]

Based on the important cell regulatory and survival aspects of *p21*, several investigators have tried to correlate *p21* expression to prognosis. Haitel and colleagues[86] analyzed nuclear staining of *p21* in clear cell RCC. Nuclear staining of *p21* was observed in nearly all cases. *p21* staining was correlated to related expression of cell-cycle regulators *p27* and pRb, both of which proved to be independent predictors of outcome. However, *p21* positivity was not related to either grade or stage and did not correlate with outcome.[86] Weiss and colleagues[87] recently reported the results of an immunohistochemical analysis of a tissue array containing 366 patients with RCC. Nuclear *p21* expression was more frequently observed in aggressive renal tumors, such as collecting duct carcinoma, and less frequently in oncocytomas. In localized disease, higher levels of nuclear *p21* was strongly associated with a better prognosis (hazard ratio = 0.27).[87]

### p27

*p27* is an important cell-cycle regulator that regulates proliferation in the G1/S checkpoint by modulating the action of cyclin-dependent kinases. Migita and colleagues[88] examined the role of *p27* alterations in clear cell RCC. Decreased *p27* expression was associated with larger tumor size

and was an independent predictor of poor disease-specific survival.[88] Hedberg and colleagues[89] assessed *p27* in a larger cohort including all histologic subtypes. Low levels of *p27* were associated with higher tumor grade and larger size. Again, decreased levels of *p27* were found to be an independent predictor of worse disease-specific survival.[89]

## Cellular Adhesion Molecules

### Epithelial Cell Adhesion Molecule

A wide variety of cellular adhesion molecules have been studied in RCC and may affect prognosis. Decreased expression of adhesion molecules are believed to play a role in the acquisition of invasive characteristics. Seligson and colleagues[90] examined the role of EpCAM. The EpCAM is seen in normal renal epithelium, however, its expression is frequently absent in clear cell carcinoma. Expression of EpCAM was an independent predictor of improved disease-specific survival in localized RCC.[90]

### EphA2

EphA2 is a different cellular adhesion molecule that may have implications in RCC. Overexpression of EphA2 has been shown to disrupt cell-cell contacts and is believed to promote invasive characteristics of tumor cells.[91] Herrem and colleagues[92] examined EphA2 expression in nephrectomy specimens with clinically localized disease. Higher levels of EphA2 were associated with larger tumor size and higher grade, and overexpression was predictive of disease-free recurrence and overall survival.[92]

## FUTURE OF MOLECULAR PROGNOSTIC MODELS

The next generation of prognostic models will incorporate the molecular biology and genetics of RCC. Once specific genetic alterations are identified that correlate with clinical prognosis, these markers will be incorporated into new, more accurate models of RCC. Incorporation of this information into future staging systems will revolutionize the way the disease process is understood. Kim and colleagues[83] began this process developing a prognostic model for survival in patients with metastatic clear cell RCC.[83] Using molecular and clinical predictors, this model was significantly more accurate than the clinical predictions alone.

## CONCLUSIONS

RCC is a complex disease comprising a family of epithelial tumors that displays a wide variety of clinical behavior. A variety of anatomic, histologic, laboratory, clinical, and molecular markers of disease aggressiveness can be used to understand the disease and to predict disease aggressiveness. By using these prognostic factors that influence outcome, patients can be better counseled regarding their disease risk, surveillance strategies can be better tailored to risk of recurrence, and high-risk patients can be better identified for adjuvant trials.

## REFERENCES

1. Hafez KS, Fergany AF, Novick AC. Nephron sparing surgery for localized renal cell carcinoma: impact of tumor size on patient survival, tumor recurrence and TNM staging. J Urol 1999;162:1930–33.
2. Lerner SE, Hawkins CA, Blute ML, et al. Disease outcome in patients with low stage renal cell carcinoma treated with nephron sparing or radical surgery. J Urol 1996;155:1868–73.
3. Frank I, Blute ML, Leibovich BC, et al. Independent validation of the 2002 American Joint Committee on cancer primary tumor classification for renal cell carcinoma using a large, single institution cohort. J Urol 2005;173:1889–92.
4. Zisman A, Pantuck AJ, Chao D, et al. Reevaluation of the 1997 TNM classification for renal cell carcinoma: T1 and T2 cutoff point at 4.5 rather than 7 cm. better correlates with clinical outcome. J Urol 2001;166:54–58.
5. Cheville JC, Blute ML, Zincke H, et al. Stage pT1 conventional (clear cell) renal cell carcinmoa: pathological features associated with cancer specific survival. J Urol 2001;166:453–56.
6. Ficarra V, Guille F, Schips L, et al. Proposal for revision of the TNM classification system for renal cell carcinoma. Cancer 2005;104:2116–23.
7. Tsui KH, Shvarts O, Smith RB, et al. Renal cell carcinoma: prognostic significance of incidentally detected tumors. J Urol 2000;163:426–30.
8. Frank I, Blute ML, Leibovich BC, et al. pT2 classification for renal cell carcinoma. Can its accuracy be improved? J Urol 2005;173:380–4.
9. Lam JS, Patard JJ, Goel RH, et al. Can pT2 classification for renal cell carcinoma be improved? An international multicenter experience. In. AUA Abstract. 2006;740.
10. Han KR, Bui MH, Pantuck AJ, et al. TNM T3a renal cell carcinoma: adrenal gland involvement is not the same as renal

fat invasion. J Urol 2003;169:899–903;discussion 903–894.
11. Thompson RH, Cheville JC, Lohse CM, et al. Reclassification of patients with pT3 and pT4 renal cell carcinoma improves prognostic accuracy. Cancer 2005;104:53–60.
12. Thompson RH, Leibovich BC, Cheville JC, et al. Should direct ipsilateral adrenal invasion from renal cell carcinoma be classified as pT3a? J Urol 2005;173:918–21.
13. Leibovich BC, Cheville JC, Lohse CM, et al. Cancer specific survival for patients with pT3 renal cell carcinoma-can the 2002 primary tumor classification be improved? J Urol 2005;173:716–19.
14. Kim HL, Zisman A, Han KR, et al. Prognostic significance of venous thrombus in renal cell carcinoma. Are renal vein and inferior vena cava involvement different? J Urol 2004;171(2 Pt 1):588–91.
15. Moinzadeh A, Libertino JA. Prognostic significance of tumor thrombus level in patients with renal cell carcinoma and venous tumor thrombus extension. Is all T3b the same? J Urol 2004;171(2 Pt 1):598–601.
16. Blute ML, Leibovich BC, Lohse CM, et al. The Mayo Clinic experience with surgical management, complications and outcome for patients with renal cell carcinoma and venous tumour thrombus. BJU Int 2004;94:33–41.
17. Pantuck AJ, Zisman A, Dorey F, et al. Renal cell carcinoma with retroperitoneal lymph nodes. Impact on survival and benefits of immunotherapy. Cancer 2003;97:2995–3002.
18. Vasselli JR, Yang JC, Linehan WM, et al. Lack of retroperitoneal lymphadenopathy predicts survival of patients with metastatic renal cell carcinoma. J Urol 2001;166:68–72.
19. Waters WB, Richie JP. Aggressive surgical approach to renal cell carcinoma: review of 130 cases. J Urol 1979;122:306–9.
20. Pantuck AJ, Zisman A, Dorey F, et al. Renal cell carcinoma with retroperitoneal lymph nodes: role of lymph node dissection. J Urol 2003;169:2076–83.
21. Joslyn SA, Sirintrapun SJ, Konety BR. Impact of lymphadenectomy and nodal burden in renal cell carcinoma: retrospective analysis of the National Surveillance, Epidemiology, and End Results database. Urology 2005;65:675–80.
22. Terrone C, Cracco C, Porpiglia F, et al. Reassessing the current TNM lymph node staging for renal cell carcinoma. Eur Urol 2006;49:324–31.
23. Canfield SE, Kamat AM, Sanchez-Ortiz RF, et al. Renal cell carcinoma with nodal metastases in the absence of distant metastatic disease (clinical stage TxN1-2M0): the impact of aggressive surgical resection on patient outcome. J Urol 2006;175(3 Pt 1):864–9.
24. Storkel S, Eble JN, Adlakha K, et al. Classification of renal cell carcinoma: Workgroup No. 1. Union Internationale Contre le Cancer (UICC) and the American Joint Committee on Cancer (AJCC). Cancer 1997;80:987–9.
25. Cheville JC, Lohse CM, Zincke H, et al. Comparisons of outcome and prognostic features among histologic subtypes of renal cell carcinoma. Am J Surg Pathol 2003;27:612–24.
26. Patard JJ, Leray E, Rioux-Leclercq N, et al. Prognostic value of histologic subtypes in renal cell carcinoma: a multicenter experience. J Clin Oncol 2005;23:2763–71.
27. Delahunt B, Eble JN, McCredie MR, et al. Morphologic typing of papillary renal cell carcinoma: comparison of

growth kinetics and patient survival in 66 cases. Hum Pathol 2001;32:590–5.

28. Chao D, Zisman A, Pantuck AJ, et al. Collecting duct renal cell carcinoma: clinical study of a rare tumor. J Urol 2002; 167:71–4.

29. Fuhrman SA, Lasky LC, Limas C. Prognostic significance of morphologic parameters in renal cell carcinoma. Am J Surg Pathol 1982;6:655–63.

30. Bretheau D, Lechevallier E, de Fromont M, et al. Prognostic value of nuclear grade of renal cell carcinoma. Cancer 1995;76:2543–9.

31. Tsui KH, Shvarts O, Smith RB, et al. Prognostic indicators for renal cell carcinoma: a multivariate analysis of 643 patients using the revised 1997 TNM staging criteria. J Urol 2000;163:1090–5;quiz 1295.

32. Gudbjartsson T, Hardarson S, Petursdottir V, et al. Histological subtyping and nuclear grading of renal cell carcinoma and their implications for survival: a retrospective nation-wide study of 629 patients. Eur Urol 2005; 48:593–600.

33. Lang H, Lindner V, de Fromont M, et al. Multicenter determination of optimal interobserver agreement using the Fuhrman grading system for renal cell carcinoma: Assessment of 241 patients with > 15-year follow-up. Cancer 2005;103:625–9.

34. Lam JS, Shvarts O, Said JW, et al. Clinicopathologic and molecular correlations of necrosis in the primary tumor of patients with renal cell carcinoma. Cancer 2005;103:2517–25.

35. Moch H, Gasser T, Amin MB, et al. Prognostic utility of the recently recommended histologic classification and revised TNM staging system of renal cell carcinoma: a Swiss experience with 588 tumors. Cancer 2000;89:604–14.

36. Frank I, Blute ML, Cheville JC, et al. An outcome prediction model for patients with clear cell renal cell carcinoma treated with radical nephrectomy based on tumor stage, size, grade and necrosis: the SSIGN score. J Urol 2002; 168:2395–400.

37. de la Taille A, Rubin MA, Buttyan R, et al. Is microvascular invasion on radical prostatectomy specimens a useful predictor of PSA recurrence for prostate cancer patients? Eur Urol 2000;38:79–84.

38. Van Poppel H, Vandendriessche H, Boel K, et al. Microscopic vascular invasion is the most relevant prognosticator after radical nephrectomy for clinically nonmetastatic renal cell carcinoma. J Urol 1997;158:45–49.

39. Goncalves PD, Srougi M, Dall'lio MF, et al. Low clinical stage renal cell carcinoma: relevance of microvascular tumor invasion as a prognostic parameter. J Urol 2004; 172:470–4.

40. Sorbellini M, Kattan MW, Snyder ME, et al. A postoperative prognostic nomogram predicting recurrence for patients with conventional clear cell renal cell carcinoma. J Urol 2005;173:48–51.

41. Farrow GM, Harrison EG Jr, Utz DC. Sarcomas and sarcomatoid and mixed malignant tumors of the kidney in adults. 3. Cancer 1968;22:556–63.

42. Goldstein NS. The current state of renal cell carcinoma grading. Union Internationale Contre le Cancer (UICC) and the American Joint Committee on Cancer (AJCC). Cancer 1997;80:977–80.

43. Cangiano T, Liao J, Naitoh J, et al. Sarcomatoid renal cell carcinoma: biologic behavior, prognosis, and response to combined surgical resection and immunotherapy. J Clin Oncol 1999;17:523–8.

44. Bertoni F, Ferri C, Benati A, et al. Sarcomatoid carcinoma of the kidney. J Urol 1987;137:25–28.

45. de Peralta-Venturina M, Moch H, Amin M, et al. Sarcomatoid differentiation in renal cell carcinoma: a study of 101 cases. Am J Surg Pathol 2001;25:275–84.

46. Uzzo RG, Cherullo EE, Myles J, Novick AC. Renal cell carcinoma invading the urinary collecting system: implications for staging. J Urol 2002;167:2392–6.

47. Terrone C, Cracco C, Guercio S, et al. Prognostic value of the involvement of the urinary collecting system in renal cell carcinoma. Eur Urol 2004;46:472–6.

48. Palapattu GS, Pantuck AJ, Dorey F, et al. Collecting system invasion in renal cell carcinoma: impact on prognosis and future staging strategies. J Urol 2003;170:768–72;discussion 772.

49. Casamassima A, Picciariello M, Quaranta M, et al. C-reactive protein: a biomarker of survival in patients with metastatic renal cell carcinoma treated with subcutaneous interleukin-2 based immunotherapy. J Urol 2005; 173:52–55.

50. Sengupta S, Lohse CM, Leibovich BC, et al. Histologic coagulative tumor necrosis as a prognostic indicator of renal cell carcinoma aggressiveness. Cancer 2005; 104:511–20.

51. Fujikawa K, Matsui Y, Oka H, et al. Serum C-reactive protein level and the impact of cytoreductive surgery in patients with metastatic renal cell carcinoma. J Urol 1999;162:1934–7.

52. Komai Y, Saito K, Sakai K, Morimoto S. Increased preoperative serum C-reactive protein level predicts a poor prognosis in patients with localized renal cell carcinoma. BJU Int 2006.

53. Symbas NP, Townsend MF, El-Galley R, et al. Poor prognosis associated with thrombocytosis in patients with renal cell carcinoma. BJU Int 2000;86:203–7.

54. Gogus C, Baltaci S, Filiz E, et al. Significance of thrombocytosis for determining prognosis in patients with localized renal cell carcinoma. Urology 2004;63:447–50.

55. Bensalah K, Leray E, Fergelot P, et al. Prognostic value of thrombocytosis in renal cell carcinoma. J Urol 2006;175 (3 Pt 1):859–63.

56. Skinner DG, Colvin RB, Vermillion CD, et al. Diagnosis and management of renal cell carcinoma. A clinical and pathologic study of 309 cases. Cancer 1971;28:1165–7.

57. Lee CT, Katz J, Fearn PA, Russo P. Mode of presentation of renal cell carcinoma provides prognostic information. Urol Oncol 2002;7:135–40.

58. Ficarra V, Prayer-Galetti T, Novella G, et al. Incidental detection beyond pathological factors as prognostic predictor of renal cell carcinoma. Eur Urol 2003;43:663–9.

59. Thompson IM, Peek M. Improvement in survival of patients with renal cell carcinoma—the role of the serendipitously detected tumor. J Urol 1988;140:487–90.

60. Mani S, Todd MB, Katz K, Poo WJ. Prognostic factors for survival in patients with metastatic renal cancer treated with biological response modifiers. J Urol 1995;154:35–40.

61. Fallick ML, McDermott DF, LaRock D, et al. Nephrectomy before interleukin-2 therapy for patients with metastatic renal cell carcinoma. J Urol 1997;158:1691–5.

62. Kim HL, Belldegrun AS, Freitas DG, et al. Paraneoplastic signs and symptoms of renal cell carcinoma: implications for prognosis. J Urol 2003;170:1742–6.

63. Kim HL, Han KR, Zisman A, et al. Cachexia-like symptoms predict a worse prognosis in localized t1 renal cell carcinoma. J Urol 2004;171:1810–3.

64. Kattan MW, Reuter V, Motzer RJ, et al. A postoperative prognostic nomogram for renal cell carcinoma. J Urol 2001;166:63–67.

65. Hupertan V, Roupret M, Poisson JF, et al. Low predictive accuracy of the Kattan postoperative nomogram for renal cell carcinoma recurrence in a population of French patients. Cancer 2006;107:2604–8.

66. Han KR, Bleumer I, Pantuck AJ, et al. Validation of an integrated staging system toward improved prognostication of patients with localized renal cell carcinoma in an international population. J Urol 2003;170(6 Pt 1):2221–4.

67. Zisman A, Pantuck AJ, Wieder J, et al. Risk group assessment and clinical outcome algorithm to predict the natural history of patients with surgically resected renal cell carcinoma. J Clin Oncol 2002;20:4559–66.

68. Zisman A, Pantuck AJ, Figlin RA, Belldegrun AS. Validation of the UCLA integrated staging system for patients with renal cell carcinoma. J Clin Oncol 2001;19:3792–3.

69. Patard JJ, Kim HL, Lam JS, et al. Use of the University of California Los Angeles integrated staging system to predict survival in renal cell carcinoma: an international multicenter study. J Clin Oncol 2004;22:3316–22.

70. Cindolo L, Patard JJ, Chiodini P, et al. Comparison of predictive accuracy of four prognostic models for nonmetastatic renal cell carcinoma after nephrectomy: a multicenter European study. Cancer 2005;104:1362–71.

71. Pantuck AJ, Zeng G, Belldegrun AS, Figlin RA. Pathobiology, prognosis, and targeted therapy for renal cell carcinoma: exploiting the hypoxia-induced pathway. Clin Cancer Res 2003;9:4641–52.

72. Linehan WM. Molecular targeting of VHL gene pathway in clear cell kidney cancer. J Urol 2003;170(2 Pt 1):593–4.

73. Lidgren A, Hedberg Y, Grankvist K, Rasmuson T, Vasko J, Ljungberg B. The expression of hypoxia-inducible factor 1alpha is a favorable independent prognostic factor in renal cell carcinoma. Clin Cancer Res 2005;11:1129–35.

74. Bui MH, Seligson D, Han KR, Pantuck AJ, Dorey FJ, Huang Y, et al. Carbonic anhydrase IX is an independent predictor of survival in advanced renal clear cell carcinoma: implications for prognosis and therapy. Clin Cancer Res 2003;9:802–11.

75. Bui MH, Visapaa H, Seligson D, Kim H, Han KR, Huang Y, et al. Prognostic value of carbonic anhydrase IX and KI67 as predictors of survival for renal clear cell carcinoma. J Urol 2004;171(6 Pt 1):2461–66.

76. Latif F, Tory K, Gnarra J, Yao M, Duh FM, Orcutt ML, et al. Identification of the von Hippel-Lindau disease tumor suppressor gene. Science 1993;260:1317–20.

77. Gnarra JR, Tory K, Weng Y, Schmidt L, Wei MH, Li H, et al. Mutations of the VHL tumour suppressor gene in renal carcinoma. Nat Genet 1994;7:85–90.

78. Yao M, Yoshida M, Kishida T, et al. VHL tumor suppressor gene alterations associated with good prognosis in sporadic clear-cell renal carcinoma. J Natl Cancer Inst 2002;94:1569–75.

79. Lane DP. Cancer p53, guardian of the genome. Nature 1992;358:15–16.

80. Zigeuner R, Ratschek M, Rehak P, et al. Value of p53 as a prognostic marker in histologic subtypes of renal cell carcinoma: a systematic analysis of primary and metastatic tumor tissue. Urology 2004;63:651–55.

81. Moch H, Sauter G, Gasser TC, et al. p53 protein expression but not mdm-2 protein expression is associated with rapid tumor cell proliferation and prognosis in renal cell carcinoma. Urol Res 1997;25 Suppl 1:S25–30.

82. Shvarts O, Seligson D, Lam J, et al. p53 is an independent predictor of tumor recurrence and progression after nephrectomy in patients with localized renal cell carcinoma. J Urol 2005;173:725–8.

83. Kim HL, Seligson D, Liu X, et al. Using tumor markers to predict the survival of patients with metastatic renal cell carcinoma. J Urol 2005;173:1496–501.

84. Brugarolas J, Moberg K, Boyd SD, et al. Inhibition of cyclin-dependent kinase 2 by p21 is necessary for retinoblastoma protein-mediated G1 arrest after gamma-irradiation. Proc Natl Acad Sci U S A 1999;96:1002–7.

85. el-Deiry WS, Tokino T, Velculescu VE, et al. WAF1, a potential mediator of p53 tumor suppression. Cell 1993;75:817–25.

86. Haitel A, Wiener HG, Neudert B, et al. Expression of the cell cycle proteins p21, p27, and pRb in clear cell renal cell carcinoma and their prognostic significance. Urology 2001;58:477–81.

87. Weiss RH, Borowsky AD, Seligson D, et al. p21 is a prognostic marker for renal cell carcinoma: implications for novel therapeutic approaches. J Urol 2007;177:63–68;discussion 68–69.

88. Migita T, Oda Y, Naito S, Tsuneyoshi M. Low expression of p27(Kip1) is associated with tumor size and poor prognosis in patients with renal cell carcinoma. Cancer 2002;94:973–9.

89. Hedberg Y, Ljungberg B, Roos G, Landberg G. Expression of cyclin D1, D3, E, and p27 in human renal cell carcinoma analysed by tissue microarray. Br J Cancer 2003;88:1417–23.

90. Seligson DB, Pantuck AJ, Liu X, et al. Epithelial cell adhesion molecule (KSA) expression: pathobiology and its role as an independent predictor of survival in renal cell carcinoma. Clin Cancer Res 2004;10:2659–69.

91. Zantek ND, Azimi M, Fedor-Chaiken M, et al. E-cadherin regulates the function of the EphA2 receptor tyrosine kinase. Cell Growth Differ 1999;10:629–38.

92. Herrem CJ, Tatsumi T, Olson KS, et al. Expression of EphA2 is prognostic of disease-free interval and overall survival in surgically treated patients with renal cell carcinoma. Clin Cancer Res 2005;11:226–31.

8

# Radical Nephrectomy for Localized Renal Cell Carcinoma

REBECCA L. O'MALLEY, MD

GUILHERME GODOY, MD

SAMIR S. TANEJA, MD

Despite impressive advances in the understanding of the tumor biology of renal cell carcinoma (RCC) and the development of medical therapies,[1] surgery remains the mainstay of treatment for cure. In 1969, Robson and colleagues[2] described the four crucial components of a perifascial, radical nephrectomy, including early ligation of the renal artery and vein, removal of all contents of Gerota's fascia, removal of the ipsilateral adrenal gland, and performance of a complete regional lymphadenectomy.[2] This surgical approach replaced the pericapsular nephrectomy and has remained the standard of care for clinically localized renal tumors until the last two decades, in which elective partial nephrectomy challenged the paradigm of complete renal excision. In this chapter, we review the outcomes of conventional radical nephrectomy and discuss the evolution of the procedure to its current form.

## OUTCOMES OF RADICAL NEPHRECTOMY

### Oncologic Outcomes

In the review of eighty-eight patients having undergone radical nephrectomy at Toronto General Hospital from 1949 to 1964, Robson and colleagues[2] found poor prognosis to be related to involvement of adjacent structures or lymph nodes, gross invasion of the renal vein or distant organs, and histologic grade. The population of treated tumors consisted of 40.9% kidney-confined, 45.5% with perirenal fat involvement, 5.7% with adrenal involvement, 0.1% with extension into adjacent organs, 22.7% with nodal positivity, 9.1% with distant metastasis, and 31% and 9.1% with renal vein and inferior vena cava involvement, respectively. Even with including the subjects lost to follow-up in the group which died of disease, the survival advantage over simple nephrectomy was evident. The 3-year, 5-year, and 10-year survival of Robson's group was 61, 52, and 49%, compared with those of the reported series of simple nephrectomy of the time at 45 to 56%, 33 to 48%, and 18 to 27%, respectively.[3]

In the decades following Robson's report, several large series demonstrated the persistent survival advantage of radical nephrectomy over simple nephrectomy for localized disease (Tables 1 and 2). The overall 5-year and 10-year survivals range from 37 to 73% and 24 to 35%, repectively.[4–8] For organ-confined disease, 5-year overall survival ranged from 65 to 93%.[2,6–13] As pathologic stage is the most important factor predictive of survival, outcomes were poorer in those with high-stage disease, culminating in a bleak 0 to 12% 10-year survival for those with metastatic disease.[2,6–13] In a retrospective comparison of patients who had undergone simple nephrectomy or radical nephrectomy, the latter showed significantly improved overall survival at three, five, and ten years of follow-up among those with low-stage disease.[14]

| Table 1. SURVIVAL IN LOW-STAGE DISEASE BY ROBSON STAGE | | | | | |
|---|---|---|---|---|---|
| | | 5-year Survival (%) | | 10-year Survival (%) | |
| Author | Total Number of Patients | Stage I | Stage II | Stage I | Stage II |
| Robson et al,[2] (1969) | 88 | 66 | 64 | 60 | 67 |
| Skinner et al,[13] (1971) | 203 | 68 | 50 | 65 | 17 |
| McNichols et al,[7] (1981*) | 506 | 67 | 51 | 56 | 28 |
| Selli et al,[8] (1983) | 115 | 93 | 63 | NA | NA |
| Golimbu et al,[11] (1986) | 326 | 88 | 67 | 66 | 35 |
| Hermanek et al,[12] (1990) | 872 | 92 | 77 | NA | NA |
| Dinney et al,[10] (1992) | 251 | 73 | 68 | NA | NA |
| Chatelain (1980) | 204 | 71 | 77 | 65 | 77 |
| Guinan et al,[6] (1995) | 2,473 | 75 | 63 | NA | NA |

NA = not available.

| Table 2. SURVIVAL IN LOW-STAGE DISEASE BY AJCC TNM STAGE | | | |
|---|---|---|---|
| | | 5-year Survival (%) | |
| Author | Total Number of Patients | T1 | T2 |
| Guliani (1990) | 200 | 80 | 68 |
| Hermanek et al,[12] (1990) | 872 | 86 | 86 |
| Giberti et al,[4] (1997) | 328 | 75 | 63 |
| Dinney et al,[10] (1992) | 251 | 76 | 77 |
| Selli et al,[8] (1983) | 115 | 95 | 92 |

AJCC = American Joint Committee on Cancer; TNM = tumor node metastasis.

Stage is the most important predictor of relapse following radical nephrectomy. The fact that locoregional recurrence is unusual in the setting of radical nephrectomy for localized disease suggests that relapse in most cases is more likely a function of disease biology and stage than surgical technique. Nonetheless, complete resection of the local tumor with wide excision of the perinephric contents is essential in avoiding locoregional recurrence. It remains unclear if inadequate local excision results in a higher risk of metastatic relapse.

The results of radical nephrectomy on the whole have improved with stage migration and the increasing detection of incidentally-detected, smaller tumors.[15] Downward size and stage migration have also allowed the emergence of a number of nephron-sparing treatments and has drawn into question the necessity of all of the conventional components of traditional radical nephrectomy as described by Robson. Although no excessive morbidity or mortality has been attributed to ipsilateral adrenalectomy or lymphadenectomy concurrently executed with radical nephrectomy,[16,17] the demonstration of the safety and effectiveness of nephron sparing and consequently adrenal and lymph node sparing procedures, in multiple large series,[18–26] draws into question the necessity of these procedures as standard practice in the treatment of all organ-confined renal tumors.

## Role of Ipsilateral Adrenalectomy

The incidence of adrenal involvement related to RCC has been investigated in autopsy series and noted to be 7 to 23% in disseminated cases, and 19% if only ipsilateral disease is included.[27] The incidence in radical nephrectomy specimens has been noted to be between 1.2 and 10%.[28–36] The frequency of solitary, synchronous, ipsilateral involvement is much lower at 2.8 to 3.3% in autopsy series[37] and 0.7 to 5% in radical nephrectomy series.[28,29,33,34,38–42] The incidence of adrenal involvement has been decreasing over time[34] and will likely continue to do so as the proportion of renal masses incidentally discovered continues to increase.

In several retrospective direct comparisons, the overall and cancer-specific survival of patients undergoing adrenalectomy at the time of nephrectomy is similar to those whose adrenals were spared.[34,38,43,44] There is a bias in that those with adrenal involvement are shown to have higher overall stage, but upon stage stratification, one large multicenter study still found no survival advantage for adrenalectomy in early-stage disease.[38] In a retrospective series of almost 400 patients, one-third of which underwent adrenalectomy and two-thirds of which had adrenal-sparing procedures, there were no recurrences in the adrenal at a median follow-up of 69 months and there was no demonstrable survival advantage afforded for those whose adrenal was removed.[45] The emerging data from large series of nephron-sparing treatments of RCC corroborate these findings, in that long-term survival and long-term outcomes are similar to those of traditional radical nephrectomy.[26,29,46–49]

Among patients with solitary adrenal involvement, the majority (60 to 100%) have upper pole renal tumors.[50] Some series have failed to demonstrate this association, but these series included either patients with micrometastatic involvement of the adrenal or patients with widespread disease elsewhere.[31,51] There is reasonable evidence to suggest as some authors have proposed that upper pole tumor location should be an indication to perform ipsilateral adrenalectomy at the time of radical nephrectomy.[35,43,47,50] It has also been observed that the majority of ipsilateral adrenal metastases (62 to 100%) occur on the left side,[31,33,41,43,47,50] but on multivariate analysis, this is not an independent risk factor.[29,33,38,52,53] Renal vein thrombus appears to consistently predict a higher risk of adrenal disease.[33,35,36] In those with adrenal metastasis, multifocality of the renal primary has been found in 16 to 45% of patients in both radical nephrectomy specimens and autopsy studies and is independently predictive.[28,29,33,35,36,53] There are also considerable data suggesting that lymph node metastasis independently predicts adrenal involvement.[36,51–53] Lymph node involvement and multifocality are very difficult to predict preoperatively and are less relevant when considering clinically localized disease.

In a review of multiple series encompassing over 3,500 patients, it was noted that 85% of those with adrenal metastasis had stage T3a or higher stage disease.[33] Multiple multivariate analyses have demonstrated that stage is an independent predictor of adrenal involvement, irrespective of size of tumor.[29,33,38,53] Those with adrenal involvement consistently have larger average size of tumor, shown to be significantly different from those without adrenal disease in some series,[34,53–55] but insignificant in others.[33,38] Many studies demonstrated that patients with renal tumors less than 5 cm very rarely have adrenal involvement.[28,36,47,50,56] Using ROC curves, Paul and colleagues[51], defined a cutoff of 6 cm for increased risk of adrenal metastasis.

As tumor size, stage, and location appear to be the primary determinants of necessity for adrenalectomy, presurgical imaging has become more relevant in planning surgery. In a retrospective review of 157 patients who underwent radical nephrectomy, Gill and colleagues[30], noted that no adrenal that was called normal on preoperative computed tomography scan (CT) report contained cancer at the time of surgery.[30] There were, however, several false positive reports of abnormal adrenals found to have benign disease at surgery, including hemorrhage, adenomas, and hyperplasia. Similar findings are echoed in many large series, demonstrating the superb sensitivity and negative predictive value of imaging techniques in evaluating the adrenal, with values of 87 to 100% and 96 to 100 %, respectively, in most studies.[28–30,32,33,35,43,57] This is particularly true when the protocol recommended by Gill and colleagues[30] consisting of overlapping or contiguous 0.8 to 1 cm axial images with a slice thickness of 0.5 to 1 cm after intravenous contrast is used.[30]

We do not routinely perform adrenalectomy at the time of radical nephrectomy for clinically localized disease. In patients with radiologic evidence of ipsilateral adrenal metastasis, poor visualization of the adrenal gland due to tumor size, or large upper pole lesions abutting the adrenal gland, ipsilateral adrenalectomy should be performed. In the vast majority of patients, prophylactic resection is not necessary.

## Role of Lymphadenectomy

The reported overall incidence of lymph node metastasis in RCC has been as low as 3.3% in surgical series and as high as 63% in autopsy series.[58] There is a tremendous variation in the incidence due in part to differences in clinical stage and grade among the populations assessed.[5,17,59] Several series have shown that the extent of the dissection, the site of dissection, and the presence of gross lymphadenopathy cause variations in the detection of occult lymph node metastases.[60–62] Terrone and colleagues[63] found a significant increase in the likelihood of lymph node disease when excising thirteen or more nodes. Current UICC recommendations suggest resection of a minimum of eight lymph nodes to determine an individual node negative although evidence for this number is lacking.

In general, the pathways of lymphatic drainage of the kidneys, first described by Parker[64] in 1935, are noted to be variable and unpredictable in both anatomical studies[64] and autopsy series.[65] The extensive neovascularization commonly associated with RCC is believed to distort the normal anatomy and render the lymphatic drainage unpredictable.[59,66] In the case of clinically localized disease, the para-aortic nodes are most essential for left-sided tumors, and the inter-aortocaval nodes are the most likely drainage site of right-sided tumors.[59]

Most practitioners agree that suspicious or palpable nodes should be excised at the time of surgery, but the predictive value of these nodes is surprisingly low, with nodes up to 2.2 cm being inflammatory in 56% of cases.[67] In a prospective randomized trial assessing the therapeutic benefit of lymphadenectomy, 16% of palpable nodes harbored metastasis compared to 1% of palpably normal lymph nodes.[68]

Overall survival and cancer-specific survival is highly correlated with lymph node meatastasis.[69] Blute and colleagues[69] found cancer-specific survivals at 1, 5, and 10 years of 52%, 21%, and 11%, respectively, with lymph node positive disease, as compared with 96%, 83%, and 73% without lymph node positive disease.[69] Nonetheless, whether lymph node dissection provides a survival advantage for all patients is unclear. In evaluating N0M0 disease submitted to extended, regional or hilar lymph node dissection, Siminovitch and colleagues[62] found no relationship between survival and extent of dissection. Giuliani and colleagues[5] demonstrated a 5-year and 10-year disease-free survival of 48% and 32%, respectively, among patients undergone extended

lymphadenectomy. This approximated the survival of patients with pT3N0M0 disease.[5] Another study demonstrated improvements in 1-year and 5-year survivals with lymphadenectomy with rates of 87% versus 57% and 44% versus 26%, respectively.[70] The solitary prospective, randomized trial evaluating lymphadenectomy has failed to show an improvement in survival when analyzing all stages combined.[68] It is likely that the failure to demonstrate improvement in survival among individuals with clinically localized disease relates to the extremely low prevalence of lymph node metastasis in this group.

In a recent large series, the incidence of lymph node metastasis was found to be 2%, 3%, and 20% among those with T1, T2, and T3-T4 stage disease, respectively.[17] A comparison of the incidence of positive lymph nodes in Robson's early series with the more recent treatment arm of the EORTC protocol 30881,[68] reveals a drop from 30 to 3.3%, likely representing downward stage migration in the current era and, perhaps, a less aggressive dissection.[71,72] If those with metastatic disease undergoing nephrectomy for cytoreduction are excluded, the incidence of lymph node disease is in the range of 3 to 10%.[5,60,68]

In a multivariate logistic regression model, Blute and colleagues[69] identified the following characteristics that were associated with increased risk of lymph node disease in nonmetastatic renal cancer: stage (T3-T4), size of the tumor (greater than 10 cm), tumor grade III-IV, presence of sarcomatoid differentiation, and presence of necrosis. The presence of two or more of these factors was associated with a 15-fold higher incidence of lymph node disease. In clinically localized disease, these risk factors are rare, making the standard inclusion of lymph node dissection unnecessary for most patients.

Although several large retrospective series have failed to demonstrate any increase in morbidity when extended lymph node dissection is performed at the time of radical nephrectomy,[13,17,58,60,68,73–76] its routine use does not appear justified in patients with early-stage disease. When palpable nodes are encountered during radical nephrectomy for organ-confined disease or when preoperative high-risk features can be identified, extended, complete lymphadenectomy is warranted.

## Laparoscopic Outcomes

The introduction of laparoscopic nephrectomy for the treatment of localized RCC by Clayman and colleagues[77] in 1991 revolutionized renal surgery for renal tumors. The technique has gained popularity and acceptance secondary to decreases in postoperative pain and analgesic requirements resulting in shorter hospital stays and faster convalescence, as well as improvements in cosmesis.[78–80]

In the absence of early randomized trials comparing open and laparoscopic radical nephrectomy, various measures of oncologic efficacy were used. Retrospective cohorts were compared to open series on the basis of surgical margins, rates of local recurrence, distant metastasis, and survival with no obvious reduction in efficacy.[81] Early series reported no difference in the size or weight of the tumors extracted[81,82] or in the incidence of positive margins when compared with open series.[83–85]

Recently, longer follow-up data has validated early observations, with local recurrence rates and survival data similar to that of traditional open surgery. Several series have reported 5-year disease-free and actuarial survival for patients with stage T1-2N0M0, ranging from 91 to 95% and 81 to 95%, respectively (Table 3).[79,81–84,86] Concerns about tumor spillage, particularly with morcellation and the risk of port site recurrence were shown to be unfounded as rates are equivalent with open surgery (Table 4). There have been only nine reported cases of port site metastases following laparoscopic nephrectomy with an overall reported incidence of 0 to 6.25% in the urologic literature for all laparoscopic surgery and 0 to 2% for laparoscopic nephrectomy specifically, which is similar to that of open nephrectomy.[80,83,87,88]

Based upon the more rapid recovery from surgery, low rates of surgical complication and the absence of any evidence suggesting oncologic compromise, laparoscopic radical nephrectomy is emerging as the standard of care for clinically localized renal tumors. Training of urologists to provide reproducible outcomes and high quality of care remains a priority.

## TECHNICAL CONSIDERATIONS

### Preoperative Evaluation

#### Host Factors

Whether a renal mass is found incidentally or due to a symptomatically provoked evaluation, initial history and physical along with selective laboratory assessment and review of imaging will direct further preoperative evaluation and subsequent treatment. Upon determination of stage and surgical resectability, the goals of preoperative assessment are three-fold: (1) to optimize cardiopulmonary and nutritional status for surgical intervention, (2) to identify and stabilize paraneoplastic syndromes, and (3) to develop a treatment plan specifically addressing timing and approach of surgical intervention.

| Table 3. ONCOLOGIC OUTCOMES OF LAPAROSCOPIC RADICAL NEPHRECTOMY | | | | | | | |
|---|---|---|---|---|---|---|---|
| Author | Total Number of Patients | Clinical Stage | Approach | Port-site Recurrence | Local Recurrence | Follow-up (mo) | 5-year CSS (%) |
| Cadeddu (1998) | 157 | T1-2N0M0 | TP | 0 | 0 | 19.2 | 91 |
| Ono et al,[99] (2001) | 147 | T1-3N0M0 | TP | 0 | 1 | 29 | 95 |
| Chan et al,[78] (2001) | 67 | T1-2N0M0 | TP | 0 | 0 | 35.6 | 95 |
| Portis et al,[81] (2002) | 64 | T1-2N0M0 | TP | 0 | 1 | 54 | 98 |
| Stifelman (2002) | 108 | T1-3N0M0 | HAL | 0 | 1 | 14 | 93 |
| Saika et al,[100] (2003) | 195 | T1N0M0 | TP | 0 | 1 | 40 | 94 |
| Permpongkosol et al,[79] (2005) | 67 | T1-2N0M0 | TP | 0 | 0 | 73 | 97 |

CSS = cancer-specific survival; HAL = hand-assisted laparoscopic; TP = transperitoneal.

| Author | Laparoscopic | | Open | |
|---|---|---|---|---|
| | Total Number of Patients | % Complications | Total Number of Patients | % Complications |
| McDougall (1996) | 12 | 36 | 12 | 40 |
| Abbou (1999) | 29 | 6.9 | 29 | 27.2 |
| Walther (1998) | 11 | 18 | 19 | 18 |
| Ono (1999) | 60 | 13 | 40 | 8 |
| Dunn (2000) | 61 | 37 | 33 | 54 |
| Shuford (2004) | 33 | 15 | 41 | 10 |

**Table 4. COMPARISON OF OPEN VERSUS LAPAROSCOPIC COMPLICATION RATESTNM**

Adapted from Shuford et al.[102]

Serum analysis including, hemogram, electrolyte, renal and liver chemistries with serum calcium will identify paraneoplastic phenomena, such as hypercalcemia, anemia, polycythemia, or Stauffer syndrome (reversible liver dysfunction), which may require treatment prior to surgery. More commonly, medical comorbidities requiring optimization are discovered. Comorbidities may influence the selection of surgical approach. Flank incision should be avoided in patients with substantial pulmonary disease, whereas transperitoneal approaches should be avoided in individuals with substantial liver disease and ascites. The presence of retroperitoneal varices due to portocaval hypertension should be considered in planning surgical approach. Those with poor preoperative nutritional status should be considered for oral and in severe cases intravenous nutritional support prior to surgery to aid in more rapid recovery and wound healing. Assessment of renal function will help define those who are likely not able to tolerate radical nephrectomy without requiring postoperative dialysis. In these patients, nephron-sparing approaches are warranted.

## Staging

Staging of renal tumors should include a complete history, physical examination, and laboratory analysis. Routine chest imaging with radiograph or CT is indicated for all patients. Bone scan is unnecessary due to low yield, unless the serum alkaline phosphatase is elevated without other explanation

(hepatobiliary disease or Stauffer syndrome) or the patient complains of skeletal pain.[89] Imaging evaluation of intracranial pathology can safely be omitted in the absence of suggestive symptomatology or overt metastatic disease.

## Tumor Factors

The CT with intravenous contrast remains the study of choice for staging and assessing renal tumors due to its superior ability to provide details allowing the differentiation of benign from malignant lesions, definition of tumor extension, and the identification and delineation of extent of venous, lymph node, and visceral organ involvement.[90] All patients should have a CT prior to surgery unless contraindicated, in which case magnetic resonance imaging (MRI) is a suitable substitute. MRI is superior to CT in defining the presence and extent of venous involvement, as well as in defining venous collateral circulation and should be considered in patients with large or centrally located tumors as well as in those with suspicious or equivocal venous findings on CT.[91] In planning laparoscopic surgery, we have found it extremely useful to identify anomalous renal vasculature prior to resection.

The current approach to individuals with localized renal tumors is based in part upon tumor and patient characteristics, and, in part, upon the experience of the surgeon. Many tumors falling in the T1 (smaller than 7 cm) designation are amenable to partial nephrectomy. For tumors less than 4 cm, there is extensive data supporting oncologic equivalence between radical and partial nephrectomy.[22,92,93] For T1b tumors (4 to 7 cm), there is emerging data that partial nephrectomy may be appropriate for selected tumors.[94–96] Several controversies arise in selecting patients for partial versus radical nephrectomy, but in general, baseline renal function, the presence of a contralateral normal renal moiety, patient risk factors, and surgical experience are likely the most important guiding factors. There is considerable emerging data that patients who undergo radical nephrectomy may be at higher risk of long-term renal dysfunction and resultant noncologic risk of mortality.[93] If this data is validated, then the rationale for elective partial nephrectomy will be much stronger in the future.

The decision to undertake a radical or partial nephrectomy is primarily based on size and location of the tumor. In cases of equivocal imaging, three-dimensional cross-sectional imaging has been shown to aid in the decision-making process.[97] Three-dimensional imaging more accurately shows the anatomic relationship of the tumor to the surrounding tissues, including better predictions of venous involvement, pelvicalyceal invasion, multifocality, and tumor extension, as well as superior delineation of anomalous vascular anatomy.[91]

As the long-term impact of radical nephrectomy on renal function is unclear in the absence of randomized trials, we have generally advocated partial nephrectomy for most lesions less than 4 cm in size and select lesions in the 4 to 7 cm size range. We recommend elective partial nephrectomy for tumors less than 7 cm, with no involvement of the renal sinus or collecting system, in individuals with a perceived minimum 10-year life expectancy. Individuals with bleeding diathesis or a need for postoperative anticoagulation may be better treated by radical extirpation. The long-term benefit of partial nephrectomy is unproven in older patients or those with comorbidity limiting longevity. In such patients, radical nephrectomy is warranted even for small lesions, particularly those that are centrally located within the kidney. The specific indications for partial nephrectomy are discussed elsewhere in the text.

## Selection of Surgical Approach

Radical nephrectomy can safely be performed by open or laparoscopic means. As previously discussed, the oncologic outcomes of laparoscopic radical nephrectomy, particularly for localized disease, appear to be equivalent to open radical nephrectomy (see Table 4).[79,81,84,98–100] Individuals with extensive previous surgery, local lymphadenopathy, bulky hilar tumors, local organ involvement, retroperitoneal varices (portocaval hypertension), or vein thrombus may be better treated through an open approach. The vast majority of individuals with clinically localized disease are candidates for laparoscopic radical nephrectomy. This decision is heavily based upon operator experience. Improved convalescence, reduction of pulmonary morbidity, reduction of postoperative pain, and the apparent equivalence of oncologic outcomes make laparoscopic radical nephrectomy highly desirable. In our program, individuals are generally offered laparoscopic radical nephrectomy first unless a contraindication exists.

### Flank Approach

Open radical nephrectomy has historically been performed by a variety of incisional approaches. Extraperitoneal approaches commonly used include retroperitoneal flank incisions, whereas transperitoneal approaches include subcostal, midline, chevron, or transthoracic incisions (Figures 1 and 2). The primary advantages of a flank approach include

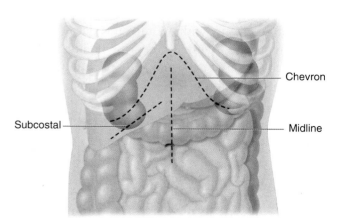

**Figure 1.** Transabdominal incisions for radical nephrectomy.

avoidance of ileus, bowel obstruction, or intraperitoneal visceral injury; early arterial access; and ease of access to the kidney in obese patients. Disadvantages of the flank approach include the necessity for pleural mobilization and diaphragm release, postoperative pulmonary compromise, potential denervation of flank musculature, and poor exposure of the medial hilum in individuals with hilar tumor, lymphadenopathy, or venous thrombus.

Flank incision can be carried out through the bed of the eleventh or twelfth rib following excision of the rib or through a supracostal incision by releasing the intercostal ligament, incising the costovertebral ligament, and disarticulating the rib (see Figure 2). Rib disarticulation and early release of the diaphragm at its insertion to the chest wall will release tension from the pleura and avoid incidental pleurotomy. In the event of pleurotomy, complete mobilization of the residual pleura from the chest wall generally allows repair and evacuation of the pneumothorax without the need of a thoracostomy tube. The peritoneum is then swept medially off the anterior surface of Gerota's fascia, and the renal hilum is developed (Figure 3). In general, flank exposure requires some mobilization of the upper or lower pole of the kidney prior to hilar control, and this is a theoretical disadvantage. Although many surgeons prefer a twelfth-rib incision to avoid extensive mobilization of the pleura, an eleventh-rib incisions allows better exposure of the hilum, upper pole tumors, and large tumors with perinephric venous collateral circulation.

Thoracoabdominal incision is carried out through the eighth to tenth intercostal space and involves entry into the chest, division of the diaphragm over the upper pole of the kidney, and entry into the peritoneal cavity (see Figure 2). Its primary advantage is in the excellent hilar exposure and access to the vena cava (right side), aorta (left side), and upper abdominal organs. As such exposure is rarely required in the setting of localized disease, this incision should not be required for early-stage disease.

## Transabdominal Approach

Transperitoneal exposure of the kidney can be performed by subcostal or midline approaches. A midline incision is typically used if radical

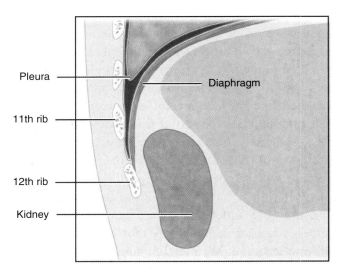

**Figure 2.** Flank incisions for radical nephrectomy and positioning of pleura, kidney and diaphragm relative to rib cage. Higher incisions require more diaphragmatic release in order to reflect the pleura. Lower incisions limit exposure of the upper pole of the kidney. Use of a thoracoabdominal incision allows excellent exposure of the upper pole of the kidney and the renal hilum, but it requires entry into the chest and incision of the diaphragm.

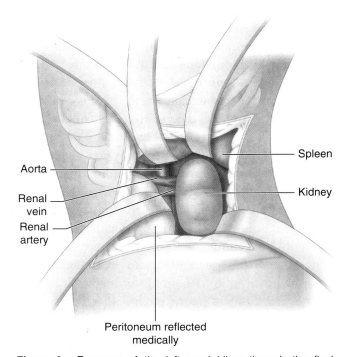

**Figure 3.** Exposure of the left renal hilum through the flank approach. Following release of the diaphragmatic insertion, the pleura is reflected upward allowing exposure of the retroperitoneum and complete division of the intercostal ligament. By disarticulating the rib, the intercostal space can be widely spread. The peritoneum is then reflected medially to expose the renal hilum.

nephrectomy is performed concomitant with other intra-abdominal procedures (see Figure 1). In such cases, extension of the incision to the xyphoid will allow adequate retraction to expose the upper pole of the kidney on either side. In the supine position, a roll placed beneath the ipsilateral rib cage can aid in overcoming the depth of the renal fossa and help deliver the kidney into the operative field.

The subcostal approach is generally preferred when transperitoneal radical nephrectomy is performed. Advantages of the approach include the ability to control the renal hilum prior to renal mobilization, access to retroperitoneal lymph nodes, and avoidance of the diaphragm and pleural cavity. Disadvantages include disturbance of the intra-abdominal contents potentially leading to ileus, bowel obstruction, or visceral injury. On the right, the liver must be retracted cephalad, the right colon reflected medially, and the duodenum rolled off the anterior surface of the venal cava and renal hilum (Kocher maneuver) (Figure 4). In cases of large upper pole

tumors, retro-hepatic kidney location, or very obese patients, extension of the incision across the midline (chevron incision) will allow better exposure.

On the left, the lateral splenic attachments must be divided and the splenic hilum rolled medially and cephalad off the surface of Gerota's fascia (Figure 5). Division of the splenocolic ligaments will facilitate this maneuver by allowing the tail of the pancreas to roll cranially. The splenic flexure and left colon are reflected medially. Obvious concerns of this exposure are the risk of splenic and pancreatic injury. Early series of transperitoneal nephrectomy reported an unacceptably high rate of incidental splenectomy. Inadvertently, traversing the left mesocolon during reflection can result in a duodenal injury at the level of the ligament of Treitz.

Once anterior exposure has been obtained, the anterior surface of the renal vein is exposed, and the vein is skeletonized and retracted cephalad. Lateral distraction of the lower pole of the kidney allows

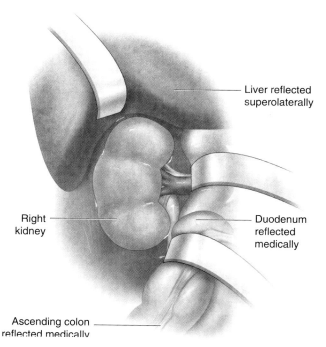

**Figure 4.** Transabdominal exposure of the right kidney. The right colon is reflected medially by incising the paracolic gutter and releasing the lateral attachments of the colon. Medial release of the hepatic flexure of the colon allows exposure of the underlying duodenum. A wide Kocher maneuver exposes the underlying vena cava and anterior renal hilum. Depending upon the position of the kidney, release of the right lobe of the liver and cranial reflection of the triangular ligament may be required to expose the upper pole and ipsilateral adrenal.

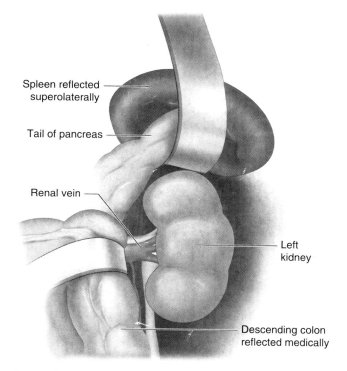

**Figure 5.** Transabdominal exposure of the left kidney. The left colon is reflected medially by incising the left paracolic gutter and lateral colonic attachments. Division of the splenocolic attachments facilitates downward reflection of the splenic flexure and cranial reflection of the tail of the pancreas and splenic hilum. Release of the lateral splenic attachments allows concomitant medial rotation of the spleen and cranial reflection of the pancreatic tail, thereby exposing the underlying renal hilum.

surgeon to develop a plane of dissection medial to the kidney and lateral to great vessels. In so doing, dissecting in a cephalad direction allows exposure of the renal artery dorsal to the renal vein. In cases of multiple renal arteries, these vessels are usually found at the lower or upper pole of the kidney and should be divided prior to the renal vein. Venous hemorrhage often occurs from the short lumbar vein entering into the dorsal surface of the left renal vein, the gonadal vein insertion in the left renal vein or vena cava, or the short right adrenal vein. Knowledge of anatomy is paramount in identifying these vessels and anomalous vessels, such as retro-aortic venous branches on the left.

Selection of open approach for radical nephrectomy is highly dependent upon surgeon experience. As mentioned previously, patient factors such as underlying pulmonary disease, ascites, portocaval hypertension, or previous intra-abdominal surgery might influence the decision for a transperitoneal or flank approach. Transperitoneal approaches are desirable, but they require a good knowledge of upper abdominal anatomic relationships.

### Laparoscopic Approach

Laparoscopic radical nephrectomy can be performed by either a transperitoneal or a retroperitoneal approach. The advantages of a retroperitoneal laparoscopic radical nephrectomy are similar to those of the extraperitoneal open approach. Our preference has been to use a transperitoneal approach because of the larger working space. With this approach, maneuvers on both the left and right mimic the open transperitoneal approach.

The patient is positioned in a modified semi-oblique flank (lateral decubitus) position allowing exposure to the abdominal wall (Figures 6 and 7). Medial reflection of the overlying bowel is essential in an early approach to the hilum. Following reflection of the bowel, full medial rotation of the table allows the bowel to fall forward, exposing Gerota's fascia overlying the renal hilum and the medial renal attachments. It has been our preference to elevate the lower pole of the kidney to distract the hilum for dissection. The lower pole and lateral renal attachments must remain intact during hilar dissection to allow

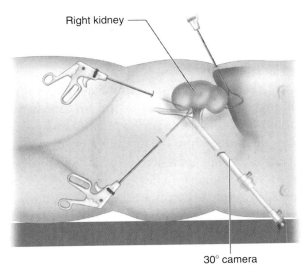

**Figure 6.** Patient and instrument positioning in right laparoscopic radical nephrectomy. Use of a 30º angle laparoscopic lens allows the laparoscope to be placed in the cranial port. Use of the lower two ports for instrumentation allows the surgeons hands to rest in a natural pronated position with elbows close to the body. We prefer a paramedian alignment of the ports to allow the lower port instruments to reach the upper pole attachments of the kidney.

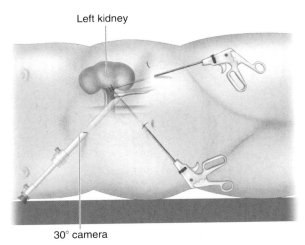

**Figure 7.** Patient and instrument positioning in left laparoscopic radical nephrectomy. Use of a 30º angle laparoscopic lens allows the laparoscope to be placed in the cranial port. Use of the lower two ports for instrumentation allows the surgeons hands to rest in a natural pronated position with elbows close to the body. We prefer a paramedian alignment of the ports to allow the lower port instruments to reach the upper pole attachments of the kidney.

stretch on the hilar vessels (Figures 8 and 9). We have used a 30º angle laparoscopic lens through the upper most port site (see Figures 6 and 7). Rotation of the scope allows cephalad visualization of the renal hilum while dissecting in line with the field of view from the lower ports (Figures 8 to 10).

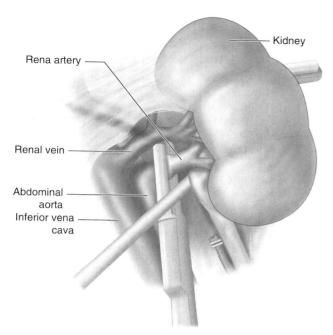

Figure 8. Stretching of the left renal hilum via distraction of the lower pole with a blunt instrument through the lower medial port during renal artery stapling in laparoscopic radical nephrectomy.

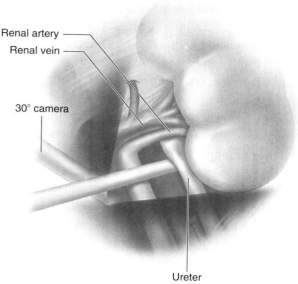

Figure 10. Visualization of the renal hilum during laparoscopic radical nephrectomy using a 30° laparoscope placed through the upper (cranial) port. The laparoscope crosses beneath the working ports and angles cranially to visualize the hilum in line with the working ports.

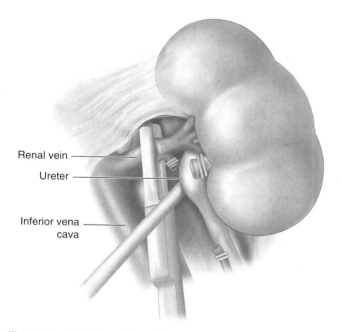

Figure 9. Stretching of the left renal hilum via distraction of the lower pole with a blunt instrument through the lower medial port during renal vein stapling in laparoscopic radical nephrectomy.

Large tumors (greater than 7 cm) can represent a challenge for laparoscopic resection due to the tendency of the kidney to fall over the hilum and the presence of large peri-hilar collateral vascularity.

In approaching such tumors, an extra port placed lateral to the working ports can allow assistant to provide lateral distraction of the kidney during hilar dissection.

## Complications of Radical Nephrectomy

Historically, the complication rate of open radical nephrectomy has been as high as 20% in the prelaparoscopic era.[101] The nature and frequency of complication varied by surgical approach. In 1983, Swanson and Borges[101] reported on the outcomes of 193 patients treated by open transperitoneal radical nephrectomy for all stages of disease. Splenic injuries were noted in 12.4% of patients, whereas vascular injuries were noted in 8.2%, including more commonly the vena cava, lumbar veins, and hepatic veins. Hemorrhage was also a significant complication in Swanson's series with a mean estimated blood loss of 2,683 mL. The rate of postoperative complications was noted to be 19.1%, including pleural effusions, infections, acute renal failure, vascular thrombosis, as well as other general complications, such as myocardial infarction, congestive heart failure, cerebrovascular accidents, and sepsis. The mortality rate was 2.1%.[101]

Recently with shifts in patient characteristics and advances in technique in addition to the advent of laparoscopic techniques, the rate of complications related to radical nephrectomy has decreased significantly. Contemporary series comparing complications of laparoscopic (transperitoneal, retroperitoneal, or hand-assisted techniques) and open radical nephrectomy, have demonstrated that morbidity is acceptable in the laparoscopic series, when compared with the open approach.[84,86,98,102,103] The rate of complications reported in laparoscopic series ranges between 16 to 37%, whereas in the open counterpart, rates range from 8 to 54% (see Table 4). A recent comparative study showed overall median rates of 15% and 10% for laparoscopic and open groups, respectively.[102] Differences in the estimated blood loss and transfusion requirements were not significant among the groups.[102] The wide variation among these studies is explained by differing criteria used to define minor and major complications in various subsets of patients along with the known selection bias of the retrospective design.

## CONCLUSIONS

Radical nephrectomy remains the standard of care for patients presenting with clinically localized disease. The original paradigm of radical nephrectomy set by Robson has been challenged in recent years. Contemporary data would suggest that regional lymphadenectomy and adrenalectomy are not necessary in the majority of individuals with localized disease. The use of partial nephrectomy in tumors less than 4 cm in size has limited the use of radical nephrectomy. In general, patients with tumors between 4 and 7 cm and reasonable longevity should be considered for partial nephrectomy as a first-line treatment. In those individuals with limited longevity, central tumor location, contraindication to partial nephrectomy, radical nephrectomy remains the appropriate treatment in patients with a normal contralateral moiety. The technique of radical nephrectomy can be performed through a variety of approaches. Laparoscopic radical nephrectomy has emerged as the technique of choice owing to a more rapid convalescence, increasing surgeon experience, and apparent equivalence of oncologic outcomes.

## REFERENCES

1. Novick AC. Kidney cancer: past, present, and future. Urol Oncol 2007;25:188–95.
2. Robson CJ, Churchill BM, Anderson W. The results of radical nephrectomy for renal cell carcinoma. J Urol 1969;101:297–301.
3. Kaufman JJ MM. Tumors of the kidney. Curr Probl Surg 1966;3–42.
4. Giberti C, Oneto F, Martorana G, et al. Radical nephrectomy for renal cell carcinoma: long-term results and prognostic factors on a series of 328 cases. Eur Urol 1997;31:40–48.
5. Giuliani L, Giberti C, Martorana G, Rovida S. Radical extensive surgery for renal cell carcinoma: long-term results and prognostic factors. J Urol 1990;143:468–73; discussion 473–4.
6. Guinan PD, Vogelzang NJ, Fremgen AM, et al. Renal cell carcinoma: tumor size, stage and survival. Members of the Cancer Incidence and End Results Committee. J Urol 1995;153(3 Pt 2):901–3.
7. McNichols DW, Segura JW, DeWeerd JH. Renal cell carcinoma: long-term survival and late recurrence. J Urol 1981;126:17–23.
8. Selli C, Hinshaw WM, Woodard BH, Paulson DF. Stratification of risk factors in renal cell carcinoma. Cancer 1983;52:899–903.
9. Chatelain C. Results of radical nephrectomy without lymphadenectomy in renal cell carcinoma. Prog Clin Biol Res 1982;100:475–80.
10. Dinney CP, Awad SA, Gajewski JB, et al. Analysis of imaging modalities, staging systems, and prognostic indicators for renal cell carcinoma. Urology 1992;39:122–9.
11. Golimbu M, Joshi P, Sperber A, et al. Renal cell carcinoma: survival and prognostic factors. Urology 1986;27:291–301.
12. Hermanek P, Schrott KM. Evaluation of the new tumor, nodes and metastases classification of renal cell carcinoma. J Urol 1990;144(2 Pt 1):238–41; discussion 241–2.
13. Skinner DG, Colvin RB, Vermillion CD, et al. Diagnosis and management of renal cell carcinoma. A clinical and pathologic study of 309 cases. Cancer 1971;28:1165–77.
14. Ramon J, Goldwasser B, Raviv G, et al. Long-term results of simple and radical nephrectomy for renal cell carcinoma. Cancer 1991;67:2506–11.
15. Motzer RJ, Bander NH, Nanus DM. Renal-cell carcinoma. N Engl J Med 1996;335:865–75.
16. Hellström PA, Bloigu R, Ruokonen AO, et al. Is routine ipsilateral adrenalectomy during radical nephrectomy harmful for the patient? Scand J Urol Nephrol 1997;31:19–25.
17. Pantuck AJ, Zisman A, Dorey F, et al. Renal cell carcinoma with retroperitoneal lymph nodes: role of lymph node dissection. J Urol 2003;169:2076–83.
18. Haber GP, Gill IS. Laparoscopic partial nephrectomy: contemporary technique and outcomes. Eur Urol 2006;49:660–5.
19. Lane BR, Gill IS. 5-Year outcomes of laparoscopic partial nephrectomy. J Urol 2007;177:70–4; discussion 74.
20. Mitchell RE, Gilbert SM, Murphy AM, et al. Partial nephrectomy and radical nephrectomy offer similar cancer outcomes in renal cortical tumors 4 cm or larger. Urology 2006;67:260–4.

21. Allaf ME, Bhayani SB, Rogers C, et al. Laparoscopic partial nephrectomy: evaluation of long-term oncological outcome. J Urol 2004;172:871–3.

22. Uzzo RG, Novick AC. Nephron sparing surgery for renal tumors: indications, techniques and outcomes. J Urol 2001;166:6–18.

23. Gill IS, Remer EM, Hasan WA, et al. Renal cryoablation: outcome at 3 years. J Urol 2005;173:1903–7.

24. Blute ML. Open partial nephrectomy for tumor in a solitary kidney: experience with 400 cases Fergany AF, Saad IR, Woo L, Novick AC, Glickman Urological Institute, Cleveland Clinic Foundation, Cleveland, OH. Urol Oncol 2006; 24:556.

25. Fergany AF, Hafez KS, Novick AC. Long-term results of nephron sparing surgery for localized renal cell carcinoma: 10-year followup. J Urol 2000;163:442–5.

26. Novick AC. Laparoscopic and partial nephrectomy. Clin Cancer Res 2004;10(18 Pt 2):6322S–7S.

27. Saitoh H, Nakayama M, Nakamura K, Satoh T. Distant metastasis of renal adenocarcinoma in nephrectomized cases. J Urol 1982;127:1092–5.

28. Autorino R, Di Lorenzo G, Damiano R, et al. Adrenal sparing surgery in the treatment of renal cell carcinoma: when is it possible? World J Urol 2003;21:153–8.

29. De Sio M, Autorino R, Di Lorenzo G, et al. Adrenalectomy: defining its role in the surgical treatment of renal cell carcinoma. Urol Int 2003;71:361–7.

30. Gill IS, McClennan BL, Kerbl K, Carbone JM, et al. Adrenal involvement from renal cell carcinoma: predictive value of computerized tomography. J Urol 1994;152:1082–5.

31. Ito A, Satoh M, Ohyama C, Saito S, et al. Adrenal metastasis from renal cell carcinoma: significance of adrenalectomy. Int J Urol 2002;9:125–8.

32. Kletscher BA, Qian J, Bostwick DG, et al. Prospective analysis of the incidence of ipsilateral adrenal metastasis in localized renal cell carcinoma. J Urol 1996;155:1844–6.

33. Moudouni SM, En-Nia I, Patard JJ, et al. Real indications for adrenalectomy in renal cell carcinoma. Scand J Urol Nephrol 2002;36:273–7.

34. Siemer S, Lehmann J, Kamradt J, et al. Adrenal metastases in 1635 patients with renal cell carcinoma: outcome and indication for adrenalectomy. J Urol 2004;171(6 Pt 1):2155–9; discussion 2159.

35. Tsui KH, Shvarts O, Barbaric Z, et al. Is adrenalectomy a necessary component of radical nephrectomy? UCLA experience with 511 radical nephrectomies. J Urol 2000; 163:437–41.

36. Wunderlich H, Schlichter A, Reichelt O, et al. Real indications for adrenalectomy in renal cell carcinoma. Eur Urol 1999;35:272–6.

37. Saitoh H, Hida M, Nakamura K, et al. Metastatic processes and a potential indication of treatment for metastatic lesions of renal adenocarcinoma. J Urol 1982;128:916–8.

38. Kozak W, Holtl W, Pummer K, et al. Adrenalectomy—still a must in radical renal surgery? Br J Urol 1996;77:27–31.

39. O'Brien WM, Lynch JH. Adrenal metastases by renal carcinoma. Incidence at nephrectomy. Urology 1987;29:605–7.

40. Paul R, Mordhorst J, Leyh H, Hartung R. Incidence and outcome of patients with adrenal metastases of renal cell cancer. Urology 2001;57:878–82.

41. Sagalowsky AI, Kadesky KT, Ewalt DM, Kennedy TJ. Factors influencing adrenal metastasis in renal cell carcinoma. J Urol 1994;151:1181–4.

42. Winter P, Miersch WD, Vogel J, Jaeger N. On the necessity of adrenal extirpation combined with radical nephrectomy. J Urol 1990;144:842–3; discussion 844.

43. Leibovitch I, Raviv G, Mor Y, et al. Reconsidering the necessity of ipsilateral adrenalectomy during radical nephrectomy for renal cell carcinoma. Urology 1995;46:316–20.

44. Robey EL, Schellhammer PF. The adrenal gland and renal cell carcinoma: is ipsilateral adrenalectomy a necessary component of radical nephrectomy? J Urol 1986;135:453–5.

45. Kobayashi T, Nakamura E, Yamamoto S, et al. Low incidence of ipsilateral adrenal involvement and recurrences in patients with renal cell carcinoma undergoing radical nephrectomy: a retrospective analysis of 393 patients. Urology 2003;62:40–5.

46. Bazeed MA, Scharfe T, Becht E, et al. Conservative surgery of renal cell carcinoma. Eur Urol 1986;12:238–43.

47. Li GR, Soulie M, Escourrou G, et al. Micrometastatic adrenal invasion by renal carcinoma in patients undergoing nephrectomy. Br J Urol 1996;78:826–8.

48. Morgan WR, Zincke H. Progression and survival after renal-conserving surgery for renal cell carcinoma: experience in 104 patients and extended follow up. J Urol 1990; 144:852–7; discussion 857–8.

49. Provet J, Tessler A, Brown J, et al. Partial nephrectomy for renal cell carcinoma: indications, results and implications. J Urol 1991;145:472–6.

50. Sandock DS, Seftel AD, Resnick MI. Adrenal metastases from renal cell carcinoma: role of ipsilateral adrenalectomy and definition of stage. Urology 1997;49:28–31.

51. Paul R, Mordhorst J, Busch R, et al. Adrenal sparing surgery during radical nephrectomy in patients with renal cell cancer: a new algorithm. J Urol 2001;166:59–62.

52. Shalev M, Cipolla B, Guille F, et al. Is ipsilateral adrenalectomy a necessary component of radical nephrectomy? J Urol 1995;153:1415–7.

53. Kuczyk M, Munch T, Machtens S, et al. The need for routine adrenalectomy during surgical treatment for renal cell cancer: the Hannover experience. BJU Int 2002;89:517–22.

54. von Knobloch R, Seseke F, Riedmiller H, et al. Radical nephrectomy for renal cell carcinoma: Is adrenalectomy necessary? Eur Urol 1999;36:303–8.

55. Yokoyama H, Tanaka M. Incidence of adrenal involvement and assessing adrenal function in patients with renal cell carcinoma: is ipsilateral adrenalectomy indispensable during radical nephrectomy? BJU Int 2005;95:526–9.

56. Antonelli A, Cozzoli A, Simeone C, et al. Surgical treatment of adrenal metastasis from renal cell carcinoma: a single-centre experience of 45 patients. BJU Int 2006;97:505–8.

57. Sawai Y, Kinouchi T, Mano M, et al. Ipsilateral adrenal involvement from renal cell carcinoma: retrospective study of the predictive value of computed tomography. Urology 2002;59:28–31.

58. Freedland SJ, Dekernion JB. Role of lymphadenectomy for patients undergoing radical nephrectomy for renal cell carcinoma. Rev Urol 2003;5:191–5.

59. Phillips CK, Taneja SS. The role of lymphadenectomy in the surgical management of renal cell carcinoma. Urol Oncol 2004;22:214–23;discussion 223–4.

60. Herrlinger A, Schrott KM, Schott G, Sigel A. What are the benefits of extended dissection of the regional renal lymph nodes in the therapy of renal cell carcinoma. J Urol 1991;146:1224–7.

61. Minervini A, Lilas L, Morelli G, et al. Regional lymph node dissection in the treatment of renal cell carcinoma: is it useful in patients with no suspected adenopathy before or during surgery? BJU Int 2001;88:169–72.

62. Siminovitch JP, Montie JE, Straffon RA. Lymphadenectomy in renal adenocarcinoma. J Urol 1982;127:1090–1.

63. Terrone C, Guercio S, De Luca S, et al. The number of lymph nodes examined and staging accuracy in renal cell carcinoma. BJU Int 2003;91:37–40.

64. Parker AE. Studies on the main posterior lymph channels of the abdomen and their connections with the lymphatics of the genitourinary system. Am J Anat 1935;56:409.

65. Johnsen JA, Hellsten S. Lymphatogenous spread of renal cell carcinoma: an autopsy study. J Urol 1997;157:450–3.

66. DeKernion JB. Lymphadenectomy for renal cell carcinoma. Therapeutic implications. Urol Clin North Am 1980;7: 697–703.

67. Studer UE, Scherz S, Scheidegger J, et al. Enlargement of regional lymph nodes in renal cell carcinoma is often not due to metastases. J Urol 1990;144(2 Pt 1):243–5.

68. Blom JH, van Poppel H, Marechal JM, et al. Radical nephrectomy with and without lymph node dissection: preliminary results of the EORTC randomized phase III protocol 30881. EORTC Genitourinary Group. Eur Urol 1999;36:570–5.

69. Blute ML, Leibovich BC, Cheville JC, et al. A protocol for performing extended lymph node dissection using primary tumor pathological features for patients treated with radical nephrectomy for clear cell renal cell carcinoma. J Urol 2004;172:465–9.

70. Peters PC, Brown GL. The role of lymphadenectomy in the management of renal cell carcinoma. Urol Clin North Am 1980;7:705–9.

71. Giannakopoulos X, Charalabopoulos K, Charalabopoulos A, et al. The role of lymphadenectomy in renal cancer surgery. An update. Exp Oncol 2004;26:261–4.

72. Mickisch G, Carballido J, Hellsten S, et al. Guidelines on renal cell cancer. Eur Urol 2001;40:252–5.

73. Ferrigni RG, Novicki DE. Chylous ascites complicating genitourinary oncological surgery. J Urol 1985;134:774–6.

74. Schafhauser W, Ebert A, Brod J, et al. Lymph node involvement in renal cell carcinoma and survival chance by systematic lymphadenectomy. Anticancer Res 1999; 19(2C):1573–8.

75. Waters WB, Richie JP. Aggressive surgical approach to renal cell carcinoma: review of 130 cases. J Urol 1979;122:306–9.

76. Carmignani G, Belgrano E, Puppo P, et al. Lymphadenectomy in renal cancer. In: Cancer of the prostate and kidney. New York: Plenum Press; 1983. p. 645–50.

77. Clayman RV, Kavoussi LR, Soper NJ, et al. Laparoscopic nephrectomy: initial case report. J Urol 1991;146:278–82.

78. Chan DY, Cadeddu JA, Jarrett TW, et al. Laparoscopic radical nephrectomy: cancer control for renal cell carcinoma. J Urol 2001;166:2095–9; discussion 2099–100.

79. Permpongkosol S, Chan DY, Link RE, et al. Laparoscopic radical nephrectomy: long-term outcomes. J Endourol 2005;19:628–33.

80. Lam JS, Shvarts O, Pantuck AJ. Changing concepts in the surgical management of renal cell carcinoma. Eur Urol 2004;45:692–705.

81. Portis AJ, Yan Y, Landman J, et al. Long-term follow up after laparoscopic radical nephrectomy. J Urol 2002; 167:1257–62.

82. Gill IS, Schweizer D, Hobart MG, et al. Retroperitoneal laparoscopic radical nephrectomy: the Cleveland clinic experience. J Urol 2000;163:1665–70.

83. Gill IS, Meraney AM, Schweizer DK, et al. Laparoscopic radical nephrectomy in 100 patients: a single center experience from the United States. Cancer 2001;92:1843–55.

84. Dunn MD, Portis AJ, Shalhav AL, et al. Laparoscopic versus open radical nephrectomy: a 9-year experience. J Urol 2000;164:1153–9.

85. Ogan K, Cadeddu JA, Stifelman MD. Laparoscopic radical nephrectomy: oncologic efficacy. Urol Clin North Am 2003;30:543–50.

86. Ono Y, Kinukawa T, Hattori R, et al. Laparoscopic radical nephrectomy for renal cell carcinoma: a five-year experience. Urology 1999;53:280–6.

87. Rassweiler J, Tsivian A, Kumar AV, et al. Oncological safety of laparoscopic surgery for urological malignancy: experience with more than 1,000 operations. J Urol 2003; 169:2072–5.

88. Tsivian A, Sidi AA. Port site metastases in urological laparoscopic surgery. J Urol 2003;169:1213–8.

89. Seaman E, Goluboff ET, Ross S, Sawczuk IS. Association of radionuclide bone scan and serum alkaline phosphatase in patients with metastatic renal cell carcinoma. Urology 1996;48:692–5.

90. Heidenreich A, Ravery V. Preoperative imaging in renal cell cancer. World J Urol 2004;22:307–15.

91. Huang GJ, Israel G, Berman A, Taneja SS. Preoperative renal tumor evaluation by three-dimensional magnetic resonance imaging: staging and detection of multifocality. Urology 2004;64:453–7.

92. Herr HW. Partial nephrectomy for unilateral renal carcinoma and a normal contralateral kidney: 10-year followup. J Urol 1999;161:33–4; discussion 34–5.

93. Lau WK, Blute ML, Weaver AL, et al. Matched comparison of radical nephrectomy vs nephron-sparing surgery in patients with unilateral renal cell carcinoma and a normal contralateral kidney. Mayo Clin Proc 2000;75:1236–42.

94. Leibovich BC, Blute ML, Cheville JC, et al. Nephron sparing surgery for appropriately selected renal cell carcinoma between 4 and 7 cm results in outcome similar to radical nephrectomy. J Urol 2004;171:1066–70.

95. Patard JJ, Shvarts O, Lam JS, et al. Safety and efficacy of partial nephrectomy for all T1 tumors based on an international multicenter experience. J Urol 2004;171(6 Pt 1):2181–5, quiz 2435.

96. Russo P, Goetzl M, Simmons R, et al. Partial nephrectomy: the rationale for expanding the indications. Ann Surg Oncol 2002;9:680–7.

97. Chernoff DM, Silverman SG, Kikinis R, et al. Three-dimensional imaging and display of renal tumors using spiral CT: a potential aid to partial nephrectomy. Urology 1994;43:125–9.

98. McDougall E, Clayman RV, Elashry OM. Laparoscopic radical nephrectomy for renal tumor: the Washington University experience. J Urol 1996;155:1180–5.

99. Ono Y, Kinukawa T, Hattori R, et al. The long-term outcome of laparoscopic radical nephrectomy for small renal cell carcinoma. J Urol 2001;165(6 Pt 1):1867–70.

100. Saika T, Ono Y, Hattori R, et al. Long-term outcome of laparoscopic radical nephrectomy for pathologic T1 renal cell carcinoma. Urology 2003;62:1018–23.

101. Swanson DA, Borges PM. Complications of transabdominal radical nephrectomy for renal cell carcinoma. J Urol 1983;129:704–7.

102. Shuford MD, McDougall EM, Chang SS, et al. Complications of contemporary radical nephrectomy: comparison of open vs. laparoscopic approach. Urol Oncol 2004;22:121–6.

103. Abbou CC, Cicco A, Gasman D, et al. Retroperitoneal laparoscopic versus open radical nephrectomy. J Urol 1999;161:1776–80.

# 9

# Surgical Management of Locally Advanced Renal Cell Carcinoma

VITALY MARGULIS, MD
CHRISTOPHER G. WOOD, MD, FACS

## INTRODUCTION

The incidence of renal cell carcinoma (RCC) has risen at a rate of approximately 3% per year since the 1970s and in 2006, approximately 12,840 patients died of RCC.[1] In addition to increased radiologic detection of "incidental" renal tumors, the incidence of advanced tumors and death from disease in patients with RCC has also increased.[2] Tumor stage, as determined by the American Joint Committee for Cancer (AJCC) primary tumor classification system (Table 1), remains the most important and widely utilized prognosticator of progression-free survival and overall survival following surgical management of RCC.[3] Contemporary literature reveals that 5-year cancer-specific survival after radical nephrectomy (RN) ranged from 75–95% for patients with organ-confined disease to 0–5% for patients with metastatic disease at presentation.[4,5] Located between these clinical extremes are patients with locally advanced renal cell carcinoma (LARCC), considered to be at significant risk for progression and death from their renal tumors due to adverse pathologic features.

Definitions of LARCC vary throughout the literature, however, authors of this text utilize the 2002 AJCC primary tumor classification to identify LARCC as non-metastatic (M0) tumors in pT3-T4 and/or N+ categories, which include features of perirenal fat and/or ipsilateral adrenal gland invasion (pT3a), associated malignant venous thrombus below (pT3b) and above (pT3c) the diaphragm, extension beyond the Gerota's fascia (pT4), and/or involvement of locoregional lymph nodes by RCC (N+). Modern series report 5-year disease-specific survival rates of 65 to 80% for tumors with perinephric fat or adrenal involvement, 40 to 60% for RCC with associated vena cava thrombus and 10 to 20% for RCC with concurrent locoregional lymph node involvement.[6–8]

Since pioneering description by Robson and colleagues, surgical removal of the primary tumor with RN has remained the only available curative option and continues to be the mainstay of treatment for patients with LARCC.[9] While basic surgical and oncologic principles established by Robson and colleagues remain unchanged, the modern surgical armamentarium for treatment of LARCC has expanded with evolution of standard open, minimally invasive and nephron-sparing techniques. Marked advances in perioperative supportive management, coupled with improved and diversified surgical approaches have allowed delivery of more complex, yet safer surgical treatment options for patients with LARCC.

In this context, we review general concepts, outcomes and controversies of the current surgical options available for management of patients with LARCC.

| Table 1. THE AMERICAN JOINT COMMITTEE ON CANCER STAGING SYSTEM FOR RENAL CELL CARCINOMA |
| --- |

**Primary tumor (T)**

TX   Primary tumor cannot be assessed (information not available)

T0   No evidence of a primary tumor

T1a   Tumor is 4 cm in diameter or smaller, limited to the kidney

T1b   Tumor is larger than 4 cm but smaller than 7 cm, limited to the kidney

T2   Tumor is larger than 7 cm, limited to the kidney

T3a   Direct tumor invasion into the adrenal gland, perinephric fat or renal sinus fat, tumor confined within Gerota's fascia

T3b   Tumor invasion of the renal vein or the inferior vena cava below the diaphragm

T3c   Tumor invasion of the vena cava above the diaphragm

T4   Tumor invasion beyond Gerota's fascia

**Regional lymph nodes (N)**

NX   Regional lymph nodes cannot be assessed

N0   No regional lymph node metastasis

N1   Metastasis to one regional lymph node

N2   Metastasis to more than one regional lymph node

**Distant metastasis (M)**

MX   Presence of distant metastasis cannot be assessed

M0   No distant metastasis

M1   Distant metastasis present; includes metastasis to non regional lymph nodes and/or to other organs

**Stage grouping**

I   T1a-T1b, N0, M0

II   T2, N0, M0

III   T1a-T3b, N1, M0 or T3a-T3c, N0, M0

IV   T4, N0-N1, M0 or Any T, N2, M0 or Any T, Any N, M1

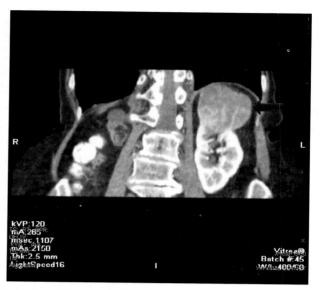

**Figure 1.** pT3a renal cell carcinoma (Red arrow – tumor within perinephric fat).

## RCC WITH PERINEPHRIC FAT INVOLVEMENT

Modern nephrectomy series demonstrate that approximately 20 to 30% of RCC are found to extend into the perinephric fat (Figure 1).[4,8] Because of large tumor bulk and frequent collateral vascularization, RCC with suspected extension into perinephric fat has traditionally been managed with standard open RN. The basic principles of this procedure include early ligation of the renal vasculature and en bloc removal of the kidney within the surrounding perinephric fat and Gerota's fascia, thus assuring negative surgical margins, while minimizing vascular and intraperitoneal dissemination of cancer cells.[9]

The surgical approach to open RN is determined by the size and location of the tumor, body habitus of the patient and surgeon preference. Larger tumors are approached through a transperitoneal or thoracoabdominal incision to allow abdominal exploration for metastatic disease and early access to the renal vessels with minimal manipulation of the tumor. Smaller tumors and renal masses in obese patients can be safely approached with extraperitoneal flank incision.[10]

Since introduction in 1990s, laparoscopic radical nephrectomy (LRN) has gained wide acceptance for management of low-volume, organ-confined RCC.[11] This procedure is performed transperitoneally, retroperitoneally or hand-assisted and offers the advantages of decreased postoperative pain, shorter hospital stay and convalescence, while maintaining oncologic efficacy.[12,13] Recently LRN has been applied to patients with locally advanced and metastatic RCC.[14–16] Several investigators have reported feasibility and oncologic efficacy of LRN, when utilized in the management of large renal tumors involving the perinephric fat.[17,18] While the maximum tumor size limit for LRN has been debated, it is most likely a function of surgeon comfort rather than a limitation of the technique. Because of a theoretically increased risk of intraperitoneal tumor spillage and possibility of port site tumor recurrence, the role of LRN has been questioned. To date these concerns remain speculative and unsubstantiated, and despite thousands of LRN procedures performed each year, only three cases of port-site metastases are reported in the urologic literature.

While elective indications for nephron-sparing surgery continue to evolve, preservation of renal function is essential, if feasible, in patients who would otherwise be rendered functionally or anatomically anephric following RN. Partial nephrectomy (PN), performed openly or laparoscopically, allows an oncologically complete local excision of RCC, while preserving a functional renal remnant. Oncologic efficacy of PN for small (< 4.0 cm) organ-confined renal tumors has been clearly established in the literature.[19] In addition, there is emerging evidence that PN can safely be performed for patients with locally advanced tumors, provided an adequate surgical margin and sufficient remaining renal parenchyma can be obtained.[20] Investigators from the Cleveland Clinic have reported 85 and 74% 5- and 10-year cancer-specific survival rates following PN for pT3a RCC.[19] Although these results compare favorably to the oncologic outcomes achieved by RN, there was an increased rate of local recurrence in the PN group, necessitating intensive post-treatment surveillance.[19]

In summary, regardless of surgical approach, RN remains the treatment of choice for RCC extending into the perinephric fat. LRN can safely be performed for the majority of pT3a RCC patients, and offers the advantage of reduced postoperative pain, shortened length of hospitalization, reduced duration of convalescence, and improved cosmesis. In select cases where nephron preservation is mandatory and feasible, PN can be performed, avoiding the complications and cost of an anephric state.

## RCC WITH IPSILATERAL ADRENAL INVOLVEMENT

As originally advocated by Robson and colleagues, the practice of routine adrenalectomy in conjunction with RN has recently been questioned. Several reports have documented relative rarity of isolated ipsilateral adrenal metastases or direct adrenal invasion by RCC in contemporary patient cohorts. Specifically, in patients without evidence of systemic metastatic disease, presence of adrenal involvement by RCC has been demonstrated in only 1 to 5% of cases.[21–25] Moreover, modern day imaging modalities, such as computed tomography and

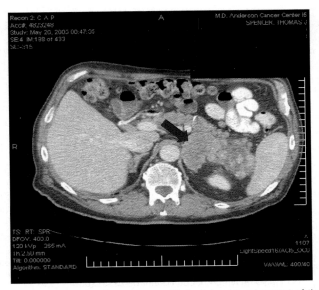

**Figure 2.**   Renal cell carcinoma with ipsilateral involvement of the adrenal gland (Red arrow).

magnetic resonance imaging, have demonstrated > 99% specificity and nearly 90% sensitivity to detect adrenal involvement preoperatively (Figure 2).[23,26] A prospective study of 511 nephrectomies performed by the investigators at UCLA revealed no survival benefit to routine adrenalectomy.[23] These results suggest that the majority of patients with RCC can be spared the potential morbidity associated with an ipsilateral adrenalectomy. However, because complete surgical removal of all malignant tissue is essential to achieve a favorable oncologic outcome, a number of predictive factors have been studied in an attempt to identify patients with a high probability of adrenal involvement. By and large, tumors with clinical features of locally advanced disease, such as large tumor bulk, presence of extrarenal tumor extension, and venous tumor thrombus, have been associated with high risk of ipsilateral adrenal involvement.[23,25,27,28] In addition, several studies have associated the location of the primary tumor in the upper pole of the kidney with an increased incidence of adrenal involvement.[22,29,30] Based on the information available, adrenalectomy should be performed if adrenal involvement is suspected on preoperative imaging or during surgical exploration and in all patients with features of locally advanced disease.

Patients with direct adrenal involvement by RCC are currently classified as pT3a, despite convincing evidence from several large single center experiences demonstrating significantly lower cancer-specific survival for patients with direct adrenal invasion than for other patients with pT3a RCC.[7,31] Patients with direct adrenal invasion have been shown to have similar disease-specific survival to patients with adjacent organ invasion (pT4), prompting adjustment of the current AJCC TNM classification.[32–35] Five-year disease-specific survival rates of 0 to 30% have been reported for surgically treated non-metastatic patients, with ipsilateral adrenal gland involvement by RCC.[32–35] While such dismal outcomes have led some investigators to question the therapeutic benefit of adrenalectomy, complete surgical excision of the cancerous kidney and adrenal gland represent the only realistic chance of cure in these patients.

Given the low prevalence of patients with ipsilateral adrenal involvement and use of modern advanced preoperative imaging, the vast majority of patients with RCC can be spared the potential morbidity associated with ipsilateral adrenalectomy. Despite poor cancer specific outcomes associated with ipsilateral adrenal involvement by RCC, a small but significant proportion of patients can expect a durable cure following complete surgical resection. As such, patients with preoperative or intraoperative evidence of adrenal involvement, as well as patients with features of LARCC should undergo nephrectomy with concomitant en bloc adrenalectomy.

## RCC WITH VENOUS TUMOR THROMBUS

The incidence of venous tumor extension in patients with RCC is reported to be between 4 and 10%.[6,36,37] In up to 25% of patients, the tumor extends above the confluence of the hepatic veins and in approximately 5%, the thrombi are supra-diaphragmatic or intracardiac (Figure 3A,B,C). The prognostic implication of the level of the tumor thrombus has been extensively studied, with most studies reporting no significant difference in survival based on the extent of the tumor thrombus.[6,38,39] Rather, oncologic outcome of patients with venous tumor thrombus correlates with biologic tumor aggressiveness, as determined by tumor grade, perinephric fat invasion, nodal and metastatic status. Most series report 30 to 70% 5-year cancer-specific survival following

complete resection of venous tumor thrombus in the absence of nodal or distant metastases, clearly establishing a role for aggressive surgical resection in these patients.[36–38,40–42]

Surgical management of patients with venous tumor thrombus continues to epitomize one of the most challenging genitourinary procedures, and even in specialized surgical centers, operations of this nature carry significant morbidity and mortality. Nonetheless, continued improvements in intraoperative monitoring, surgical technique, and prudent use of sophisticated vascular bypass techniques have lessened the incidence of profound hemodynamic changes that can lead to death, visceral injury and

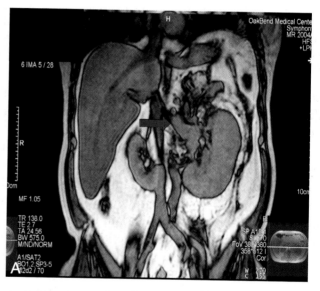

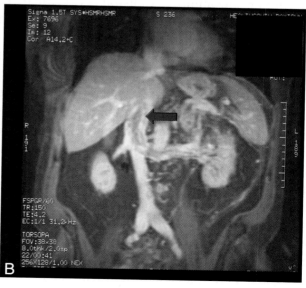

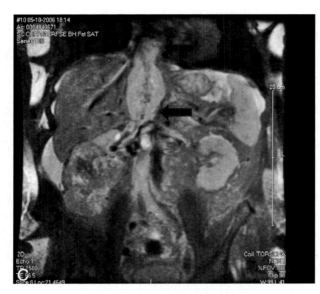

**Figure 3.** *A*, pT3b renal cell carcinoma. (Red arrow – tumor thrombus within the left renal vein). *B*, pT3b renal cell carcinoma (Red arrow – tumor thrombus within the infradiaphragmatic vena cava). *C*, pT3c renal cell carcinoma (Red arrows – tumor thrombus within the supradiaphragmatic vena cava).

| Table 2. VENOUS TUMOR THROMBUS CLASSIFICATION | |
|---|---|
| Level | Venous tumor thrombus extent |
| I | Renal vein |
| II | Infrahepatic vena cava |
| III | Retrohepatic vena cava |
| IV | Supradiaphragmatic vena cava, intracardiac |

coagulopathy, and have allowed progressively more difficult thrombus cases to be managed with lower complication rates.[6,42–45]

Basic oncologic principles of RN as set forth by Robson and colleagues, apply to the management of patients with a venous tumor thrombus and include complete renal arterial control, early isolation of the tumor thrombus within the venous system, followed by removal of the kidney within the Gerota's fascia and complete extraction of the neoplastic thrombus.[9] Preoperative assessment of the tumor thrombus extension is critical to surgical planning and the success to the operation (Table 2). The introduction and refinement of magnetic resonance imaging and transesophageal echocardiography resulted in a shift away from invasive procedures such as vena cavography, while allowing safe and accurate assessment of thrombus extent. Magnetic resonance imaging is 90 to 100% accurate in determination of the venous tumor thrombus extent, differentiates between benign and neoplastic thrombus and allows simultaneous evaluation for presence of systemic metastatic disease.[6,46] Transesophageal echocardiography is safe and well tolerated by patients; preoperatively it can be used, in equivocal cases, to confirm the extent of the tumor thrombus, assess for invasion of the caval wall by the thrombus and study the patency of the intrahepatic veins.[47]

Accurate knowledge of the tumor thrombus extent determines whether or not vascular bypass techniques will be necessary for safe thrombus extraction. Tumor thrombi with a definite infra hepatic cranial margin can be safely managed without the need for a vascular bypass. When a bypass is unlikely, an anterior subcostal or midline abdominal incision is utilized. In these cases, after the tumor bearing kidney has been mobilized, the neoplastic thrombus is isolated within the venous system by sequentially controlling the infrarenal vena cava, contralateral renal vein, and suprarenal vena cava.[6,48] Following cavotomy and removal of the tumor thrombus, the vena caval lumen is flushed and inspected for residual tumor fragments or irregularities that may require biopsy. In some instances the tumor thrombus can be milked easily into the renal vein and a vascular clamp or a staple line applied proximally without extensive vena cava dissection.

In patients with retrohepatic or a more caudal thrombus extent, surgery should be done in a location and setting where the options of cardiopulmonary bypass and deep hypothermic circulatory arrest are readily available. When a vascular bypass is indicated or possible, a midline abdominal and a median sternotomy incision, a "chevron" incision or a thoracoabdominal approach is necessary.[37,42,43,49] With application of liver transplant and vascular techniques, the majority of patients with high but infradiaphragmatic venous thrombi may be managed without utilizing cardiopulmonary bypass.[37,45] After arterial ligation and renal mobilization, surgeons use liver transplant techniques for a complete hepatic mobilization to expose and completely dissect the retrohepatic vena cava and use the Pringle maneuver to control the hepatic inflow.[50] Once complete caval control is established above and below the tumor thrombus, surgeons routinely assess patient's ability to tolerate caval cross-clamping, as sudden occlusion of the vena cava can compromise venous return with a subsequent decrease in cardiac output, hypotension and hypoperfusion of vital organs. During this portion of the procedure, transesophageal echography provides a noninvasive assessment of patient hemodynamics, while continuously monitoring the tumor thrombus location. In patients who cannot safely tolerate caval cross-clamping, veno-venous bypass is initiated by cannulating the vena cava below the distal aspect of the tumor thrombus, and returning the effluent into the right atrium or into the right brachial vein.

An alternative surgical approach to patients with a high retrohepatic venous thrombus is complete cardiopulmonary bypass with or without circulatory arrest.[43,44,51] The advantages of cardiopulmonary bypass and circulatory arrest include careful, controlled dissection in an essentially bloodless surgical field. However, because of the need for anticoagulation and the negative implications of hypothermic circulatory arrest on the coagulation system, mesenteric perfusion and neurologic function, surgeons reserve the use of this technique for patients with broad tumor infiltration of the suprahepatic caval wall or patients with atrial extension of the tumor thrombus.[6,42] If cardiopulmonary bypass is deemed necessary, the kidney and tumor mass are completely mobilized as previously described, so that the only remaining attachment is through the vein and the thrombus. When the renal tumor is extremely large, it is occasionally useful to remove the kidney, improving retroperitoneal exposure and access. The aortic arch and right atrial appendage are cannulated, and extracorporeal circulation is instituted. Once the patient is cooled down to the core temperature of 18°C, total circulatory exsanguination is accomplished, producing circulatory arrest. At 18°C, 45 to 60 minutes of ischemia time are well tolerated by the nervous system and is more than an adequate time necessary for thrombus extraction in well-planned procedures. An atriotomy and cavotomy are made, and the tumor thrombus en bloc with the renal mass and a large ellipse of vena cava are removed. After closure of the atriotomy and

cavotomy and achieving meticulous hemostasis, cardiopulmonary bypass is reinstituted. Once a normal core body temperature is achieved, regular sinus rhythm returns spontaneously or defibrillation is necessary.[43,51]

Occasionally, resection of the venous wall is necessary when the tumor directly invades the wall of the vena cava.[52] A pericardial patch may be used for reconstruction of the caval defect.[53] Alternatively, a total replacement of the IVC using an expanded polytetrafluoroethylene tubular graft is a feasible option, with acceptable long-term patency rates.[54]

Patients with non-metastatic RCC and associated neoplastic venous thrombus can expect excellent long-term survival, provided complete removal of all malignant tissue can be achieved. Extent of the venous thrombus does not carry significant prognostic information, but dictates the surgical approach and technical details. Marked advancements in preoperative imaging, intraoperative monitoring and anesthetic techniques, and prudent application of vascular bypass procedures have dramatically improved the feasibility and safety of surgical management of patients with RCC-associated venous tumor thrombi.

## RCC WITH DIRECT INVASION OF ADJACENT ORGANS

Tumor invasion beyond Gerota's fascia into adjacent organs (pT4), without concomitant metastatic disease, is a relatively unusual. Large retrospective series report a 5 to 15% incidence of pT4 RCC, the majority of which were associated with synchronous metastases.[4,33] Published literature addressing the group of patients with non-metastatic RCC with adjacent organ involvement is scant and contradictory, but most reports suggest that < 5% of patients survive 5 years after surgery.[4,55,56] Invasion of liver, spleen, and bowel mesentery by RCC have been reported, however, colon, pancreas, and diaphragm appear to be the most frequently involved viscera (Figure 4).[57]

Because surgical removal of the primary tumor remains the mainstay of treatment for localized RCC, and a fundamental part of an integrated

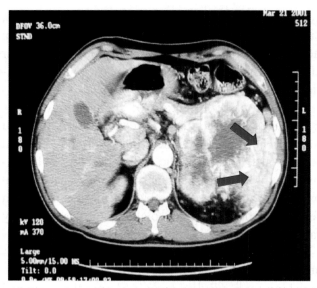

**Figure 4.** pT4 renal cell carcinoma (Red arrows – tumor invasion of the spleen).

multi-modality treatment plan for patients with advanced RCC, we evaluated oncologic efficacy of an aggressive surgical approach in pT4 patients at the M.D. Anderson Cancer Center. Several important observations were made.[57] First, a significant proportion of patients were clinically overstaged, in view of the fact that 60% of patients, thought to have invasion of adjacent organs clinically, were down-staged during final pathologic evaluation. Second, neither preoperative radiologic imaging, nor intraoperative surgical assessment could accurately differentiate between true pathologic involvement of adjacent viscera and benign desmoplastic adhesions. Moreover, 13 patients pathologically down-staged after surgical resection to < pT4 stage, demonstrated expected stage-appropriate disease-specific survival, and 5 (42%) pT4 patients were alive at a median follow-up of 38 months. Finally, compared to the RN series reported in the literature, concomitant resection of adjacent organs at the time of nephrectomy was associated with an increased blood loss and hospital stay, however, all patients in our series recovered from the procedure with similar morbidity and no mortality.[4,33]

Based on the above observations, we advocate aggressive surgical resection with en bloc removal of all affected organs in patients with adjacent organ involvement by RCC.

## RCC WITH LOCOREGIONAL LYMPH NODE INVOLVEMENT

The original description of RN by Robson and colleagues included routine extensive lymph node dissection of the paraaortic and paracaval lymph nodes from the crus of the diaphragm to the bifurcation of the aorta.[9] The applicability of this dictum, written in the era of poor preoperative imaging and high proportion of advanced disease at presentation, has been questioned in the modern era of small incidentally discovered RCC and sophisticated radiologic staging modalities.

Nodal involvement is one of the main factors influencing the prognosis of patients with cancer and RCC is no exception. Life expectancy decreases considerably when lymph node metastases are present, with overall 5-year survival rates of 11 to 35% reported in the literature.[58–60] The reported incidence of locoregional lymph node metastasis associated with RCC varies significantly throughout the modern literature, but largely depends on the primary tumor stage, presence of associated lymphadenopathy, and the extent of the lymphadenectomy performed.[61–63] In general, lymph node dissection at the time of RN has resulted in finding of metastatic lymph nodes in 5 to 22% of patients without associated systemic metastatic disease.[58,64] Up to 45% of patients with LARCC disease have been found to have malignant lymph node deposits, compared to 5% of patients with organ-confined RCC.[60,61,63,65] Moreover, with modern imaging techniques, unsuspected nodal involvement in patients with no radiologic or clinical evidence of lymphadenopathy is extremely rare (1 to 3%).[60,61] As such, patients with organ-confined RCC and no evidence of lymphadenopathy are unlikely to have associated lymph node metastasis and can be spared the potential morbidity of lymphadenectomy at the time of RN. Conversely, patients with LARCC and patients with radiologic or intraoperative finding of lymphadenopathy are at increased risk of harboring metastatic lymph node deposits (Figure 5).

While the prognostic value provided by lymph node dissection is unquestionable, the extent and therapeutic benefit of lymphadenectomy at the time

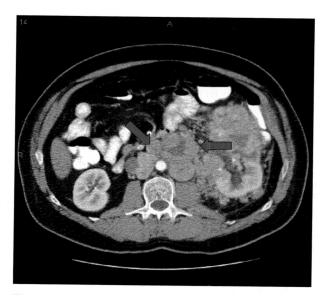

**Figure 5.** Renal cell carcinoma with locoregional lymph node metastases (Red arrows – precaval and interaortocaval lymphadenopathy).

of RN have been debated. The anatomic boundaries of lymph node dissection at the time of RN have not been standardized and current AJCC TNM tumor classification does not specify the minimal amount of lymph nodes necessary for accurate staging.[3] In patients with non-metastatic RCC treated with nephrectomy and lymph node dissection, Terrone and colleagues[63] have found that patients with < 13 lymph nodes recovered had a 3.4% risk of being staged node positive, whereas patients with at least 13 nodes recovered had a 10.5% risk of being staged node positive. These authors suggest that limited lymph node sampling during RN is insufficient, and recommend removal of the paraaortic and paracaval lymph nodes from the crus of the diaphragm to the bifurcation of the aorta to adequately stage patients.

Therapeutic benefit of lymph node dissection has unequivocally been demonstrated in several urologic malignancies, including bladder, testicular, and penile carcinomas, but remains a matter of debate in renal cancer.[66–68] Several retrospective studies have suggested a survival advantage to performing routine lymph node dissection at the time of RN, whereas other studies have revealed that routine lymphadenectomy does not improve survival.[60,65,69–72] The only randomized prospective clinical study to evaluate the role of routine lymphadenectomy at the

time of RN for RCC was conducted by European Organization for Research and Treatment of Cancer (EORTC 30881).[61] In this trial, 772 patients with clinical T1-3N0M0 RCC were randomized to RN only or RN and lymph node dissection. Although the study has not reached maturity, preliminary results failed to demonstrate any significant differences in cancer-specific survival between the study groups. Because only 3% of patients who underwent lymph node dissection at the time of RN had lymph node metastases, and very few patients (17%) progressed to died from RCC, conclusions about therapeutic efficacy of lymph node dissection are difficult to draw.[61]

Several recent reports presented a more convincing evidence of therapeutic efficacy of lymph node dissection in patients with clinically positive lymph nodes. Numerous single center reports have established that patients with suspected lymph node involvement at the time of RN (TxN1-2M0), who underwent lymph node dissection had significantly longer survival than node positive patients whose nodal tissue was left in situ.[58,59,73] Although retrospective in nature, these studies suggest that the biology and outcomes of lymph node positive RCC patients can be altered by surgical removal of cancerous lymph nodes, and make a strong case for lymphadenectomy when nodal involvement is suspected.

In conclusion, there is mounting evidence that oncologic outcome of RCC can be altered by removal of involved lymph nodes at the time of RN. As such, RCC patients with clinical suspicion of lymph node involvement should be managed with RN and extended lymphadenectomy. On the other end of the spectrum are the patients with organ-confined RCC and no clinical evidence of lymphadenopathy, who are unlikely to harbor metastatic lymph nodes and in whom a lymph node dissection can be safely omitted. In between these extremes are patients with LARCC and no clinical evidence of lymph node enlargement, large percentage of who harbor micro-metastatic lymph node disease. The question of therapeutic relevance of lymph node dissection in this group of patients can only be answered in a context of prospective randomized clinical study.

## CONCLUSION

Patients with LARCC harbor adverse pathologic features and are at significant risk of disease relapse. Despite the trend toward less invasive and less extirpative approaches, complete resection of all cancerous tissue is critical for long-term survival of LARCC patients. Significant advances in anesthetic, radiologic, and surgical techniques have empowered urologic oncologists to deliver more complex, yet safer surgical treatment options for patients with advanced RCC. Nonetheless, it is evident that aggressive surgical resection alone is not sufficient to prevent disease recurrence in a significant number of patients with LARCC. As such, there is a clear-cut need for improved ability to predict individual tumor's behavior and for development of effective systemic adjuvant therapies to treat disease relapse. As we move into the future, combined and structured analysis of clinical information, histopathologic criteria, molecular and genetic markers of disease will enable stratification of LARCC patients into sophisticated risk categories, and ultimately permit delivery of individualized therapies for targeted patient populations.[74–77]

## REFERENCES

1. Jemal A, Siegel R, Ward E, et al. Cancer statistics 2006. CA Cancer J Clin 2006;56:106.
2. Hock LM, Lynch J, Balaji KC. Increasing incidence of all stages of kidney cancer in the last 2 decades in the United States: an analysis of surveillance, epidemiology and end results program data. J Urol 2002;167:57.
3. Greene FL. American Joint Committee on Cancer. American Cancer Society: AJCC cancer staging manual. 6th ed. New York: Springer-Verlag; 2002. p. xiv, 421.
4. Lam JS, Belldegrun AS, Pantuck AJ. Long-term outcomes of the surgical management of renal cell carcinoma. World J Urol 2006;24:255.
5. Motzer RJ, Bacik J, Schwartz LH, et al. Prognostic factors for survival in previously treated patients with metastatic renal cell carcinoma. J Clin Oncol 2004;22:454.
6. Blute ML, Leibovich BC, Lohse CM, et al. The Mayo Clinic experience with surgical management, complications and outcome for patients with renal cell carcinoma and venous tumour thrombus. BJU Int 2004;94:33.
7. Han KR, Bui MH, Pantuck AJ, et al. TNM T3a renal cell carcinoma: adrenal gland involvement is not the same as renal fat invasion. J Urol 2003;169:899.
8. Tsui KH, Shvarts O, Smith RB, et al. Prognostic indicators for renal cell carcinoma: a multivariate analysis of 643 patients using the revised 1997 TNM staging criteria. J Urol 2000;163:1090.
9. Robson CJ, Churchill BM, Anderson W. The results of radical nephrectomy for renal cell carcinoma. J Urol 1969;101:297.
10. Mickisch GH. Principles of nephrectomy for malignant disease. BJU Int 2002;89:488.
11. Clayman RV, Kavoussi LR, Soper NJ, et al. Laparoscopic nephrectomy. N Engl J Med 1991;324:1370.
12. Clayman RV. Laparoscopic radical nephrectomy: oncologic efficacy. J Urol 2005;173:1201.
13. Permpongkosol S, Chan DY, Link RE, et al. Laparoscopic radical nephrectomy: long-term outcomes. J Endourol 2005; 19:628.
14. Walther MM, Lyne JC, Libutti SK, et al. Laparoscopic cytoreductive nephrectomy as preparation for administration of systemic interleukin-2 in the treatment of metastatic renal cell carcinoma: a pilot study. Urology 1999;53:496.
15. Matin SF, Madsen LT, Wood CG. Laparoscopic cytoreductive nephrectomy: the M.D. Anderson cancer center experience. Urology 2006;68:528.
16. Pautler SE, Walther MM. Laparoscopic radical nephrectomy for advanced kidney cancer. Curr Urol Rep 2002;3:21.
17. Cadeddu JA, Ono Y, Clayman RV, et al. Laparoscopic nephrectomy for renal cell cancer: evaluation of efficacy and safety: a multicenter experience. Urology 1998; 52:773.
18. Stifelman MD, Handler T, Nieder AM, et al. Hand-assisted laparoscopy for large renal specimens: a multi-institutional study. Urology 2003;61:78.
19. Fergany AF, Hafez KS, Novick AC. Long-term results of nephron sparing surgery for localized renal cell carcinoma: 10-year follow up. J Urol 2000;163:442.
20. Hafez KS, Fergany AF, Novick AC. Nephron sparing surgery for localized renal cell carcinoma: impact of tumor size on patient survival, tumor recurrence and TNM staging. J Urol 1999;162:1930.
21. Kletscher BA, Qian J, Bostwick DG, et al. Prospective analysis of the incidence of ipsilateral adrenal metastasis in localized renal cell carcinoma. J Urol 1996;155:1844.
22. Shalev M, Cipolla B, Guille F, et al. Is ipsilateral adrenalectomy a necessary component of radical nephrectomy? J Urol 1995;153:1415.
23. Tsui KH, Shvarts O, Barbaric Z, et al. Is adrenalectomy a necessary component of radical nephrectomy? UCLA experience with 511 radical nephrectomies. J Urol 2000; 163:437.
24. Kuczyk M, Munch T, Machtens S, et al. The need for routine adrenalectomy during surgical treatment for renal cell cancer: the Hannover experience. BJU Int 2002;89:517.
25. Siemer S, Lehmann J, Kamradt J, et al. Adrenal metastases in 1635 patients with renal cell carcinoma: outcome and indication for adrenalectomy. J Urol 2004;171:2155.
26. Sawai Y, Kinouchi T, Mano M, et al. Ipsilateral adrenal involvement from renal cell carcinoma: retrospective study of the predictive value of computed tomography. Urology 2002;59:28.

27. Sagalowsky AI, Kadesky KT, Ewalt DM, et al. Factors influencing adrenal metastasis in renal cell carcinoma. J Urol 1994;151:1181.

28. Antonelli A, Cozzoli A, Simeone C, et al. Surgical treatment of adrenal metastasis from renal cell carcinoma: a single-centre experience of 45 patients. BJU Int 2006;97:505.

29. Sandock DS, Seftel AD, Resnick MI. Adrenal metastases from renal cell carcinoma: role of ipsilateral adrenalectomy and definition of stage. Urology 1997;49:28.

30. Leibovitch I, Raviv G, Mor Y, et al. Reconsidering the necessity of ipsilateral adrenalectomy during radical nephrectomy for renal cell carcinoma. Urology 1995;46:316.

31. Thompson RH, Leibovich BC, Cheville JC, et al. Should direct ipsilateral adrenal invasion from renal cell carcinoma be classified as pT3a? J Urol 2005;173:918.

32. Siemer S, Lehmann J, Loch A, et al. Current TNM classification of renal cell carcinoma evaluated: revising stage T3a. J Urol 2005;173:33.

33. Thompson RH, Cheville JC, Lohse CM, et al. Reclassification of patients with pT3 and pT4 renal cell carcinoma improves prognostic accuracy. Cancer 2005;104:53.

34. Leibovich BC, Cheville JC, Lohse CM, et al. Cancer specific survival for patients with pT3 renal cell carcinoma-can the 2002 primary tumor classification be improved? J Urol 2005;173:716.

35. Ficarra V, Novara G, Iafrate M, et al. Proposal for reclassification of the TNM staging system in patients with locally advanced (pT3-4) renal cell carcinoma according to the cancer-related outcome. Eur Urol 2006.

36. Zisman A, Wieder JA, Pantuck AJ, et al. Renal cell carcinoma with tumor thrombus extension: biology, role of nephrectomy and response to immunotherapy. J Urol 2003;169:909.

37. Parekh DJ, Cookson MS, Chapman W, et al. Renal cell carcinoma with renal vein and inferior vena caval involvement: clinicopathological features, surgical techniques and outcomes. J Urol 2005;173:1897.

38. Sweeney P, Wood CG, Pisters LL, et al. Surgical management of renal cell carcinoma associated with complex inferior vena caval thrombi. Urol Oncol 2003;21:327.

39. Kim HL, Zisman A, Han KR, et al. Prognostic significance of venous thrombus in renal cell carcinoma. Are renal vein and inferior vena cava involvement different? J Urol 2004;171:588.

40. Skinner DG, Pritchett TR, Lieskovsky G, et al. Vena caval involvement by renal cell carcinoma. Surgical resection provides meaningful long-term survival. Ann Surg 1989;210:387.

41. Swierzewski DJ, Swierzewski MJ, Libertino JA. Radical nephrectomy in patients with renal cell carcinoma with venous, vena caval, and atrial extension. Am J Surg 1994;168:205.

42. Lubahn JG, Sagalowsky AI, Rosenbaum DH, et al. Contemporary techniques and safety of cardiovascular procedures in the surgical management of renal cell carcinoma with tumor thrombus. J Thorac Cardiovasc Surg 2006;131:1289.

43. Novick AC, Kaye MC, Cosgrove DM, et al. Experience with cardiopulmonary bypass and deep hypothermic circulatory arrest in the management of retroperitoneal tumors with large vena caval thrombi. Ann Surg 1990;212:472.

44. Wotkowicz C, Libertino JA, Sorcini A, et al. Management of renal cell carcinoma with vena cava and atrial thrombus: minimal access vs median sternotomy with circulatory arrest. BJU Int 2006;98:289.

45. Ciancio G, Soloway MS. Renal cell carcinoma with tumor thrombus extending above diaphragm: avoiding cardiopulmonary bypass. Urology 2005;66:266.

46. Goldfarb DA, Novick AC, Lorig R, et al. Magnetic resonance imaging for assessment of vena caval tumor thrombi: a comparative study with venacavography and computerized tomography scanning. J Urol 1990;144:1100.

47. Glazer A, Novick AC. Preoperative transesophageal echocardiography for assessment of vena caval tumor thrombi: a comparative study with venacavography and magnetic resonance imaging. Urology 1997;49:32.

48. Bachmann A, Seitz M, Graser A, et al. Tumour nephrectomy with vena cava thrombus. BJU Int 2005;95:1373.

49. Nesbitt JC, Soltero ER, Dinney CP, et al. Surgical management of renal cell carcinoma with inferior vena cava tumor thrombus. Ann Thorac Surg 1997;63:1592.

50. Delis S, Dervenis C, Lytras D, et al. Liver transplantation techniques with preservation of the natural venovenous bypass: effect on surgical resection of renal cell carcinoma invading the inferior vena cava. World J Surg 2004;28:614.

51. Marshall FF, Dietrick DD, Baumgartner WA, et al. Surgical management of renal cell carcinoma with intracaval neoplastic extension above the hepatic veins. J Urol 1998;139:1166.

52. Ciancio G, Soloway M. Resection of the abdominal inferior vena cava for complicated renal cell carcinoma with tumour thrombus. BJU Int 2005;96:815.

53. Marshall FF, Reitz BA. Supradiaphragmatic renal cell carcinoma tumor thrombus: indications for vena caval reconstruction with pericardium. J Urol 1985;133:266.

54. Caldarelli G, Minervini A, Guerra M, et al. Prosthetic replacement of the inferior vena cava and the iliofemoral vein for urologically related malignancies. BJU Int 2002;90:368.

55. Hayakawa M, Nakajima F, Higa I, et al. [Study on clinical courses of 7 patients undergone resection of adjacent organs in the treatment of locally extensive renal cell carcinoma]. Nippon Hinyokika Gakkai Zasshi 1995;86:1302.

56. Fukuda M, Satomi Y, Nakahashi M, et al. [Treatment and prognosis of T 4 renal cell carcinoma]. Nippon Hinyokika Gakkai Zasshi 1999;90:753.

57. Margulis V, Sanchez-Ortiz R, Tamboli P, et al. Renal cell carcinoma clinically involving adjacent organs - our experience with aggressive surgical management. Cancer 2007, in press.

58. Pantuck AJ, Zisman A, Dorey F, et al. Renal cell carcinoma with retroperitoneal lymph nodes: role of lymph node dissection. J Urol 2003;169:2076.

59. Canfield SE, Kamat AM, Sanchez-Ortiz RF, et al. Renal cell carcinoma with nodal metastases in the absence of distant metastatic disease (clinical stage TxN1-2M0): the impact of aggressive surgical resection on patient outcome. J Urol 2006;175:864.

60. Minervini A, Lilas L, Morelli G, et al. Regional lymph node dissection in the treatment of renal cell carcinoma: is it useful in patients with no suspected adenopathy before or during surgery? BJU Int 2001;88:169.

61. Blom JH, van Poppel H, Marechal JM, et al. Radical nephrectomy with and without lymph node dissection: preliminary results of the EORTC randomized phase III protocol 30881. EORTC Genitourinary Group. Eur Urol 1999; 36:570.

62. Blute ML, Leibovich BC, Cheville JC, et al. A protocol for performing extended lymph node dissection using primary tumor pathological features for patients treated with radical nephrectomy for clear cell renal cell carcinoma. J Urol 2004;172:465.

63. Terrone C, Guercio S, De Luca S, et al. The number of lymph nodes examined and staging accuracy in renal cell carcinoma. BJU Int 2003;91:37.

64. Vasselli JR, Yang JC, Linehan WM, et al. Lack of retroperitoneal lymphadenopathy predicts survival of patients with metastatic renal cell carcinoma. J Urol 2001;166:68.

65. Siminovitch JP, Montie JE, Straffon RA. Lymphadenectomy in renal adenocarcinoma. J Urol 1982;127:1090.

66. Skinner EC, Stein JP, Skinner DG. Surgical benchmarks for the treatment of invasive bladder cancer. Urol Oncol 2007; 25:66.

67. Carver BS, Sheinfeld J. Germ cell tumors of the testis. Ann Surg Oncol 2005;12:871.

68. Kroon BK, Horenblas S, Lont AP, et al. Patients with penile carcinoma benefit from immediate resection of clinically occult lymph node metastases. J Urol 2005;173:816.

69. Peters PC, Brown GL. The role of lymphadenectomy in the management of renal cell carcinoma. Urol Clin North Am 1980;7:705.

70. Herrlinger A, Schrott KM, Schott G, et al. What are the benefits of extended dissection of the regional renal lymph nodes in the therapy of renal cell carcinoma. J Urol 1991;146:1224.

71. Giberti C, Oneto F, Martorana G, et al. Radical nephrectomy for renal cell carcinoma: long-term results and prognostic factors on a series of 328 cases. Eur Urol 1997;31:40.

72. Schafhauser W, Ebert A, Brod J, et al. Lymph node involvement in renal cell carcinoma and survival chance by systematic lymphadenectomy. Anticancer Res ????;19:1573.

73. Karakiewicz PI, Trinh QD, Bhojani N, et al. Renal cell carcinoma with nodal metastases in the absence of distant metastatic disease: prognostic indicators of disease-specific survival. Eur Urol 2006.

74. Kattan MW, Reuter V, Motzer RJ, et al. A postoperative prognostic nomogram for renal cell carcinoma. J Urol 2001; 166:63.

75. Frank I, Blute ML, Cheville JC, et al. An outcome prediction model for patients with clear cell renal cell carcinoma treated with radical nephrectomy based on tumor stage, size, grade and necrosis: the SSIGN score. J Urol 2002; 168:2395.

76. Zisman A, Pantuck AJ, Wieder J, et al. Risk group assessment and clinical outcome algorithm to predict the natural history of patients with surgically resected renal cell carcinoma. J Clin Oncol 2002;20:4559.

77. Lam JS, Leppert JT, Figlin RA, et al. Role of molecular markers in the diagnosis and therapy of renal cell carcinoma. Urology 2005;66:1.

# 10

# Adjuvant Therapy in Renal Cell Carcinoma

AHMAD RAHMAN, MB, BS

TIM EISEN, PHD, FRCP

Renal cell carcinoma (RCC) is treated by curative nephrectomy in early stage disease, but 20% of patients will ultimately develop metastatic lesions.[1] The median time to relapse postnephrectomy is 15 to 18 months and the 5-year survival rate for stage IV metastatic RCC is estimated to be less than 10%.[2,3] Thus, patients who have a significant risk of relapse postnephrectomy have a great need for effective adjuvant therapy to improve disease-free and overall survival.

In this chapter, we will review the rationale and the possible selection of patients for adjuvant treatment. We then go on to discuss the spectrum of therapeutic options and the current data supporting each of those options. Some treatments that have been proven in the advanced disease setting are now coming forward to the adjuvant setting. Having outlined the current trials portfolio, we will end by discussing other potential adjuvant therapy strategies.

## RISK STRATIFICATION

Any potential therapeutic option would need to balance the risk to benefit ratio in an asymptomatic patient with a significant risk of recurrence. To select patients appropriately for adjuvant therapy, one must identify the population with a significant risk of recurrence. Different strategies have been used to stratify patients' risk, leading to the creation of a number of nomograms. (Table 1) These are important tools, aiding patient counseling, treatment decisions, and entry into clinical trials.

For instance, the University of California Los Angeles Integrated Staging System[4,5] stratified patients with metastatic and nonmetastatic disease into low-, intermediate-, and high-risk groups. Patients in the nonmetastatic high-risk group had a high systemic failure rate. Validation of this algorithm[6] was done using an international database of more than 1,000 patients with localized RCC (Table 1). In the future, it may be possible to use molecular biomarkers as an adjunct or even a replacement for clinical prognostic indicators. Clearly, this must remain entirely speculative at present. A number of good candidate molecular markers have been identified, including proliferation and cell-cycle regulators, such as protein tyrosine phosphatase, P21

| Table 1. RENAL CELL CARCINOMA PREDICTION NOMOGRAM VARIABLES | | | |
|---|---|---|---|
| Memorial Sloan–Kettering Cancer Center[7] | Modified UCLA integrated staging system [4,5,6] | SSIGN score algorithm[8] | Mayo et al[9] |
| Symptoms, histology, tumor size, tumor stage | Stage, Fuhrman nuclear grade, ECOG performance status | Tumor stage, Node stage, metastasis stage, tumor size, Fuhrman nuclear grade, presence of necrosis | clinical presentation, grade, Stage, tumor size |

ECOG = Eastern Cooperative Oncology Group; SSIGN = Mayo Clinic stage, size, grade, and necrosis score; UCLA = University of California at Los Angeles.

and P53; apoptosis markers, such as AKT1, BCL2, and BACS; growth signals, such as SRC, TTF1β, and epidermal growth factor; and perhaps most promisingly at present, angiogenic markers, such as vascular endothelial growth factor (VEGF), VEGF receptors, platelet-derived growth factor (PDGF), PDGF receptors, and hypoxia-inducible factor (HIF). The majority of data at present relate to VEGF and the VEGF-signalling system. In this regard, the discovery that Von Hippel-Lindau (VHL) protein expression correlates with survival[10] is notable. Similarly, the discovery that VEGF levels appear to correlate with survival in papillary and clear cell renal cell carcinoma[11] is consistent with the important role of the VEGF-signalling system in renal cell carcinoma. Whether these potential prognostic markers will in fact prove useful clinically will depend on prospective studies, preferably in the context of randomized clinical trials.

## RADIOTHERAPY

Theoretically, the concept of sterilizing the tumor bed following resection of a high-risk renal cell carcinoma may be attractive. However, renal cell carcinomas may be very resistant to radiotherapy. Three studies are worth noting in this context. The first randomized 72 patients to observation of adjuvant radiotherapy at 50 Gy in 20 fractions following resection of a stage II or III tumor. Some 26 months after follow-up, the survival in the radiotherapy group was 50% compared with 62% in the observation group.[12] The second study retrospectively assessed the results for 186 patients who had received a nephrectomy for locally advanced renal cell carcinoma. In all, 114 patients received postoperative radiotherapy of 50 Gy to the renal bed, 72 patients received standard follow-up. In this retrospective analysis, there was no statistically significant difference in overall disease-free survival (overall survival 37.9 vs 35.5%, disease-free survival 29.5 vs 31.3% at 5 years). Of considerable importance was the fact that local relapse was evenly distributed between the two groups, suggesting that radiotherapy had little effect in controlling local relapse let alone distant metastases.[13] There was also a trial of neoadjuvant radiotherapy in

which 38 patients were randomized to 33 Gy of preoperative radiotherapy followed by nephrectomy and 50 patients to nephrectomy alone. At 5-year follow-up, the overall survival in the radiotherapy and nephrectomy group was 47%, whereas the overall survival in the nephrectomy alone group was 63%. Although this difference is not statistically significant, there is clearly no evidence of any radiotherapy benefits.[14]

## CHEMOTHERAPY

RCC is a notoriously chemorefractory tumor. Response rates in metastatic RCC are generally poor varying between 2 and 6%.[15] Multidrug resistance is thought to be mediated by p-glycoprotein.[16] Both renal proximal tubules and renal cell carcinoma express high levels of this peptide. Calcium-channel blockers or other drugs that interfere with the function of p-glycoprotein can diminish resistance to vinblastine and anthracycline in human renal cell carcinoma cell lines. However, these agents have been shown to improve the efficacy of vinblastine in metastatic RCC.

A phase II study[17] combining gemcitabine and fluorouracil (FU) in metastatic RCC showed a partial response rate of 17% with a significantly longer mean progression-free survival of 28.7 weeks compared with historical controls. 5-FU has been shown to have a response rate of 10% but when used in combination with interferon (IFN)-α and prednisolone has had a response rate of 23% in one study.[18]

The efficacy of chemotherapy has as also been investigated in the adjuvant setting. One trial looked at VAU therapy[19] (vinblastine, adriamycin, and tegafur-uracil [UFT]) given postoperatively to 31 patients with stage I, II, or III RCC. The 1-year survival of patients was 100%, and the 3- and 5-year survival values were 96%. These results were significantly better ($p < .01$) than the respective values (81%, 72%, and 60%) obtained for the historical controls. This trial has subsequently been criticized for the low overall risk of patients receiving adjuvant treatment and for the limited sample size.

Currently, there is no evidence to support the use of adjuvant chemotherapy in RCC.

## IMMUNOTHERAPY

### Vaccine Therapy

The activity of interleukin (IL)-2 and IFN-α; in renal cell carcinoma suggests that RCC may be sensitive to immune-based strategies.

Cancer vaccine therapy aims to heighten antitumor immunity, for example, by bolstering the number of tumor-reactive effector T lymphocytes through immunization and stimulating a long-lasting T-cell memory.

There appears to be a special immunological window of opportunity after resection, when residual tumor mass is at its lowest and the host immune system has been relieved of suppression related to tumor bulk.[20]

However, harnessing the immune system to achieve effective control still faces a number of challenges as tumor cells often evade immune surveillance by a variety of mechanisms; not only are tumor antigens downregulated but also most are immunogenically weak. The tumor microenvironment inhibits T-cell activation and function, in addition to accruing immunosuppressive cells. In addition, patients with RCC characteristically exhibit gross immunologic dysfunction,[20] and proteins secreted in RCC (granulocyte colony–stimulating factor, VEGF, and IL-10) have immunoregulatory properties, dampening the antitumor response.

### Active Specific Immunotherapy

A prospective randomized trial[21] investigated the role of adjuvant active specific immunotherapy in 120 consecutive patients with RCC (pT1-3b pN0 or pN+) after radical nephrectomy. Patients were randomized to observation versus intradermal injection of irradiated tumor cells either on a single agent or were boosted with adjuvant Bacillus Calmette-Guerin. Following a median follow-up of 61 months, there was no statistical difference in overall or disease-free survival.

### Autologous Renal Tumor Cell Vaccine

An adjuvant vaccine trial[22] using an autologous cell lysate incubated in tocopherol and IFN-γ demonstrated a striking 5-year progression-free survival in patients with T3 N0 M0 disease (vaccine arm 68.2% vs historical controls 19.4%). Patients were injected subdermally every 4 weeks for 6 months, and treatment was well tolerated warranting further investigation. In a subsequent phase III trial,[23] 558 patients scheduled for radical nephrectomy were randomized to receive autologous renal tumor cell vaccine or observation alone. At 5-year and 70-month follow-up, the hazard ratios for tumor progression were 1.58 (95% confidence interval [CI] = 1.05 to 2.37) and 1.59 (1.07–2.36), respectively, in favor of the vaccine arm. Progression-free survival at 5 years and 70 months were 77.4% and 72%, respectively, in the vaccine group, compared with 67.8% and 59.3%, respectively, in the control group. Treatment was well tolerated and was demonstrated by only 12 adverse events in the vaccine arm. This study has been criticized for the significant proportion of patients lost with randomization (32%) particularly from the vaccine arm and with the absence of overall survival rates in initial reports. An intention to treat analysis may reduce the clinical significance of this therapeutic approach and further confirmatory studies are required.

### Heat-Shock Proteins

An alternative vaccine approach is to use heat-shock proteins (HSP). They are ubiquitous proteins found in all cells and defend the cell during injury. Acting as chaperones, they guide newly synthesized cellular proteins to fold into their functional conformations. The antitumor possibilities stem from the complex formed between HSP and the antigens they chaperone, which is highly immunogenic.[24] This heat-shock peptide–protein complex (HSPPC) can in turn direct certain immune pathways to target malignant cells, such as T- and natural killer (NK) cell activation, maturation of dendritic cells, and cytokine secretion.

Laboratory mice vaccinated with attenuated tumor cells exhibited specific future protection against similar live tumor cells. Further experiments showed HSP to play a role in protective immunity. Mice tumor models demonstrated tumor shrinkage when treated with HSPPCs, and in those with minimal residual disease, there was long-lasting protection from recurrence.

HSPPCs can be purified to extract the peptide library corresponding to the tissue of origin. Autologous HSPPCs have the advantage of high specificity for tumors in individual patients and are able to bypass the immune tolerance of certain tumors.

Oncophage, a HSPPC-96 vaccine, was the first such autologous treatment in RCC made from surgically resected tumor. Phase I trials in patients with pretreated metastatic RCC showed that Oncophage was well tolerated, with low-grade fevers and injection-site reactions most commonly being reported. A phase II study[25] of Oncophage with the addition of IL-2 for those who progressed on vaccine treatment, enrolled 61 patients with metastatic RCC. From the 61 patients who received at least one vaccine dose, there were two partial responses and one complete response, and 18 had stable disease. Of those who progressed, 7 of the 16 had stable disease after receiving IL-2. Median progression-free survival was 18 weeks for the whole group and 25 weeks in those who received both treatments.

A phase III multicenter, randomized, open-label trial[26] of Oncophage in patients with nonmetastatic RCC at high risk of relapse following nephrectomy has recently reported. Patients were randomized 1:1 to Oncophage postsurgery or surgery alone. In March 2006, a provisional analysis of the trial data suggested a trend toward Oncophage increasing recurrence-free survival but against overall survival. However, an independent review by the trial's Clinical Events Committee determined that the study did not meet its end points and that the number of events were insufficient for analysis. The trial protocol had required patients to be disease-free at baseline; however, it was brought to light that 124 of the 728 patients actually had identifiable disease at this point. Of the 218 events reported by investigators, 92 were from this group, which was ineligible for the trial. A subsequent review of the data at an international expert panel meeting found that in the full analysis set (representing the true adjuvant patient population intended for the trial), a trend toward recurrence-free survival and against overall survival was demonstrated. As of May 2006, there were 27 deaths in the observation arm and 33 in the Oncophage arm. However, there was a significant improvement in recurrence-free survival in a subgroup of better prognosis patients. This group of 361 patients compromising 60% of the total full analysis set included those whose disease was stage I-II (high grade) and stage III T1-3a (low grade) as defined by the American Joint Committee on Cancer. These patients showed the most significant response to Oncophage versus observation with respect to recurrence-free survival (hazard ratio = 0.567; $p$ = .018). Treatment was generally well tolerated, with most adverse events related to the actual injection or being constitutional in nature (headache, fatigue, or rash).[27]

## WX-G250 Monoclonal Antibody Therapy

Tumors in laboratory animals have been shown to shrink after administration of serum derived from immunocompetent animals immunized with tumor antigens. Experiments have shown that antibodies directed against tumors can guide toxic substances or radionulides to it and promote antibody-dependent cellular cytotoxicity. A number of monoclonal antibodies have already been licensed for use in the treatment of cancer.

Carbonic anhydrase (CA) IX is expressed in 94% of clear cell RCC cases but not in normal renal tissue.[28] Its normal function is to regulate intra- and extracellular pH of cells by catalyzing the reversible conversion of carbon dioxide and water to carbonic acid[29.] It may also be a prognostic marker for response to IL-2.

In vitro studies have shown potent and durable immune effector activity when combining WX-G250 and cytokines. This led to the hypothesis that adding cytokines like IL-2 with WX-G250 might have a synergistic effect in treating RCC. One such trial[30] in metastatic RCC had shown an overall clinical benefit rate (objective response or stable disease at 6 months) of 25 % and a median survival time of 22 months. WX-G250 in combination with IFN-α showed a tumor response and/or disease stabilization in 42% of the 26 evaluable patients.

WX-G250 (cG250, Rencarex) is a chimeric IgG monoclonal antibody that binds to CA IX. Phase I studies have demonstrated WX-G250 to be safe and well tolerated both as monotherapy and in combination with IL-2 and IFN-α.

In phase II studies, weekly intravenous WX-G250 was administered in patients with metastatic RCC.[31] Stable disease was noted in 11 of the 36 patients, as well as one complete response (CR) and partial response (PR), and the treatment was well tolerated.

A multicenter phase III trial of adjuvant WX-G250 versus placebo, Adjuvant Rencarex Immunotherapy trail to Study Efficacy, is currently enrolling. Its aim is to evaluate the disease-free survival and overall survival of patients treated with WX-G250 who have nonmetastatic clear cell RCC at high risk of relapse after nephrectomy and lymphadenectomy. It aims to recruit more than 800 patients with an Eastern Cooperative Oncology Group (ECOG) score of 0 and no macro- or microscopic residual disease. Participants will receive a once-weekly infusion of WX-G250 or placebo for 24 weeks. Those randomized to the treatment arm will receive a loading dose of 50 mg WX-G250 in week 1, followed by weekly doses of 20 mg during weeks 2 to 24.

## IFN

Interferons are known to have antiproliferative, antiangiogenic and immunomodulatory properties. They have been shown to have a direct antiproliferative effect on renal tumor cells in vitro and enhance expression of major histocompatibility complex molecules.

IFN-$\alpha$ has been shown to be active in metastatic RCC unlike IFN-$\beta$ and $\gamma$ with an overall response rate of 14.5% (range 0 to 30%) in a review[32] of 648 patients with metastatic RCC.

A randomized trial investigated the efficacy of adjuvant IFN-$\alpha$ postradical nephrectomy versus nephrectomy only in Robson Stage II and III RCC.[33] Over a 62-month surveillance period, 51 of the 123 patients in the treatment arm had a recurrence of RCC compared with 38 of 124 patients in the control arm. At 5 years, the probability of event-free and overall survival was 0.671 and 0.665, respectively, for the control arm compared with 0.567 and 0.66, respectively, for the treatment arm. The differences were not statistically significant.

In a multicenter phase III trial,[34] 283 patients with pT3-4a and/or node-positive disease were randomized postradical nephrectomy and lymphadenectomy to IFN-$\alpha$, administered daily for 5 days every 3 weeks for up to 12 cycles, or observation. After a median follow-up of 10.4 years, median survival in the observation arm was 7.4 years and 5.1 years in the treatment arm ($p = .09$), and recurrence-free survival was 3.0 years in the observation arm and 2.2 years in the IFN arm ($p = .33$). The authors, therefore, concluded that treatment with IFN did not confer survival or relapse-free survival advantage in the adjuvant setting.

Preclinical studies have shown synergy between IFNs and cytotoxic drugs, and the use of chemotherapy in combination with IFN has also been investigated in the adjuvant setting. A study of 32 patients postnephrectomy receiving IFN-$2\alpha$ and vinblastine found no statistical difference in progression-free survival or death when compared with 30 patients observed after nephrectomy alone.[35] A trial of 10 patients with pT3N0M0 RCC who received radical nephrectomy were randomly assigned to receive treatment with either IFN-$\alpha$ alone or IFN-$\alpha$ and vinblastine.[36] There were no statistical differences in time to progression and survival rate between the two groups when compared with a nonrandomized cohort. Despite its modest activity in metastatic patients, it appears to have none in the adjuvant setting.

## IL-2

IL-2 is normally produced by the body during an immune response and activates both T and NK cells.[37] Phase II studies using high-dose bolus intravenous IL-2 (600,000 to 720,000 IU/kg) in patients with metastatic RCC showed an overall objective response rate of 14%. In addition, there were 12 (5%) CRs and 24 (9%) PRs with a median duration of response of 54 months in 255 assessable patients. Median survival of all patients was 16.3 months.[38,39] On the basis of these data, IL-2 was approved by the food and drug administration (FDA) for use in metastatic RCC. The only predictive prognostic factor for response was performance status. Treatment was associated with severe acute toxicities, including capillary leak, hypotension requiring inotropes and oliguria and a significant number of patients will require intensive care unit support. In all, 4% patients died of adverse events judged to be possibly or probably treatment related.

A multicenter, prospective, randomized phase III trial compared IL-2 (600,000 U/kg) versus observation in patients with high-risk RCC following nephrectomy, including resected locally advanced (T3b-4 or N1-3) or metastatic (M1) RCC and treatment naïve.[40] This was discontinued early as its interim analysis determined that the treatment arm would fail to reach its 2-year survival goal of 30% improvement in disease-free survival despite full accrual. At this time point, 15 of the 21 (71%) patients in the treatment arm and 16 of the 23 (69%) patients in the observation arm experienced relapse. There was no difference in disease-free survival or overall survival even when patients with metastasectomy were included in the analysis.

## IL-2, IFN-α 2a, 5-FU

A prospective randomized trial[41] investigated the efficacy of adjuvant immunochemotherapy in high-risk patients following radical nephrectomy for RCC. In all, 203 patients with RCC were stratified into three risk groups:

1. tumor extending into renal vein/vena cava or invading beyond Gerota's fascia (pT3b/c pN0 or pT4 pN0),
2. locoregional lymph node infiltration (pN+), and
3. complete resection of tumor relapse or solitary metastasis (R0)

Subjects were then randomized to either 8 weeks of IL-2, subcutaneous IFN-α2a, and intravenous 5-FU or observation. Overall survival after a median follow-up of 4.3 years was lower in the treatment arm with 2-, 5-, and 8-year survival rates of 81%, 58%, and 58%, respectively, and 91%, 76%, and 66% in the observation arm ($p = .0278$). Relapse-free survival rates at 2, 5, and 8 years were calculated at 54%, 42%, and 39% in the treatment arm, and at 62%, 49%, and 49% in the observation arm ($p = .02398$), respectively. The authors concluded that the overall survival was inferior in the combination arm and that there was no benefit seen in relapse-free survival. A further randomized phase III trial (EORTC 30955/HYDRA) compared observations with a single cycle of the Atzpodien regimen and results are awaited.

The disappointing results produced during the investigation of cytokine agents in the adjuvant setting has led to investigators to shift attention to other treatment modalities in the hope of demonstrating a clinical benefit. (Table 2)

## SIGNALLING INHIBITORS

Most sporadic clear cell renal cancers, accounting for 80% of all renal cell cancers, have hypermethylation or silencing of the *VHL* gene.[42–44] Its normal function is to regulate intracellular hypoxia-induced factor-1[45] α by controlling the ubiquitination and subsequent breakdown by the proteasome. In the absence of *VHL* function, hypoxia-induced factor-1 α expression, as well as activation of hypoxia-sensitive genes, increases. The consequence is an increase in the levels of VEGF, transforming growth factor–α (TGF-α), platelet-derived growth factor–β (PDGF-β), and other gene products.[45,46] As overproduction of these growth factors are thought to be integral to transformation,

| First Author | Agent | Result |
|---|---|---|
| Pizzocaro[32] | Interferon | No clinical benefit |
| Messing[33] | Interferon | No clinical benefit |
| Clark[39] | Interleukin-2 | No clinical benefit |
| Migilari[34] | Interferon/vinblastine | No clinical benefit |
| Jeon[35] | Interferon/vinblastine | No clinical benefit |
| Atzpodien[40] | Interleukin-2, interferon α2a, 5-fluorouracil | No clinical benefit |

Table 2. ADJUVANT CYTOKINE TRIALS IN RENAL CELL CARCINOMA

growth, and dissemination of renal cell carcinoma, it follows that inhibiting their activity may provide an effective therapeutic option. (Figure 1)

## Sorafenib (BAY 43-9006)

Sorafenib (Nexavar; Bayer) is an orally administered small-molecule inhibitor of multiple tyrosine kinases.[47]

Phase I studies resulted in a phase II dose of 400 mg twice daily continuously.[48] At this dose, almost complete inhibition of externally regulated kinases (ERK) phosphorylation was reported in peripheral blood lymphocytes, a marker for raf kinase inhibition, with partial inhibition at 200 mg twice daily. The most significant dose-limiting toxicity was hand-foot skin reaction with diarrhea, fatigue and

hypertension also being noted, all of which were reversible with drug discontinuation.

A randomized phase II discontinuation study of sorafenib was undertaken where 202 patients with metastatic renal cell cancer received single agent sorafenib for a 12-week run-in period.[49] Those patients with stable disease after this period were then randomly assigned to sorafenib or oral placebo for another 12 weeks. Patients who drew placebo were switched to sorafenib if they progressed. During the run-in period, 73 patients had tumor shrinkage of $\geq 25\%$, and at 12 weeks, 65 patients had stable disease. Median progression-free survival from randomization was significantly longer in the sorafenib arm (24 weeks) versus placebo (6 weeks; $p = .0087$), in the 28 patients who had progressed on placebo, and to whom sorafenib was readministered until progression, for a median of 24 weeks. Most adverse events were manageable (skin rash/desquamation, fatigue, and hand-foot skin reaction), and hypertension responded well to diuretics/$\beta$-blockers.

On the basis of these data, a large placebo-controlled, double-blind, randomized phase III trial[50] investigated the efficacy of sorafenib in patients who had progressed on or after first-line treatment, usually immunotherapy. In all, 93% had prior nephrectomies; 99% had received prior systemic therapies, including IL-2 (44%), and an IFN (68%). A progression-free survival advantage was reported in treatment arm of 24 versus 12 weeks ($p < .000001$) across all patient subsets, as well as a 39% prolongation of overall survival despite only a 2% response evaluation criteria in solid tumors (RECIST)–defined response rate. Once a progression-free survival was shown in interim analysis, patients who drew placebo were allowed to receive sorafenib thus confounding overall survival data.

The most common adverse events were diarrhea, rash/desquamation, fatigue, hand-foot skin reaction, alopecia, and nausea/vomiting. The incidence of grade 3/4 adverse events was reported as 38% for sorafenib versus 28% for placebo. Grade 3 and 4 adverse events were unusual; only hand-foot skin reaction occurred at 5% or greater frequency in the sorafenib arm.

On the basis of the above trials, the FDA approved sorafenib for the treatment of patients with advanced renal cell carcinoma.

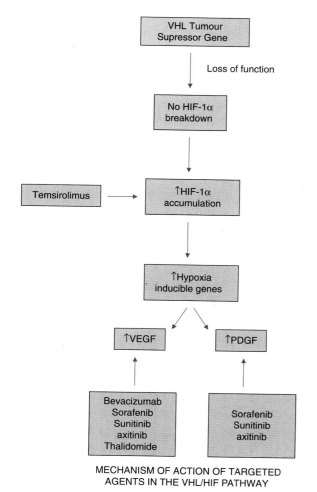

MECHANISM OF ACTION OF TARGETED AGENTS IN THE VHL/HIF PATHWAY

**Figure 1.** Mechanism of action of targeted agents in the Von Hippel-Lindau/hypoxia-inducible factor pathway.

| Table 3. ONGOING RENAL CELL CARCINOMA ADJUVANT TRIALS | | | | | |
|---|---|---|---|---|---|
| Trial | EAU STAR | ECOG ASSURE | MRC/EORTC SORCE | MD ANDERSON | ARISER |
| Study design | Sunitinib vs Placebo | Placebo vs Sunitinib vs Sorafenib | Sorafenib 3 yr vs sorafenib 1 yr and placebo 2 yr vs placebo 3 yr | Thalidomide vs observation | WX-G250 vs placebo |
| Class | TKI | TKI | TKI | Immunomodulatory | Vaccine |
| 1° End point | DFS | DFS | DFS | RFS | DFS |
| Patient target | 250 | 1,332 | 1,656 | 46+ | 800 |
| Risk Group | High | High | High/intermediate | High | High |
| Inclusion Histology | Not yet final | All | All | All | Clear Cell |
| Duration | 1 yr | 1 yr | 3 yr | 2 yr | 24 weeks |

ARISER = Adjuvant Rencarex Immunotherapy trail to Study Efficacy; TKI, tyrosine kinase inhibitor.

## Sunitinib (Sutent)

Sunitinib malate (SU11248; Pfizer) is a novel, oral, potent, and selective multitargeted tyrosine kinase inhibitor. It inhibits vascular endothelial growth factor receptors (VEGFR), KIT, FLT-3, and platelet-derived growth factor receptor (PDGFR). PDGF is associated with growth stimulation by binding to three different tyrosine kinase receptor isoforms, in particular PDGFR α.[51] In human RCC, higher levels of expression of this receptor were found in grade 3 and 4 tumors and also correlated with tumor progression.

A number of phase I trials have been conducted with sunitinib.[52–56] In most patients, therapeutic plasma concentrations (50 to 100 ng/mL) were achieved with daily doses ≥ 50 mg. Postdrug exposure and increased levels of VEGF were noted. Dose-limiting toxicity included fatigue, cytopenias, diarrhea, and skin toxicity, which were reversible upon discontinuation of treatment. A daily dose of 50 mg administered on a 4-weeks-on/2-weeks-off schedule was taken forward into phase II trials.

Two phase II, single-arm, open-label, multicenter trials have looked at the activity of sunitinib in patients with cytokine-refractory metastatic RCC.[57]

The most common adverse events in both trials were fatigue, diarrhea, stomatitis, neutropenia, elevation of lipase, and anemia, the majority being grade 1 or 2.

In an initial study[58] of sunitinib in 63 cytokine-refractory metastatic RCC, patients with all histological subtypes, 25 (40%) achieved partial responses with another 17 (27%) demonstrated stable disease lasting ≥ 3 months. Median time to progression in the 63 patients was 8.7 months.

A further study[59] enrolled 106 patients who had undergone a prior nephrectomy with clear cell histology who had radiological evidence of progression by RECIST/ World Health Organization criteria during or within 9 months of completion of one cytokine treatment. Investigators reported a partial response in 36 patients (34%) and a median progression-free survival of 8.3 months.

The US FDA approved sunitinib based on the high response rate and duration of response as a result of these trails for the treatment of metastatic RCC as second-line therapy in patients who had progressed after a trial of immunotherapy in January 2006.

A multicenter, open-label,[60] phase III randomized trial of 750 patients comparing the efficacy of sunitinib versus IFN-α as first-line therapy in metastatic clear cell RCC has recently reported. Patients received either sunitinib at 50 mg daily for 4 weeks followed by 2-weeks-off treatment per every 6 week cycle or IFN-α at a dose of 9 MU given subcutaneously three times weekly. The primary end point of the study was progression-free survival and secondary points included overall survival, overall response rate, safety, and patient-reported outcomes. In a planned interim analysis assessed by a third party independent review, the median progression-free survival was greater in the sunitinib group (11 months) than the IFN-α group (5 months, hazard ratio = 0.415; $p < .0001$). The response rate was calculated at 31% in the sunitinib arm versus 6% for the

IFN-$\alpha$ cohort ($p < .001$). Toxicities were similar to phase II studies with the most common adverse events including fatigue, hand-foot skin reaction, skin rash, and diarrhea. Patients also reported a significantly better quality of life in the sunitinib than those receiving IFN-$\alpha$. The authors of the study conclude that based on the results of the interim analysis that sunitinib is standard therapy for first-line treatment of metastatic RCC.

## CURRENT ADJUVANT TRIALS WITH SIGNALLING INHIBITORS

### MRC/EORTC SORCE Trial

The SORCE trial will investigate the utility of sorafenib and optimal duration of response in the adjuvant setting. Led by the Medical Research Council (MRC), 1,656 patients with high or intermediate risk resected RCC will be randomized 2:3:2 postnephrectomy to sorafenib for 3 years, sorafenib for 1 year followed by placebo for 2 years or placebo for 3 years. In addition investigators will also search for biological parameters which may predict which patients benefit from adjuvant sorafenib, for example tumors that exhibit deregulated VEGF/PDGF signalling.

### ECOG ASSURE Trial

The ASSURE study is a randomized double-blind multicenter phase III trial being conducted by the ECOG Intergroup. The primary end point is to compare disease-free survival. Overall survival is a secondary end point. Patients who are at high or intermediate risk of recurrence following resection of a primary RCC will be randomized into one of three treatment groups:

1. once daily oral sunitinib for four weeks (days 1 to 28) and a twice daily oral placebo for sorafenib for 6 weeks (days 1 to 42),
2. twice daily oral sorafenib for 6 weeks (days 1 to 42) and oral placebo for sunitinib (days 1 to 28), and
3. oral placebo for sorafenib as in arm one and oral placebo for sunitinib as in arm.

### EAU STAR Trial

The STAR study will be run by the European Association of Urology and will randomize around 250 patients to placebo or to sunitinib 50 mg daily each treatment for 1 year. This study will be confined to patients at high risk of relapse following resection, and the relatively small numbers of the trial may, therefore, be adequate to detect a significant benefit in a population who are extremely likely to relapse. The primary end point will be disease-free survival, and secondary end points will include overall survival and safety.

Tyrosine kinases inhibitors are sufficiently well tolerated to be taken as adjuvant treatment for prolonged periods. Although they have been a welcome addition to the armory in RCC, the duration of response is limited with an average time to progression of 6 to 12 months. Further research into translational work is needed to select the most appropriate targeted therapy based on an individual patient's own molecular markers and individual's tumor and *VHL* gene characteristics.

## THALIDOMIDE

Angiogenesis is recognized to be a key factor in tumor progression. Thalidomide is an immunomodulatory agent[61] that inhibits VEGF and cytokine production (TNF $\alpha$) and stimulates T-cell responses. It has been shown to eradicate tumors in mice models, to induce apoptosis of neovasculature, and is currently being used in the clinic to treat myeloma and Kaposi's sarcoma, a vascular tumor.

In a randomized phase II study comparing thalidomide with medroxyprogesterone acetate, there was no significant evidence of thalidomide benefit, and there was significant toxicity.[62] Interest in thalidomide remains as the occasional good response, and prolonged stabilization has been noted. However, the lack of any randomized data supporting activity in the advanced disease state is not encouraging.

At present, a single-center trial comparing adjuvant thalidomide with observation is enrolling patients.[63] Following nephrectomy, patients are randomized to observation or thalidomide, 300 mg for 2 years. The trial includes all RCC histologies, and there were 23 patients in both the observation and thalidomide arm. After a median follow-up of 18 months, there were seven recurrences and two disease-related deaths in the thalidomide arm compared with six recurrences and five disease-related deaths in the observation arm. No significant difference in recurrence-free survival was observed between the thalidomide arm (mean 24.7 months) and observation (31 months) (hazard ratio = 1.04, 95% CI = 0.34 to 3.14; $p = .945$). Of note however, patients in the adjuvant thalidomide arm had a significantly improved disease-specific survival (mean 40.1 months) compared with the observation arm (mean 37.1 months) (hazard ratio = 0.086, 95% CI = 0.008 to 0.981; $p = .048$). These results must be weighed against the toxicity of treatment. Only one participant in the thalidomide arm tolerated treatment for 2 years without dose reduction, and two patients had to stop treatment with the first month due to toxicity. Thalidomide derivatives are known to have different toxicity profiles and may merit further investigation in adjuvant therapy.

## POSSIBLE ADJUVANT AGENTS IN RCC

### Bevacizumab

Bevacizumab is a recombinant monoclonal anti-VEGF antibody that binds and neutralizes all biologically active isoforms of VEGF. It has shown activity as a single-agent treatment. In a randomized phase II trial[64] comparing 5 mg/kg with 10 mg/kg bevacizumab and with placebo, patients with refractory metastatic RCC in the treatment arm had a significantly prolonged time to disease progression in the high-dose bevacizumab group compared with the placebo group (4.8 vs 2.5 months, hazard ratio = 2.55; $p < .001$), but this did not translate into a survival benefit. Treatment resulted in relatively minor toxic effects, with hypertension and asymptomatic proteinuria predominating. The lack of an overall survival benefit in this trial and the small size of the increase in the time to progression may reflect the crossover design and the rigorous indications for declaring progression and removing a patient from the study (an increase in diameter of any single lesion by as

little as 12% could constitute tumor progression). A randomized phase III trial has recently finished accrual and will investigate IFN-$\alpha$ as a single agent or in combination with bevacizumab in treatment naïve patients with metastatic RCC.

### Mammalian Target of Rapamycin Inhibitors

The mammalian target of rapamycin (mTOR) pathway (phosphoinositide 3-kinase/Akt pathway) plays a key role in cell growth regulation, protein degradation, and angiogenesis. Its dysregulation has been implicated in cancer; therefore, inhibitors of this pathway provide a novel therapeutic option in RCC.

There are at least four mTOR inhibitors currently in clinical development: rapamycin, RAD001, temsirolimus, AP23573.

Rapamycin (Sirolimus; Wyeth Pharmaceuticals) is a macrolide antibiotic, which was originally developed as an antifungal agent. However, it was abandoned when it was found that it had potent immunosuppressive and antiproliferative properties. It is already in current use for the prevention of organ rejection in patients with kidney transplants due to its ability to suppress T-cell activation. Rapamycin also induces G1 cell cycle growth arrest in certain tumor cell lines, which led to further investigation of its anticancer potential.

CCI-779 (temsirolimus, Wyeth) is a derivative of rapamycin with identical specificity and potency for mTOR but with a longer half-life. Phase I studies showed partial responses and disease stabilization in several patients with advanced RCC. Interestingly, few immunosuppressive effects were seen, and the maximum tolerated dose was not reached specifying a high therapeutic index. A phase II trial[65] of 111 pretreated patients with advanced renal cell carcinoma demonstrated a median survival of 15 months and median time to progression of almost 6 months. The objective response rate was only 7%; however, disease stabilization was noted in roughly 50% of patients. A retrospective analysis of patients in a poor risk category (low hemoglobin, multiple-organ metastases sites, and high low-density lipoprotein–cholesterol) found that temsirolimus-treated patients had a 1.7-fold longer median overall survival (from 5 months to 8.2 months) than similar risk patients treated with IFN-α.

A phase III trial[66] in treatment naïve advanced RCC with poor risk features and treatment naïve were assigned patients to three arms. The first arm received IFN-α up to 18 mg three times weekly subcutaneously, the second intravenous temsirolimus 25 mg intravenously once weekly, and the last arm received both drugs at lower doses (temsirolimus 15 mg intravenously weekly and IFN 6 mg subcutaneously thrice weekly) at the same schedule to limit toxicity. An interim analysis showed a similar number of deaths across all study arms, but median overall survival was 7.3 months (IFN-α), 10.9 months (temsirolimus), and 8.4 months in the combined arm. Treatment with single agent temsirolimus resulted in a 49% increase in median overall survival. The most common grade 3 and 4 toxicities were shortness of breath, fatigue, and anemia, observed in all arms.

Both bevacizumab and temsirolimus are intravenous agents and are therefore less attractive as adjuvant therapies.

## CONCLUSIONS

Although there are promising new therapeutic agents in renal cell carcinoma, none have been clinically proven in the adjuvant setting. The adjuvant investigation of treatment in renal cell carcinoma has not produced evidence of benefit to date. The field has been made difficult by the proliferation of small studies. Now the ability to conduct large randomized trials in the adjuvant setting is being investigated, and a number of large studies are currently recruiting around the world. Data are awaited from completed studies such as the EORTC30955-HYDRA study comparing observation with a single cycle of the atzpodien regimen. Looking ahead, gene array analysis may enable the rapid acquisition of data relating to molecular markers as correlates for disease progression, treatment efficacy, and overall survival. This will aid the field and selection of patients for adjuvant treatments. It should not be forgotten that immunotherapy may well still have an important, although limited, role to play in advanced disease, and this role may also extend to the adjuvant setting.

Vaccines potentially hold great promise, and further prospective randomized studies are warranted. It is important to note that until there is robust long-term evidence of efficacy and safety for any of these new approaches, observation remains the standard of care in patients at risk of relapse following radical nephrectomy for renal cell carcinoma.

## REFERENCES

1. Jemal A, Siegel R, Ward E, et al. Cancer statistics. CA Cancer J Clin 2006;56:106–30.
2. Rabinovitch RA, Zelefsky MJ, Gaynor JJ, et al. Patterns of failure following surgical resection of renal cell carcinoma: implications for adjuvant local and systemic therapy. J Clin Oncol 1994;12:206–12.
3. Motzer RJ, Bander NH, Nanus DM. Renal-cell carcinoma. N Engl J Med 1996;335:865–75.
4. Zisman A, Pantuck AJ, Chao D, et al. Reevaluation of the 1997 TNM classification for renal cell carcinoma: T1 and T2 cutoff point at 4.5 rather than 7 cm better correlates with clinical outcome. J Urol 2001;166:54–8.
5. Zisman A, Pantuck AJ, Dorey F, et al. Improved prognostication of renal cell carcinoma using an integrated staging system. J Clin Oncol 2001;19:1649–57.
6. Han KR, Bleumer I, Pantuck AJ, et al. Validation of an integrated staging system toward improved prognostication of patients with localized renal cell carcinoma in an international population. J Urol 2003;170:2221–4.
7. Kattan MW, Reuter V, Motzer RJ. A postoperative prognostic nomogram for renal cell carcinoma. J Urol 2001;166:63–7.
8. Frank I, Blute ML, Cheville JC. An outcome prediction model for patients with clear cell renal cell carcinoma treated with radical nephrectomy based on tumor stage, size, grade and necrosis: the SSIGN score. J Urol 2002; 168: 2395–400.
9. Leibovich BC, Blute ML, Cheville JC, et al. Prediction of progression after radical nephrectomy for patients with clear cell renal cell carcinoma. Cancer 2003;97:1663–1671.
10. Schraml P, Hergovitz A, Hatz F, et al. Relevance of nuclear and cytoplasmic von Hippel Lindau protein expression for renal carcinoma orogression. Am J Pathol 2003;163:1013–20.
11. Jacobsen J, Grankvist K, Rasmuson T, et al. Different isoform patterns for vascular endothelial growth factor between clear cell and papillary renal cell carcinoma. BJU Int 2006;97:1102–8.
12. Kjaer M, Frederiksen PL, Engelholm SA. Post-operative radiotherapy in stage II and III renal adenocarcinoma. A randomised trial by the Copenhagen Renal Cancer Study Group. Int J Radiat Oncol Biol Phys. 1987;13: 665–72.
13. Makarewicz R, Zarzycka M, Kulinska G, Windorbska W. The value of post-operative radiotherapy in advanced renal cell carcinoma. Neoplasma 1998;45:380–3.
14. Gez E, Libes M, Bar-Deroma R, et al. Postoperative irradiation in localised renal cell carcinoma: the Rambam Medical Centre experience. Tumori 2002;88:500–2.

15. Yagoda A, Abi-Rached B, Petrylak D. Chemotherapy for advanced renal-cell carcinoma: 1983–1993. Semin Oncol 1995;22:42–60.

16. Asakura T, Imai A, Ohkubo-Uraoka N. Relationship between expression of drug-resistance factors and drug sensitivity in normal human renal proximal tubular epithelial cells in comparison with renal cell carcinoma. Oncol Rep 2005;14:601–7.

17. Rini BI, Vogelzang NJ, Dumas MC, et al. Phase II trial of weekly intravenous gemcitabine with continuous infusion fluorouracil in patients with metastatic renal cell cancer. J Clin Oncol 2000;18:2419–26.

18. Haarstad H, Jacobsen AB, Schjolseth SA, et al. Interferon-α, 5- FU and prednisone in metastatic renal cell carcinoma: a phase II study. Ann Oncol 1994;5:245–8.

19. Masuda F, Nakada J, Kondo I. Adjuvant chemotherapy with vinblastine adriamycin and UFT for renal-cell carcinoma. Cancer Chemother Pharmacol 1992;30:477–9.

20. Derweesh IH, Tannenbaum CS, Rayman PA. Mechanisms of immune dysfunction in renal cell carcinoma. Cancer Treat Res 2003;116:29–51.

21. Galligioni E, Quaia M, Merlo A. Adjuvant immunotherapy treatment of renal carcinoma patients with autologous tumor cells and Bacillus Calmette-Guerin: five-year results of a prospective randomized study. Cancer 1996;77:2560–6.

22. Repmann R, Goldschmidt AJ, Richter A. Adjuvant therapy of renal cell carcinoma patients with an autologous tumor cell lysate vaccine: a 5-year follow-up analysis. Anticancer Res 2003;23:969–74.

23. Jocham D, Richter A, Hoffmann L. Adjuvant autologous renal tumour cell vaccine and risk of tumour progression in patients with renal-cell carcinoma after radical nephrectomy: phase III, randomized controlled trial. Lancet 2004;363:594–99.

24. Srivastava PK. Immunotherapy for human cancer using heat shock protein-peptide complexes. Curr Oncol Rep 2005;7:104–8.

25. Assiki VJ, Daliani D, Pagliaro L. Phase II study of autologous tumor derived heat shock protein-peptide complex vaccine (HSPPC-96) for patients with metastatic renal cell carcinoma [abstract]. Proc Am Soc Clin Oncol 2003;22:386.

26. Antigenics Reports Phase 3 Results for Oncophage in Kidney Cancer.

27. Oosterwijk E, Ruiter DJ, Hoedemaeker PJ, et al. Monoclonal antibody G 250 recognizes a determinant present in renal-cell carcinoma and absent from normal kidney. Int J Cancer 1986;38:489–94.

28. Ivanov S, Liao SY, Ivanova A, et al. Expression of hypoxia-inducible cell-surface transmembrane carbonic anhydrases in human cancer. Am J Pathol 2001;158:905–19.

29. Bleumer I, Oosterwijk E, Oosterwijk-Wakka JC, et al. A clinical trial with chimeric monoclonal antibody WX-G250 and low dose interleukin-2 pulsing scheme for advanced renal cell carcinoma. J Urol 2006;175:57–62.

30. Bleumer I, Knuth A, Oosterwijk E. A phase II trial of chimeric monoclonal antibody G250 for advanced renal cell carcinoma patients. Br J Cancer 2004;90:985–90.

31. Bleumer I, Oosterwijk E, De Mulder P. Immunotherapy for renal cell carcinoma. Eur Urol 2003;44:65–75.

32. Pizzocaro G, Piva L, Colavita M. Interferon adjuvant to radical nephrectomy in Robson stages II and III renal cell carcinoma: a multicentric randomized study. J Clin Oncol 2001;19:425–31.

33. Messing EM, Manola J, Wilding G. Phase III study of interferon α as adjuvant treatment for resectable renal cell carcinoma: an Eastern Cooperative Oncology Group/Intergroup trial. J Clin Oncol 2003;21:1214–22.

34. Migliari R, Muscas G, Solinas A. Is there a role for adjuvant immunochemotherapy after radical nephrectomy in pT2-3N0M0 renal cell carcinoma? J Chemother 1995;7:240-45.

35. Jeon SH, Chang SG, Kim JI. The role of adjuvant immunotherapy after radical nephrectomy and prognostic factors in pT3N0M0 renal cell carcinoma. Anticancer Res 1999;19:5593–7.

36. van Spronsen DJ, Mulders PF, De Mulder PH. Novel treatments for metastatic renal cell carcinoma. Crit Rev Oncol Hematol 2005;55:177–91.

37. Fyfe G, Fisher RI, Rosenberg SA, et al. Results of treatment of 255 patients with metastatic renal cell carcinoma who received high-dose recombinant interleukin2 therapy. J Clin Oncol 1995;13:688–96.

38. Fisher RI, Rosenberg SA, Fyfe G. Long-term survival update for high-dose recombinant interleukin-2 in patients with renal cell carcinoma. Cancer J Sci Am 2000;6 Suppl 1:S55–7.

39. Clark JI, Atkins MB, Urba WJ, et al. Adjuvant high-dose bolus interleukin-2 for patients with high-risk renal cell carcinoma: a cytokine working group randomized trial. J Clin Oncol 2003;21:3133–40.

40. Atzpodien J, Schmitt E, Gertenbach U, et al. Adjuvant treatment with interleukin-2- and interferon-α 2a-based chemoimmunotherapy in renal cell carcinoma post tumour nephrectomy: results of a prospectively randomised trial of the German Cooperative Renal Carcinoma Chemoimmunotherapy Group (DGCIN). Br J Cancer 2005;92:843–6.

41. Gallou C, Joly D, Mejean A. Mutations of the VHL gene in sporadic renal cell carcinoma: definition of a risk factor for VHL patients to develop an RCC. Hum Mutat 1999;13:464–75.

42. Schraml P, Struckmann K, Hatz F. VHL mutations and their correlation with tumour cell proliferation, microvessel density, and patient prognosis in clear cell renal cell carcinoma. J Pathol 2002;196:186–93.

43. Herman JG, Latif F, Weng Y. Silencing of the VHL tumor-suppressor gene by DNA methylation in renal carcinoma. Proc Natl Acad Sci U S A 1994;91:9700–4.

44. Krieg M, Haas R, Brauch H. Up-regulation of hypoxia-inducible factors HIF-1α and HIF-2α under normoxic conditions in renal carcinoma cells by von Hippel-Lindau tumor suppressor gene loss of function. Oncogene 2000;19:5435–43.

45. Kourembanas S, Hannan RL, Faller DV. Oxygen tension regulates the expression of the platelet-derived growth factor-B chain gene in human endothelial cells. J Clin Invest 1990;86:670–4.

46. Gnarra JR, Zhou S, Merrill MJ. Post-transcriptional regulation of vascular endothelial growth factor mRNA by the product of the VHL tumor suppressor gene. Proc Natl Acad Sci U S A 1996;93:10589–94.

47. Wilhelm SM, Carter C, Tang L, et al. BAY 43-9006 exhibits broad spectrum oral antitumor activity and targets the RAF/MEK/ERK pathway and receptor tyrosine kinases involved in tumor progression and angiogenesis. Cancer Res 2004;64:7099–109.

48. Strumberg D, Richly H, Hilger RA, et al. Phase I clinical and pharmacokinetic study of the novel Raf kinase and vascular endothelial growth factor receptor inhibitor BAY 43-9006 in patients with advanced refractory solid tumors. J Clin Oncol 2005;23:965–72.

49. Ratain MJ, Eisen T, Stadler WM, et al. Phase II olacebo-controlled randomized discontinuation trial of sorafenib in patients with metastatic renal cell carcinoma. J Clin Oncol 2005;24:2505–12.

50. Escudier B, Eisen T, Stadler WM, et al. sorafenib in advanced clear-cell renal-cell carcinoma. N Engl J Med 2007; 356:125–34.

51. Sun L, Tran N, Tang F. Synthesis and biological evaluations of 3-substituted indolin-2-ones: a novel class of tyrosine kinase inhibitors that exhibit selectivity toward particular receptor tyrosine kinases. J Med Chem 1998;41:2588–603.

52. Demetri GD, Desai J, Fletcher JA. SU11248, a multi-targeted tyrosine kinase inhibitor, can overcome imatinib (IM) resistance caused by diverse genomic mechanisms in patients (pts) with metastatic gastrointestinal stromal tumor (GIST) [abstract 3001]. Proc Am Soc Clin Oncol 2005;22:14S.

53. Fiedler W, Serve H, Dohner H. A phase 1 study of SU11248 in the treatment of patients with refractory or resistant acute myeloid leukemia (AML) or not amenable to conventional therapy for the disease. Blood 2005;105:986–93.

54. Manning WC, Bello CL, Deprimo SE. Pharmacokinetic and pharmacodynamic evaluation of SU11248 in a phase I clinical trial of patients with imatinib-resistant GIST [abstract 768]. Proc Am Soc Clin Oncol 2003;22:14S.

55. Rosen L, Mulay M, Long J. Phase I trial of SU011248, a novel tyrosine kinase inhibitor in advanced solid tumors [abstract 765]. Proc Am Soc Clin Oncol 2003;22:14S.

56. Faivre S, Delbaldo C, Vera K. Safety, pharmacokinetic, and antitumor activity of SU11248, a novel oral multitarget tyrosine kinase inhibitor, in patients with cancer. J Clin Oncol 2006;24:25–35.

57. Motzer RJ, Hutson TE, Tomczak P, et al. Sunitinib versus interferon α in metastatic renal-cell carcinoma. N Engl J Med 2007;356:115–24.

58. Motzer R, Michaelson MD, Redman BG. Activity of SU11248, a multitargeted inhibitor of vascular endothelial growth factor receptor and platelet-derived growth factor receptor, in patients with metastatic renal cell carcinoma. J Clin Oncol 2006;24:1–8.

59. Motzer RJ, Rini B, Bukowski RM. Sunitinib in patients with metastatic renal cell carcinoma. JAMA 2005; 295:2516–2524.

60. Motzer RJ, Hutson TE, Tomczak P, et al. Phase III randomized trial of sunitinib malate (SU11248) versus interferon-α (IFN-α) as first-line systemic therapy for patients with metastatic renal cell carcinoma (mRCC). N Engl J Med.

61. D'Amato RJ, Loughnan MS, Flynn E, et al. Thalidomide is an inhibitor of angiogenesis. Proc Natl Acad Sci U S A 1994; 91:4082–5.

62. Lee C, Patel PM, Selby PJ, Hancock BW, et al. J Clin Oncol 2006;24:898–903.

63. Sanchez-Ortiz R, Tamboli P, Lozano M, et al. Adjuvant thalidomide improves disease specific survival for patients with renal cell carcinoma at high risk for relapse following surgery[abstract 14586]. J Clin Oncol 2006.

64. Yang JC, Haworth L, Sherry RM, et al. A randomized trial of bevacizumab, an anti-vascular endothelial growth factor antibody, for metastatic renal cancer. N Engl J Med 2003;349:427–34.

65. Atkins MB, Hidalgo M, Stadler WM, et al. Randomized phase II study of multiple dose levels of CCI-779, a novel mammalian target of rapamycin kinase inhibitor, in patients with advanced refractory renal cell carcinoma. J Clin Oncol 2004;22:909–18.

66. Hudes G, Carducci M, Tomczak P, et al. A phase III, randomized, 3-arm study of temsirolimus (TEMSR) or interferon-α (IFN) or the combination of TEMSR = IFN in the treatment of first-line poor-prognosis patients with advanced renal cell carcinoma [abstract LBA4]. J Clin Oncol 2006;24 Suppl 18:2S.

# 11

# Prognostic Factors in Metastatic Renal Cell Carcinoma

TONI K. CHOUEIRI, MD

The identification of prognostic factors in patients with advanced renal cell carcinoma (RCC) represents an area of expanding interest. Extensive data published in the last 20 years have led to the establishment of integrated clinical models as the main tools used for disease prognostication. The Memorial Sloan Kettering Cancer Center model represents the most commonly used clinical model based on the large number of patients included and its recent external validation by the Cleveland Clinic group. A group of international investigators are compiling a comprehensive database of > 4,000 patients with metastatic renal cell carcinoma to provide and validate a single model that can be used to predict survival. Although integrated staging systems have improved patient stratification and risk-directed therapies in advanced RCC, the use of molecularly targeted approaches in RCC has made possible the discovery of potential tumor molecular markers. The aim of the current review is to provide an overview, an update and future directions on prognostic factors for metastatic RCC.

Despite recent major therapeutic advances, the natural history of renal cell carcinoma (RCC) remains variable, and an important consideration for the evaluation of new treatments is the role of prognostic factors (PF), which are loosely defined as patient or tumor characteristics associated with clinical outcome. It is acknowledged that prognostic factors relate to the natural history of a disease (in the absence of treatment and/or not affected by treatment), and that predictive factors describe features associated with outcome to a given therapy. The term prognostic factors will be used here in a general sense to describe factors associated with clinical outcome in RCC. Knowledge of PF can help direct treatment strategies to the patients who are most likely to benefit from such treatment. In addition, knowledge of PF can aid in the interpretation of clinical trial results and help distinguish the extent to which a certain therapy is altering the natural history of the disease. A number of patient- and disease-related factors are recognized as being important PF in this disease. Several clinical, histologic, immune, and, more recently, molecular markers have been identified. The following sections summarize the factors that have been suggested to be of important and independent prognostic value in metastatic RCC.

## PATIENT- AND DISEASE-RELATED CLINICAL PROGNOSTIC FACTORS

Patient and disease characteristics are clinical factors that have been extensively studied as potential PF in metastatic RCC. These include demographics, presenting symptoms, disease history, previous treatment, sites and number of metastases, and laboratory parameters. Only studies that used multivariate analysis and provided independent information will be cited. Table 1 summarizes the results of the main published studies that have examined these factors.[1–11] It is important to keep in mind that all the studies were retrospective in nature and that many included data from different agents, which were often investigational in nature at that time. However, most patients included were initially part of well-designed prospective clinical trials, and the statistical methods were, in

| Table 1. SELECTED MULTIVARIATE ANALYSES OF PATIENT- AND DISEASE-RELATED PROGNOSTIC IN METASTATIC RCC | | | | |
|---|---|---|---|---|
| **Investigator (Institution)** | **Treatment Period** | **N** | **Therapy Received** | **Adverse Prognostic Factors** |
| Elson et al[1] (ECOG) | 1975 to 1984 | 610 | Chemotherapy | ECOG PS > 1, recent weight loss, prior chemotherapy, DFI ≤ 1 yr, >1 metastatic site |
| DeForges et al[2] (IGR) | 1971 to 1986 | 134 | Unspecified | Metastases at diagnosis, presence of liver metastases, lung lesions > 2 cm and/or ≥ 5, ESR ≥ 100, weight loss >10% |
| Palmer et al[3] (CETUS corporation) | 1986 to 1990 | 327 | Interleukin-2 | ECOG PS ≥ 1, DFI ≤ 2 yr, > 1 metastatic site |
| Fossa et al[4] (multiinstitutional) | 1975 to 1990 | 295 | Immunotherapy Chemotherapy | ECOG PS > 1, weight loss > 10%, DTI < 1 yr, elevated ESR |
| Motzer et al[5] (MSKCC) | 1975 to 1996 | 670 | Immunotherapy Chemotherapy | ECOG PS > 1, absence of nephrectomy, Low hemoglobin, LDH > 300 U/L, corrected calcium > 10 mg/dL |
| Motzer et al[6] (MSKCC) | 1975 to 1996 | 463 | Interferon-α | ECOG PS > 1, time from diagnosis to start of therapy < 1 yr, Low hemoglobin, LDH > 1.5 ULN, corrected calcium > 10 mg/dL |
| Negrier et al[7] (Group Francais d'Immunotherapie) | 1970 to 1980 | 782 | Immunotherapy | Presence of liver metastases, > 1 metastatic site, DFI < 1 year, elevated neutrophils count > 7500 k/μL |
| Atzpodien et al[8] (DGCIN) | 1988 to 1998 | 425 | Immunotherapy Chemotherapy | Neutrophil counts > 6500 k/μL, LDH > 220 U/L, CRP ≥ 11, DFI < 3 yr, ≥ 3 metastatic sites, presence of bone metastases |
| Mekhail et al[9] (Cleveland Clinic) | 1987 to 2002 | 353 | Immunotherapy Chemotherapy | Time from diagnosis to therapy < 1 yr, low hemoglobin, LDH > 1.5 ULN, corrected calcium > 10 mg/dL, prior radiotherapy, > 1 metastatic site |
| Choueiri et al[10] (Cleveland Clinic) | 1987 to 2002 | 257 | Immunotherapy Chemotherapy | Low hemoglobin, left kidney, > 2 metastatic sites, ECOG PS ≥ 1 |
| Choueiri et al[11] (Cleveland Clinic) | 2003 to 2006 | 120 | Anti-VEGF agents | Time from diagnosis to study entry < 2 yr, > 2 metastatic sites platelets count > 300 k/μL, Neutrophils count > 4.5 k/μL, abnormal serum calcium |
| Motzer et al[84] (MSKCC) | 2004 to 2005 | 375 | Sunitinib | ECOG PS 1, time from diagnosis to treatment < 1 year, and corrected calcium > 10 mg/dL |

CRP = C-reactive protein; DFI = disease-Free interval; DGCIN = German Cooperative Renal Carcinoma Chemo-Immunotherapy Trials Group; ECOG PS = Eastern Cooperative Oncology Group Performance Status; ESR = erythrocyte sedimentation rate; IGR = Institut Gustave Roussy; LDH = lactate dehydrogenase; MSKCC = Memorial Sloan Kettering Cancer Center; N = number of patients; OS = overall survival; PFS = progression-free survival; RCC = renel cell carcinoma; VEGF = vascular endothelial growth factor.

general, based on sound analysis. In addition, not all factors were tested in each study, and the evidence for their relevance as a PF comes from a limited number of published reports.

## Demographics

Most studies have found that factors such as age and race are not associated with survival in metastatic RCC. Only 1 early study of 101 patients suggested that men have a better prognosis than women, but this conclusion has not been validated in larger and more recent studies.[12]

## Performance Status

Performance status (PS) is a measure of overall well being and is used routinely as a selection criterion for clinical trials. Most commonly used PS scales in cancer are the Eastern Cooperative Oncology Group (ECOG) score and the Karnofsky Performance Status. ECOG score ranges from 0 to 5 (5 indicates death) with asymptomatic patients having an ECOG PS of 0 and completely bedridden patient have an ECOG PS of 4. PS is the most consistently reported factor associated with survival in advanced RCC (see Table 1). Patients with good PS are reported to have a median survival of 10 to 21 months as opposed to 2 to 7 months in patients with poor PS[1,3,5,9] A few other studies did not find PS to be significant on multivariate analysis when correcting for other PF.[13]

## Disease-related Factors

Several aspects of metastatic RCC have been studied as potential PF. These include sites and number of metastatic lesions, time from initial diagnosis to metastatic disease, and location (right vs left) of the primary tumor. Some studies have found the presence of visceral (lung, liver, and adrenals), bone, and brain metastases to be associated with poor survival,[1,2,9,13,14] whereas others have found no relationship between these sites and prognosis.[5,15] A more reliable finding is the number of metastatic sites, which provides a rough estimate of tumor burden. Most studies have found that patients with higher number of metastatic sites (2 vs more than 2)

are independently associated with at least 2 fold greater probability of death (see Table 1). Similarly, patients with a short metastasis-free interval were found to have twice the risk of death. However, several different cut points were used in these studies to define a short metastasis-free interval, with some authors including metastases within 2 to 3[3,8] or 1 year of diagnosis[6,9] or synchronous metastases.[2]

In addition to the extent of metastatic disease and metastasis-free interval, laterality of primary tumor was also examined in few studies. One study suggested that right-sided tumors may have 3-fold survival benefit compared with left-sided tumors.[10] No clear anatomic explanation for this finding exists, and it may simply be due to an unknown confounding factor that was not accounted for on multivariate analysis. This has not been consistently found in other analyses.

## Prior Treatment

Factors such as prior chemotherapy, radiotherapy, and nephrectomy were examined in several studies as possible PF correlating with survival. Prior radiotherapy was generally not found to be associated with poor survival when considering other factors. However, 1 recent study found that patients with prior radiation had significantly lower survival rates than patients with no history of radiation.[9] Similarly, prior chemotherapy was found to be of prognostic significance in one large study.[1] Another landmark study found it also to be associated with poor survival but did not include it as a factor on multivariate analysis.[5]

Although of favorable prognostic significance in many studies,[5] prior nephrectomy was not found to be of major importance when adjusted for other factors in several other studies.[1-4] Nevertheless, 2 prospective randomized controlled trials have shown a clear survival advantage for patients undergoing cytoreductive nephrectomy, and therefore, nephrectomy has become a standard procedure in advanced disease if the patient is medically fit to undergo surgery.[16]

Finally, metastasectomy was found recently, even if negative margins were not achieved surgically, to be a powerful PF in metastatic RCC (median survival of 27.2 vs 20.6 months in patients with vs without metastatectomy, respectively, $p = .02$). However, most patients who underwent surgery had a good performance status, suggesting a careful patient selection for any surgical procedure at this stage of the disease.[17]

## Laboratory Parameters

Investigators have evaluated the effects of several hematologic and biochemical parameters on survival in patients with advanced RCC. Erythrocyte sedimentation rate (ESR), C-reactive protein (CRP), hemoglobin, and white blood cells / platelet parameters were evaluated as markers of inflammation with a potential role as PF. Elevated ESR and CRP were found consistently to be independent poor PF depending on the threshold value used.[4,8,13,18] Anemia has also consistently been found to be an independent PF for an adverse outcome. Patients with pretreatment hemoglobin below the lower limit of laboratory normal values were found to have twice the risk of death than patients with normal hemoglobin in several large studies.[5,9] Patients with thrombocytosis (defined as platelet counts > 400,000/µL), another potential marker of inflammation, have been reported to have a negative survival outcome mostly in patients with localized RCC. Overall, studies have been inconsistent in the metastatic setting, especially when other markers of inflammation were considered. However, a recent large retrospective study of 700 patients showed that thrombocytosis at study entry conferred a 2-fold increase risk of death in patients with metastatic RCC.[19] The exact mechanism producing secondary thrombocytosis (and anemia) in association with RCC is unclear, but this could be a reflection of an overproduction of interleukins (IL) and other growth factors by the tumor.[20,21] In turn, platelet overproduction can enhance the adherence and penetration of malignant cells through the endothelial wall,[22] and platelet granules contain a variety of angiogenic factors such as vascular endothelial growth factor (VEGF), PDGF, transforming growth factor β, and others that have been implicated in various steps of tumor progression.[23,24]

Biochemical factors that have been studied include pretreatment serum lactate dehydrogenase (LDH) and serum calcium (corrected for albumin).

Several large studies found that these 2 parameters impact survival. Corrected serum calcium > 10 mg/dL and LDH > 1.5 times the upper limit of normal have been associated with a 2 to 3 fold higher risk of death.[5,8,9] Other biochemical factors have been studied and found not to be of prognostic value, including serum alkaline phosphatase, creatinine, γ glutamyl-transferase, and triglycerides.

## CLINICAL PROGNOSTIC MODELS

Once PF are identified on multivariate analysis, these factors can be used to stratify patients into subgroups that can be analyzed for survival, leading to the development of prognostic survival models. Several groups have developed prognostic models that can be used to predict survival and stratify patients into distinct risk groups.

Since the first large-scale comprehensive prognostic model proposed by Elson and colleagues in 610 patients treated primarily with chemotherapy,[1] numerous stratification models for metastatic RCC have been defined. PS, nephrectomy status, disease-free interval, hemoglobin, LDH, corrected calcium, and inflammation markers were the most frequently identified risk factors in major studies of previously untreated RCC patients (see Table 1). To date, several investigators favor the Memorial Sloan Kettering Cancer Center (MSKCC) risk stratification model proposed in 2002, which included over 400 patients treated with interferon-α based therapies. This model was originally published in 1999 and included 670 patients treated with cytokines (interferon-α and/or IL-2), chemotherapy, and hormonal therapy.[5] The 2002 model[6] attempted to reduce heterogeneity caused by various therapies and account for the role of cytoreductive nephrectomy in the metastatic setting in patients with good PS. In this model, LDH (> 1.5 times normal), high corrected calcium, low serum hemoglobin, low Karnofsky PS, and time from diagnosis to start of therapy (less than 1 year) were found as independent adverse prognostic factors for overall survival. Subsequently, 3 risk groups with statistically significant survival differences have been described (30, 14, and 5 months for good, intermediate, and poor risk, respectively) (Figure 1). This model was recently externally validated in 353 patients treated

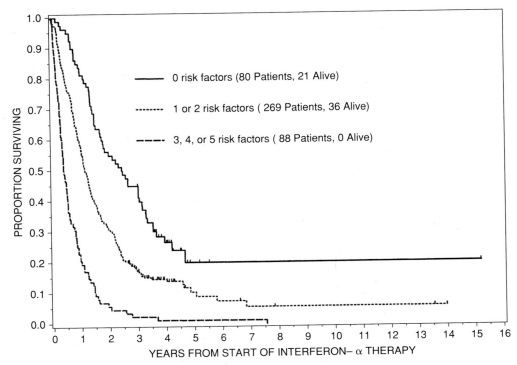

**Figure 1.**   Risk stratification according to Memorial Sloan Kettering Cancer Center criteria.[6]

on clinical trials at Cleveland Clinic.[9] Investigators from this institution identified 2 additional independent PF (prior radiotherapy and number of metastatic sites). Table 2 provides survival data according to MSKCC and Cleveland Clinic models.

Two additional prognostic models in patients receiving cytokines as first-line therapy have been published. The French model (Group Francais d'Immunotherapie) analyzed 782 patients and validated 5 previously reported PF (PS, number of metastatic sites, disease-free interval, biologic signs of inflammation, and hemoglobin levels) associated with survival.[7] In addition, 4 independent factors were reported that were predictive of rapid disease progression while receiving cytokine therapy: presence of hepatic metastases, less than 1 year interval from renal tumor to metastases, more than 1 metastatic site, and elevated neutrophil counts. Patients who had ≥ 3 of these factors had > 80% chance of rapid progression (within 3 months). The authors recommended that these patients not receive cytokine regimens. The second model proposed by Atzpodien and colleagues reported a comprehensive prognostic system of pretreatment clinical parameters in 425 patients.[8] Neutrophil count was found to be the major prognostic factor (hazard ratio = 1.9), whereas serum levels of LDH and CRP, time between diagnosis of tumor and onset of metastatic disease, number of metastatic sites, and bone metastases were significant but somewhat less important prognostic variables within the multiple risk factor model (hazard ratio ≤ 1.5).

Other authors have looked at long-term survivors (defined as ≥ 5 years since the diagnosis of metastatic disease) to try to identify patient characteristics associated with this particular outcome. Comparing 31 long-term survivors with 226 patients who died within 2 years of metastatic RCC diagnosis revealed similar parameters as associated with good outcome: baseline hemoglobin level, number of involved sites, and ECOG PS were found to be predictors of long-term survival.[10]

As new therapies are being introduced and major developments have been made in managing this tumor, the treatment of metastatic RCC has experienced a major shift. Therapy targeted against the VEGF pathway is now a standard of care in metastatic renal cell carcinoma. Although these

| Table 2. RENAL CELL CARCINOMA SURVIVAL BY RISK GROUPS IN PREVIOUSLY UNTREATED PATIENTS ACCORDING TO MEMORIAL SLOAN KETTERING CANCER CENTER AND CLEVELAND CLINIC MODELS[6,9] | | | | |
| --- | --- | --- | --- | --- |
| | MSKCC (*N* = 437) | | Cleveland Clinic (*N* = 308) | |
| Risk Group | No. of Adverse Factors (% of patients included) | Median Survival (mo) | No. of Adverse Factors (% of patients included) | Median Survival (mo) |
| Favorable Risk | 0 (18%) | 30 | 0–1 (37%) | 26 |
| Intermediate Risk | 1–2 (62%) | 14 | 2 (35%) | 14 |
| Poor Risk | > 2 (20%) | 5 | > 2 (28%) | 7 |

MSKCC = Memorial Sloan Kettering Cancer Center.

recent trials have enrolled patients and/or reported results according to existing classification schemas, such schemas have been developed from patients treated with cytokines or other earlier therapies, and it is unclear if the same factors previously reported continue to be relevant to patients treated with current VEGF-targeted therapy. Therefore, identification of relevant clinical factors in the anti-VEGF era is warranted. Studies of PF in this context are evolving. Potential presunitinib predictors of progression-free survival (PFS) in 168 patients treated on 2 phase II trials with sunitinib were examined.[25] Hemoglobin (< normal) was found to be the sole independent PF. Similarly, a retrospective study of 43 patients treated with 3 anti-VEGF agents reported a shorter time to progression (TTP) in patients with low hemoglobin and liver metastases.[26] More recently, 120 metastatic RCC patients who received bevacizumab, sorafenib, sunitinib, or axitinib on 1 of 8 prospective clinical trials at Cleveland Clinic were examined. Multivariate analysis identified time from diagnosis to current treatment < 2 years, baseline platelet and neutrophil counts > 300 K/µL and > 4.5 K/µL, respectively, baseline corrected serum calcium < 8.5 or > 10.0 mg/dL, and initial ECOG performance status > 0 as independent adverse PF for PFS. Using these factors, 3 prognostic subgroups were formed based on the number of adverse PF present. Median PFS in patients with 0 or 1 adverse PF was 20.1 months compared with 13 months in patients with 2 adverse PF and 3.9 months in patients with more than 2 adverse PF.[11] Patient baseline characteristics ECOGPS (Ovsl), time from diagnosis to treatment (≥ 1 year vs < 1 year), and corrected calcium (≤ 10 vs > 10

mg/dL) were found to be independent pre-therapy features associated with progression free survival (PFS) in patients receiving frontline sunitinib therapy. A nomogram (concordance index = 0.63) was developed from pretreatment clinical features to predict the probability of acheiving 12-month progression-free survival.[84] Further model development and assessment of features predictive of overall survival (as opposed to PFS) will be done when additional follow-up for patients receiving anti-VEGF agents is collected.

## PREVIOUSLY TREATED PATIENTS

The clinical prognostic models that have been developed related to previously untreated patients but are often applied to previously treated patients. Such models may not apply uniformly in these 2 distinct populations. Data are scant regarding prognostication in previously treated patients and 1 study of 137 patients found adverse risk factors to include low performance status, low hemoglobin level, and high corrected calcium. Median survival was 22 months in patients with zero risk factors, 11.9 months in patients with 1 risk factor and only 5.4 months in patients with 2 or more risk factors.[27] Two other studies, in this particular patient population, including the largest experience in 300 patients who failed immunotherapy are listed in Table 3.[28,29]

## HISTOLOGIC PROGNOSTIC FACTORS

Several studies have examined the impact of histology on survival. Tumors containing a sarcomatoid

**Table 3. STUDIES OF PROGNOSTIC FACTORS IN PREVIOUSLY TREATED RCC PATIENTS**

| | Motzer et al[27] | Bou Merhi et al[28] | Escudier et al[29] |
|---|---|---|---|
| No. of patients | 137 | 85 | 300 |
| % of patients with 1 prior therapy only | 121/137 (88) | 100 | 100 |
| % clear cell histology | 83/90* (92) | 85 | 93 |
| % prior nephrectomy | 74 | 85 | 94 |
| Median survival (mo) | 12.7 | 16.5 | 12.6 |
| % pts with cytokines | 80 | NR | 100 |
| Time from nephrectomy/ diagnosis to metastases | – | – | + |
| Hemoglobin | + | + | – |
| Alkaline Phosphatase | + | – | + |
| Corrected Calcium | + | + | + |
| LDH | – | – | + |
| Performance Status | – | – | – |
| No. of Metastatic Sites | – | – | + |

*Histology was reviewed for 90 patients.

+ = factors associated with an adverse outcome; – = factors not associated with an adverse outcome; LDH = lactate dehydrogenase; NR = not reported; RCC = renal cell carcinoma.

component appear to have a worse prognosis with some studies reporting a 3-fold increase in the risk of death.[25,30,31] Other studies have found aneuploid tumors to be negatively correlated with survival,[32] although contradictory results have challenged this view.[33] Because RCC is a heterogeneous tumor, the validity of determining that the tumor is aneuploid or not depends largely on the number and quality of samples taken.[34] Investigations of tumor grade have had mixed results. Earlier studies and 1 recent study[15,17] found patients with higher grade to have a poorer prognosis than patients with well-differentiated tumors. However, other studies showed no effect when adjusted for other factors on multivariate analysis.[35] The problem with tumor grading remains in the subjectivity associated with its evaluation and the various systems used.[36] Another issue is the missing data on a significant numbers of patients in many large studies leading to the evaluation of tumor grade solely on univariate analysis.[9]

The presence of histologic necrosis in the primary tumor of patients with RCC has been suggested to be an important predictor of survival. However, a recent study of more than 300 patients showed that the presence of this histologic finding was an independent predictor of poor survival in patients with localized but not metastatic disease.[37]

Recent studies underscore the importance of histologic classification of into clear cell and nonclear cell subtypes. The majority of RCC are of clear cell type (70 to 80%). The remaining cases consist of papillary RCC, chromophobe RCC, collecting duct carcinoma, and medullary carcinoma. When confined to the kidney, papillary RCC and chromophobe RCC generally have a better prognosis than clear cell or collecting duct RCC. A retrospective review of 64 metastatic nonclear cell RCC found a median overall survival of 9.4 months. Survival was longer for patients with chromophobe tumors compared with other histologies. Overall, patients with nonclear cell histologies appear to be resistant to systemic therapies, which suggests that histology should be considered in guiding treatment decisions.[38] A recent study reported that patients with nonclear cell histology or with papillary or granular features, and no alveolar features in the pathologic specimen, respond poorly to IL-2.[39] This concept of divergent outcomes in different histologic subtypes in RCC coupled with understanding the role of *VHL* gene and the downstream signals in clear cell RCC led to the development of novel anti-VEGF agents most active in patients with clear cell histology.

## IMMUNE FACTORS

The ability to mount an effective immune response to RCC was shown to depend on the activation of T lymphocytes following presentation of tumor-associated antigens by antigen-presenting cells.[40] A prospective study examined several specific and nonspecific immune parameters in patients before nephrectomy. Treated patients who relapsed during the 3-year follow-up exhibited significantly reduced proportion of CD80[+] and CD10/80[+] cells at diagnosis compared to those who are disease free.[41] Other investigators have found that the absolute numbers of CD4[+] and CD8[+] B and T lymphocytes prior to starting therapy and the CD4[+]/CD8[+] ratio during treatment to be an important PF.[42,43] The prognostic values of IL-6 and IL-10 (both secreted by RCC) were also explored in several studies. IL-6 is a multifunctional cytokine with several immunoregulatory effects, and IL-10 is an immunosuppressive cytokine with a direct effect on IL-2 production and an inhibitory effect on the maturation of predendritic cells. One study showed that high pretreatment serum IL-10 levels (> 1pg/mL) are associated with poor survival after correcting for the effects of elevated ESR, LDH, and anemia.[44] Three other studies reported elevated serum IL-6 to have a negative impact on survival.[45,46,47] Donskov and colleagues explored immunologic variables derived from blood (neutrophil counts) and tumor analyses (intratumoral neutrophils and CD57 (+) natural killer cell count) and found them to significantly add to prognostic models based on clinical risk factors only, in patients treated with IL-2–based regimens.[48]

Recently, B7-H1 molecule has been implicated as a potent negative regulator of T-cell–mediated immunity, functioning as an inhibitor of antitumoral immune response. RCC as well as many other tumor types aberrantly express B7-H1, possibly contributing to cancer progression through impairment of host T cell–mediated immunity.[49] Investigators studied B7-H1 expression in 196 primary metastatic RCC tumors and found that patients with high expression of B7-H1 (> 10%) on primary tumor cells and/or lymphocytes were 4 fold more likely to die of RCC

compared with patients with low B7-H1 expression. The risk persisted in multivariate analysis after adjusting for tumor size, grade, and necrosis.[50] One can hypothesize that B7-H1 blockade may increase immunotherapy response, including patients treated for metastases after cytoreductive nephrectomy.

Overall, these markers of immune function are considered to be of interest from research perspective only and are not currently used in patient management. The main limitation of all these analyses is the nonspecific nature of the immune readouts; the sometimes specialized assays needed and further the diminishing role of immunotherapy in metastatic RCC.

## MOLECULAR MARKERS

The next generation of prognostic models expects to incorporate the advancements of molecular biology and genetics. Methods based on gene arrays, which screen for differential expression of thousands of genes, have identified large numbers of new, potentially important prognostic markers.[51] Similarly, protein expression is a natural extension to the efforts in molecular staging. Sections of the microarray permit the rapid analysis of hundreds of DNA, RNA, and protein molecular markers in the same set of specimens, which can be correlated to clinical data with respect to disease outcome.

Kim and colleagues have recently demonstrated that molecular characterization improves upon the UISS (UCLA integrated staging system), which represents a purely clinical prognostic model based on T category, histologic grade, and performance status.[52] Immunohistochemical analysis of Ki-67, *TP53*, gelsolin, carbonic anhydrase (CA) IX, CA XII, PTEN (phosphatase and tensin homologue deleted on chromosome 10), epithelial cell adhesion molecule (EpCAM), and vimentin was performed on a tissue microarray, using clear cell RCC from 318 patients (localized and metastatic RCC). Markers examined in this study were selected based on previous reports linking the markers to the development of malignancies.[52] However, these clinical/molecular nomograms need to be validated on independent patient populations prior to being applied to patient care.

| Table 4. RECENTLY-INVESTIGATED PROGNOSTIC MOLECULAR MARKERS IN METASTATIC RENAL CELL CARCINOMA | | | |
|---|---|---|---|
| VHL and Hypoxia-Inducible Factors | Regulators of Apoptosis | Regulators of Cell Cycle | Adhesion Molecules |
| HIF-1α | TP53 | P27 | EpCAM |
| CA IX | bcl-2 | PTEN | EphA2 |
| VHL alteration (mutation/methylation) | Survivin | — | Vascular-cell adhesion molecule-1 |
| VEGF and VEGF receptors | Smac/DIABLO | — | — |

CA = carbonic anhydrase; EpCAM = epithelial cell adhesion molecule; HIF-1 = Hypoxia-inducible factor-1; PTEN = phosphatase and tensin; RCC = renal cell carcinoma.

Currently, there are a variety of molecular targets that have been identified to be important in RCC biology. Molecular markers of known importance include hypoxia-inducible factors, cell cycle regulators, mediators of cellular proliferation, cellular adhesion molecules, and a variety of other molecules (Table 4).

## Hypoxia-inducible Factor

The hypoxia-inducible pathway plays a crucial role in angiogenesis, epithelial proliferation, and apoptosis of common cancers and contributes to the ability of cancers to adapt to hypoxic environment and resist radiation and chemotherapy.[53] Hypoxia-inducible factor-1 (HIF-1) is a heterodimer of HIF-1α and HIF-1β. Upregulation of HIF-α is significantly associated with an upregulation of vascular endothelial growth factor VEGF, PDGF, and others, which promotes angiogenesis and tumor growth.[54] The role of HIF-1α in determining prognosis was recently examined in a cohort of 92 patients (36% with stage IV disease) undergoing nephrectomy. HIF-1α was differentially expressed between histologic subtypes, with clear cell displaying greater expression compared with either papillary or chromophobe subtypes. For clear cell RCC, increased HIF-1α expression was an independent favorable predictor of survival.[55] However, in a more comprehensive and larger study specifically in stage IV disease, HIF-1 alpha "overexpression" was found to be an unfavorable independent prognostic factor for patients with metastatic clear cell RCC.[85] Patients with tumors exhibiting high HIF-1 alpha expression (> 35% by IHC) had significantly worse survival (median of 13 months) than patients with low expression (median of 24 months, P = 0.005).

Additionally, Patel et al reported on the predictive value of HIF expression in pre-treatment tumor specimens by Western analysis in a small cohort of 43 clear-cell RCC patients treated with sunitinib.[86] Patients with tumors exhibiting high HIF-2α expression had > 90% chance of responding to sunitinib compared to 27% of patients whose tumors had low expression and 13% of patients with tumors showing no expression (p-value < 0.0001). Additional studies are needed to confirm the predictive value of HIF-2 for sunitinib and other VEGF-targeted agents in patients with metastatic RCC.

## Carbonic Anhydrase IX

Carbonic anhydrase (CA) IX, a member of the carbonic anhydrase family, regulates pH during hypoxia and is a product of the HIF complex overexpression. Bui and colleagues reported that 94% of clear cell RCC tumor samples stained positive for CA IX, and that overall expression of CA IX decreased with development of metastasis.[56] High CA IX staining (> 85% staining by IHC) was found to be an independent favorable prognostic indicator of survival in patients with metastatic clear cell RCC. Furthermore, high CA IX may be associated with a better response to IL-2–based therapy.[57] Patients with high CA IX expression were twice as likely to have a response to treatment. This may explain the poor response of papillary and chromophobe subtypes to IL-2 immunotherapy because these 2 histologic subtypes express low or no levels of CA IX.[57]

## VHL Gene Alteration

The prognostic capability of *VHL* alterations was studied in 187 patients and found that *VHL* alteration was an independent predictor of cancer-free survival and disease-specific survival for patients with stages I to III but not stage IV RCC.[58] Nevertheless, 1 study with 88 clear cell RCC failed to demonstrate a survival impact from VHL mutational status,[59] and the other one also failed to detect an association between VHL alteration and response to immunotherapy.[60] However, only one study to date examined the predictive value of VHL status after VEGF-targeted therapy. A study of 43 patients with metastatic RCC patients receiving anti-VEGF therapies and showed that VHL methylation or a mutation predicted to truncate or shift the VHL reading frame had a median TTP of 13.3 months vs 7.4 months in patients with none of these features ($p = .06$).[26] Choueiri et al reported on the VHL status of 123 patients with metastatic, clear-cell RCC with who received VEGF-targeted agents.[87] Based on VHL status inactivation (mutated or methylated gene vs. wild type), responses to VEGF-targeted agents were not different. Interestingly, patients with "loss of function" (LOF) mutations (defined as frameshift, nonsense, splice and in-frame deletions/insertions) had an improved response ($p = .03$) independent of other prognostic variables. As *VHL* potentially mediates hundreds of genes relevant to RCC biology and response to therapy, gene status is likely only 1 factor in determining outcome. Further, the complex biology of the *VHL*/HIF interaction and subsequent gene transcription will require functional studies of specific *VHL* gene mutations to correlate genotype with phenotype. Additional large-scale studies are ongoing to examine the impact of *VHL* gene alteration in relation to the outcome of patients receiving VEGF-targeted agents.

## Vascular Endothelial Growth Factor

VEGF is a key regulator of endothelial cells derived from arteries, veins, and lymphatics and is a downstream product of the HIF pathway.[61] One study found serum VEGF to be associated with cancer-specific survival but not metastatic status or histologic subtype.[62] Another study found VEGF to have a significant correlation with survival on univariate analysis only.[47] Investigators have evaluated survival and metastatic pattern in clear cell RCC

and found that VEGFR-1 and VEGFR-2 (and not VEGF) in the tumor-associated endothelium predicted hematogenous spread in multivariate analysis. On contrary, low VEGFR-3 expression was retained as an independent predictor of lymph node involvement with a 4-fold increase in risk of lymphatic spread. When evaluating disease-specific survival, VEGF, VEGFR-1, and VEGFR-2 in the tumor epithelium and low expression of VEGFR-3 in tumor-associated endothelium were significant in univariate analysis; nevertheless, only low endothelial expression of VEGFR-3 was retained as an independent predictor of survival in multivariate analysis. These findings require independent validation but may suggest that decreased expression of VEGFR-3 is an independent predictor of both nodal involvement and poor disease-free survival.[63] A biomarker analysis from a phase II sunitinib trial in cytokine-refractory metastatic disease found significantly larger changes in VEGF, sVEGFR-2, and sVEGFR-3 levels at Day 28 in patients exhibiting a response compared with stable disease or disease progression.[88] Similarly, data from the a trial of pazopanib, another potent VEGF receptor inhibitor, showed that a more profound sVEGFR-2 levels decrease after 2 weeks of therapy of therapy predicted a better outcome in terms of response and PFS.[89]

Several other molecular markers have been studied in RCC. Regulators of apoptosis such as *TP53*,[64–67] bcl-2,[68–70] Survivin,[71–74] and *Smac/DIABLO*,[75,76] have been cited as potential markers of interest in this disease. Similarly, decreased expression (by IHC) of cell cycle regulators such as *p27*[77,78] and *PTEN*[52,79,80] showed an association with a poor outcome in RCC. Finally, adhesion molecules such as EpCAM,[81] receptor tyrosine kinase (EphA2),[82] and vascular cell adhesion molecule-1[83] were investigated in few studies and found to be of prognostic value, although their particular relevance to the metastatic setting is not well established.

By better understanding the genetic alterations at the molecular level, clinicians will be able to tailor treatment type. These tumor-specific treatment plans will be more effective at targeting the genotypic alterations unique to each cancer with less systemic side effects.

## CONCLUSIONS

Metastatic RCC remains a largely incurable disease. Prognostic models based on pretreatment clinical characteristics are widely used in this disease. However, more recent advances in understanding the underlying molecular mechanisms in RCC are being accompanied by a gradual transition from the use of solitary clinical factors as prognostic markers to incorporation of molecular and genetic markers. These markers will eventually enhance our ability to predict the behavior of tumors in a patient and to stratify individuals into more accurate risk categories. This may help select patients for new therapeutic strategies and continue to transform the management of this malignancy in the future.

## REFERENCES

1. Elson PJ, Witte RS, Trump DL. Prognostic factors for survival in patients with recurrent or metastatic renal cell carcinoma. Cancer Res 1988;48(24 Pt 1):7310–3.
2. de Forges A, Rey A, Klink M, et al. Prognostic factors of adult metastatic renal carcinoma: a multivariate analysis. Semin Surg Oncol 1988;4:149–54.
3. Palmer PA, Vinke J, Philip T, et al. Prognostic factors for survival in patients with advanced renal cell carcinoma treated with recombinant interleukin-2. Ann Oncol 1992;3:475–80.
4. Fossa SD, Kramar A, Droz JP. Prognostic factors and survival in patients with metastatic renal cell carcinoma treated with chemotherapy or interferon-α. Eur J Cancer 1994;30A:1310–4.
5. Motzer RJ, Mazumdar M, Bacik J, et al. Survival and prognostic stratification of 670 patients with advanced renal cell carcinoma. J Clin Oncol 1999;17:2530–40.
6. Motzer RJ, Bacik J, Murphy BA, et al. Interferon-α as a comparative treatment for clinical trials of new therapies against advanced renal cell carcinoma. J Clin Oncol 2002;20:289–96.
7. Negrier S, Escudier B, Gomez F, et al. Prognostic factors of survival and rapid progression in 782 patients with metastatic renal carcinomas treated by cytokines: a report from the Groupe Francais d'Immunotherapie. Ann Oncol 2002;13:1460–8.
8. Atzpodien J, Royston P, Wandert T, Reitz M. Metastatic renal carcinoma comprehensive prognostic system. Br J Cancer 2003;88:348–53.
9. Mekhail TM, Abou-Jawde RM, Boumerhi G, et al. Validation and extension of the memorial sloan-kettering prognostic factors model for survival in patients with previously untreated metastatic renal cell carcinoma. J Clin Oncol 2005;23:832–41.
10. Choueiri TK, Rini BI, Garcia JA, et al. Prognostic factors associated with long-term survival in previously untreated metastatic renal cell carcinoma. Ann Oncol. 2007;18:249–55 [Epub 2006 Oct 23].
11. Choueiri TK, Garcia JA, Elson P, et al. Clinical factors associated with outcome in patients with metastatic clear-cell renal cell carcinoma treated with vascular endothelial growth factor-targeted therapy. Cancer 2007 [Epub ahead of print].
12. Klugo RC, Detmers M, Stiles RE, et al. Aggressive versus conservative management of stage IV renal cell carcinoma. J Urol 1977;118:244–6.
13. Lopez Hanninen E, Kirchner H, Atzpodien J. Interleukin-2 based home therapy of metastatic renal cell carcinoma: risks and benefits in 215 consecutive single institution patients. J Urol 1996;155:19–25.
14. Landonio G, Baiocchi C, Cattaneo D, et al. Retrospective analysis of 156 cases of metastatic renal cell carcinoma: evaluation of prognostic factors and response to different treatments. Tumori 1994;80:468–72.
15. Neves RJ, Zincke H, Taylor WF. Metastatic renal cell cancer and radical nephrectomy: identification of prognostic factors and patient survival. J Urol 1988;139:1173–6.
16. Flanigan RC, Mickisch G, Sylvester R, et al. Cytoreductive nephrectomy in patients with metastatic renal cancer: a combined analysis. J Urol 2004;171:1071–6.
17. Vogl UM, Zehetgruber H, Dominkus M, et al. Prognostic factors in metastatic renal cell carcinoma: metastasectomy as independent prognostic variable. Br J Cancer 2006;95:691–8.
18. Ljungberg B, Grankvist K, Rasmuson T. Serum acute phase reactants and prognosis in renal cell carcinoma. Cancer 1995;76:1435–9.
19. Suppiah R, Shaheen PE, Elson P, et al. Thrombocytosis as a prognostic factor for survival in patients with metastatic renal cell carcinoma. Cancer 2006;107:1793–800.
20. Hollen CW, Henthorn J, Koziol JA, Burstein SA. Elevated serum interleukin-6 levels in patients with reactive thrombocytosis. Br J Haematol 1991;79:286–90.
21. Hollen CW, Henthorn J, Koziol JA, Burstein SA. Serum interleukin-6 levels in patients with thrombocytosis. Leuk Lymphoma 1992;8:235–41.
22. Karpatkin S, Pearlstein E. Role of platelets in tumor cell metastases. Ann Intern Med 1981;95:636–41.
23. Mohle R, Green D, Moore MA, et al. Constitutive production and thrombin-induced release of vascular endothelial growth factor by human megakaryocytes and platelets. Proc Natl Acad Sci U S A 1997;94:663–8.
24. O'Byrne KJ, Dobbs N, Propper D, et al. Vascular endothelial growth factor platelet counts, and prognosis in renal cancer. Lancet 1999;353:1494–5.
25. Mani S, Todd MB, Katz K, Poo WJ. Prognostic factors for survival in patients with metastatic renal cancer treated with biological response modifiers. J Urol 1995;154:35–40.
26. Rini BI, Jaeger E, Weinberg V, et al. Clinical response to therapy targeted at vascular endothelial growth factor in metastatic renal cell carcinoma: impact of patient characteristics and Von Hippel-Lindau gene status. BJU Int 2006;98:756–62.
27. Motzer RJ, Bacik J, Schwartz LH, et al. Prognostic factors for survival in previously treated patients with metastatic renal cell carcinoma. J Clin Oncol 2004;22:454–63.
28. Boumerhi G, Mekhail TM, Abou-Jawde, RM, et al. Prognostic factors for survival in previously treated patients (pts)

with metastatic renal cell cancer (RCC) [abstract 1647]. Proc Am Soc Clin Oncol 2003;22:16S.

29. Escudier B, Choueiri TK, Oudard S, et al. Prognostic factors in metastatic renal cell carcinoma after failure of immunotherapy: new paradigm from a large phase III trial with Neovastat. J Urol 2007;178:1901–05.

30. Kanamaru H, Sasaki M, Miwa Y, et al. Prognostic value of sarcomatoid histology and volume-weighted mean nuclear volume in renal cell carcinoma. BJU Int 1999;83:222–6.

31. Cheville JC, Lohse CM, Zincke H, et al. Sarcomatoid renal cell carcinoma: an examination of underlying histologic subtype and an analysis of associations with patient outcome. Am J Surg Pathol 2004;28:435–41.

32. Ljungberg B, Mehle C, Stenling R, Roos G. Heterogeneity in renal cell carcinoma and its impact no prognosis–a flow cytometric study. Br J Cancer 1996;74:123–7.

33. Eskelinen M, Lipponen P, Nordling S. Prognostic evaluation of DNA flow cytometry and histo-morphological criteria in renal cell carcinoma. Anticancer Res 1995;15(5B):2279–83.

34. Ruiz-Cerda JL, Hernandez M, Sempere A, et al. Intratumoral heterogeneity of DNA content in renal cell carcinoma and its prognostic significance. Cancer 1999;86:664–71.

35. Citterio G, Bertuzzi A, Tresoldi M, et al. Prognostic factors for survival in metastatic renal cell carcinoma: retrospective analysis from 109 consecutive patients. Eur Urol 1997;31:286–91.

36. Lanigan D, Conroy R, Barry-Walsh C, et al. A comparative analysis of grading systems in renal adenocarcinoma. Histopathology 1994;24:473–6.

37. Lam JS, Shvarts O, Said JW, et al. Clinicopathologic and molecular correlations of necrosis in the primary tumor of patients with renal cell carcinoma. Cancer 2005;103:2517–25.

38. Motzer RJ, Bacik J, Mariani T, et al. Treatment outcome and survival associated with metastatic renal cell carcinoma of non-clear-cell histology. J Clin Oncol 2002;20:2376–81.

39. Upton MP, Parker RA, Youmans A, et al. Histologic predictors of renal cell carcinoma response to interleukin-2-based therapy. J Immunother 2005;28:488–95.

40. Altman A, Coggeshall KM, Mustelin T. Molecular events mediating T cell activation. Adv Immunol 1990;48:227–360.

41. Lauerova L, Dusek L, Spurny V, et al. Relation of prenephrectomy CD profiles and serum cytokines to the disease outcome and response to IFN-α/IL-2 therapy in renal cell carcinoma patients. Oncol Rep 2001;8:685–92.

42. Gohring B, Riemann D, Rebmann U, et al. Prognostic value of the immunomonitoring of patients with renal cell carcinoma under therapy with IL-2/IFN-α-2 in combination with 5-FU. Urol Res 1996;24:297–303.

43. Hernberg M, Muhonen T, Pyrhonen S. Can the CD4+/CD8+ ratio predict the outcome of interferon-α therapy for renal cell carcinoma? Ann Oncol 1997;8:71–7.

44. Wittke F, Hoffmann R, Buer J, et al. Interleukin 10 (IL-10): an immunosuppressive factor and independent predictor in patients with metastatic renal cell carcinoma. Br J Cancer 1999;79:1182–4.

45. Ljungberg B, Grankvist K, Rasmuson T. Serum interleukin-6 in relation to acute-phase reactants and survival in patients with renal cell carcinoma. Eur J Cancer 1997;33:1794–8.

46. Blay JY, Negrier S, Combaret V, et al. Serum level of interleukin 6 as a prognosis factor in metastatic renal cell carcinoma. Cancer Res 1992;52:3317–22.

47. Negrier S, Perol D, Menetrier-Caux C, et al. Interleukin-6, interleukin-10, and vascular endothelial growth factor in metastatic renal cell carcinoma: prognostic value of inter-leukin-6—from the Groupe Francais d'Immunotherapie. J Clin Oncol 2004;22:2371–8.

48. Donskov F, von der Maase H. Impact of immune parameters on long-term survival in metastatic renal cell carcinoma. J Clin Oncol 2006;24:1997–2005.

49. Mazanet MM, Hughes CC. B7-H1 is expressed by human endothelial cells and suppresses T cell cytokine synthesis. J Immunol 2002;169:3581–8.

50. Thompson RH, Gillett MD, Cheville JC, et al. Costimulatory molecule B7-H1 in primary and metastatic clear cell renal cell carcinoma. Cancer 2005;104:2084–91.

51. Tan MH, Rogers CG, Cooper JT, et al. Gene expression profiling of renal cell carcinoma. Clin Cancer Res 2004;10 (18 Pt 2):6315S–21S.

52. Kim HL, Seligson D, Liu X, et al. Using tumor markers to predict the survival of patients with metastatic renal cell carcinoma. J Urol 2005;173:1496–501.

53. Harris AL. Hypoxia—a key regulatory factor in tumour growth. Nat Rev Cancer 2002;2:38–47.

54. Iliopoulos O. Molecular biology of renal cell cancer and the identification of therapeutic targets. J Clin Oncol 2006;24:5593–600.

55. Lidgren A, Hedberg Y, Grankvist K, Rasmuson T, Vasko J, Ljungberg B. The expression of hypoxia-inducible factor 1α is a favorable independent prognostic factor in renal cell carcinoma. Clin Cancer Res 2005;11:1129–35.

56. Bui MH, Seligson D, Han KR, et al. Carbonic anhydrase IX is an independent predictor of survival in advanced renal clear cell carcinoma: implications for prognosis and therapy. Clin Cancer Res 2003;9:802–11.

57. Atkins M, Regan M, McDermott D, et al. Carbonic anhydrase IX expression predicts outcome of interleukin 2 therapy for renal cancer. Clin Cancer Res 2005;11:3714–21.

58. Yao M, Yoshida M, Kishida T, et al. VHL tumor suppressor gene alterations associated with good prognosis in sporadic clear-cell renal carcinoma. J Natl Cancer Inst 2002;94:1569–75.

59. Tan MH, Teh BT. The von Hippel-Lindau gene mutation is associated with the good-prognosis profiling subtype of clear cell renal cell carcinoma [abstract 4532]. Proc Am Soc Clin Oncol 2006;24:18S.

60. Kim J, Kim H, Jung C, et al. Somatic VHL alteration and its impact on prognosis in patients with clear cell renal cell carcinoma [abstract 4602]. Proc Am Soc Clin Oncol 2005;23:16S.

61. Ferrara N, Gerber HP, LeCouter J. The biology of VEGF and its receptors. Nat Med 2003;9:669–76.

62. Partard J, Rioux-Leclercq N, Bensalah K, Fergelot P. Biological significance of serum VEGF measurement in renal cell carcinoma [abstract 4596]. Proc Am Soc Clin Oncol 2006;24:18S.

63. Lam JS, Leppert JT, Yu H, et al. Expression of the vascular endothelial growth factor family in tumor dissemination and disease free survival in clear cell renal cell carcinoma [abstract 4538]. Proc Am Soc Clin Oncol 2005;23:16S.

64. Lane DP. Cancer. p53, guardian of the genome. Nature 1992;358:15–6.

65. Moch H, Sauter G, Gasser TC, et al. p53 protein expression but not mdm-2 protein expression is associated with rapid tumor cell proliferation and prognosis in renal cell carcinoma. Urol Res 1997;25 Suppl 1:25S–30S.

66. Zigeuner R, Ratschek M, Rehak P, et al. Value of p53 as a prognostic marker in histologic subtypes of renal cell carcinoma: a systematic analysis of primary and metastatic tumor tissue. Urology 2004;63:651–5.

67. Shvarts O, Seligson D, Lam J, et al. p53 is an independent predictor of tumor recurrence and progression after nephrectomy in patients with localized renal cell carcinoma. J Urol 2005;173:725–8.

68. Vasavada SP, Novick AC, Williams BR. P53, bcl-2, and Bax expression in renal cell carcinoma. Urology 1998;51:1057–61.

69. Itoi T, Yamana K, Bilim V, et al. Impact of frequent Bcl-2 expression on better prognosis in renal cell carcinoma patients. Br J Cancer 2004;90:200–5.

70. Lee CT, Genega EM, Hutchinson B, et al. Conventional (clear cell) renal carcinoma metastases have greater bcl-2 expression than high-risk primary tumors. Urol Oncol 2003;21:179–84.

71. Verhagen AM, Coulson EJ, Vaux DL. Inhibitor of apoptosis proteins and their relatives: IAPs and other BIRPs. Genome Biol 2001;2:REVIEWS3009.

72. Okada H, Mak TW. Pathways of apoptotic and non-apoptotic death in tumour cells. Nat Rev Cancer 2004;4:592–603.

73. Mahotka C, Krieg T, Krieg A, et al. Distinct in vivo expression patterns of survivin splice variants in renal cell carcinomas. Int J Cancer 2002;100:30–6.

74. Parker AS, Kosari F, Lohse CM, et al. High expression levels of survivin protein independently predict a poor outcome for patients who undergo surgery for clear cell renal cell carcinoma. Cancer 2006;107:37–45.

75. Srinivas S GA. Randomized trial of high and low dose thalidomide in metastatic renal carcinoma [abstract 2403]. Proc Am Soc Clin Oncol 2002;21:147b.

76. Mizutani Y, Nakanishi H, Yamamoto K, et al. Downregulation of Smac/DIABLO expression in renal cell carcinoma and its prognostic significance. J Clin Oncol 2005;23:448–54.

77. Migita T, Oda Y, Naito S, Tsuneyoshi M. Low expression of p27(Kip1) is associated with tumor size and poor prognosis in patients with renal cell carcinoma. Cancer 2002;94:973–9.

78. Hedberg Y, Ljungberg B, Roos G, Landberg G. Expression of cyclin D1, D3, E, and p27 in human renal cell carcinoma analysed by tissue microarray. Br J Cancer 2003;88:1417–23.

79. Hay N. The Akt-mTOR tango and its relevance to cancer. Cancer Cell 2005;8:179–83.

80. Pantuck AJ, Seligson DB, Wu H. Characterization of the mTOR pathway in renal cell carcinoma and its use in predicting patient selection for agents targeting this pathway [abstract 350]. J Urol 2005;173:.

81. Seligson DB, Pantuck AJ, Liu X, et al. Epithelial cell adhesion molecule (KSA) expression: pathobiology and its role as an independent predictor of survival in renal cell carcinoma. Clin Cancer Res 2004;10:2659–69.

82. Herrem CJ, Tatsumi T, Olson KS, et al. Expression of EphA2 is prognostic of disease-free interval and overall survival in surgically treated patients with renal cell carcinoma. Clin Cancer Res 2005;11:226–31.

83. Vasselli JR, Shih JH, Iyengar SR, et al. Predicting survival in patients with metastatic kidney cancer by gene-expression profiling in the primary tumor. Proc Natl Acad Sci U S A 2003;100:6958–63.

84. Motzer RJ, Figlin RA, Hutson TE, et al. Sunitinib versus interferon-alfa as first-line treatment of metastatic renal cell carcinoma (mRCC), updated results and analysis of prognostic factors. J Clin Oncol 2007;25:Abstr 5024.

85. Klatte T, Seligson DB, Riggs SB, Leppert JT, Berkman MK, Kleid MD, et al. Hypoxia-inducible factor 1 alpha in clear cell renal cell carcinoma. *Clin Cancer Res* 2007;13(24): 7388–93.

86. Patel PH CR, Ishill NM, et al. 2008. Hypoxia-inducible factor (HIF) 1a and 2a levels in cell lines and human tumor predicts response to sunitinib in renal cell carcinoma (RCC). *Journal of Clinical Oncology, 2008 ASCO Annual Meeting Proceedings Part I*. 2008;26:Abstract 5008.

87. Choueiri TK, Vaziri SA, Jaeger E, et al. von Hippel-Lindau gene status and response to vascular endothelial growth factor targeted therapy for metastatic clear cell renal cell carcinoma. J Urol. 2008;180 (3):860-5; discussion 865–6. Epub 2008 Jul 17.

88. Deprimo SE, Bello CL, Smeraglia J, Baum CM, Spinella D, Rini BI, et al. Circulating protein biomarkers of pharmacodynamic activity of sunitinib in patients with metastatic renal cell carcinoma: modulation of VEGF and VEGF-related proteins. *J Transl Med* 2007;5:32.

89. Hutson T, Davis ID, Macheils JH, et al,. Biomarker analysis and final efficacy and safety results of a phase II renal cell carcinoma trial with pazopanib (GW786034), a multi-kinase angiogenesis inhibitor. *Journal of Clinical Oncology, 2008 ASCO Annual Meeting Proceedings Part I* 2008;26:5046:Abstract 5046.

# 12

# Immunobiology of Metastatic Renal Cell Carcinoma

RENEE N. SALAS, BS

JENNIFER S. KO, MD

JAMES H. FINKE, PHD

There is accumulating evidence that the immune system recognizes and can eliminate transformed tumor cells and can thus contribute to the prevention of clinically apparent cancer, as well as the eradication of established tumors.[1] Several cancer types, including renal cell carcinoma (RCC), are reported to have an increased incidence in patients who are pharmacologically immunosuppressed.[2,3] In fact, paraneoplastic autoimmunity in patients with cancer receiving immunotherapy is associated with an improved overall survival.[4–6] Additionally, CD8 effector T-cell subsets in the tumor microenvironment of several solid tumor cancers have been linked to improve overall patient survival.[7–10] RCC is understood to be particularly immunogenic. The curative potential of cytokine therapy in a small but definite subset of patients reaffirms the potential immunogenicity of this cancer.[11] The unique biology of RCC that allows the tumor to thrive in the face of immune recognition will be the focus of this chapter.

## THE IMMUNE SYSTEM

Myeloid cells include those white blood cells that are not lymphoid, namely, monocytes/macrophages, dendritic cells (DCs), and granulocytes—all of which have phagocytic capabilities. DCs are specialized antigen-presenting cells (APCs) that are pivotal in directing antitumor immunity. They are required to activate naive resting T cells against new antigens because they express several costimulatory molecules and cytokines necessary for such T-cell activation (Figure 1). They are generated in the bone marrow and mostly differentiate along the myeloid-lineage pathway from common myeloid precursors. This differentiation occurs under the control of several soluble growth factors such as GM-CSF, IL-3, stem cell factor, and fms-related tyrosine kinase-3 ligand. DCs emerge from the bone marrow and are seeded throughout the body in a relatively immature state that allows them to have strong phagocytic antigen processing capabilities and weak antigen presenting/T cell stimulating capabilities.

Macrophages and DCs process and present phagocytosed materials on their cell surface along with major histocompatibility complex (MHC) molecules (see Figure 1). Once the DC contacts these various foreign products in the tissues, it becomes activated and matures such that it can no longer uptake and process antigen. At this point, in time, it migrates to draining lymph nodes and strongly activates T cells.[12] T-cell recognition of MHC and these antigens allow for T-cell activation, thus, initiating the transition from an innate to an adaptive immune response. The context in which antigen is presented to T cells determines the flavor of the adaptive immune response. This can be described in terms of the T-helper (Th) cells that direct it and the manner in which the response attacks the immune insult. Th1 and Th2 responses were the first described, and they generate a

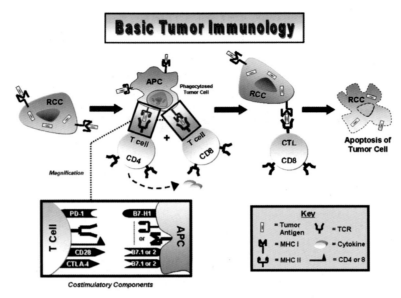

**Figure 1.**   Basic tumor immunology: induction of T-cell responses against tumor cells. Renal cell carcinoma cells (RCCs) present their own tumor antigen on major histocompatibility complex (MHC) I. It is believed that antigen-presenting cells (APCs), such as dendritic cells, ingest and process either tumor cells and/or tumor antigens. These processed antigens can then be presented to naive CD4 and CD8 T cells and induce an antitumor T-cell response, which is also called cross-priming. When an APC stimulates a CD4 helper T cell, it produces cytokines, which result in the proliferation and differentiation of both CD4 and CD8 cells. The costimulator molecules, such as B7, expressed on the APCs can also provide the second signal for the differentiation of T cells when they come into contact with CD28 on the T cell as shown in the magnification view insert. The T-cell receptor in conjunction with either CD4 or CD8 depending on the cell type bind with either MHC II or MHC I, respectively, on the APC. A suppressive costimulatory molecule includes cytotoxic T lymphocyte associated-4 on the T cell with B7 costimulators on the APC. In addition, as discussed later in relation to RCC, T cells also express the programmed death receptor-1 that binds with B7-H1 expressed on such cells as APCs and results in a negative signal. The CD8 cell differentiates into an activated tumor specific cytotoxic T lymphocyte, which recognizes the tumor cell without any requirement for CD4 T cells or costimulation. This results in apoptosis of the tumor cell. Although theoretically this process should allow a host to eradicate malignancies, numerous defects in the process occur and will be further discussed in relation to RCC.

cell-mediated and humoral immune response, respectively, with distinct cytokine profiles. The emergence of the T regulatory (Treg) cell as a CD4 subset has gained momentum recently.[13] Notably, Treg cells are elevated in several types of cancer and are thought to suppress an antitumor adaptive immune response.[14] Transforming growth factor (TGF)-β has been shown to be a suppressor of Th1 and Th2 cell differentiation and to drive the development of Treg cells.[15]

In tumor tissues, it is thought that debris from dying tumor cells can be picked up by DCs and presented on DC surfaces (see Figure 1). Necrotic cells and cytokines present in the tumor microenvironment may activate these DCs and induce them to stimulate an antitumor T-cell response. Indeed, clones of T cells recognizing tumor-associated antigens can be found in patients with cancer. Yet the ineffectiveness of immune containment of cancer, combined with several reported defects in T cells

and DCs in patients with cancer compared with normal hosts, suggest that problems with tumor immunity begin very early in the scheme of tumor progression. These immune cell types and concepts will be further explored in relation to the immunobiology of RCC.

## Overview of the RCC Immune Environment

Existing research has made general observations relating to immune cell variations in patients with RCC. Examination of TILs present within 25 RCC tumors found that the lymphocytic infiltration was composed of approximately 45% CD4/CD8 T cells, 29% CD14 macrophages, and 24% CD56 NK cells.[16] Another study examining the peripheral blood and tumors of 47 patients with RCC reported decreased circulating levels of CD4/CD45RA naive and CD4/CD45RO memory

T cells, CD16 NK cells, and DCs.[17] In addition, the study reported an increase in circulating lymphocytes expressing CD4 and CD8 antigens, as well as activation of CD3/HLA-DR lymphocytes and CD56 NK cells. Lastly, the tumor samples were also found to be deficient in CD16/CD56 NK and DCs.

Moving beyond this general characterization, investigations into the presence of immune cells within RCC tumors and outcome have been reported. One study found that increased CD4 and decreased CD8 cells in patient's peripheral blood with stage III and IV RCC was a favorable prognostic factor.[18] However, a study of 306 patients with RCC nephrectomy found that patients whose tumors were infiltrated with mononuclear cells were at a significantly increased risk of dying from RCC when compared with patients without infiltration.[16] A subsequent study found that intratumoral CD4 T-lymphocyte infiltration to be associated with poor cancer-specific survival.[19] The results of these initial reports characterizing RCC tumor infiltrating leukocytes have been somewhat counterintuitive and lead one to speculate that the mere presence of cells is not sufficient for a true understanding of the immunobiology (Figure 2).

Instead, the nature and function of these immune cells must be characterized.

## Evidence for Immune Dysfunction in Patients With RCC

### T-Helper 2 Cytokine Bias

CD4 helper T cells differentiate into 2 distinct subsets of effector cells, referred to as Th1 and Th2, which have characteristic cytokine profiles and functions.[20] Th1 cytokines include IFN-γ and IL-12 and activate a cell-mediated immune response. Conversely, Th2 cytokines include IL-4, IL-5, IL-6, and IL-10 that lead to a humoral immune response. Although a Th1 adaptive immune response is the desired and appropriate antitumor response, several studies have shown that patients with RCC T cells are selectively deficient in one or many of the functions necessary for the generation of a Th1 response. Results of several studies have shown that biasing toward a Th2 T helper cell response takes place in the presence of RCC tumors.[21,22] This tendency also correlated with stage and grade such that higher staged/graded tumors were associated with a

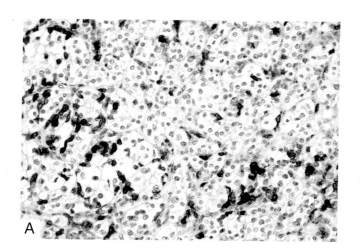
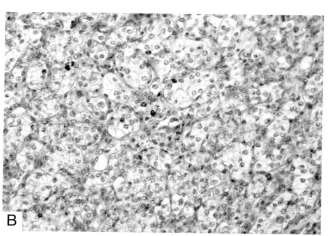

**Figure 2.** Clear cell renal cell carcinoma cell (RCC) with CD3 and FoxP3 antibody staining. *A,* RCC clear cell tumor specimen at 200 magnification stained with an antibody specific for CD3 exhibiting that the tumor specimen is diffusely infiltrated with CD3(+) lymphocytes. *B,* RCC clear cell tumor specimen at 200 magnification stained with an antibody specific for FoxP3, a marker specific for natural T regulatory cells, exhibiting the presence of scattered FoxP3(+) lymphocytes. However, although gathering this information is necessary, research has revealed that the mere presence of immune cells such as these is not sufficient to truly understand the immunobiology of RCC. Instead, the nature and function of the immune cells, such as the ability of the immune cell to be directed at RCC antigens, need to be understood. (Picture compliments of Dr. Ming Zhou, Department of Pathology at the Cleveland Clinic Foundation).

stronger Th2 bias. Further analysis of Th1 and Th2 associated genes, cytokines/chemokines, and their respective receptors revealed that patients whose RCC tumor environments are biased toward a Th1 immune response have a more favorable prognosis.[23] Evaluations of peripheral blood T-cell responses have produced similar results.[24] In addition, patients with RCC T cells produce markedly reduced levels of cytokines and proliferate less in response to nonspecific T-cell activation as compared with normal blood donors.[25] Thus, it appears that RCC creates a Th2 biased milieu, which perpetuates the immunosuppressive environment.

### Increased Sensitivity of T Cells to Apoptosis

The reduction in the Th1 response in patients with RCC may be partly explained by the demonstration that Th1 CD4 T cells with specificity for tumor expressed antigens display an increased sensitivity to apoptosis. One study using MHC class II tetramers and tumor peptides has demonstrated that although CD4 T cells specific for the RCC antigens, melanoma antigenic epitope-6 and EphA2 were detectable in the peripheral blood of patients with RCC; many of these cells stained positive for annexin V suggesting that they were undergoing apoptosis.[26] In fact, a significant number of the bulk T-cell population infiltrating renal tumors appear to undergo apoptosis.[27]

## Mechanism of Immune Suppression by RCC Tumors

Despite the expression of molecules that is capable of activating the host immune response, RCC tumors still grow to overwhelm their hosts. Studies investigating tumor immune cell infiltrates suggest that this may be partially due to tumor-induced immune suppression mediated by soluble products (eg, gangliosides) and costimulatory molecules expressed by RCC. In addition, suppressive immune cell types have been identified and found to be interacting in this complex network. Figure 3 diagrams the complex relationships believed to be present in the RCC environment.

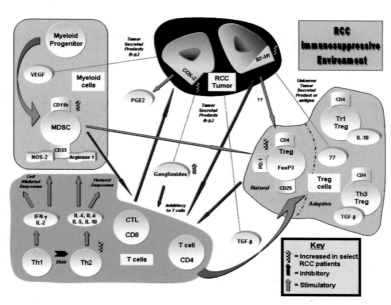

**Figure 3.** The immunosuppressive environment in renal cell carcinoma (RCC). A few of the known mechanisms through which RCC tumor cells generate an immunosuppressive environment are through the secretion of tumor secreted products and the expression of antigens. For example, RCC produces vascular endothelial growth factor, which has been shown to induce myeloid-derived suppressor cells (MDSCs) from myeloid progenitors. Subsequently, the MDSCs suppress T-cell function and promote natural T regulatory (Treg) cell formation. There is also a bias toward a T-helper (Th) 2 cell response in poorer stages that diminishes the activity of cell-mediated, and thus tumor directed, immunity. The cytokines produced by the Th2 cells further mediate the immunosuppressive activity of the MDSCs on T cells through the enzyme arginase 1. In addition, one of the secreted factors that RCC produces is transforming growth factor-B, which induces the transformation of T cells into natural Treg cells. The natural Treg cells in turn suppress T-cell function. It is currently not known if there is a secreted product or an antigen by the tumor that promotes the development of the adaptive Treg cells in RCC. Tumor expression of cyclooxygenase-2 and production of prostaglandin E2 is believed to contribute to the immunosuppression though the elucidation of that role is still under investigation. Lastly, gangliosides and B7-H1 are both known to be inhibitory to T-cell function.

## Suppressive RCC Molecules

### Gangliosides

Gangliosides can be defined as sialic acid containing glycosphingolipids, and there are multiple species of gangliosides, which are classified based on the number and location of the sialic acid subgroups.[28,29] Gangliosides are ubiquitous and found in the lipid raft portions of cell membranes where they play a role in cell development, growth, and communication via the regulation of various signaling events.[30] Renal tumor cells produce excessive amounts of gangliosides (GM2, GM1 and GD1a), which are likely shed into the tumor microenvironment.[31-33] There have been several immunosuppressive functions attributed to gangliosides including T-cell apoptosis,[34-36] inhibition of T-cell proliferation,[37] suppression of T-cell production of IFN-γ,[32,38] and impairment of antigen presentation by DC.[39]

The RCC derived gangliosides that induce apoptosis and suppress a Th1 response have not been well defined. However, recent findings suggest that GM2 is one tumor-derived ganglioside with immunosuppressive activity. This conclusion is supported by the demonstration that many clear cell RCC tumors express GM2 as do 5 RCC lines tested via immunostaining with anti-GM2 specific antibody.[32] Furthermore, the addition of antibodies specific for GM2 to the T-cell ganglioside cultures blocked the ability of gangliosides isolated from RCC tissue to induce apoptosis and inhibited IFN-γ production by greater than 50%. Thus, it appears that GM2 is shed from RCC tissue and can bind to T cells and initiate T-cell apoptosis.

## B7-H1

### B7-H1 Expression and Immunoregulatory Properties

B7-H1 represents a cell surface glycoprotein belonging to the B7 family of costimulatory molecules that is known to have regulatory effects on T and B cells.[40,41] B7-H1 is normally restricted to macrophage lineage cells yet has wide mRNA expression in murine and human lines and has constitutive expression on the human maternal-fetal interface.[42] Recently, B7-H1 has been observed in both murine and human microvascular endothelial cells (ECs) in basal states and induced and/or upregulated by cytokines in mice and humans.[43,44] In addition, vascular endothelial growth factor (VEGF) has been shown to upregulate B7-H1 on myeloid DCs.[45] B7-H1 protein is also aberrantly expressed on a variety of human tumors including glioblastoma, melanoma, and cancers arising from the lung, ovary, colon, head and neck, and breast.[40,41] Lastly, the receptor for B7-H1 is programmed death receptor-1 (PD-1, CD279) and is expressed on T cells, B cells, and myeloid cells.[46,47] Although B7-H1 is reported to either inhibit or simulate T-cell function, most studies suggest that its interaction with the PD-1 receptor results in immune suppression.[46,48]

### Clinical Significance of B7-H1 and B7-H4 Expression in RCC

In RCC, expression of B7-H1 has been found in both primary and metastatic lesions and is associated with a poor prognosis.[49-51] In a study of 196 tumors of clear cell RCC, over half of the tumors express B7-H1, whereas normal renal cortex did not. When total B7-H1 expression by tumors or infiltrating lymphocytes was compared with patient outcome (median follow-up of 2.1 years), B7-H1 expression either on cell type or on both cell types was associated with an increased risk of death from RCC. Combined high-aggregate intratumoral expression was most strongly associated with an increased risk of death ($p \leq .001$) and the association remained significant after adjusting for various other histologic prognostic factors one at a time.

In a similar study by the same group, B7-H4, another negative T-cell regulator of the B7 family, was found in over half of the RCC tumors analyzed. Expression was found on tumor cells and tumor-associated ECs.[52] B7-H4 expression was also associated with adverse clinical and pathologic features (including lymphocytic infiltration), as well as an increased risk of death from RCC and disease progression after surgical removal of localized RCC. Patients with B7-H4 and B7-H1 positive tumors were over 4 times more likely to die from RCC compared with patients with negative or singly positive tumors. Interestingly, this study also showed that B7-H4 expression was found on over 80% of tumor vasculature versus 6.5% on adjacent normal renal vessels. IL-10 typically present in the tumor microenvironment was shown to induce B7-H4 on APCs,[53] thus, providing a possible mechanism to further suppress T-cell function. Lastly, TIL expression of PD-1 is also associated with high-risk tumors and a greater risk of cancer specific death,[54] suggesting that interactions between immunosuppressive molecules on tumors and TILs can and do take place to limit effector T-cell function. This could partly help to explain why CD4 tumor infiltration is associated with poor outcome in patients with RCC, considering that these cells are dysfunctional.[9,55,56] Animal studies have shown that administration of monoclonal anti-B7-H1 antibody can enhance the survival of mice previously injected with B7-H1 tumors and also increase the antitumor activity resulting from immunotherapy.[57–59] Thus, blocking B7-H1 may be a relevant strategy for improving the development of an effective antitumor immune response in patients with metastatic RCC.

### Cyclooxygenase-2 and Prostaglandin E2

Cyclooxygenase-2 (COX-2) is an early response gene that has been linked to carcinogenesis and found to be induced by tumor promoters, cytokines, growth factors, and hypoxia. The enzyme has been identified in neoplastic cells, microvascular ECs, and stromal fibroblasts.[60] In RCC, studies have reported COX-2 expression in tumors ranging between approximately 50 to 100% and have found correlations of COX-2 with parameters such as tumor cell proliferation, apoptosis, angiogenesis, expression of matrix metalloproteinase-2, as well as increased MVD, stage and grade, tumor progression, and survival.[61–64] In addition, it was reported that macrophages found in cystic RCC regression, and in necrotic rims with hypoxic endothelia, express COX-2. This suggests that COX-2 could provide a mechanism via which tumors are able to overcome hypoxia and continue to compound immune suppression.[65,66] One of the well described downstream products of COX-2 is prostaglandin $E_2$ ($PGE_2$), which has been shown to stimulate tumor cell growth and migration, inhibit tumor cell apoptosis, lead to neovascularization, and increase EC migration.[67,68] More specifically, though it has been well accepted for some time that PGE plays a role in the regulation of both cellular and humoral immune responses.[69] RCC has been found to induce PBMCs, especially monocytes, to produce $PGE_2$.[21,70,71] Clinical trial experience with celecoxib in patients with RCC is limited, but early interpretations thus far suggest that the selection of patients based on an abundant expression of COX-2 in their tumors (3+ score) is necessary to examine an effect.[72] A further analysis of the contribution of COX-2, and its downstream molecule $PGE_2$, to immunosuppression and tumor escape is important, especially if celecoxib proves effective in the subset of patients with 3+ COX2 expression.

## SUPPRESSIVE IMMUNE CELLS

The 2 main suppressive immune cell types believed to further compound suppression of the host immune system against RCC are Treg cells and myeloid-derived suppressor cells (MDSCs) (Table 1).

### T Regulatory Cells

#### Phenotype and Function of Treg cells

Treg cells are potent inhibitors of T-cell immunity that are first postulated back in the 1970s, faded from popularity, and then had a resurgence of interest as of late—especially in the field of cancer research.[13,73] Treg cells can be divided into 2 subsets: natural/intrinsic and adaptive/induced subsets. The natural subset, characterized as CD4(+), interleukin (IL)-2 receptor-$\alpha$ or CD25(+), and nuclear transcription factor forkhead box P3 (+) (FoxP3), is believed to be a distinct T-cell lineage originating from the thymus and to compose about 1 to 3% of CD4(+) T cells in healthy humans.[74,75] Once activated through T-cell receptor and IL-2 in an antigen-specific manner, they are postulated to suppress immune function through the antigen-independent inhibition of IL-2 production in target

## Table 1. MAJOR IMMUNOSUPPRESSIVE CELL TYPES RELEVANT TO RENAL CELL CARCINOMA

| Cell Type | Cellular Markers | Mechanism of Effect/Cytokines Produced | Relevant RCC Data |
|---|---|---|---|
| Natural Tregs | CD3(+)/CD4(+) CD25(hi+)/FoxP3(+) | Immunosuppression mainly through intercellular contact | • Tumor derived TGF-β produces Tregs[112]; • Increased Treg levels in blood[75,83]; • Decreased Treg levels in patients with objective response to high-dose IL-2[75]; • Increased Treg levels after high-does IL-2 without correlation to response[85]; • Decreased Tregs with DAB389IL-2[86] |
| Adaptive Tregs Tr1 | CD4(+) otherwise not conclusively characterized by markers | IL-10(+), TGF-β (+) IL-2(–), IL-4(–) | Intratumoral cells that could possibly be Tr1 cells vs activated T cells associated with poor outcome and death[84] |
| Th3 | CD4(+) otherwise not conclusively characterized by markers | TGF-β(+) | Peripheral blood Th3 response not seen against MAGE-6 peptides[113] |
| Myeloid-derived suppressor cells | CD15(+), CDIIb(+), CD33(+), HLA-DR(–), CD14(–), Lin(–) and lack of other mature myeloid cell markers | Nitric oxide synthase 2 (upregulated by Th1 cytokines), Arginase 1 (upregulated by Th2 cytokines) | • Increased MDSCs in blood and increased arginase activity[25,71]; • Mature DCs in tumor correlate with improved survival[110]; • Administration of ATRA decreases levels of MDSCs[88] |

ATRA = all-trans-retinoic acid; CD = cytoplasmic domain; DC = dendritic cell; FOX = forkhead box; HLA = human leukocyte antigen; IL = interleukin; MAGE = melanoma antigenic epitope; MDSC = myeloid-derived suppressor cell; RCC = renal cell carcinoma; TGF = transforming growth factor; Treg = T regulatory cell.

T effector cells.[76] This Treg subset is the most characterized and understood of the Treg cells. The adaptive subset is not characterized by a specific marker but instead by a representative immunosuppressive cytokine profile.[77] In a general sense, Tr1 Treg cells produce IL-10 but not IL-4, whereas Th3 Treg cells produce TGF-β. Adaptive Treg cells are believed to originate from Th0 cells after interaction with DCs. Studies using murine models have supported the notion that Treg cells are immunosuppressive and that their removal improves immunity against and rejection of tumors.[78,79] In mouse tumor models, Treg depletion in vivo can enhance antitumor immunity resulting from vaccination and blockade of the suppressive costimulatory molecule, cytotoxic T lymphocyte-associated antigen 4.[80]

## Importance of Treg Cells in Human Cancer and RCC

Accumulation of Treg cells in the tumor microenvironment has been shown to correlate inversely with patient survival in several tumor types.[10,81,82] In a study of ovarian cancer, an increase in Treg numbers was associated with inhibition of tumor specific cytotoxic T cell activity and cytokine production.[10] Patients with metastatic RCC have been found to have a statistically significant increase in CD4(+)CD25(high) Treg cells in their peripheral blood.[75,83] These Treg cells were confirmed to have suppressive function by their ability to inhibit T effector (CD4+CD25–) cell proliferation. Furthermore, increased Treg (CD4+CD25+FOXP3+) numbers in the peripheral blood of patients with metastatic RCC correlate with poor clinical outcome. However, an increase in this cell population within tumors was not found to be significantly associated with poor outcome and death from RCC in another study.[84] Instead, it found infiltrating CD4(+)CD25(+)FOXP3(−) in about 84% of the tumor samples and a correlation of this cell type with poor outcome. When these intratumoral cells were analyzed by flow cytometry, they were seen to have increased production of IL-10 suggesting that they could possibly be Treg cells of the Tr1 phenotype.

Interestingly, the dependence of Treg cells on high levels of IL-2 contradicts the fact that high-dose IL-2 therapy is able to produce a complete durable response in selected patients with metastatic RCC. However, when this was analyzed further in patients receiving high-dose IL-2 therapy, it was found that patients who achieved an objective clinical response had a statistically significant decrease of Treg cells when compared with normal donors.[75] Another study reported opposing results and found an increase in Treg levels after treatment with high-dose IL-2 and reported no correlation with response.[85] Thus clarification is needed, and the potential mechanism underlying this finding will need further elucidation.

Therapeutic avenues targeting Treg cells are beginning to be examined. One study used DAB389IL-2, a recombinant IL-2 diphtheria toxin conjugate, to remove Treg cells in human cancer patients and reported an effective decrease in peripheral blood Treg cells.[86] In the same study, it was also shown that a reduction of Treg cells leads to an augmented T-cell response to tumor antigens following vaccination. Thus, the literature on the involvement of Treg cells in RCC provides evidence that they are directly contributing to the immunosuppressive environment that is allowing tumor cells to thrive. Additional studies are needed to further define strategies that may reduce Treg numbers and Treg function and further assess the impact that Treg reduction may have on promoting tumor immunity and improved clinical outcome. Lastly, there is some suggestion that sunitinib, which blocks signaling through multiple receptor tyrosine kinases including VEGF and PDGF, may decrease

the percentage of FoxP3(+) Treg cells within the PBMC of patients with metastatic RCC. Additionally, in 3 of 5 patients tested to date, the function of Treg cells remaining after treatment may be impaired as well (Finke and colleagues, manuscript in preparation). In vitro studies exhibited that the isolated cells had a decreased capacity to suppress the proliferation of effector cells defined as CD4(+)CD25(−). Whether sunitinib induced changes in Treg cells correlate to improved immune reactivity and clinical outcome is still under investigation.

## Dendritic Cell Dysfunction

Several lines of evidence suggest that tumor induced alterations in myeloid cell differentiation lead to a reduction in functionally competent DCs, as well as an accumulation of tolerogenic DCs and suppressive myeloid cells.[87] These cells ultimately impair antitumor effector T-cell function indirectly and directly. Patients with RCC have reduced numbers of Lin(−)/HLA-DR(+) circulating DCs with an associated increase in Lin(−)/DR(−)/CD33(+) MDSCs.[88] In addition, when DC populations were examined in a series of RCC tissues, mature DCs represented less than 1% of the leukocytes and were more abundant outside of the tumor than within. These immature DCs failed to stimulate an allogeneic mixed leukocyte reaction suggesting possible anergy at a minimum.[89] Thus, lack of mature DCs for the initiation of an appropriate antitumor adaptive immune response appears to play a fundamental role in RCC immunosubversion.

Additionally, tumors often secrete products that either inhibit DC maturation or confer a mature but regulatory phenotype to DCs. RCC tumors are known to secrete several factors that could combine to result in the accumulation of immature myeloid DCs such as VEGF, IL-6, TGF-β, GM-CSF, M-CSF, and gangliosides.[90–97] TILs in the tumor microenvironment may also secrete IL-10 and IL-4, which then become available to influence myeloid cell development.[22,92,98] Products, such as prostaglandins, IL-10, TGF-β, and VEGF, in the tumor microenvironment can condition DCs to be regulatory and induce the formation of adaptive Treg cells.[99–101] In vitro (human) and in vivo (mouse) studies have shown that VEGF inhibits the formation of functionally mature DCs[101,102] and correlates with an increase in immature MDSCs.[101,103]

## Myeloid-Derived Suppressor Cells

These cells collectively called MDSCs or immature myeloid cells describe a heterogenous group that includes all cells of myeloid lineage [CD33(+)] that are not effective APC [HLA-DR(−) or low and B7 (−) or low] and are capable of inhibiting T-cell function.[87] In the mouse tumor model, MDSCs are identified by the coexpression of CD11b (Mac-1) and GR-1 (Ly6G), and they inhibit CD8 T-cell production of IFN-$\gamma$ in response to MHC I presented antigen in a cell-contact and reactive oxygen species dependent manner.[90,104] Thus, they are macrophages, granulocytes, and DCs at various levels of maturation and activation, which are present in the bone marrow and spleens of normal mice, yet accumulate excessively in the spleens and lymph nodes of tumor-bearing mice.[90] Lastly, MDSCs may also lead to CD8 T-cell tolerance and Treg formation in tumor-bearing mice.[105,106]

MDSCs have also been described in the peripheral blood of human cancer patients.[25,88,107,108] MDSCs most closely resembling granulocytes have been seen in patients with RCC peripheral blood.[25] When MDSCs are activated by T cells, it is believed they in turn inhibit T-cell proliferation through 2 distinct enzymes.[109] The first is nitric oxide synthase 2, which is upregulated by Th1 cytokines, and the second is arginase 1, which is upregulated by Th2 cytokines and leads to a depletion of arginine and an upregulation of ornithine. Thus, a study examining the blood of 123 patients with metastatic RCC found elevated levels of MDSCs with an associated increase in arginase activity and decrease in CD3 $\zeta$chain expression.[25] The MDSCs were shown to nonspecifically impair T-cell function in vitro. This was confirmed by a second study in mRCC, which also reported elevated levels of MDSCs, lower levels of mature DCs, and patient mononuclear cells

that had decreased ability to stimulate an allogeneic T-cell response or autologous T cells to tetanus toxoid.[88] Lastly, another report that examined tumor specimens of cytokine treated patients with RCC and found that an increased infiltration of mature DCs (CD83+) correlated with better survival.[110] Means with which to eliminate MDSCs has been examined, and all-trans-retinoic acid (ATRA) has been reported in murine models to lead to the maturation of MDSCs.[111] This was used in one of the previously described human clinical trials and found that some of the described deficits, including the elevation of MDSCs, could be reversed with administration of ATRA.[88]

## CONCLUSION

RCC is a prototypical model of a malignancy that interacts heavily with its host's immune system. The current understanding of the immunobiology of RCC overwhelmingly points to the complex interplay between RCC tumors and host immune cells and suggests that the mere presence of immune cells in renal cell tumors is likely to have little significance when compared with the effector capacity of those cells that are present. There are currently many unanswered questions, and the mechanisms by which immune dysfunction are created and perpetuated are still being defined. The ability to characterize and individualize the specific mechanisms by which each patient's tumor is evading his or her immune system will allow more directed and theoretically more efficacious therapy. In the age of targeted therapy, understanding the intersection of angiogenesis and immune function will be vital to direct further combination treatment with other methods of immunotherapy.

## REFERENCES

1. Dunn GP, Old LJ, Schreiber RD. The three Es of cancer immunoediting. Annu Rev Immunol 2004; 22:329–60.
2. Birkeland SA, Storm HH, Lamm LU, et al. Cancer risk after renal transplantation in the Nordic countries, 1964–1986. Int J Cancer 1995; 60:183–9.
3. Birkeland SA, Lokkegaard H, Storm HH. Cancer risk in patients on dialysis and after renal transplantation. Lancet 2000; 355:1886–7.

4. Gogas H, Ioannovich J, Dafni U, et al. Prognostic significance of autoimmunity during treatment of melanoma with interferon. N Engl J Med 2006; 354:709–18.

5. Graus F, Dalmou J, Rene R, et al. Anti-Hu antibodies in patients with small-cell lung cancer: association with complete response to therapy and improved survival. J Clin Oncol 1997; 15:2866–72.

6. Darnell RB, DeAngelis LM. Regression of small-cell lung carcinoma in patients with paraneoplastic neuronal antibodies. Lancet 1993; 341:21–2.

7. Sato E, Olson SH, Ahn J, et al. Intraepithelial CD8+ tumor-infiltrating lymphocytes and a high CD8+/regulatory T cell ratio are associated with favorable prognosis in ovarian cancer. Proc Natl Acad Sci U S A 2005; 102:18538–43.

8. Pages F, Berger A, Camus M, et al. Effector memory T cells, early metastasis, and survival in colorectal cancer. N Engl J Med 2005; 353:2654–66.

9. Nakano O, Sato M, Naito Y, et al. Proliferative activity of intratumoral CD8(+) T-lymphocytes as a prognostic factor in human renal cell carcinoma: clinicopathologic demonstration of antitumor immunity. Cancer Res 2001; 61: 5132–6.

10. Curiel TJ, Coukos G, Zou L, et al. Specific recruitment of regulatory T cells in ovarian carcinoma fosters immune privilege and predicts reduced survival. Nat Med 2004; 10:942–9.

11. Yang JC, Childs R. Immunotherapy for renal cell cancer. J Clin Oncol 2006; 24:5576–83.

12. Kindt TJ OB. Kuby immunology. New York (NY): W .H. Freedman and Company; 2007.

13. O'Garra A, Vieira P. Regulatory T cells and mechanisms of immune system control. Nat Med 2004; 10:801–5.

14. Knutson KL. Strong-arming immune regulation: suppressing regulatory T-cell function to treat cancers. Future Oncol 2006; 2:379–89.

15. Sakaguchi S. Regulatory T cells: key controllers of immunologic self-tolerance. Cell 2000; 101:455–8.

16. Webster WS, Lohse CM, Thompson RH, et al. Mononuclear cell infiltration in clear-cell renal cell carcinoma independently predicts patient survival. Cancer 2006; 107:46–53.

17. Porta C, Bonomi L, Lillaz B, et al. Renal cell carcinoma-induced immunosuppression: an immunophenotypic study of lymphocyte subpopulations and circulating dendritic cells. Anticancer Res 2007; 27(1A):165–73.

18. Igarashi T, Takahashi H, Tobe T, et al. Effect of tumor-infiltrating lymphocyte subsets on prognosis and susceptibility to interferon therapy in patients with renal cell carcinoma. Urol Int 2002; 69:51–6.

19. Bromwich EJ, McArdle PA, Canna K, et al. The relationship between T-lymphocyte infiltration, stage, tumour grade and survival in patients undergoing curative surgery for renal cell cancer. Br J Cancer 2003; 89:1906–8.

20. Reiner SL. Development in motion: helper T cells at work. Cell 2007; 129:33–6.

21. Smyth GP, Stapleton PP, Barden CB, et al. Renal cell carcinoma induces prostaglandin E2 and T-helper type 2 cytokine production in peripheral blood mononuclear cells. Ann Surg Oncol 2003; 10:455–62.

22. Onishi T, Ohishi Y, Imagawa K, et al. An assessment of the immunological environment based on intratumoral cytokine production in renal cell carcinoma. BJU Int 1999; 83:488–92.

23. Kondo T, Nakazawa H, Ito F, et al. Favorable prognosis of renal cell carcinoma with increased expression of chemokines associated with a Th1-type immune response. Cancer Sci 2006; 97:780–6.

24. Tatsumi T, Herrem CJ, Olson WC, et al. Disease stage variation in CD4+ and CD8+ T-cell reactivity to the receptor tyrosine kinase EphA2 in patients with renal cell carcinoma. Cancer Res 2003; 63:4481–9.

25. Zea AH, Rodriguez PC, Atkins MB, et al. Arginase-producing myeloid suppressor cells in renal cell carcinoma patients: a mechanism of tumor evasion. Cancer Res 2005; 65:3044–8.

26. Tatsumi Tea. CD4+ T cell-mediated immunity to cancer. Cancer immunotherapy at the crossroads; how tumor evade immunity and what can be done. : Humana Press; 2004. p. 67.

27. Uzzo RG, Rayman P, Kolenko V, et al. Mechanisms of apoptosis in T cells from patients with renal cell carcinoma. Clin Cancer Res 1999; 5:1219–29.

28. Sorice M, Parolini I, Sansolini T, et al. Evidence for the existence of ganglioside-enriched plasma membrane domains in human peripheral lymphocytes. J Lipid Res 1997; 38:969–80.

29. Ritter G, Livingston PO. Ganglioside antigens expressed by human cancer cells. Semin Cancer Biol 1991; 2:401–9.

30. Zhang X, Kiechle FL. Review: Glycosphingolipids in health and disease. Ann Clin Lab Sci 2004; 34:3–13.

31. Hoon DS, Okun E, Neuwirth H, et al. Aberrant expression of gangliosides in human renal cell carcinomas. J Urol 1993; 150:2013–8.

32. Biswas K, Richmond A, Rayman P, et al. GM2 expression in renal cell carcinoma: potential role in tumor-induced T-cell dysfunction. Cancer Res 2006; 66:6816–25.

33. Hakomori S, Handa K. Glycosphingolipid-dependent crosstalk between glycosynapses interfacing tumor cells with their host cells: essential basis to define tumor malignancy. FEBS Lett 2002; 531:88–92.

34. Kudo D, Rayman P, Horton C, et al. Gangliosides expressed by the renal cell carcinoma cell line SK-RC-45 are involved in tumor-induced apoptosis of T cells. Cancer Res 2003; 63:1676–83.

35. Garcia-Ruiz C, Colell A, Paris R, Fernandez-Checa JC. Direct interaction of GD3 ganglioside with mitochondria generates reactive oxygen species followed by mitochondrial permeability transition, cytochrome c release, and caspase activation. FASEB J 2000; 14:847–58.

36. Chahlavi A, Rayman P, Richmond AL, et al. Glioblastomas induce T-lymphocyte death by two distinct pathways involving gangliosides and CD70. Cancer Res 2005; 65:5428–38.

37. Ladisch S, Li R, Olson E. Ceramide structure predicts tumor ganglioside immunosuppressive activity. Proc Natl Acad Sci U S A 1994; 91:1974–8.

38. Irani DN, Lin KI, Griffin DE. Brain-derived gangliosides regulate the cytokine production and proliferation of activated T cells. J Immunol 1996; 157:4333–40.

39. Tourkova IL, Shurin GV, Chatta GS, et al. Restoration by IL-15 of MHC class I antigen-processing machinery in human dendritic cells inhibited by tumor-derived gangliosides. J Immunol 2005; 175:3045–52.

40. Greenwald RJ, Freeman GJ, Sharpe AH. The B7 family revisited. Annu Rev Immunol 2005; 23:515–48.

41. Flies DB, Chen L. The new B7s: playing a pivotal role in tumor immunity. J Immunother 2007; 30:251–60.
42. Petroff MG, Chen L, Phillips TA, et al. B7 family molecules are favorably positioned at the human maternal-fetal interface. Biol Reprod 2003; 68:1496–504.
43. Eppihimer MJ, Gunn J, Freeman GJ, et al. Expression and regulation of the PD-L1 immunoinhibitory molecule on microvascular endothelial cells. Microcirculation 2002; 9:133–45.
44. Mazanet MM, Hughes CC. B7-H1 is expressed by human endothelial cells and suppresses T cell cytokine synthesis. J Immunol 2002; 169:3581–8.
45. Curiel TJ, Wei S, Dong H, et al. Blockade of B7-H1 improves myeloid dendritic cell-mediated antitumor immunity. Nat Med 2003; 9:562–7.
46. Freeman GJ, Long AJ, Iwai Y, et al. Engagement of the PD-1 immunoinhibitory receptor by a novel B7 family member leads to negative regulation of lymphocyte activation. J Exp Med 2000; 192:1027–34.
47. Nishimura H, Honjo T. PD-1: an inhibitory immunoreceptor involved in peripheral tolerance. Trends Immunol 2001; 22:265–8.
48. Carter L, Fouser LA, Jussif J, et al. PD-1:PD-L inhibitory pathway affects both CD4(+) and CD8(+) T cells and is overcome by IL-2. Eur J Immunol 2002; 32:634–43.
49. Thompson RH, Kuntz SM, Leibovich BC, et al. Tumor B7-H1 is associated with poor prognosis in renal cell carcinoma patients with long-term follow-up. Cancer Res 2006; 66:3381–5.
50. Thompson RH, Gillett MD, Cheville JC, et al. Costimulatory B7-H1 in renal cell carcinoma patients: Indicator of tumor aggressiveness and potential therapeutic target. Proc Natl Acad Sci U S A 2004; 101:17174–9.
51. Thompson RH, Webster WS, Cheville JC, et al. B7-H1 glycoprotein blockade: a novel strategy to enhance immunotherapy in patients with renal cell carcinoma. Urology 2005; 66 Suppl 5:10–4.
52. Krambeck AE, Thompson RH, Dong H, et al. B7-H4 expression in renal cell carcinoma and tumor vasculature: associations with cancer progression and survival. Proc Natl Acad Sci U S A 2006; 103:10391–6.
53. Kryczek I, Wei S, Zou L, et al. Cutting edge: induction of B7-H4 on APCs through IL-10: novel suppressive mode for regulatory T cells. J Immunol 2006; 177:40–4.
54. Thompson RH, Dong H, Lohse CM, et al. PD-1 is expressed by tumor-infiltrating immune cells and is associated with poor outcome for patients with renal cell carcinoma. Clin Cancer Res 2007; 13:1757–61.
55. Coulie PG, Connerotte T. Human tumor-specific T lymphocytes: does function matter more than number? Curr Opin Immunol 2005; 17:320–5.
56. Kramer G, Steiner GE, Paiha S, et al. Human accessory cells activate fresh, normal, tumor-distant T lymphocytes but not tumor-infiltrating T lymphocytes to lyse autologous tumor cells in a primary cytotoxic T lymphocyte assay in renal cell carcinoma. Eur Urol 2001; 40:427–33.
57. Hirano F, Kaneko K, Tamura H, et al. Blockade of B7-H1 and PD-1 by monoclonal antibodies potentiates cancer therapeutic immunity. Cancer Res 2005; 65:1089–96.
58. Iwai Y, Ishida M, Tanaka Y, et al. Involvement of PD-L1 on tumor cells in the escape from host immune system and tumor immunotherapy by PD-L1 blockade. Proc Natl Acad Sci U S A 2002; 99:12293–7.
59. Dong H, Strome SE, Salomao DR, et al. Tumor-associated B7-H1 promotes T-cell apoptosis: a potential mechanism of immune evasion. Nat Med 2002; 8:793–800.
60. Gately S. The contributions of cyclooxygenase-2 to tumor angiogenesis. Cancer Metastasis Rev 2000; 19:19–27.
61. Chen Q, Shinohara N, Abe T, et al. Significance of COX-2 expression in human renal cell carcinoma cell lines. Int J Cancer 2004; 108:825–32.
62. Hashimoto Y, Kondo Y, Kimura G, et al. Cyclooxygenase-2 expression and relationship to tumor progression in human renal cell carcinoma. Histopathology 2004; 44:353–9.
63. Yoshimura R, Matsuyama M, Kawahito Y, et al. Study of cyclooxygenase-2 in renal cell carcinoma. Int J Mol Med 2004; 13:229–33.
64. Miyata Y, Koga S, Kanda S, et al. Expression of cyclooxygenase-2 in renal cell carcinoma: correlation with tumor cell proliferation, apoptosis, angiogenesis, expression of matrix metalloproteinase-2, and survival. Clin Cancer Res 2003; 9:1741–9.
65. Hemmerlein B, Galuschka L, Putzer N, et al. Comparative analysis of COX-2, vascular endothelial growth factor and microvessel density in human renal cell carcinomas. Histopathology 2004; 45:603–11.
66. Yang X, Sheares KK, Davie N, et al. Hypoxic induction of cox-2 regulates proliferation of human pulmonary artery smooth muscle cells. Am J Respir Cell Mol Biol 2002; 27:688–96.
67. Uefuji K, Ichikura T, Mochizuki H. Cyclooxygenase-2 expression is related to prostaglandin biosynthesis and angiogenesis in human gastric cancer. Clin Cancer Res 2000; 6:135–8.
68. Masferrer JL, Leahy KM, Koki AT, et al. Antiangiogenic and antitumor activities of cyclooxygenase-2 inhibitors. Cancer Res 2000; 60:1306–11.
69. Goodwin JS, Ceuppens J. Regulation of the immune response by prostaglandins. J Clin Immunol 1983; 3:295–315.
70. Menetrier-Caux C, Bain C, Favrot MC, et al. Renal cell carcinoma induces interleukin 10 and prostaglandin E2 production by monocytes. Br J Cancer 1999; 79:119–30.
71. Ochoa AC, Zea AH, Hernandez C, Rodriguez PC. Arginase, prostaglandins, and myeloid-derived suppressor cells in renal cell carcinoma. Clin Cancer Res 2007; 13(2 Pt 2): 721s–6s.
72. Rini BI, Weinberg V, Dunlap S, et al. Maximal COX-2 immunostaining and clinical response to celecoxib and interferon α therapy in metastatic renal cell carcinoma. Cancer 2006; 106:566–75.
73. Gershon RK, Kondo K. Cell interactions in the induction of tolerance: the role of thymic lymphocytes. Immunology 1970; 18:723–37.
74. Fontenot JD, Rudensky AY. A well adapted regulatory contrivance: regulatory T cell development and the forkhead family transcription factor Foxp3. Nat Immunol 2005; 6:331–7.

75. Cesana GC, DeRaffele G, Cohen S, et al. Characterization of CD4+CD25+ regulatory T cells in patients treated with high-dose interleukin-2 for metastatic melanoma or renal cell carcinoma. J Clin Oncol 2006; 24:1169–77.

76. Thornton AM, Shevach EM. CD4+CD25+ immunoregulatory T cells suppress polyclonal T cell activation in vitro by inhibiting interleukin 2 production. J Exp Med 1998; 188:287–96.

77. Lan RY, Ansari AA, Lian ZX, Gershwin ME. Regulatory T cells: development, function and role in autoimmunity. Autoimmun Rev 2005; 4:351–63.

78. Onizuka S, Tawara I, Shimizu J, et al. Tumor rejection by in vivo administration of anti-CD25 (interleukin-2 receptor α) monoclonal antibody. Cancer Res 1999; 59:3128–33.

79. Sutmuller RP, van Duivenvoorde LM, van Elsas A, et al. Synergism of cytotoxic T lymphocyte-associated antigen 4 blockade and depletion of CD25(+) regulatory T cells in antitumor therapy reveals alternative pathways for suppression of autoreactive cytotoxic T lymphocyte responses. J Exp Med 2001; 194:823–32.

80. Curiel TJ. Tregs and rethinking cancer immunotherapy. J Clin Invest 2007; 117:1167–74.

81. Bates GJ, Fox SB, Han C, et al. Quantification of regulatory T cells enables the identification of high-risk breast cancer patients and those at risk of late relapse. J Clin Oncol 2006; 24:5373–80.

82. Kobayashi N, Hiraoka N, Yamagami W, et al. FOXP3+ regulatory T cells affect the development and progression of hepatocarcinogenesis. Clin Cancer Res 2007; 13:902–11.

83. Griffiths RW, Elkord E, Gilham DE, et al. Frequency of regulatory T cells in renal cell carcinoma patients and investigation of correlation with survival. Cancer Immunol Immunother 2007.

84. Siddiqui SA, Frigola X, Bonne-Annee S, et al. Tumor-infiltrating Foxp3-CD4+CD25+ T cells predict poor survival in renal cell carcinoma. Clin Cancer Res 2007; 13:2075–81.

85. van Dervliet HJ, Koon HB, Yue SC, et al. Effects of the administration of high-dose interleukin-2 on immunoregulatory cell subsets in patients with advanced melanoma and renal cell cancer. Clin Cancer Res 2007; 13:2100–8.

86. Dannull J, Su Z, Rizzieri D, et al. Enhancement of vaccine-mediated antitumor immunity in cancer patients after depletion of regulatory T cells. J Clin Invest 2005; 115:3623–33.

87. Talmadge JE. Pathways mediating the expansion and immunosuppressive activity of myeloid-derived suppressor cells and their relevance to cancer therapy. Clin Cancer Res 2007; 13(18 Pt 1):5243–8.

88. Mirza N, Fishman M, Fricke I, et al. All-trans-retinoic acid improves differentiation of myeloid cells and immune response in cancer patients. Cancer Res 2006; 66:9299–307.

89. Troy AJ, Summers KL, Davidson PJ, et al. Minimal recruitment and activation of dendritic cells within renal cell carcinoma. Clin Cancer Res 1998; 4:585–93.

90. Gabrilovich D. Mechanisms and functional significance of tumor-induced dendritic-cell defects. Nat Rev Immunol 2004; 4:941–52.

91. Koo AS, Armstrong C, Bochner B, et al. Interleukin-6 and renal cell cancer: production, regulation, and growth effects. Cancer Immunol Immunother 1992; 35:97–105.

92. Maeurer MJ, Martin DM, Castelli C, et al. Host immune response in renal cell cancer: interleukin-4 (IL-4) and IL-10 mRNA are frequently detected in freshly collected tumor-infiltrating lymphocytes. Cancer Immunol Immunother 1995; 41:111–21.

93. Gastl GA, Abrams JS, Nanus DM, et al. Interleukin-10 production by human carcinoma cell lines and its relationship to interleukin-6 expression. Int J Cancer 1993; 55:96–101.

94. Junker U, Knoefel B, Nuske K, et al. Transforming growth factor β1 is significantly elevated in plasma of patients suffering from renal cell carcinoma. Cytokine 1996; 8:794–8.

95. Knoefel B, Nuske K, Steiner T, et al. Renal cell carcinomas produce IL-6, IL-10, IL-11, and TGF-β1 in primary cultures and modulate T lymphocyte blast transformation. J Interferon Cytokine Res 1997; 17:95–102.

96. Menetrier-Caux C, Montmain G, Dieu MC, et al. Inhibition of the differentiation of dendritic cells from CD34(+) progenitors by tumor cells: role of interleukin-6 and macrophage colony-stimulating factor. Blood 1998; 92:4778–91.

97. Steiner T, Junker U, Wunderlich H, Schubert J. Are renal cell carcinoma cells able to modulate the cytotoxic effect of tumor infiltrating lymphocytes by secretion of interleukin-6? Anticancer Res 1999; 19(2C):1533–6.

98. Menetrier-Caux C, Thomachot MC, Alberti L, et al. IL-4 prevents the blockade of dendritic cell differentiation induced by tumor cells. Cancer Res 2001; 61:3096–104.

99. Bergmann C, Strauss L, Zeidler R, et al. Expansion of human T regulatory type 1 cells in the microenvironment of cyclooxygenase 2 overexpressing head and neck squamous cell carcinoma. Cancer Res 2007; 67:8865–73.

100. Ghiringhelli F, Puig PE, Roux S, et al. Tumor cells convert immature myeloid dendritic cells into TGF-β-secreting cells inducing CD4+CD25+ regulatory T cell proliferation. J Exp Med 2005; 202:919–29.

101. Gabrilovich D, Ishida T, Oyama T, et al. Vascular endothelial growth factor inhibits the development of dendritic cells and dramatically affects the differentiation of multiple hematopoietic lineages in vivo. Blood 1998; 92:4150–66.

102. Gabrilovich DI, Chen HL, Girgis KR, et al. Production of vascular endothelial growth factor by human tumors inhibits the functional maturation of dendritic cells. Nat Med 1996; 2:1096–103.

103. Almand B, Resser JR, Lindman B, et al. Clinical significance of defective dendritic cell differentiation in cancer. Clin Cancer Res 2000; 6:1755–66.

104. Kusmartsev S, Nefedova Y, Yoder D, Gabrilovich DI. Antigen-specific inhibition of CD8+ T cell response by immature myeloid cells in cancer is mediated by reactive oxygen species. J Immunol 2004; 172:989–99.

105. Huang B, Pan PY, Li Q, et al. Gr-1+CD115+ immature myeloid suppressor cells mediate the development of tumor-induced T regulatory cells and T-cell anergy in tumor-bearing host. Cancer Res 2006; 66:1123–31.

106. Kusmartsev S, Nagaraj S, Gabrilovich DI. Tumor-associated CD8+ T cell tolerance induced by bone marrow-derived immature myeloid cells. J Immunol 2005; 175:4583–92.

107. Schmielau J, Finn OJ. Activated granulocytes and granulocyte-derived hydrogen peroxide are the underlying mechanism of suppression of t-cell function in advanced cancer patients. Cancer Res 2001; 61:4756–60.

108. Goddard DS, Yamanaka K, Kupper TS, Jones DA. Activation of neutrophils in cutaneous T-cell lymphoma. Clin Cancer Res 2005; 11:8243–9.

109. Bronte V, Serafini P, Mazzoni A, et al. L-arginine metabolism in myeloid cells controls T-lymphocyte functions. Trends Immunol 2003; 24:302–6.

110. Kobayashi M, Suzuki K, Yashi M, et al. Tumor infiltrating dendritic cells predict treatment response to immunotherapy in patients with metastatic renal cell carcinoma. Anticancer Res 2007; 27:1137–41.

111. Kusmartsev S, Cheng F, Yu B, et al. All-trans-retinoic acid eliminates immature myeloid cells from tumor-bearing mice and improves the effect of vaccination. Cancer Res 2003; 63:4441–9.

112. Liu VC, Wong LY, Jang T, et al. Tumor evasion of the immune system by converting CD4+CD25− T cells into CD4+CD25+ T regulatory cells: role of tumor-derived TGF-β. J Immunol 2007; 178:2883–92.

113. Tatsumi T, Kierstead LS, Ranieri E, et al. Disease-associated bias in T-helper type 1 (Th1)/Th2 CD4(+) T-cell responses against MAGE-6 in HLA-DRB10401(+) patients with renal cell carcinoma or melanoma. J Exp Med 2002; 196:619–28.

# 13

# Immunotherapy in Metastatic Renal Cell Carcinoma

**DAVID MCDERMOTT, MD**

RCC evokes an immune response, which has occasionally resulted in spontaneous and dramatic remissions.[1–3] In an attempt to reproduce or accentuate this response, various immunotherapeutic strategies have been used, including nonspecific stimulators of the immune system, specific antitumor immunotherapy, adoptive immunotherapy, the induction of a graft-versus-tumor response via allogeneic hematopoietic stem cell transplantation, and the administration of partially purified or recombinant cytokines.[4–14] Although many such therapies display antitumor activity, research over the past two decades has tended to focus on various cytokines whose protein structure and biologic properties are more clearly defined.

Although a number of cytokines have shown antitumor activity in RCC, the most consistent results have been reported with interferon-α (IFN-α) and interleukin-2 (IL-2). Although IFN-α has produced modest benefits in unselected patients, randomized clinical trials have shown a small survival benefit with manageable toxicity when compared with nonIFN-α control arms.[15–23] High-dose bolus IL-2 was granted Food and Drug Administration approval based on its ability to produce durable complete responses in a small number of patients with metastatic RCC. However, the substantial toxicity and limited efficacy that is associated with IL-2 has narrowed its application to highly selected patients treated at specialized centers.[24–28]

As we enter the era of targeted therapy, this chapter will examine the evolving role of immunotherapy in patients with RCC, with a particular focus on the phase III trials that have helped to define the proper use of cytokine therapy. Given the limitations of immunotherapy, this review will also discuss improvements in patient selection and investigational approaches to immunotherapy that may lead future improvements in patient outcome.

## IFN-α

IFN-α is a naturally occurring glycoprotein produced in response to viral infections and foreign antigens. It has been investigated in a variety of diseases with postulated mechanisms of action including immunomodulation, antiproliferative activity, and inhibition of angiogenesis. In advanced RCC, both recombinant IFN-α 2a (Roferon, Hoffmann-La Roche, Basel, Switzerland) and IFN-α 2b (Intron A, Schering Plough International, Kenilworth, NJ, USA) have undergone extensive clinical evaluation. Results of these investigations are thoroughly described in several reviews.[15–18] There is no clinically meaningful difference between these two IFNs, and thus the generic IFN-α will be used to describe these data. Despite the use of a variety of preparations, doses, and schedules, most studies have shown modest antitumor activity, with the overall response rate being approximately 10 to 15%. Responses are often delayed in onset, with median time to response being approximately 4 months. Most responses are partial and short-lived (median response duration, 6 to 7 months). Approximately 2% of patients have had complete responses, with only an occasional patient having a response persist in excess of 1 year after therapy. Although no clear dose–response relationship exists, daily doses in the 5- to 10-MU range (MU = million units) appear to have the highest therapeutic index. The toxicity of IFN includes flu-like symptoms such as fever, chills, myalgias, and fatigue, as well as weight loss, altered taste, depression, anemia, leucopenia, and elevated liver function tests. Most side effects, especially the flu-like symptoms, tend to diminish with time during chronic therapy.[15–23]

To investigate a possible survival benefit to IFN-α in RCC, several randomized trials have been performed. Table 1 is a summary of randomized trials that have investigated the effect of IFN-α on overall survival (OS) in metastatic RCC patients. One study randomized 350 patients with metastatic RCC to receive IFN-α 10 MU 3×/week (TIW) × 12 weeks or medroxyprogesterone (MPA) 300 mg daily × 12 weeks.[21] Patients in each treatment arm were well balanced with respect to prognostic characteristics in RCC, including performance status, time from first diagnosis of RCC to treatment, number of metastatic sites, and nephrectomy status. This trial was closed at an interim analysis when the stopping boundary for a survival advantage of IFN-α had been reached. Intent-to-treat analysis reported a significant OS advantage for patients randomized to IFN-α, with a hazard ratio of 0.72 ($p = .017$). The median OS was 8.5 months in the IFN arm and 6.0 months in the MPA arm.

Another study randomized 160 patients with advanced, progressive RCC to receive IFN-α 18 MU TIW plus vinblastine 0.1 mg/kg IV q3 weeks or the same dose and schedule of vinblastine alone.[22] The primary endpoint of this trial was OS, with 80% power to detect a difference in median OS of 12 months vs 8

months. Patients in each treatment arm were well balanced with respect to characteristics known to be prognostic for OS in RCC. A significant OS advantage was reported for the IFN-α arm with a median OS of 15.8 months vs 8.8 months for the vinblastine arm ($p = .0049$). Significant differences in overall response rates (16.5% vs 2.4%; $p = .0025$), complete response rates (8.9% vs 1.2%), and median time to disease progression (3 months vs 2 months; $p = .0001$) were also observed, all favoring the IFN-α arm.

In addition, a meta-analysis reviewed 53 randomized controlled trials involving 6,117 patients treated between 1995 and 2004 with IL-2 or IFN-α in metastatic RCC.[23] There were four trials ($n = 644$ patients) that randomized patients to IFN-α versus a nonIFN-α control arm, including the two largest trials noted above. The weighted median survival improvement with IFN-α treatment versus control was 3.8 months ($p = .007$) with an odds ratio for death at 1 year of 0.56 for IFN-α (95% CI 0.40 to 0.77). There was no evidence of dose–response relationship and no correlation between response rate and OS.

More recent studies have delineated some limits to the antitumor effects of IFN-α. For example, a French Immunotherapy Group phase III trial comparing IFN-α with both IL-2 and IL-2 plus IFN-α reported a response rate of only 7.5% for the IFN arm with a 1-year event-free survival rate of only 12%.[29] In addition, a Southwest Oncology Group (SWOG) study comparing IFN-α alone with debulking nephrectomy followed by IFN-α reported tumor responses in less than 5% of patients receiving either treatment approach.[30]

Given the modest survival impact of IFN-α seen in phase III studies and its widespread application

| Author | Trial Design | Number of Patients | Response Rate Advantage for IFN-α (%) | Overall Survival Impact |
|---|---|---|---|---|
| Ritchie[6] | IFN-α versus medroxyprogesterone | 335 | 10 | 2.5 months. Advantage for IFN-α ($p = .017$) |
| Pyrhonen[22] | IFN-α plus vinbla stine versus vinblastine | 160 | 14 | 7.0 months. Advantage for IFN-α ($p = .0049$) |
| Coppin[23] | Meta-analysis of randomized, controlled trials of IFN-α | 4216 (42 trials) | 11 | 3.8 months. Advantage for IFN-α ($p = .0005$) |

**Table 1. INTERFERON-α IN METASTATIC RENAL CELL CARCINOMA**

IFN-α = interferon-α.

worldwide, regulatory agencies have supported the use of IFN as control arm for randomized trials investigating targeted therapies that are reported elsewhere in this text. The results of these investigations will certainly narrow the future use of IFN as a single agent.

## IL-2

IL-2 is an important member of a class of glycoproteins that regulate lymphocyte function and growth. It is produced in response to infection and essential for discriminating between self and foreign antigens. Although the mechanism of action of IL-2 is not completely understood, antitumor effects in murine models have been linked to the direct killing of tumor cells by activated T cells and natural killer cells.[13,14]

High-dose bolus IL-2 was granted Food and Drug Administration approval based on its ability to produce durable complete responses in a small number of patients with metastatic RCC. However, the substantial toxicity and limited efficacy that are associated with IL-2 have narrowed its application to highly selected patients treated at specialized centers.[24–28] In an attempt to reduce toxicity, several investigators evaluated regimens that contained lower doses of IL-2.[31–33] Attempts were also made to improve treatment efficacy by adding IFN-α 2b (IFN-α) and then fluorouracil to lower-dose IL-2 regimens. These regimens were reported to produce response rates and survival comparable with those reported for high-dose IL-2 with much less toxicity but possibly less durable benefit. In recent years, the relative merits of these low- and high-dose IL-2 regimens have been clarified by the results of four randomized trials. More significantly, laboratory investigations associated with this clinical research suggest that the potential exists for identifying predictors of response (or resistance) and thus limiting IL-2 therapy to those most likely to benefit.

## RANDOMIZED TRIALS OF IL-2 WITH OR WITHOUT IFN-α

The French Immunotherapy Group conducted a large-scale, phase III randomized trial that compared intermediate-dose IL-2 administered by continuous intravenous (IV) infusion plus subcutaneous IFN-α with either IL-2 or IFN-α administered

alone.[29] A total of 425 patients were enrolled. The three treatment groups were well balanced for age and sex, as well as known predictors of response and survival. The response rate and 1-year event-free survival were significantly greater for the combined IL-2 and IFN-α arm than for either of the single-agent arms although there was no significant difference in OS among the three groups. Of note, responses were seen in only 6.5 and 7.5% of patients receiving IL-2 or IFN-α alone, respectively, with only 2.9 and 6.1% of these patients still responding at the week 25 evaluations. Although more antitumor activity was seen with the combination arm, this was largely due to the rather limited activity of the single-agent regimens. How an intermediate-dose combination of IL-2 and IFN-α would compare with high-dose IL-2 alone remained to be established.

The National Cancer Institute Surgery Branch investigators performed a randomized trial comparing standard high-dose IV bolus IL-2 and a low-dose IV bolus IL-2 regimen developed by Yang and colleagues.[38] After randomizing 117 patients, a third arm was added that involved subcutaneous IL-2 administered according to the regimen described by Sleijfer and colleagues.[31] Results were analyzed and reported according to groups that were concurrently randomized. Among the 306 patients concurrently assigned to either high- or low-dose IV IL-2, the response rate was significantly higher with high-dose therapy (21% vs 13%), with a trend toward more durable responses. Duration of response was superior in patients who received the high-dose IV IL-2 compared with those who received the low-dose IV IL-2. There were no differences in OS. Although toxic effects were also significantly greater in the high-dose group (particularly hypotension), there were no deaths attributable to IL-2 in either arm, and patient assessments of quality of life were found to be roughly equivalent. Among the patients concurrently assigned to either subcutaneous IL-2 or high-dose IV IL-2, a higher response rate was seen with high-dose IV IL-2 (21% vs 10%), but the difference was of borderline statistical significance. Once again, there were no differences in OS.

In an effort to determine the value of outpatient subcutaneous IL-2 and IFN-α relative to high-dose IV IL-2, the Cytokine Working Group (CWG) performed a phase III trial in which patients were randomized to receive either outpatient IL-2 and IFN-α every 6 weeks or standard high-dose inpatient IL-2 every 12 weeks.[39] A total of 193 patients were enrolled, and 192 patinets were evaluable for toxicity and tumor response. The response rate for high-dose IL-2 was 23% (22/96) vs 10% (9/96) for IL-2 and IFN-α ($p = .018$). Eight patients achieved a complete response receiving high-dose IL-2 versus three patients receiving low-dose IL-2 and IFN-α. The median response durations were 24 months for high-dose IL-2 and 15 months for IL-2 and IFN-α ($p = .18$). Median OSs were 17.5 and 13 months ($p = .12$), favoring high-dose IL-2. Of note, responses to high-dose IL-2 were seen with equal frequency across the stratification criteria, whereas low-dose IL-2 and IFN-α appeared to produce fewer responses in patients with liver and/or bone metastases and in those who had not undergone previous nephrectomy to remove the primary tumor.

Last, a more recent phase III trial by the French Immunotherapy Group studied the impact of low-dose cytokine therapy on survival in patients with intermediate likelihood of response to IL-2 and IFN-α[40] as defined in previous studies with these cytokines.[29] Untreated patients with Karnofsky performance status of 80 or greater and more than one site of metastatic disease were randomized to receive MPA (control group), subcutaneous IFN-α, subcutaneous IL-2, or the combination of IFN-α and IL-2. A total of 492 patients were randomized, and the treatment groups were well balanced for predictors of response and survival. Although significant toxicity was more common in the IL-2 and IFN-α arm, median OS did not differ between the arms. The investigators concluded that subcutaneous IFN-α and IL-2 should no longer be recommended in patients with metastatic RCC and intermediate prognosis. Investigators from the CWG have reanalyzed the results of their phase III trial in the subset of patients who would have fallen into the "intermediate" prognosis group defined by the French Immunotherapy Group (unpublished data). Most patients treated in the CWG study (80%) were in either the intermediate or poor prognosis group. In this subset, high-dose IL-2 continued to produce a significant improvement in response rate (25% vs 10%, $p = .017$) and durable complete response (7 vs 0, $p = .014$) compared

with IL-2 and IFN-α. Furthermore, all 10 patients taking high-dose IL-2 were progression free at 3 years in this intermediate-risk group, whereas three intermediate-risk patients were progression free in IL-2 and IFN-α group ($p = .08$).

Taken together, these studies suggest that high-dose IV bolus IL-2 is superior in terms of response rate and possibly response quality to regimens that involve low-dose cytokines (Table 2). The superiority of high-dose IL-2 is particularly apparent in patients with tumor metastases in immune sequestered sites, such as liver or bone, who have their primary tumor in place, or who fall into the intermediate- or poor-risk groups defined by the French Immunotherapy Group. Consequently, although low-dose cytokine therapy has a limited role in metastatic RCC, high-dose IV IL-2 should be a therapeutic option for appropriately selected patients with access to such therapy. However, given the toxicity and limited efficacy of high-dose IV IL-2 therapy, additional efforts should be directed at better defining the patient population for whom this therapy is appropriate.

## OTHER CYTOKINES

In addition to IFN-α and IL-2, other immunotherapeutic agents have been evaluated in patients with such as IFN-γ, IL-4, IL-6, pegylated IFN, and GM-CSF, have produced only occasional responses when administered as single agents [1,41–46] Based on interesting preclinical data, investigators have combined GM-CSF with IL-2 and IFN-α, but this approach is yet to lead to significant clinical benefit.[47–48]

A few durable responses have been observed in phase I trials with recombinant human IL-12 (rhIL-12) administered either intravenously or subcutaneously; however, in general, antitumor activity in these studies has been less than predicted by preclinical models. In two such studies that included 71 patients with advanced RCC, IL-12 produced one complete and one partial response.[49,50]

A peculiar schedule dependency associated with IL-12 whereby a single "test dose" increases a patient's tolerance to subsequent therapy and possibly reduces antitumor effects has made clinical development of this agent more complicated.[51] Novel schedules of IL-12 have been explored in an effort to sustain

| Table 2. SELECTED RANDOMIZED TRIALS OF CYTOKINE THERAPY IN METASTATIC RENAL CELL CARCINOMA | | | | | | | |
|---|---|---|---|---|---|---|---|
| Trial | Treatment Regimens | N | Response Rate (%) | p Value | Durable Complete Response (%) | Overall Survival (months) | Overall Survival Difference |
| FIG[19] | CIV IL-2 | 138 | 6.5 | < 0.01 | 1 | 12 | NS |
| | LD SC IFN-α | 147 | 7.5 | < 0.01 | 2 | 13 | NS |
| | CIV IL-2 + IFN-α | 140 | 18.6 | < 0.01 | 5 | 17 | NS |
| NCI SB[24] | HD IV IL-2 | 156 | 21 | 0.05 | 8 | NR | NS |
| | LD IV IL-2 | 150 | 13 | 0.05 | 3 | NR | NS |
| | HD IV IL-2 | 95 | 23 | 0.05 | 7 | 17.5 | NS |
| CWG[25] | LD SC IL-2/ IFN-α | — | 10 | 0.02 | NR | 13 | NS |
| | HD IV IL-2 | — | 23 | 0.02 | NR | 17.5 | NS |

CIV = continuous IV infusion; CWG = Cytokine Working Group; FIG = French Immunotherapy Group; HD = high dose; IFN-α = interferon-α; IL-2 = interleukin-2; IV = intravenous; LD = low dose; NCI SB = National Cancer Institute Surgery Branch; NS = not statistically significant; SC = subcutaneous.

its biologic activity.[52] These studies have shown a correlation with the ability to sustain IFN-α production and antitumor effects. Although the addition of low-dose IL-2 to IL-12 has been able to sustain IFN-α production in the majority of patients, the antitumor effect of this combination has remained modest.[53] Efforts are currently in progress to use IL-12 ± IL-2 as immune adjuvants in combination with dendritic-cell-based vaccines in patients with RCC.

## ADJUVANT THERAPY

In an effort to apply the clinical activity observed with cytokines to patients with earlier stages of disease, a variety of adjuvant trials have been performed. The Eastern Cooperative Oncology Group completed a trial comparing adjuvant IFN-α with observation in patients with high-risk resected RCC. Eligible patients were to be T3b-c, T4, and/or N1-N3. Patients were randomly assigned to receive either a year of IFN-α or routine observation. With a minimum follow-up of 36 months and a mean of 68 months overall, no statistically significant difference in disease-free survival was observed between the treatment arms.[54] A similar study performed by the EORTC also showed no benefit for the adjuvant administration of IFN-α.[55]

The CWG performed a trial randomly assigning patients who satisfied these high-risk staging criteria (stage T3b-4, N1-3, or resected metastatic disease)

to either a single cycle of high-dose IL-2 or observation (with IL-2-based therapy at the time of recurrence).[56] This study took several years to accrue 69 patients and ultimately was closed early after an interim analysis determined that the anticipated 30% improvement in disease-free survival for the patients receiving high-dose IL-2 could not be achieved.

Thus, there is currently no evidence to support the use IFN-α or IL-2 in the adjuvant setting in patients with high-risk renal cancer. These studies have been compromised by the inability to clearly define a population at high risk of recurrence and the increasing lack of availability of such high-risk patients. Furthermore, there is a growing uncertainty as to whether the biology (in particular susceptibility to cytokine-based therapy) of tumors metastasizing to regional nodes is identical to that of tumors that metastasize systemically.[57] Until this crucial issue can be sorted out, it will remain difficult to translate advances in the treatment of patients with stage IV disease to the adjuvant setting.

## IMPACT OF NEPHRECTOMY BEFORE CYTOKINE THERAPY

Historically, patients with metastatic RCC at the time of initial presentation have not been routinely subjected to resections of their primary tumor. However, recent studies have suggested that the effectiveness of immunotherapy in patients with metastatic RCC may be enhanced following cytoreductive nephrectomy.[30,58] For example, the SWOG randomly assigned 246 patients presenting with metastatic disease to receive IFN-α either alone (5 MU/m[2] TIW) or following debulking nephrectomy.[30] Although few responses to IFN-α were observed on either treatment arm, the median OS was significantly longer for patients undergoing cytoreductive nephrectomy (12.5 vs 8.1 months). Other investigators have confirmed these results[59–61] suggesting that bulky primary tumors may facilitate disease progression at least in part through immune suppression.

## PREDICTORS OF CLINICAL BENEFIT FROM CYTOKINE-BASED THERAPY

Many groups have attempted to determine reliable predictors of response and survival for patients with metastatic RCC who were receiving immunotherapy.[24,29,60–67] Factors that have been variably associated with response to IL-2 include performance status,[24] number of organs with metastases (one versus two or more),[29] absence of bone metastases, previous nephrectomy,[61] degree of treatment-related thrombocytopenia, absence of previous IFN therapy,[62] thyroid dysfunction,[63] lymphocyte count,[64] rebound lymphocytosis,[65] and erythropoietin production.[66]

It has been shown in patients receiving IFN-α that poor survival is associated with low Karnofsky performance status, high serum lactate dehydrogenase, low hemoglobin, high "corrected" serum calcium, and time from initial RCC diagnosis to start of therapy of less than 1 year. In a cohort of 453 patients who received IFN-α as initial therapy, the median survival for the favorable- (no risk factors), intermediate- (one or two risk factors), and poor (three or more risk factors)-risk groups were 30, 14, and 5 months, respectively. Negrier and colleagues[20] also identified independent predictors of rapid disease progression, defined as progression within 10 weeks of initiation of therapy. These included greater than one metastatic site, disease-free interval of less than 1 year, and presence of liver metastases or mediastinal nodes, as well as type of immunotherapy used. Patients with liver metastases, more than one site of disease, and disease-free interval of less than 1 year had a lower response rate and a median

survival of only 6 months even though receiving combination IL-2 and IFN-α therapy. Figlin and colleagues identified previous nephrectomy and time from nephrectomy to relapse as important predictors of survival in patients receiving IL-2-based therapy.[68] In their series, patients who received systemic immunotherapy for metastatic disease more than 6 months after nephrectomy had the best median survival and had a 3-year survival rate of 46%. These clinical predictors may simply identify patients with more rapidly progressing disease who are unlikely to receive a long enough duration of cytokines to realize a potential benefit. These clinical factors offer little if any true biologic insight into mechanisms of resistance.

## PATHOLOGIC AND MOLECULAR PREDICTORS OF RESPONSE TO IL-2

### Influence of Histologic Subtype

Responses to immunotherapy are most frequently seen in patients with RCC of clear cell histology.[69–71] This observation was detailed in a retrospective analysis of pathology specimens obtained from 231 patients (163 primary and 68 metastatic tumor specimens) who had received IL-2 therapy on CWG clinical trials.[71] For patients with primary tumor specimens available for review, the response rate to IL-2 was 21% (30 of 146) for patients with clear cell histology primary tumors compared with 6% for patients with nonclear cell histology (1 responder in 17 patients). Among the patients with clear cell carcinoma, response to IL-2 was also associated with the presence of alveolar features and the absence of papillary or granular features. The response rate in patients whose primary tumors had "good" predictive features (eg, more than 50% alveolar and no granular or papillary features) was 39% (14 of 36). In addition, patients with primary tumors who contained "intermediate" predictive features (eg, alveolar but not papillary features and less than 50% granular features) had a response rate of 19% (15 of 77). Patients with tumors who contained "poor" predictive features (eg, more than 50% granular or any papillary features) had a response rate of 3% (1 of 33). When this model was then applied to the 68 patients with specimens from metastatic sites, those patients who were treated without resection of their primary tumors, five tumor responses were seen in the 20 patients with "good" predictive features, whereas no tumor responses were seen in the 16 patients in the poor predictive group, thus, supporting the validity of the model developed from the primary kidney tumor specimens. Median survivals for all patients with clear cell tumors by risk group were 2.87, 1.36, and 0.87 years, respectively ($p < .001$). As a result of these data, it may be appropriate for patients whose primary tumor is of nonclear cell histology or of clear cell histology but with "poor" predictive features to forgo IL-2-based treatment altogether. However, given that even in the most favorable predictive group more than 50% of patients failed to respond to IL-2 therapy, additional investigations into tumor-associated predictors of responsiveness to IL-2 are necessary.

## IMMUNOHISTOCHEMICAL MARKERS

Some investigators have begun to examine tumor tissue to identify immunohistochemical markers that might predict the outcomes of patients with RCC. Carbonic anhydrase IX (CAIX) has been identified as one potential marker. Bui and colleagues[72] used a monoclonal antibody designed to detect CAIX expression to perform an immunohistochemical analysis of paraffin-embedded RCC specimens. More than 90% of RCC tumors express CAIX, and expression decreases with advancing stage. High CAIX expression in primary tumors was seen in 79% of patients and was associated with improved survival and possibly response to IL-2-based therapy. In addition, all long-term responders to IL-2-based treatment had high CAIX expression. In this study, low CAIX expression was associated with a worse outcome for patients with locally advanced RCC and was an independent predictor of outcome in patients with metastatic disease.

Building on this work, Atkins and colleagues[73] performed a nested case-control study within the larger cohort of patients whose pathology was analyzed. CAIX expression levels were correlated with response to IL-2, pathologic risk categorization, and survival. As in the report by Bui and colleagues[72], the percentage of CAIX-positive tumor cells was used to separate high (> 85%) and low (< 85%) expressors. In

all, 27 (41%) of 66 selected patients had responded to IL-2-based regimens, with 20 (30%) remaining alive at a median follow-up of 2.6 years. In all, 24 (36%), 31 (47%), and 11 (17%) were classified into good-, intermediate-, and high-risk groups, respectively, according to the pathology model described above. In all, 41 specimens (62%) had high CAIX expression. In all, 21 (78%) of 27 responding patients had high CAIX expression compared with 20 (51%) of 39 nonresponders (odds ratio = 3.3; $p = .04$). Median survivals were 3 years and 1 year for high and low CAIX expressors, respectively ($p = .04$). Even though tumor responses were seen in six patients with low CAIX staining, survival greater than 5 years was only seen in the patients with high CAIX-expressing tumors. High CAIX staining was associated with better pathology features noted above but remained an independent predictor of response. A two-compartment model was proposed in which one group of patients with either good pathology or intermediate pathology and high CAIX expression contained 26 (96%) of 27 responders compared with only 18 (46%) of 39 nonresponders (odds ratio = 30; $p < .01$). Significant survival benefit was also seen for this group ($p < .01$).

The fact that this analysis enriched for responding patients makes it inappropriate to report response rates. However, if this model were applied to an unselected population renal cancer patients receiving IL-2 therapy, one would estimate that approximately half of the patients would be in each risk group and that the response rate would be 35 to 40% for the good-risk group and less than 5% for the poor-risk group. Although this model and these assumptions require prospective validation, it emphasizes the potential for using pathologic and molecular features of the tumor to identify optimal patients to receive IL-2 therapy. Additional studies to explain these preliminary observations and correlate results with previously described clinical features are necessary.

## MOLECULAR MARKERS

Gene expression profiling of tumor specimens to identify new proteins or patterns of gene expression that might be associated with IL-2 responsiveness may eventually help to further narrow the application of IL-2 therapy to those who will benefit the most.

Using this approach, Pantuck and colleagues were able to identify a set of 73 genes whose expression distinguished complete responders from nonresponders after IL-2 therapy.[74] In their hands, complete responders to IL-2 have a signature gene and protein expression pattern that includes CAIX, PTEN, and CXCR4. Although this approach requires prospective validation, it may become a powerful aid for clinicians in selecting appropriate treatment options.

## CURRENT INVESTIGATION

As the list of effective therapies for metastatic RCC grows, improvements in patient selection will be necessary to ensure that patients who might attain a durable remission with IL-2 will not miss this opportunity. This year, the CWG launched the high-dose IL-2 "Select" Trial. The primary objective of this study is to determine, in a prospective fashion, if the predictive model proposed by Atkins and colleagues[73] can identify a group of patients with advanced RCC who are significantly more likely to respond to high-dose IL-2-based therapy ("good" risk) than a historical, unselected patient population. New factors (including baseline immune function, immunohistochemical markers, and gene expression patterns) that might be associated with response to high-dose IL-2 therapy will also be explored in an attempt to more narrowly limit the application of IL-2 to those patients most likely to benefit.

Combination of cytokines with targeted therapy may also have merit through additive or synergistic effects. Bevacizumab and IL-2 are being combined in an ongoing CWG trial. Preliminary results suggest that these two agents can be given safely in combination, but efficacy data is pending. Sorafenib and IFN have been combined in two separate single-arm phase II trials.[75,76] These trials reported objective response rates of 18 and 35%. Toxicity observed was typical of that observed with each single agent with a notable reduction in hand foot syndrome compared with sorafenib monotherapy data. The benefit/toxicity ratio of this combination regimen awaits further investigation. In addition, two completed large phase III trials of IFN plus bevacizumab versus IFN alone will define the activity of this combination regimen compared with cytokine monotherapy.

## INVESTIGATIONAL IMMUNOTHERAPY

Metastatic RCC has long been a testing ground for novel immunotherapy.[77] Several such approaches, including vaccination and allogeneic bone marrow transplant, have been tested over the past two decades. Vaccination therapy has shown generation of potentially relevant immune responses although clinical benefits and objective responses have not been consistently observed.[77–82] Allogeneic bone marrow transplant attempts to induce a graft-versus-tumor effect in the patient through transfer of sibling's bone marrow stem cells. Although initial reports were encouraging, further clinical trials have emphasized the potential toxicity and limited applicability of this approach.[11,12] Active investigation into immunotherapeutic approaches in metastatic RCC are still being pursued although it is clear that such approaches must now be clinically developed accounting for the clinical effectiveness and widespread use of targeted therapy.

## CONCLUSIONS

RCC has long been considered an immunologically influenced malignancy and thus served as a platform for the clinical testing of anticancer immunotherapy. Based upon reported defects in immune function in RCC, several immunotherapeutic approaches have been investigated in this disease. The nonspecific cytokines IL-2 and IFN-α have undergone the most testing, producing modest benefits for unselected patients. More significantly, investigations associated with these trials suggest that the potential exists for identifying predictors of response (or resistance) and limiting IL-2 therapy to those most likely to benefit. When attempting to determine initial therapy for a patient with metastatic RCC, the data currently available suggest that patients with good or intermediate clinical prognostic features, clear cell histology, and high CAIX expression in their tumors are more likely to benefit from high-dose IL-2 therapy and should be presented with this treatment option. Additional immunotherapeutic strategies have been tested in metastatic RCC, but definitive evidence of clinical benefit is lacking. It is clear that further study to optimize the antitumor effect of immunotherapy in metastatic RCC is needed.

# REFERENCES

1. Gleave ME, Ehilali M, Fradet Y, et al.; Canadian Urologic Oncology Group. Interferon gamma-1b compared with placebo in metastatic renal-cell carcinoma. N Engl J Med 1998;338:1265.

2. Oliver RT, Nethersell AB, Bottomley JM. Unexplained spontaneous regression and alpha-interferon as treatment for metastatic renal carcinoma. Br J Urol 1989;63:128.

3. Vogelzang NJ, Priest ER, Borden L. Spontaneous regression of histologically proved pulmonary metastases from renal cell carcinoma: a case with 5-year followup. J Urol 1992;148:1247.

4. Marten A, Flieger D, Renoth S, et al. Therapeutic vaccination against metastatic renal cell carcinoma by autologous dendritic cells: preclinical results and outcome of a first clinical phase I/II trial. Cancer Immunol Immunother 2002;51:637.

5. Chang AE, Li Q, Jiang G, et al. Phase II trial of autologous tumor vaccination, anti-cd3-activated vaccine-primed lymphocytes, and interleukin-2 in stage IV renal cell cancer. J Clin Oncol 2003;21:884.

6. Fishman M, Seigne J. Immunotherapy of metastatic renal cell cancer. Cancer Control 2002;9:293.

7. Gitlitz BJ, Belldegrun AS, Figlin RA. Vaccine and gene therapy of renal cell carcinoma. Semin Urol Oncol 2001; 19:141.

8. Lesimple T, Moison A, Guille F, et al. Treatment of metastatic renal cell carcinoma with activated autologous macrophages and granulocyte–macrophage colony-stimulating factor. J Immunother 2000;23:675.

9. Schwabb T, Heaney JA, Schned AR, et al. A randomized phase II trial comparing two different sequence combinations of autologous vaccine and human recombinant interferon gamma and human recombinant interferon alpha2B therapy in patients with metastatic renal cell carcinoma: clinical outcome and analysis of immunological parameters. J Urol 2000;163:1322.

10. Childs R, Chernoff A, Contentin N, et al. Regression of metastatic renal-cell carcinoma after nonmyeloablative allogeneic peripheral-blood stem-cell transplantation. N Engl J Med 2000;343:750.

11. Childs R, Srinivasan R. Advances in allogeneic stem cell transplantation: directing graft-versus-leukemia at solid tumors. Cancer J Sci Am 2002;8:2.

12. Rini BI, Zimmerman T, Stadler WM, et al. Allogeneic stem-cell transplantation of renal cell cancer after nonmyeloablative chemotherapy: feasibility, engraftment, and clinical results. J Clin Oncol 2002;20:2017.

13. Rosenberg SA, Mule JJ, Spiess PJ, et al. Regression of established pulmonary metastatses and subcutaneous tumor mediated by the systemic administration of high-dose recombinant interleukin-2. J Exp Med 1985;161:1169–88.

14. Mule JJ, Yang JC, Lafreniere RL, et al. Identification of cellular mechanisms operational in vivo during the regression of established pulmonary metastases by the systemic administration of high-dose recombinant interleukin-2. J Immunol 1987;139:285–94.

15. Neidhart JA. Interferon therapy for the treatment of renal cancer. Cancer 1986;57:1696–9.

16. Muss HB. Interferon therapy for renal cell carcinoma. Semin Oncol 1987;14:36–42.

17. Parton M, Gore M, Eisen T. Role of cytokine therapy in 2006 and beyond for metastatic renal cell cancer. J Clin Oncol 2006;24:5584–92.

18. McDermott DF, Rini BI. Immunotherapy for metastatic renal cell carcinoma. Br J Urol 2007;99:1282–8.

19. Muss HB, Costanzi JJ, Leavitt R, et al. Recombinant alfa interferon in renal cell carcinoma: a randomized trial of two routes of administration. J Clin Oncol 1987; 5:286–91.

20. Negrier S, Caty A, Lesimple T, et al. Treatment of patients with metastatic renal carcinoma with a combination of subcutaneous interleukin-2 and Interferon alfa with or without fluorouracil. J Clin Oncol 2000;18:4009–15.

21. Medical Research Council and Collaborators. Interferon alfa and survival in metastatic renal carcinoma: early results of a randomised controlled trial. Lancet 1999;353:14–17.

22. Pyrhonen S, Salminen E, Ruutu M, et al. Prospective randomized trial of interferon alfa-2a plus vinblastine versus vinblastine alone in patients with advanced renal cell cancer. J Clin Oncol 1999;17:2859–67.

23. Coppin C, Porzsolt F, Awa A, et al. Immunotherapy for advanced renal cell cancer. Cochrane Database Syst Rev 2005:CD001425.

24. Fyfe G, Fisher RI, Rosenberg SA, et al. Results of treatment of 255 patients with metastatic renal cell carcinoma who received high-dose recombinant interleukin-2 therapy. J Clin Oncol 1995;13:688–96.

25. Fisher RI, Rosenberg SA, Fyfe G. Long-term survival update for high-dose recombinant interleukin-2 in patients with renal cell carcinoma. Cancer J Sci Am 2000;6:S55–7.

26. Rosenberg SA, Yang JC, White DE, et al. Durability of complete responses in patients with metastatic cancer treated with high-dose interleukin-2. Identification of the antigens mediating response. Ann Surg 1998;228:307–19.

27. Belldegrun A, Webb DE, Austin HA III, et al. Renal toxicity of interleukin-2 administration in patients with metastatic renal cell cancer: effect of pre-therapy nephrectomy. J Urol 1989;141:499–503.

28. Margolin KA, Rayner AA, Hawkins MJ, et al. Interleukin-2 and lymphokine-activated killer cell therapy of solid tumors: analysis of toxicity and management guidelines. J Clin Oncol 1989;7:486–98.

29. Negrier S, Escudier B, Lasset C, et al. Recombinant human interleukin-2, recombinant human interferon alfa-2a, or both in metastatic renal-cell carcinoma: groupe francais d'immunotherapie. N Engl J Med 1998;338:1272–8.

30. Flanigan RC, Salmon SE, Blumenstein BA, et al. Nephrectomy followed by interferon alfa-2b compared with interferon alfa-2b alone for metastatic renal-cell cancer. N Engl J Med 2001;345:1655.

31. Sleijfer DT, Janssen RA, Buter J, et al. Phase II study of subcutaneous interleukin-2 in unselected patients with advanced renal cell cancer on an outpatient basis. J Clin Oncol 1992;10:1119–23.

32. Lopez Hanninen E, Kirchner H, Atzpodien J. Interleukin-2 based home therapy of metastatic renal cell carcinoma: risks and benefits in 215 consecutive single institution patients. J Urol 1996;155:19–25.

33. Yang JC, Topalian SL, Parkinson D, et al. Randomized comparison of high-dose and low-dose intravenous interleukin-2 for the therapy of metastatic renal cell carcinoma: an interim report. J Clin Oncol 194;12:1572–6.

34. Atzpodien J, Lopez Hanninen E, Kirchner H, et al. Multi-institutional home-therapy trial of recombinant human interleukin-2 and interferon alfa-2 in progressive metastatic renal cell carcinoma. J Clin Oncol 1995;13:497–501.

35. Figlin RA, Belldegrun A, Moldawer N, et al. Concomitant administration of recombinant human interleukin-2 and recombinant interferon alfa-2A: an active outpatient regimen in metastatic renal cell carcinoma. J Clin Oncol 1992;10:414–21.

36. Vogelzang NJ, Lipton A, Figlin RA. Subcutaneous interleukin-2 plus interferon alfa-2a in metastatic renal cancer: an outpatient multicenter trial. J Clin Oncol 1993;11:1809–16.

37. Atzpodien J, Kirchner H, Hanninen EL, et al. Interleukin-2 in combination with interferon alpha and 5-fluorouracil for metastatic renal cell cancer. Eur J Cancer 1993;29A Suppl 5:S6–8.

38. Yang JC, Sherry RM, Stienberg SM, et al. A three-arm randomized comparison of high and low dose intravenous and subcutaneous interleukin-2 in the treatment of metastatic renal cancer. J Clin Oncol 2003;21:3127.

39. McDermott DF, Regan MM, Clark JI, et al. A randomized phase III trial of high-dose interleukin-2 versus subcutaneous interleukin-2 and interferon in patients with metastatic renal cell carcinoma. J Clin Oncol 2005; 23:133–41.

40. Negrier S, Perol D, Ravaud C, et al. Do cytokines improve survival in patients with metastatic renal cell carcinoma of intermediate prognosis? Results of the prospectively randomized PERCY Quattro trial. Am Soc Clin Oncol Proc 2005;4:511.

41. Margolin K, Aronson FR, Sznol M, et al. Phase II evaluation of thrice-daily intravenous bolus interleukin-4 in advanced renal cell and malignant melanoma. J Immunother 1994;15:147.

42. Weiss GR, Margolin KA, Sznol M, et al. A phase II study of the continuous intravenous infusion of interleukin-6 for metastatic renal cell carcinoma. J Immunother Emphasis Tumor Immunol 1995;18:52.

43. Motzer RJ, Rakhit A, Thompson J, et al. Phase II trial of branched peginterferon-alpha 1a (40 kDa) for patients with advanced renal cell carcinoma. Ann Oncol 2002;11:1799–805.

44. Rini BI, Stadler WM, Spielberger RI, et al. Granulocyte-macrophage-colony stimulating factor in metastatic renal cell carcinoma: a phase II trial. Cancer 1998;82:1352–8.

45. Wos E, Olencki T, Tuason L, et al. Phase II trial of subcutaneously administered granulocyte-macrophage colony-stimulating factor in patients with metastatic renal cell carcinoma. Cancer 1996;77:1149–53.

46. Verra N, Jansen R, Groenewegen G, et al. Immunotherapy with concurrent subcutaneous GM-CSF, low-dose IL-2 and IFN-α in patient with progressive metastatic renal cell carcinoma. Br J Cancer 2003;88:1346–51.

47. Ryan CW, Vogelzang NJ, Dumas MC, et al. Granulocyte-macrophage-colony stimulating factor in combination immunotherapy for patients with metastatic renal cell carcinoma: results of two phase II clinical trials. Cancer 2000;88:1317–24.

48. Smith JW II, Durk RA, Baher AG, et al. Immune effects of escalating doses of granulocyte-macrophage colony-stimulating factor added to a fixed, low-dose, inpatient interleukin-2 regimen: a randomized phase I trial in patients with metastatic melanoma and renal cell carcinoma. J Immunother 2003; 26:130–8.

49. Atkins MB, Robertson MJ, Gordon M, et al. Phase I evaluation of intravenous recombinant human interleukin-12 (RHIL-12) in patients with advanced malignancies. Clin Cancer Res 1997;3:409–17.

50. Motzer RJ, Rakhit A, Schwartz LH, et al. Phase I trial of subcutaneous recombinant human interleukin-12 in patients with advanced renal cell carcinoma. Clin Cancer Res 1998;4:1183.

51. Leonard JP, Sherman ML, Fisher GL, et al. Effects of single-dose IL-12 (IL-12) exposure on IL-12-associated toxicity and interferon-γ production. Blood 1997;90:2541–8.

52. Gollob JA, Mier JW, Veenstra K, et al. Phase I trial of twice weekly intravenous interleukin-12 in patients with metastatic renal cell cancer or malignant melanoma: ability to maintain IFN-γ induction is associated with clinical response. Clin Cancer Res 2000;6:1678–2.

53. Gollob JA, Veenstra KG, Parker RA, et al. Phase I trial of concurrent twice-weekly rhIL-12 plus low-dose IL-2 in patients with melanoma or renal cell carcinoma. J Clin Oncol 2003;21:2564.

54. Messing EM, Manola J, Wilding G, et al. Phase III study of interferon alfa-NL as adjuvant treatment for respectable renal cell carcinoma: an eastern cooperative oncology group/intergroup trial. J Clin Oncol 2003;21:1214–22.

55. Porzsolt F. Adjuvant therapy of renal cell cancer with interferon alfa-2a. Proc Am Soc Clin Oncol 1992;11:202.

56. Clark JI, Atkins MB, Urba WJ, et al. Adjuvant high-dose bolus interluekin-2 in patients with high-risk renal cell carcinoma — a Cytokine Working Group Phase III Trial. J Clin Oncol 2003;21:3133.

57. Pantuck AJ, Zisman A, Dorey F, et al. Renal cell carcinoma with retroperitoneal lymph nodes. Impact on survival and benefits of immunotherapy. Cancer 2003;97:2995–3002.

58. Mickisch GH, Garin A, Van Poppel H, et al. Radical nephrectomy plus interferon-alfa-based immunotherapy compared with interferon alfa alone in metastatic renal-cell carcinoma: a randomized trial. Lancet 2001;358:966.

59. McDermott D, Parker R, Youmans A, et al. The effect of recent nephrectomy on treatment with high-dose interleukin-2 (HD IL-2) or subcutaneous (SC) IL-2/interferon alfa-2b (IFN) in patients with metastatic renal cell carcinoma (renal cell carcinoma). Proc Am Soc Clin Oncol 2003;22:385.

60. Negrier S, Escudier B, Gomez F, et al. Prognostic factors of survival and rapid progression in 782 patients with metastatic renal carcinomas treated by cytokines: a report from the Groupe Francias d'Immunotherapie. Ann Oncol 2002;13:1460–8.

61. Figlin R, Gitlitz B, Franklin J, et al. Interleukin-2-based immunotherapy for the treatment of metastatic renal cell carcinoma: an analysis of 203 consecutively treated patients. Cancer J Sci Am 1997;3:S92.

62. Royal RE, Steinberg SM, Krouse RS, et al. Correlates of response to IL-2 therapy in patients treated for metastatic renal cancer and melanoma. Cancer J Sci Am 1996;2:91.

63. Atkins MB, Mier JW, Parkinson DR, et al. Hypothyroidism after treatment with interleukin-2 and lymphokine-activated killer cells. N Engl J Med 1988;318:1557–63.

64. Fumagalli LA, Vinke J, Hoff W, et al. Lymphocyte counts independently predict overall survival in advanced cancer patients: a biomarker for IL-2 immunotherapy. J Immunother 2003;26:394–402.

65. West WH, Tauer KW, Yanelli JR, et al. Constant-infusion recombinant interleukin-2 in adoptive immunotherapy of advanced cancer. N Engl J Med 1987;316:898–905.

66. Janik JE, Sznol M, Urba WJ, et al. Erythropoietin production. A potential marker for interleukin-2/interferon-responsive tumors. Cancer 1993;72:2656–9.

67. Donskov F, van der Masse H. Impact of immune parameters on long-term survival in metastatic renal cell carcinoma. J Clin Oncol 2006;24:1997–2005.

68. Leibovich BC, Han KR, Bui MH, et al. Scoring algorithm to predict survival after nephrectomy and immunotherapy in patients with metastatic renal cell carcinoma: a stratification tool for prospective clinical trials. Cancer 2003;98:2566–75.

69. Cangiano T, Liao J, Naitoh J, et al. Sarcomatoid renal cell carcinoma: biologic behavior, prognosis, and response to combined surgical resection and immunotherapy. J Clin Oncol 1999;17:523.

70. Motzer RJ, Bacil J, Mariani T, et al. Treatment outcome and survival associated with metastatic renal cell carcinoma of non-clear-cell histology. J Clin Oncol 2002;20:2376.

71. Upton MP, Parker RA, Youmans A, et al. Renal cell carcinoma: histologic predictors of cytokine response. J Immunother 2005;28:488–95.

72. Bui MHT, Seligson D, Han K, et al. Carbonic anhydrase IX is an independent predictor of survival in advanced renal cell carcinoma: implications for prognosis and therapy. Clin Cancer Res 2003;9:802–11.

73. Atkins M, Regan M, McDermott D, et al. Carbonic anhydrase IX expression predicts outcome of interleukin-2 therapy for renal cancer. Clin Cancer Res 2005;11:3714–21.

74. Pantuck AJ, Fang Z, Liu X, et al. Gene expression and tissue microarray analysis of interleukin-2 complete responders in patients with metastatic renal cell carcinoma. Proc Am Soc Clin Oncol 2005;4:535.

75. Gollob JA, Richmond T, Jones JL, et al. Phase II trial of sorafenib plus interferon-alpha 2b (IFN-alpha2b) as first- or second-line therapy in patients with metastatic renal cell cancer. J Clin Oncol 2007;25:3288–95.

76. Ryan CW, Goldman BH, Lara PN Jr, et al. Sorafenib plus interferon alpha2b (IFN) as first-line therapy for advanced renal cell carcinoma, SWOG 0412. J Clin Oncol 2007; 25:3296–301.

77. Yang JC, Childs R. Immunotherapy for renal cell cancer. J Clin Oncol 2006;24:5576–83.

78. Escudier B, Pluzanska A, Koralewski P, et al. Bevacizumab plus interferon alfa-2a for treatment of metastatic renal cell carcinoma: a randomized, double-blind Phase III trial. Lancet 2007;320:2103–2111.

79. Rini BI, Halabi S, Rosenberg JE, et al. CALGB 90206: A Phase III trial of bevacizumab plus interferon.

80. Avigan D. Fusions of breast cancer and dendritic cells as a novel cancer vaccine. Clin Breast Cancer 2003;(3 Suppl 4): S158–63.

81. Oosterwijk-Wakka JC, Tiemessen DM, Bleumer I, et al. Vaccination of patients with metastatic renal cell carcinoma with autologous dendritic cells pulsed with autologous tumor antigens in combination with interleukin-2: a phase 1 study. J Immunother 2002;25:500–8.

82. Wierecky J, Muller MR, Wirths S, et al. Immunologic and clinical responses after vaccinations with peptide-pulsed dendritic cells in metastatic renal cancer patients. Cancer Res 2006;66:5910–8.

83. Yang JC, Haworth L, Sherry RM, et al. A Randomized trial of bevacizumab, an anti-vascular endothelial growth factor antibody, for metastatic renal cancer. New Engl J Med 2003;349:427–34.

84. Motzer RJ, Hutson TE, Tomczak P, et al. Sunitinib versus interferon alfa in metastatic renal-cell carcinoma. New Engl J Med 2007;356:115–24.

85. Escudier B, Eisen T, Stadler W, et al. Sorafenib in advanced clear-cell renal-cell carcinoma. N Engl J Med. 2007;356:125–34.

# 14

# Angiogenesis Biology in Metastatic Renal Cell Carcinoma

**CHIRAG J. AMIN, MD**
**W. KIMRYN RATHMELL, MD, PHD**

Angiogenesis has been considered to play a crucial role in understanding the pathophysiology of cancer growth in general, and renal cell carcinoma (RCC) is a unique example of the importance of this hallmark of cancer. In the past 20 years, the pathophysiology of RCC has been investigated by many researchers, dissecting the molecular and genetic pathways of RCC. Investigations into the cancer biology of RCC, in particular the importance of angiogenesis in this tumor, have now led to the development of several molecularly targeted agents with efficacy in a disease historically resistant to systemic therapy. This chapter will focus on the molecular mechanisms of increased angiogenesis in RCC. Special attention will be given to the activation of the hypoxia response pathway by mutations of the von Hippel–Lindau (*VHL*) tumor suppressor gene, which results in the transcriptional activation of a variety of genes important in angiogenesis and tumor progression, in particular, vascular endothelial growth factor (VEGF) via the hypoxia-inducible factors (HIF-1$\alpha$ and HIF-2$\alpha$).

## RCC: AN ARCHETYPE LESION FOR TUMOR ANGIOGENESIS

Renal cell carcinoma, in particular the clear cell histology subtype, almost universally develops highly vascular features in both the primary and metastatic sites of disease (Figure 1). This long-held observation led to the initial suggestion that liberation of an angiogenic factor may be uniquely correlated with this disease.[1] The highly vascular nature of RCC lesions makes them more prone to treatment-specific complications, such as the risk of a bleeding diathesis from surgical resection of the tumor itself or even anticoagulation (because of its inherent high incidences of venous thrombosis). More recently, however, this unique characteristic of RCC has launched an explosion in research aimed at understanding the genetics and biology of RCC. Most importantly, the expanded appreciation of the distinctive biology of RCC tumor angiogenesis has invited the development of therapeutic agents targeting this biology from several mechanistic approaches.

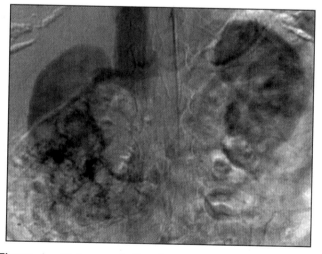

**Figure 1.** Hypervascularity of renal cell carcinoma (RCC) tumors. This angiogram acquired before renal mass embolization shows the highly vascular nature of this right-sided RCC compared with both the normal right kidney parenchyma and the left kidney. Rathmell et al.[91]

191

These developments, to be discussed in a later chapter, have led to a revolution in the treatment of RCC.

## VHL GENE INACTIVATION IN RCC

Inactivation of the *VHL* gene was first identified in association with RCC through linkage studies in patients with the autosomal dominant VHL syndrome, which predisposes to the development of clear cell type RCC, as well as central nervous system hemangioblastoma, retinal angiomas, and pheochromocytoma.[2–7] In sporadic (noninherited) clear cell RCC, *VHL* gene allele deletion (loss of heterozygosity) has been reported in 84 to 98% of sporadic renal tumors, and examination of RCC tumors for mutation in the remaining *VHL* allele has been observed in 34 to 57% of clear cell RCC tumors.[4,8–11] *VHL* gene inactivation in RCC may also occur through gene silencing by methylation.[10–13] Taken together, the above data suggest that biallelic *VHL* gene inactivation occurs.in the majority of clear cell RCC tumors. There is no evidence that nonclear cell RCC tumors harbor mutations in the *VHL* gene.[14]

### *VHL* Activity in Regulating Angiogenesis

The *VHL* gene encodes a 213 amino acid protein (pVHL), which plays an integral role in regulating the normal cellular response to oxygen ($O_2$)

deprivation. In conditions of physiologic $O_2$ availability and normal *VHL* gene function, pVHL is the substrate recognition component of an ubiquitin ligase complex that targets a family of protein transcription factors, the hypoxia-inducible factors (HIF-1$\alpha$ and HIF-2$\alpha$) for proteasome-mediated proteolysis (Figure 2A).[15–17] Under conditions of cellular hypoxia, the pVHL–HIF interaction is disrupted, thus, leading to brisk stabilization of the HIF transcription factors (Figure 2B). Elevated levels of the HIF factors can be detected within minutes of a hypoxic insult, and when $O_2$ levels are restored, pVHL-mediated HIF degradation clears the transcription factor with similar efficiency, making this molecular switch an effective method of transducing a hypoxic event in real time. With defective *VHL* gene and protein function, as in the vast majority of clear cell RCC tumors, the interaction between pVHL and HIF is disrupted even in the presence of adequate $O_2$ supplies. In this situation, HIF factors are never subjected to proteolysis and are thus constitutively activated (Figure 2B). Activated HIF translocates into the nucleus and leads to the transcription of a large repertoire hypoxia-inducible genes.[18] Several hypoxia-inducible genes induced by this process have been identified as critical mediators of the tumorigenesis process, perhaps most notably the VEGF.[18]

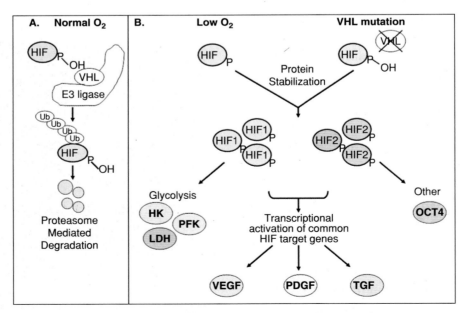

**Figure 2.** Von Hippel–Lindau (VHL) pathway of hypoxia-inducible factors (HIF) regulation. *A*, Von Hippel–Lindau protein (pVHL) targets proline-hydroxylated HIF factors for degradation when oxygen is available. *B*, In hypoxic conditions or when VHL is absent, HIF escapes proteolysis and accumulates to high levels and functions to transcriptionally activate a large repertoire of hypoxia response genes, several of which are critical mediators of angiogenesis. Reproduced with permission from Rathmell and Godley.[91]

## HIF ACTIVITY IN RCC

### HIF-1$\alpha$ and HIF-2$\alpha$: Transcriptional Activators of the Hypoxia Response

A key player in angiogenesis in RCC is the family of hypoxia-inducible factors, HIF-1$\alpha$ and HIF-2$\alpha$. Transcriptionally active HIF is a heterodimeric transcription factor that is activated by the stabilization of the $\alpha$-domain subunit of the complex in response to hypoxia. The $\beta$-subunit is also called the aryl hydrocarbon nuclear transferase (ARNT) and is a stable and ubiquitously expressed nuclear protein that participates with either HIF-$\alpha$ subunit to activate transcription.[19–21] When activated, the HIF complex binds to a conserved hypoxic response element (5'-RCGTG-3') in the enhancer regions of hypoxia-responsive genes resulting in many effects besides angiogenesis, including cell migration, energy metabolism, transcriptional and translational regulation, and other processes integral to survival in a hypoxic environment (Figure 3).[22–25]

HIF is a member of the Per-ARNT-Sim (PAS) family of heterodimeric basic helix-loop-helix transcription factors and consists of an oxygen-sensitive $\alpha$-subunit and constitutively expressed $\beta$-subunit.[26–28] The HIF $\alpha$-subunits are subdivided into at least three family members sharing homology including HIF-1$\alpha$, HIF-2$\alpha$, and HIF-3$\alpha$ (The role of HIF-3$\alpha$ is still being defined and will not be significantly addressed in the scope of this discussion). HIF-1$\alpha$ has been found to derive from chromosome 14q21–q24, and the $\beta$-subunit is mapped to human chromosome 1q21.[24] Although HIF-1$\alpha$ is present throughout many tissues, the expression of HIF-2$\alpha$ has been more limited and may be restricted to certain tissues, including hepatocytes, glial cells, and endothelial cells.[26,29]

### HIF-1$\alpha$ and HIF-2$\alpha$: Oxygen-dependent Regulatory Mechanisms

HIF-$\alpha$ subunits are dependent on the oxidative state of the cell through an oxygen-dependent post-transcriptional modification of HIF-$\alpha$. HIF-$\alpha$ subunits have two independent subdomains in the mid-portion of the molecule termed the oxygen-dependent degradation domains (ODD), N-ODD and C-ODD, respectively.[27] Moreover, these domains overlap two transactivation domains called the NAD and CAD (N- or C-terminal transactivation domain, respectively) that show destabilization in normoxia.[30–32] Under conditions of normoxia, a family of iron-dependent prolyl hydroxylases (PHDs) hydroxylate two key proline residues in the N-ODD and C-ODD region, Pro402 and Pro564 in HIF-1$\alpha$ and Pro405 and Pro531 in HIF-2$\alpha$.[33,34] The dominant prolyl hydroxylase activity has been mapped to the HIF prolyl hydroxylase gene, *Egl-9*.[35,36] Hydroxylation increases the affinity of HIF-$\alpha$ to the pVHL complex, which proceeds to undergo proteolysis via the ubiquitin–proteasome pathway.[16,27,37] The activity of the CAD domain itself is also regulated by oxygen conditions. In conditions of normoxia, an asparagine (Asn) residue in the HIF-$\alpha$ subunit (Asn803 in HIF-1$\alpha$ and Asn851 in HIF-2$\alpha$) is hydroxylated by the factor inhibiting HIF-1 (FIH-1) enzyme.[27,38] This prevents the binding of transcriptional co-activators p300 and cAMP response element–binding protein.[39–41] Therefore, the regulation of HIF is dependent by two oxygen-dependent mechanisms, *Egl-9* and FIH-1. Thus, in hypoxic conditions, HIF-$\alpha$ proteolysis is inhibited, and the CAD domain is released from the Asn hydroxylation permitting activity of the transcriptional unit.

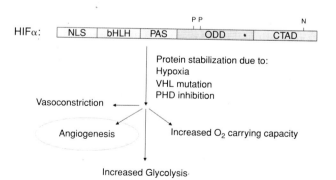

**Figure 3.** Hypoxia-inducible factors (HIF) functional domains and activities. The HIF factors are conventional bHLH/PAS domain transcription factors. The stability of the protein is regulated by proline residues located in a portion of the N-terminal activation domain (NAD) subject to oxygen-dependent hydroxylation. The protein has an additional C-terminal activation domain (CAD), which is further regulated by posttranslational hydroxylation of a critical asparagines residue. Stabilization and activation of this transcription factor induce the transcription of genes involved in mediating multiple aspects of the cellular response to hypoxia. One particularly critical aspect of this response is the promotion of angiogenesis.

## HIF-1α and HIF-2α: Roles in Angiogenesis and Tumor Development

The distinctions between the roles of the two dominant HIF factors remain an active area of investigation. The two major HIF proteins have not only different tissue distributions but also have overlapping, but not identical, patterns of transcriptional activation and tumor promotion.[42,43] Comparative studies have shown that although HIF-1α is primarily responsible for the normal cellular response to hypoxia, HIF-2α is primarily responsible for the transactivation cyclin D1, transforming growth factor-α (TGF-α), and VEGF in the renal tumor setting.[44,45]

Ultimately, HIF factors along with transcriptional co-activators function to induce the transcription of a number of genes involved in promoting endothelial cell growth in the tumor vicinity. The majority of this chapter will focus on the activity of HIF at the VEGF locus leading to the unregulated expression of VEGF.[38,46–48] VEGF performs much of its pro-angiogenic effect through co-operative mechanisms involving many other molecules, many of which are additionally targets of HIF activation. These factors contributing to renal tumor angiogenesis include angiopoietin-1 (Ang-1) and angiopoietin-4 (Ang-4), basic fibroblast growth factor (bFGF), and hepatocyte growth factor, which are pro-angiogenic factors and transcriptional target genes of HIF activity.[49] Specifically, the angiopoietins collaborate with VEGF during angiogenesis, with Ang-1 performing an antiapoptotic role in vessel development and promoting vessel stability.[50] Angiopoietin-2 (Ang-2), however, antagonizes the role of Ang-1, and its expression in the remaining internal vessels and in the angiogenic vessels at the tumor margin suggests a critical role of this destabilizing activity in facilitating the formation of fresh vessel growth promoted by VEGF. Additionally, erythropoietin is a well-established transcriptional target of HIF activation and accounts for the paraneoplastic polycythemia observed in RCC.[22,51,52] In addition to stimulating erythroid progenitor differentiation, the erythropoietin receptor is also found in the endothelial cells, and engagement of the receptor by erythropoietin can promote endothelial cell growth and vessel migration.[53,54]

Tumor vasculature is composed of a tubular structure lined by endothelial cells, which form the primary barrier between blood components and tissues. This endothelial lining is maintained by supporting cells, called pericytes, which provide the structural integrity of the vessel, mediate the permeability of the vessel, and provide critical survival signals essential to maintain the endothelial network. Although the leading edge of an angiogenic sprout is purely endothelial, the growth and proliferation of pericytes must extend along a newly formed vessel to maintain the structure of the vessel, provide a barrier to leakage, and afford the vascular tension necessary in a functioning vessel. This complex process requires the coordinated involvement of many secreted factors to complete the essential steps of endothelial cell stimulation and recruitment (mediated by VEGF signaling), pericyte recruitment (dependent on a titrated balance of Ang-1 and Ang-2, as well as platelet-derived growth factor receptor (PDGF-R) activation on the pericytes themselves), and capillary wall remodeling (also primarily mediated by VEGF signaling).

During the initial growth in angiogenesis, vessels dilate and become more permeable in response to VEGF, which must overcome the antagonistic effects of Ang-1 and the junctional molecules VE cadherin and platelet endothelial cell adhesion molecules. Ang-2 and proteinases mediate dissolution of the existing basement membrane and the interstitial matrix.[55] Matrix metalloproteinases (MMPs) have received a new focus on their importance in this process, especially in pericyte recruitment. MMPs have been shown to directly promote pericyte invasion by extracellular matrix degradation, stimulation of pericyte proliferation and protection against apoptosis, activation of pericytes through the release of growth factor bound to the extracellular matrix, and propagation of angiogenic signaling as a cofactor.[56] Moreover, other factors are also pivotal in this process. PDGF-B has been found to recruit smooth muscle cells, and TGF-b1 and Ang-1/Tie2 have been noted to stabilize the interaction between endothelial and smooth muscle cells. In addition, VEGF, Ang-1, and bFGF all have roles that are important for endothelial survival.[55]

These events occur in an ordered and synchronized manner in normal tissue angiogenesis. However, in tumors, and in particular RCC, these events are disorganized and result in the formation of a chaotic tumor vasculature with highly permeable vessels because of failed capillary wall fusion, haphazard endothelial branches, dilated caliber vessels, and areas of disorganized pericyte participation.

## ALTERNATIVE MECHANISMS OF HIF ACTIVATION IN RCC

Although one would assume that the loss of *VHL* is the sole cause of angiogenesis in RCC, newer data is showing that there are multiple mechanisms, which could lead to the highly vascular characteristics of RCC. HIF upregulation may, in fact, be a central event in the tumorigenesis of all RCC subtypes (Figure 4). An additional familial syndrome that includes development of clear cell RCC as a component of its spectrum is tuberous sclerosis.[57] Mutation in either of the genes that contribute to tuberous sclerosis (TSC-1 or TSC-2) promotes the development of clear cell RCC albeit with low penetrance. Nonetheless, one effect of loss of TSC-1 or TSC-2 is the disruption of the complex of these two proteins and release of the inhibition of the mammalian target of rapamycin (mTOR), an important regulator of HIF-1α protein synthesis. The end effect is an increase in HIF-1α in affected cells and renal tumors.[58–61] This important observation has led to the development of inhibitors of mTOR as potentially valuable therapeutic agents in RCC as is discussed in a subsequent chapter.

Further, Kim and colleagues[62] studied HIF expression in small renal cortical tumors from patients with a variety of familial forms of RCC.

Chromophobe and chromophobe/oncocytic tumors from Birt–Hogg–Dube (BHD) syndrome (patients with germline mutation in the BHD gene) displayed consistent, strong HIF-2α expression, and many people also reported increased expression of HIF-1α. Type 1 papillary tumors from patients with germline activating mutations of the MET oncogene additionally displayed HIF-2α expression in roughly half of cases, with a further half of these tumors also showing HIF-1α expression. The findings in type 1 papillary tumors are complemented by findings from Toro and colleagues[63] regarding type 2 papillary tumors with mutation in fumarate hydratase. Loss of functional fumarate hydratase leads to accumulation of fumarate in the cell, which triggers the inhibition of PHD enzymatic activity, thus, preventing pVHL-mediated degradation of HIF-α.[64] As expected, clear cell tumors from patients with germline *VHL* mutation showed consistent and simultaneous expression of HIF-1α and HIF-2α.

## VEGF: BASIC PRINCIPLES

### VEGF Activities Promoting Angiogenesis

The above data provide compelling evidence for *VHL* gene inactivation in the majority of clear cell RCC tumors leading to overexpression of VEGF and other factors as a driving force in renal tumor angiogenesis. In 1948, Michaelson[65] reported on the finding of a soluble "angiogenic factor X" that could promote the growth of vessels in the developing retina. In his seminal observation, regional tissues liberated a substance that promoted the expansion of existing blood vessel networks (angiogenesis), supported the formation of new vessels (neovascularization), and directed this process along a substrate gradient to reach a region in need of vascular supply. The angiogenic factor identified promoting this process is VEGF.

VEGF is also referred to as VPF (vascular permeability factor) and functions as a critical regulator of endothelial cell physiology. VEGF was identified in 1989 as a secreted mitogen of endothelial growth.[66,67] This secreted ligand has attracted major attention as the dominant factor regulating angiogenesis in both normal development and tumor growth. This factor exerts its mitogenic growth

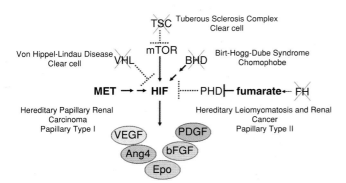

**Figure 4.** Genetic mechanisms of hypoxia-inducible factors (HIF) activation in renal cell carcinoma (RCC). In heritable forms of renal cell carcinoma, multiple genetic events converge in function to cause increased levels of HIF factors. Reprinted with permission from Rathmell, et al.[92]

promoting influence not on the tumor cells themselves (except in rare circumstances) but instead on the vascular endothelial cells, promoting both proliferation and new vessel formation. In addition to effects on proliferation, the activity of VEGF in promoting angiogenesis includes stimulating endothelial cell migration. This secreted ligand has many functions. It initiates endothelial destabilization, which results in increased permeability. Moreover, it allows endothelial cells to proliferate and migrate, or sprout, toward a localized focus of VEGF production (Figure 5). This mitogenic ligand–mediated response occurs in many physiological processes in which expansion of blood and nutrient delivery are necessary, including development, wound healing, maternal–fetal placenta formation, and uterine decidua formation, as well as pathologic processes such as diabetic retinopathy, tissue recovery from ischemic insult, and cancer.

In the development of cancer, because oxygen diffusion is limited to little more than 1 mm of tissue penetration, collections of cancer cells any larger than this must recruit and acquire the means of delivering oxygen and nutrients to deeper layers, and

HIF factor stabilization plays a critical role in promoting this process (Figure 6A). In the context of RCC, normoxic HIF activation is a central tenet of the tumorigenesis process of this tumor; thus, endothelial cell recruitment and vascularization are promoted throughout the tumor without the usual hypoxia directive (Figure 6B). The process of renal tumor angiogenesis, like other processes that integrate endothelial cell vascular network expansion, is dependent on secreted VEGF to promote existing vessel ingrowth into the tumor, as well as potentially neovascularization.

Like enhanced cellular proliferation, evasion of cell death, independence from growth factor requirement, insensitivity to antigrowth signals, and tissue invasion, the ability of a tumor to promote its own angiogenesis is one of the critical hallmarks of cancer.[68] Because of the importance of VEGF in this critical role, it has become a central player in the arena of targeted drug development for many tumors, particularly RCC. For years, the influence of angiogenesis and the impact on oxygen and nutrient delivery to rapidly growing tumors has been a basic factor of tumor biology as it impacts such key clinically relevant factors such as drug delivery, surgical resection strategies, and sensitivity to radiation therapy.

## VEGF: Protein Structure and Isoforms

VEGF actually refers to a family of related peptides, each with restricted tissue expression and receptor specificity. VEGF-A is structurally related to the platelet-derived growth factor family, sharing homology with both PDGF-A and PDGF-B. The original VEGF-A was identified as a secreted peptide from bovine pituitary follicular cells as a 45 kD protein although the apparent molecular mass is approximately 20 kD under reducing conditions.[69]

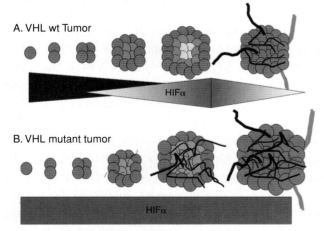

**Figure 5.** Hypoxia-inducible factors (HIF)-mediated promotion of tumor angiogenesis. *A,* During periods of cellular growth, local areas of regional hypoxia cause cellular upregulation of HIF factors. As HIF factors accumulate, they induce the expression of genes such as vascular endothelial growth factor (VEGF), which promotes angiogenesis into the affected areas. Upon revascularization of these areas and the return of access to oxygen supplies, HIF factors are destabilized and angiogenic factors decline. In this setting, HIF factors play a role in promoting vascularization of tumor tissue in areas of regional hypoxia, permitting continued growth. *B,* In renal cell carcinoma (RCC), HIF activation occurs independently of oxygen levels providing a constant stimulus for tumor-related angiogenesis.

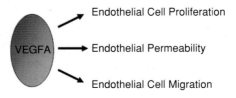

**Figure 6.** Vascular endothelial growth factor (VEGF) activities in angiogenesis. VEGF-A promotes several diverse effects on vascular development including increased proliferation, migration, and effects on vessel permeability.

The active portion of the protein is a 26 amino acid signal sequence at the amino terminus of the multiple isoforms of the protein that were eventually identified.

The VEGF-A gene is located at 6p21.3.[70] A pro-angiogenic gene transcript was cloned by Leung and colleagues,[66] identifying the first of a family of isoforms encoding the primary protein of 165 amino acids (VEGF165). Human VEGF-A has at least nine isoforms subtypes because of the alternative splicing of a single gene (Figure 7).[71] In addition to VEGF165, these include two common 121 amino acid (VEGF121) and 189 amino acid (VEGF189) forms, these latter two isoforms result from a deletion of 44 amino acids and insertion of 24 amino acids at residue 116, respectively. A 145 amino acid isoform (VEGF145) was identified that lacked exon 7 by Poltorak and colleagues[72] in carcinoma cell lines. The various isoforms all arise from one 8-exon gene through alternative splicing.[73]

The activity of the various isoforms continues to be an area of active investigation. Each of the VEGF-A isoforms has affinity for the primary VEGF receptors, VEGFR-1 and VEGFR-2 (Figure 8). Certain isoforms act in a dominant negative fashion, for example VEGF165b. This isoform binds to VEGFR-2 with the same affinity as VEGF165 but fails to activate the downstream signaling pathways.[74] Additionally, support from a variety of murine models suggests that the various isoforms play

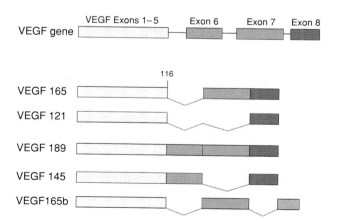

**Figure 7.** Vascular endothelial growth factor (VEGF) isoforms. The VEGF-A gene locus is composed of eight exons, which are spliced differentially to form various isoforms that differ in receptor binding affinity, secreted volume of distribution, and activity at the receptors.

distinct roles in vascular patterning and arterial development. Related family members, VEGF-B, VEGF-C, and VEGF-D, interact with a similar group of related receptors and are primarily involved in lymphatic vessel development.[75,76] Although investigations continue to examine potential activities of these proteins in tumor biology, a definitive role for these related proteins in tumor development or maintenance has not been conclusively reported.

## VEGF REGULATION IN RCC

### Cellular Sources of VEGF

Outside of RCC, VEGF is primarily produced and secreted by fibroblast cells. Primary evidence for this was provided by an elegant experiment performed by Fukumura and colleagues[77] in which a line of transgenic mice was established expressing the green fluorescent protein (GFP) under the control of the VEGF promoter. The mice showed GFP expression around healing wound margins and in the granulation tissue of superficial wounds. Solid tumors implanted in the transgenic mice led to the accumulation of GFP expression around the tumor resulting from induction of host VEGF promoter activity, and with time, the fluorescent cells could be seen throughout the tumor mass. In both implanted tumor and spontaneous tumor models in this system, GFP expression remained primarily limited to stromal cells or fibroblasts. In this investigation limited to transcriptionally affected VEGF regulation, for the first time, the cells that initiate and direct vessel formation were identified in a visual way.

In RCC, VEGF is produced by the tumor cells, with its effects on local tumor vascular components. Additionally, increased levels of VEGF can be observed to be generally higher in the serum of patients with RCC suggesting that the effects of VEGF expression by the tumor may be more widespread.[78] Much of what we understand about tumor angiogenesis comes from the studies of solid tumors with regional areas of hypoxia; therefore, RCC provides a unique clinical and biologic situation in which the hypoxic repertoire and pro-angiogenic factors, in particular, are highly upregulated even in the presence of oxygen.

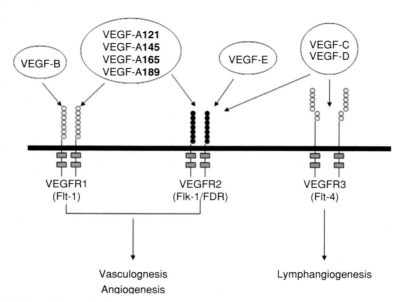

**Figure 8.**   Vascular endothelial growth factor (VEGF): receptor interactions. VEGFR-1 and VEGFR-2 are the primary VEGF receptors mediating the effects of angiogenesis. These are engaged by specific isoforms of VEGF-A, whereas other variants of VEGF display differential affinities for the different VEGF receptors and are primarily involved in the development of the lymphatic system.

## VEGF: Transcriptional Regulation

Inappropriate activation of the hypoxia response pathway, as discussed previously via *VHL* mutation and HIF factor transcriptional activation, is a major mechanism of VEGF transcriptional regulation in RCC.[79,80] On the basis of nuclear run-off transcriptional assays, the transcriptional rate for VEGF is increased 2- to 3-fold by hypoxia.[81] Interestingly, an analysis of HIF-1α versus HIF-2α activity in the transcriptional regulation of VEGF: HIF-1α appeared to be the major contributor to VEGF upregulation in response to a hypoxic stimulus and HIF-2α provided the dominant transcriptional activation of VEGF when the expression was mediated by *VHL* loss. This remains an active area of investigation and is clearly an important contributor to the highly angiogenic nature of RCC.

## VEGF Receptor Activation

The secreted VEGF protein is a potent mitogen of capillary and vascular endothelial cells.[66,69] It is, perhaps, the only chemokine with direct activity to stimulate proliferation of endothelial cells, promoted through binding and dimerization of cell surface transmembrane receptors. The receptors that bind VEGF-A are mainly classified into FLT1 (VEGFR-1) and KDR/FLK1 (VEGFR-2). These receptors are only present on the endothelial cells, and the evidence suggests that the isoforms of VEGF compete for binding on the receptor. Specifically, VEGF145, the major tumor-associated isoform, will inhibit the binding of VEGF165 to the KDR/FLK1 receptor. Both VEGF145 and VEGF189 will bind efficiently to the extracellular matrix and thus spatially fixing them as chemokines to direct vessel formation. As an elegant demonstration of the pro-angiogenic activity of VEGF145, Poltorak and colleagues[72] injected purified VEGF145 into mouse skin showing that this protein acting alone can induce angiogenesis. When nonproliferating endothelial cells in culture are deprived of oxygen and nutrients, VEGF acts independently of its mitogenic activity to stimulate elongation, network formation, and branching morphogenesis.[82] In solid tumors that are exposed to chronic or intermittent hypoxic conditions, Helmlinger proposed that autocrine endothelial VEGF production contributes to the formation of tumor blood vessels and promotes tumor growth. Investigations of oxygen gradients of tissue and cell culture have shown the induction of a VEGF gradient, followed by establishment of new vascular networks. The addition of an antiVEGF neutralizing antibody abolished vascular network formation, thus, establishing the role of this important protein in network formation.[82]

In addition to its role as a mitogen and chemokine, the VEGF family regulates the permeability of both mature and developing vessels.[83–88] VEGF increases the permeability of endothelial cells in a dose-dependent manner. These activities are additionally mediated through interactions with the FLT1 and KDR/FLK1 receptor family. Receptor activation and signal transduction via the phosphoinosital-3-kinase (PI-3 kinase) signaling cascade were required for the permeablization of these cells as inhibitors of PI-3 kinase and mitogen-activated protein kinase both were inhibitory of this process in vitro.[89] Microvessel hyperpermeability is the critical step for the abnormal transport of molecules and cells across the blood vessel wall and therefore is the crucial step for many diseases including tumor growth and metastasis.[90] Understanding the mechanisms of microvessel hyperpermeability from various approaches is important in combating these malignant diseases.

## SUMMARY: RCC AS A PROTOTYPICAL MODEL FOR BIOLOGY-DRIVEN THERAPEUTIC DEVELOPMENT

Renal cell carcinoma presents a unique clinical setting in which a tumor type nearly universally usurps a pro-angiogenic cellular homeostatic mechanism. Through mutations in *VHL* or other genetic events that result in the dysregulated expression of the hypoxia-inducible transcription factors HIF-1α and/or HIF-2α, a large cohort of hypoxia-responsive genes is induced, including VEGF as one of the classic transcriptional targets.[80] Cell culture model systems of RCC have shown a direct link between *VHL* mutation and upregulation of VEGF. RCC cells in which *VHL* is mutated express abundant levels of VEGF mRNA and protein, and reconstitution of these cells with a wild type *VHL* cDNA restores predicted patterns of VEGF hypoxia-responsive regulation.[18] Thus, increased expression of VEGF and the consequences of that increased expression are expected and

predictable events in the development of most RCC. Furthermore, with the development of effective agents targeting the angiogenesis signaling pathway, inhibition of VEGF has been aggressively pursued as a therapeutic target in RCC.

## REFERENCES

1. Bard RH, Mydlo JH, Freed SZ. Detection of tumor angiogenesis factor in adenocarcinoma of kidney. Urology 1986; 27:447–50.
2. Richards FM, Phipps ME, Latif F, et al. Mapping the von Hippel-Lindau disease tumour suppressor gene: identification of germline deletions by pulsed field gel electrophoresis. Hum Mol Genet 1993;2:879–82.
3. Crossey PA, Foster K, Richards FM, et al. Molecular genetic investigations of the mechanism of tumourigenesis in von Hippel-Lindau disease: analysis of allele loss in VHL tumours. Hum Genet 1994;93:53–8.
4. Gnarra JR, Lerman MI, Zbar B, Linehan WM. Genetics of renal-cell carcinoma and evidence for a critical role for von Hippel-Lindau in renal tumorigenesis. Semin Oncol 1995;22:3–8.
5. Maher ER, Bentley E, Yates JR, et al. Mapping of von Hippel-Lindau disease to chromosome 3p confirmed by genetic linkage analysis. J Neurol Sci 1990;100:27–30.
6. Seizinger BR, Rouleau GA, Ozelius LJ, et al. Von Hippel-Lindau disease maps to the region of chromosome 3 associated with renal cell carcinoma. Nature 1988;332:268–9.
7. Vance JM, Small KW, Jones MA, et al. Confirmation of linkage in von Hippel-Lindau disease. Genomics 1990;6:565–7.
8. Gnarra JR, Tory K, Weng Y, et al. Mutations of the VHL tumour suppressor gene in renal carcinoma. Nat Genet 1994;7:85–90.
9. Shuin T, Kondo K, Torigoe S, et al. Frequent somatic mutations and loss of heterozygosity of the von Hippel-Lindau tumor suppressor gene in primary human renal cell carcinomas. Cancer Res 1994;54:2852–5.
10. Herman JG, Latif F, Weng Y, et al. Silencing of the VHL tumor-suppressor gene by DNA methylation in renal carcinoma. Proc Natl Acad Sci U S A 1994;91:9700–4.
11. Kondo K, Yao M, Yoshida M, et al. Comprehensive mutational analysis of the VHL gene in sporadic renal cell carcinoma: relationship to clinicopathological parameters. Genes Chromosomes Cancer 2002;34:58–68.
12. Brauch H, Hoeppner W, Jahnig H, et al. Sporadic pheochromocytomas are rarely associated with germline mutations in the VHL tumor suppressor gene or the ret protooncogene. J Clin Endocrinol Metab 1997;82:4101–4.
13. Clifford SC, Prowse AH, Affara NA, et al. Inactivation of the von Hippel-Lindau (VHL) tumour suppressor gene and allelic losses at chromosome arm 3p in primary renal cell carcinoma: evidence for a VHL-independent pathway in clear cell renal tumourigenesis. Genes Chromosomes Cancer 1998;22:200–9.
14. Kenck C, Wilhelm M, Bugert P, et al. Mutation of the VHL gene is associated exclusively with the development of non-papillary renal cell carcinomas. J Pathol 1996;179:157–61.

15. Kibel A, Iliopoulos O, DeCaprio JA, Kaelin WG Jr. Binding of the von Hippel-Lindau tumor suppressor protein to elongin B and C. Science 1995;269:1444–6.

16. Maxwell PH, Wiesener MS, Chang GW, et al. The tumour suppressor protein VHL targets hypoxia-inducible factors for oxygen-dependent proteolysis. Nature 1999;399: 271–5.

17. Cockman ME, Masson N, Mole DR, et al. Hypoxia inducible factor-alpha binding and ubiquitylation by the von Hippel-Lindau tumor suppressor protein. J Biol Chem 2000; 275:25733–41.

18. Iliopoulos O, Levy AP, Jiang C, et al. Negative regulation of hypoxia-inducible genes by the von Hippel-Lindau protein. Proc Natl Acad Sci U S A 1996;93:10595–9.

19. Gruber M, Simon MC. Hypoxia-inducible factors, hypoxia, and tumor angiogenesis. Curr Opin Hematol 2006; 13:169–74.

20. Wang GL, Semenza GL. Purification and characterization of hypoxia-inducible factor 1. J Biol Chem 1995; 270:1230–7.

21. Wenger RH, Kvietikova I, Rolfs A, et al. Hypoxia-inducible factor-1 alpha is regulated at the post-mRNA level. Kidney Int 1997;51:560–3.

22. Rathmell WK, Simon MC. VHL: oxygen sensing and vasculogenesis. J Thromb Haemost 2005.

23. Semenza GL. Hypoxia-inducible factor 1: master regulator of $O_2$ homeostasis. Curr Opin Genet Dev 1998;8:588–94.

24. Semenza GL. Hypoxia-inducible factor 1 and the molecular physiology of oxygen homeostasis. J Lab Clin Med 1998;131:207–14.

25. Semenza GL. Regulation of mammalian $O_2$ homeostasis by hypoxia-inducible factor 1. Annu Rev Cell Dev Biol 1999;15:551–78.

26. Haase VH. Hypoxia-inducible factors in the kidney. Am J Physiol Renal Physiol 2006;291:F271–81.

27. Schofield CJ, Ratcliffe PJ. Oxygen sensing by HIF hydroxylases. Nat Rev Mol Cell Biol 2004;5:343–54.

28. Wenger RH, Stiehl DP, Camenisch G. Integration of oxygen signaling at the consensus HRE. Sci STKE 2005; 2005:re12.

29. Wiesener MS, Jurgensen JS, Rosenberger C, et al. Widespread hypoxia-inducible expression of HIF-2alpha in distinct cell populations of different organs. Faseb J 2003;17:271–3.

30. Pugh CW, O'Rourke JF, Nagao M, et al. Activation of hypoxia-inducible factor-1; definition of regulatory domains within the alpha subunit. J Biol Chem 1997; 272:11205–14.

31. Kallio PJ, Wilson WJ, O'Brien S, et al. Regulation of the hypoxia-inducible transcription factor 1alpha by the ubiquitin-proteasome pathway. J Biol Chem 1999; 274:6519–25.

32. Huang LE, Gu J, Schau M, Bunn HF. Regulation of hypoxia-inducible factor 1alpha is mediated by an $O_2$-dependent degradation domain via the ubiquitin-proteasome pathway. Proc Natl Acad Sci U S A 1998;95:7987–92.

33. Ivan M, Kondo K, Yang H, et al. HIFalpha targeted for VHL-mediated destruction by proline hydroxylation: implications for $O_2$ sensing. Science 2001;292:464–8.

34. Jaakkola P, Mole DR, Tian YM, et al. Targeting of HIF-alpha to the von Hippel-Lindau ubiquitylation complex by $O_2$-regulated prolyl hydroxylation. Science 2001; 292:468–72.

35. Epstein AC, Gleadle JM, McNeill LA, et al. C. elegans EGL-9 and mammalian homologs define a family of dioxygenases that regulate HIF by prolyl hydroxylation. Cell 2001;107:43–54.

36. Bruick RK, McKnight SL. A conserved family of prolyl-4-hydroxylases that modify HIF. Science 2001;294:1337–40.

37. Ohh M, Park CW, Ivan M, et al. Ubiquitination of hypoxia-inducible factor requires direct binding to the beta-domain of the von Hippel-Lindau protein. Nat Cell Biol 2000;2:423–7.

38. Lando D, Peet DJ, Whelan DA, et al. Asparagine hydroxylation of the HIF transactivation domain a hypoxic switch. Science 2002;295:858–61.

39. Kim WY, Kaelin WG. Role of VHL gene mutation in human cancer. J Clin Oncol 2004;22:4991–5004.

40. Kallio PJ, Okamoto K, O'Brien S, et al. Signal transduction in hypoxic cells: inducible nuclear translocation and recruitment of the CBP/p300 coactivator by the hypoxia-inducible factor-1alpha. Embo J 1998;17:6573–86.

41. Ema M, Hirota K, Mimura J, et al. Molecular mechanisms of transcription activation by HLF and HIF1alpha in response to hypoxia: their stabilization and redox signal-induced interaction with CBP/p300. Embo J 1999; 18:1905–14.

42. Hu CJ, Wang LY, Chodosh LA, et al. Differential roles of hypoxia-inducible factor 1alpha (HIF-1alpha) and HIF-2alpha in hypoxic gene regulation. Mol Cell Biol 2003;23:9361–74.

43. Covello KL, Simon MC, Keith B. Targeted replacement of hypoxia-inducible factor-1alpha by a hypoxia-inducible factor-2alpha knock-in allele promotes tumor growth. Cancer Res 2005;65:2277–86.

44. Sowter HM, Raval RR, Moore JW, et al. Predominant role of hypoxia-inducible transcription factor (HIF)-1alpha versus HIF-2alpha in regulation of the transcriptional response to hypoxia. Cancer Res 2003;63:6130–4.

45. Raval RR, Lau KW, Tran MG, et al. Contrasting properties of hypoxia-inducible factor 1 (HIF-1) and HIF-2 in von Hippel-Lindau-associated renal cell carcinoma. Mol Cell Biol 2005;25:5675–86.

46. Forsythe JA, Jiang BH, Iyer NV, et al. Activation of vascular endothelial growth factor gene transcription by hypoxia-inducible factor 1. Mol Cell Biol 1996;16:4604–13.

47. Dames SA, Martinez-Yamout M, De Guzman RN, et al. Structural basis for HIF-1 alpha /CBP recognition in the cellular hypoxic response. Proc Natl Acad Sci U S A 2002;99:5271–6.

48. Kobayashi A, Numayama-Tsuruta K, Sogawa K, Fujii-Kuriyama Y. CBP/p300 functions as a possible transcriptional coactivator of Ah receptor nuclear translocator (ARNT). J Biochem 1997;122:703–10.

49. Yamakawa M, Liu LX, Belanger AJ, et al. Expression of angiopoietins in renal epithelial and clear cell carcinoma cells: regulation by hypoxia and participation in angiogenesis. Am J Physiol Renal Physiol 2004;287:F649–57.

50. Holash J, Maisonpierre PC, Compton D, et al. Vessel cooption, regression, and growth in tumors mediated by angiopoietins and VEGF. Science 1999;284:1994–8.

51. Maran J, Prchal J. Polycythemia and oxygen sensing. Pathol Biol (Paris) 2004;52:280–4.

52. Varma S, Cohen HJ. Co-transactivation of the 3' erythropoietin hypoxia inducible enhancer by the HIF-1 protein. Blood Cells Mol Dis 1997;23:169–76.

53. Heeschen C, Aicher A, Lehmann R, et al. Erythropoietin is a potent physiologic stimulus for endothelial progenitor cell mobilization. Blood 2003;102:1340–6.

54. Anagnostou A, Lee ES, Kessimian N, et al. Erythropoietin has a mitogenic and positive chemotactic effect on endothelial cells. Proc Natl Acad Sci U S A 1990;87:5978–82.

55. Carmeliet P, Jain RK. Angiogenesis in cancer and other diseases. Nature 2000;407:249–57.

56. Chantrain CF, Henriet P, Jodele S, et al. Mechanisms of pericyte recruitment in tumour angiogenesis: a new role for metalloproteinases. Eur J Cancer 2006;42:310–8.

57. Bernstein J, Robbins TO. Renal involvement in tuberous sclerosis. Ann N Y Acad Sci 1991;615:36–49.

58. Brugarolas JB, Vazquez F, Reddy A, et al. TSC2 regulates VEGF through mTOR-dependent and -independent pathways. Cancer Cell 2003;4:147–58.

59. Parry L, Maynard JH, Patel A, et al. Analysis of the TSC1 and TSC2 genes in sporadic renal cell carcinomas. Br J Cancer 2001;85:1226–30.

60. Brugarolas J, Kaelin WG Jr. Dysregulation of HIF and VEGF is a unifying feature of the familial hamartoma syndromes. Cancer Cell 2004;6:7–10.

61. Liu MY, Poellinger L, Walker CL. Up-regulation of hypoxia-inducible factor 2alpha in renal cell carcinoma associated with loss of TSC-2 tumor suppressor gene. Cancer Res 2003;63:2675–80.

62. Kim CM, Vocke C, Torres-Cabala C, et al. Expression of hypoxia inducible factor-1alpha and 2alpha in genetically distinct early renal cortical tumors. J Urol 2006;175:1908–14.

63. Toro JR, Nickerson ML, Wei MH, et al. Mutations in the fumarate hydratase gene cause hereditary leiomyomatosis and renal cell cancer in families in North America. Am J Hum Genet 2003;73:95–106.

64. Pollard PJ, Briere JJ, Alam NA, et al. Accumulation of Krebs cycle intermediates and over-expression of HIF1alpha in tumours which result from germline FH and SDH mutations. Hum Mol Genet 2005;14:2231–9.

65. Michaelson IC. The mode of development of the vascular system of the retina, with some observations on its significance for certain retinal diseases. Trans Ophthalmol Soc U K 1948;68:137–80.

66. Leung DW, Cachianes G, Kuang WJ, et al. Vascular endothelial growth factor is a secreted angiogenic mitogen. Science 1989;246:1306–9.

67. Keck PJ, Hauser SD, Krivi G, et al. Vascular permeability factor, an endothelial cell mitogen related to PDGF. Science 1989;246:1309–12.

68. Hanahan D, Weinberg RA. The hallmarks of cancer. Cell 2000;100:57–70.

69. Ferrara N, Henzel WJ. Pituitary follicular cells secrete a novel heparin-binding growth factor specific for vascular endothelial cells. Biochem Biophys Res Commun 1989;161:851–8.

70. Vincenti V, Cassano C, Rocchi M, Persico G. Assignment of the vascular endothelial growth factor gene to human chromosome 6p21.3. Circulation 1996;93:1493–5.

71. Takahashi H, Shibuya M. The vascular endothelial growth factor (VEGF)/VEGF receptor system and its role under physiological and pathological conditions. Clin Sci (Lond) 2005;109:227–41.

72. Poltorak Z, Cohen T, Sivan R, et al. VEGF145, a secreted vascular endothelial growth factor isoform that binds to extracellular matrix. J Biol Chem 1997;272:7151–8.

73. Tischer E, Mitchell R, Hartman T, et al. The human gene for vascular endothelial growth factor. Multiple protein forms are encoded through alternative exon splicing. J Biol Chem 1991;266:11947–54.

74. Ferrara N, Davis-Smyth T. The biology of vascular endothelial growth factor. Endocr Rev 1997;18:4–25.

75. Paavonen K, Mandelin J, Partanen T, et al. Vascular endothelial growth factors C and D and their VEGFR-2 and 3 receptors in blood and lymphatic vessels in healthy and arthritic synovium. J Rheumatol 2002;29:39–45.

76. Kukk E, Lymboussaki A, Taira S, et al. VEGF-C receptor binding and pattern of expression with VEGFR-3 suggests a role in lymphatic vascular development. Development 1996;122:3829–37.

77. Fukumura D, Xavier R, Sugiura T, et al. Tumor induction of VEGF promoter activity in stromal cells. Cell 1998;94:715–25.

78. Edgren M, Lennernas B, Larsson A, Nilsson S. Serum concentrations of VEGF and b-FGF in renal cell, prostate and urinary bladder carcinomas. Anticancer Res 1999;19:869–73.

79. Tsuzuki Y, Fukumura D, Oosthuyse B, et al. Vascular endothelial growth factor (VEGF) modulation by targeting hypoxia-inducible factor-1alpha—> hypoxia response element—> VEGF cascade differentially regulates vascular response and growth rate in tumors. Cancer Res 2000;60:6248–52.

80. Shweiki D, Itin A, Soffer D, Keshet E. Vascular endothelial growth factor induced by hypoxia may mediate hypoxia-initiated angiogenesis. Nature 1992;359:843–5.

81. Levy AP, Levy NS, Wegner S, Goldberg MA. Transcriptional regulation of the rat vascular endothelial growth factor gene by hypoxia. J Biol Chem 1995;270:13333–40.

82. Helmlinger G, Endo M, Ferrara N, et al. Formation of endothelial cell networks. Nature 2000;405:139–41.

83. Senger DR, Perruzzi CA, Feder J, Dvorak HF. A highly conserved vascular permeability factor secreted by a variety of human and rodent tumor cell lines. Cancer Res 1986;46:5629–32.

84. Collins PD, Connolly DT, Williams TJ. Characterization of the increase in vascular permeability induced by vascular permeability factor in vivo. Br J Pharmacol 1993;109:195–9.

85. Dvorak HF, Brown LF, Detmar M, Dvorak AM. Vascular permeability factor/vascular endothelial growth factor, microvascular hyperpermeability, and angiogenesis. Am J Pathol 1995;146:1029–39.

86. Roberts WG, Palade GE. Increased microvascular permeability and endothelial fenestration induced by vascular endothelial growth factor. J Cell Sci 1995;108(Pt 6):2369–79.

87. Wu HM, Huang Q, Yuan Y, Granger HJ. VEGF induces NO-dependent hyperpermeability in coronary venules. Am J Physiol 1996;271:H2735–9.

88. Hippenstiel S, Krull M, Ikemann A, et al. VEGF induces hyperpermeability by a direct action on endothelial cells. Am J Physiol 1998;274:L678–84.

89. Lal BK, Varma S, Pappas PJ, et al. VEGF increases permeability of the endothelial cell monolayer by activation of PKB/akt, endothelial nitric-oxide synthase, and MAP kinase pathways. Microvasc Res 2001;62:252–62.

90. Bates DO, Lodwick D, Williams B. Vascular endothelial growth factor and microvascular permeability. Microcirculation 1999;6:83–96.

91. Rathmell WK, Wright TM, Rini BI. Molecularly targeted therapy in renal cell carcinoma. Expert Rev Anticancer Ther 2005;5:1031–40.

92. Rathmell WK, Martz CA, Rini BI. Renal cell carcinoma. Curr Opin Oncol 2007 [in press].

# 15a

# Antivascular Endothelial Growth Factor Therapy In Metastatic Renal Cell Carcinoma

## Vascular Endothelial Growth Factor Ligand-Binding Agents

BRIAN I. RINI, MD

W. KIMRYN RATHMELL, MD, PHD

As described elsewhere, the biology of renal cell carcinoma (RCC) leads to overexpression of vascular endothelial growth factor (VEGF). As such, approaches to block the signaling of this most potent proangiogenic protein have emerged. Methods to neutralize the circulating VEGF protein through an antibody or aptamer have undergone clinical testing in RCC.

## VEGF

The molecular underpinnings of RCC tumorigenesis suggest that the vascularity of these tumors provides a provocative target for therapy. New vessel formation is an important factor in development and wound healing, in the mature animal, the formation of new vessels is an event essentially relegated to pathologic conditions, and thus is an attractive mechanism to disrupt. Cancer cells in general require access to blood vessels for continued growth and the establishment of further metastatic sites. To obtain nutrients for their growth, cancer cells co-opt host vessels, sprout new vessels from existing ones, and/or recruit endothelial cells from the bone marrow.[1] This process is further deranged by the absence of functional hypoxia signaling in RCC and instead the unregulated constitutive activation of the hypoxia response even with immediately available oxygen. In addition, the vasculature formed by this aberrant developmental process is structurally and functionally abnormal, typically dilated, and highly permeable with global disorganization. Therefore, this unique vasculature may provide a unique target for inhibitory therapy.[2]

A large amount of data has supported the importance of VEGF and its cognate receptors in tumor angiogenesis. VEGF is elevated in the serum of patients with nonsmall cell lung, colorectal, breast, ovarian, uterine, and RCC.[3–8] As detailed in Chapter 14, a variety of mechanisms account for the increase in VEGF, with activation of the hypoxic response pathway via the transcription factors hypoxia-inducible factor 1 (HIF1$\alpha$) and HIF2$\alpha$ as the classic mechanism of tumor-specific dysregulation.

RCC presents a unique clinical setting in which a tumor type nearly universally usurps a proangiogenic cellular homeostatic mechanism. Through mutations in *VHL* and the subsequent dysregulated expression of the hypoxia-inducible transcription factors HIF1α and/or HIF2α, a large cohort of hypoxia-responsive genes is induced, including VEGF as one of the classic transcriptional targets.[9] Additionally, RCC cells in which *VHL* is mutant express abundant levels of VEGF messenger RNA (mRNA) and protein, and reconstitution of these cells with a wild-type *VHL* complementary DNA restores predicted patterns of VEGF hypoxia-responsive regulation.[10] Thus, increased expression of VEGF and the consequences of that increased expression are expected and predictable events in the development of most RCC.

## CLINICAL APPROACHES TO VEGF LIGAND IN RCC

### Anti-VEGF Antibody (Bevacizumab)

A recombinant humanized monoclonal antibody against VEGF (rhuMAb VEGF, bevacizumab, Avastin®; Genentech, South San Francisco, CA) binds and neutralizes all biological active isoforms of VEGF (also known as VEGF-A), but not other members of the VEGF family, such as VEGF-B, VEGF-C, and VEGF-D.[11] The antibody was engineered by combining VEGF-binding residues from the antigen-binding loops of a murine-neutralizing antibody with the framework of a human immunoglobulin G (IgG1).[11] This humanized antibody implies the minimum mouse part from a specific murine antibody is engineered onto a human antibody; generally humanized antibodies are 5 to 10% mouse and 90 to 95% human and generally encounter minimal, if any, host immune response (Figure 1). Results from clinical studies have also shown a rise in serum concentrations of endogenous VEGF over baseline after single and multiple intravenous (IV) administration(s) of bevacizumab at doses > 1 mg/kg.[12] The binding of this antibody to circulating human VEGF results in decreased clearance of the protein overall, which may account in part for the rise in serum levels.[13] Thus, the neutralizing activity is not mediating clearance of the protein, but rather the available protein is unable to engage the cognate receptors.

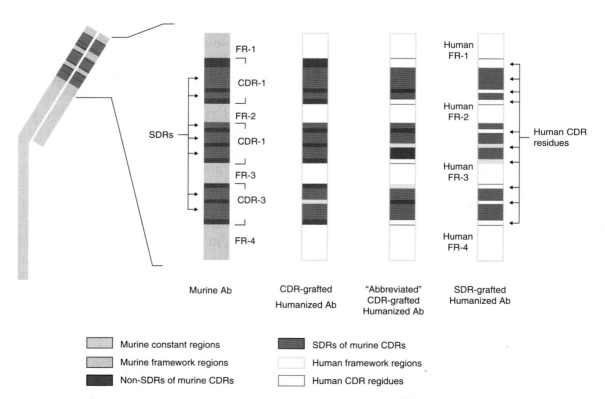

**Figure 1.**   Schematic representation of the humanization protocols of the variable light (VL) region of an antibody, showing the VL region of a murine, complementarity-determining region (CDR)–grafted, "abbreviated" CDR-grafted, and specificity-determining residue–grafted humanized antibody. Reproduced with permission from Kashmiri et al.[36]

In vitro studies have demonstrated that bevacizumab causes decreased survival of human vascular endothelial cells (HUVEC) and decreases VEGF-induced HUVEC permeability.[14] This humanized antibody was demonstrated to inhibit bovine capillary endothelial cell proliferation in response to VEGF and has showed antitumor effects in sarcoma and breast cancer cell lines.[11] In addition, preclinical studies have shown that bevacizumab has activity against metastases.[15] For example, the murine antibody (A4.6.1), from which the humanized antibody was derived, prevented lung metastases from Wilms tumors implanted into kidneys of nude mice.[16] In a study of human rectal cancer, a single infusion of bevacizumab was associated with decreased microvessel density, tumor perfusion, vascular volume, and interstitial fluid pressure.[17]

Bevacizumab in metastatic RCC was initially investigated in a randomized phase 2 trial in which 116 patients with treatment-refractory, metastatic clear cell RCC were randomized to receive placebo, low-dose (3 mg/kg) bevacizumab, or high-dose (10 mg/kg) bevacizumab every 2 weeks.[18] There were four objective partial responses (10%) in the high-dose bevacizumab arm. A substantial proportion of additional patients had tumor shrinkage not meeting objective response criteria, and the strict progression criteria resulted in several patients declared as disease progression with a lower total tumor burden than baseline. The effect of treatment on individual patients tumor burden represented graphically demonstrates that response occurs in the first cycles of administration followed generally by a period of disease stability.[19] The overall antitumor effect lead to a significant prolongation of time to progression in the high-dose bevacizumab arm compared with placebo (4.8 vs 2.5 months; $p < .001$).

The toxicity associated with neutralizing the activity of this critical signaling molecule has been thus far predictable and manageable. In the high-dose bevacizumab arm, hypertension of any grade occurred in 36% of patients, and grade 3 hypertension was observed in 21% of patients. Hypertension mechanism is not well described and is generally managed with standard antihypertensives of a variety of mechanisms. Asymptomatic proteinuria without renal insufficiency was also observed in 64% of patients. These toxic effects were reversible with cessation of therapy. Preclinical studies show that VEGF maintains tumor vessel morphology even in established

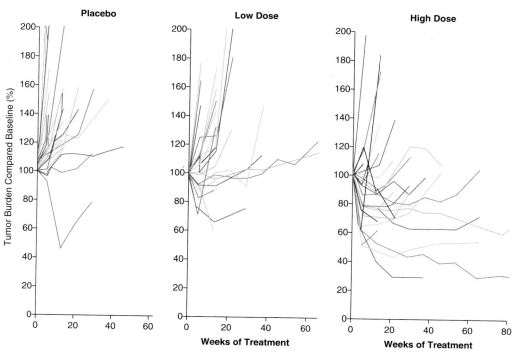

**Figure 2.** Total measured tumor burdens (sum of products of perpendicular diameters) depicted as percentage of baseline burden for each patient with metastatic renal cancer during treatment with either placebo, 3 mg/kg of bevacizumab, or 10 mg/kg of bevacizumab. Reproduced with permission from Yang.[19]

vascularized tumors, prompting a rationale for patients to continue receiving anti-VEGF therapy.[20] Follow-up from the above trial demonstrated four patients who have continued with therapy without progression for 3 to 5 years.[19] Toxic effects in these patients were limited to proteinuria with normal renal function.

A further concerning toxicity is the increased risk for life-threatening bleeding for patients receiving bevacizumab. The destabilizing effect on abnormal vasculature and probable impacts on wound healing have provoked minor restrictions on the use of this drug. This is seen in the increased rate of epistaxis observed in all studies using bevacizumab. Life-threatening bleeding has to date not been associated with the use of this drug in RCC specifically. However, it requires careful consideration for patients requiring therapeutic anticoagulation or planned surgical procedures. Because the half-life of bevacizumab is approximately 20 days, advanced preparation is required before anticipated surgical procedures. Further, as angiogenesis is implicated in would healing, delay in restarting bevacizumab after major surgical procedures is warranted.

Bevacizumab has been further investigated in RCC in combination with an antiepidermal growth factor receptor (EGFR) strategy. Preclinical investigation in human RCC xenograft models of bevacizumab and erlotinib, a small molecule EGFR inhibitor, has demonstrated a potential benefit of combination therapy on tumor growth inhibition.[21] A clinical trial in metastatic RCC with bevacizumab, 10 mg/kg intravenously every 2 weeks, in combination with erlotinib, 150 mg/d, reported a 25% partial response rate.[22] However, recent findings from a randomized, multicenter, double-blind phase 2 trial further evaluating bevacizumab with or without erlotinib as first-line therapy for metastatic RCC showed that patients in both arms had similar progression-free survival (PFS) and response rates. The bevacizumab monotherapy arm demonstrated a 14% objective response rate and an 8.5 median PFS. These data suggest that erlotinib does not add to the efficacy of bevacizumab, and perhaps that the single-agent activity of bevacizumab had been underestimated in the previous trial.

Two phase 3 trials have investigated the addition of bevacizumab to an initial systemic therapy, interferon-α, in RCC.[23] In a CALGB trial, patients with metastatic clear cell RCC without prior systemic therapy were randomized to either low-dose interferon-α 2b (Intron A, Schering-Plough, Kenilworth, NJ), 9 MU subcutaneously three times weekly, or the same dose and schedule of interferon-α 2b in combination with bevacizumab, 10 mg/kg intravenously every 2 weeks. The primary end point of the trial is overall survival, designed to detect an improvement in median survival from 13 months for interferon-α alone to 17 months for the combination. Results from this and an identical European trial demonstrated a prolonged PFS in the bevacizumab-containing arm (Table 1).[24] Importantly, this trial collected baseline tumor samples from the vast majority of patients. Analysis of tumor genomic changes (eg, *VHL* status) and RNA/protein expression is planned and will be associated with clinical outcome. Such an analysis is vital to further understand the molecular features of tumors that make them respond to a specific therapeutic targeting approach.

Combination studies are also evaluating the feasibility of combining bevacizumab with an inhibitor of the tyrosine kinase portion of the VEGF receptor, sorafenib (Nexavar®, Bayer Pharmaceuticals, West Haven, CT, and Onyx Pharmaceuticals, Richmond, CA). The rationale for this type of vertical inhibition of the VEGF axis is more complete VEGF blockade. Two separate trials are underway.[27] Preliminary results suggest that less than full monotherapy doses are tolerable with notable hand foot syndrome and hypertension limiting dose escalation. Other toxicities include fatigue, diarrhea, elevated lipase levels, proteinuria, and thrombocytopenia. Two phase 1 trials of bevacizumab in combination with another VEGF receptor (VEGFR) inhibitor, sunitinib malate (Sutent®, Pfizer Inc, New York, NY), are also underway.

## VEGF-Trap

VEGF-Trap (Regeneron Pharmaceuticals, Tarrytown, NY and Sanofi-Aventis, Bridgewater, NJ) is a fusion protein composed of the human VEGFR-1 (Flt-1) extracellular immunoglobulin (Ig) domain 2, and the VEGFR-2 (KDR) extracellular Ig domain 3 fused to human IgG1 Fc molecule (Figure 3).[28] VEGF-Trap thus acts as a soluble decoy receptor to bind VEGF and disrupt subsequent VEGF signaling. VEGF-Trap binds to VEGF with great affinity ($K_d \approx 1$ pM). This molecular approach thus neutralizes all forms of VEGF. VEGF-Trap also binds another angiogenic protein, placental growth factor. In cultured endothelial cell assays, VEGF-Trap has demonstrated inhibition of VEGF-induced VEGFR-2 phosphorylation and endothelial cell proliferation. In xenograft models, VEGF-Trap–treated mice exhibited significant inhibition of tumor growth and tumor-associated angiogenesis in implanted rat C6 glioma, human A673 rhabdomyosarcoma, and mouse B16 melanoma tumors compared with vehicle-treated controls.[28,29] A murine xenograft model using human Wilms tumor cell line derived from embryonic renal cells (SK-NEP-1 cells) demonstrated involution of existing mature vasculature and apoptosis of endothelial cells coincident with regression of established tumors after VEGF-Trap treatment.[30] A significant regression of established tumors was demonstrated in VEGF-Trap treated animals (mean tumor weight decreased by 79.3% by day 36; $p < .0002$).

Two phase 1 studies with VEGF-Trap have been reported in patients with refractory solid tumors. In the first trial, 38 patients, including nine patients with metastatic RCC, received subcutaneous dose(s) of VEGF-Trap followed 4 weeks later by 6 weekly injections (escalating dose levels of 0.025, 0.05, 0.1, 0.2, 0.4, and 0.8 mg/kg) or 6 twice weekly (0.8 mg/kg) injections.[31] Drug-related grade 3 adverse events included hypertension and proteinuria, strongly suggesting these toxicities reflect a class effect of VEGF neutralization. No anti–VEGF-Trap antibodies were detected. Although no objective responses have been observed in this trial, 14 of 24 assessable patients, including five of six patients at the highest dose level, have maintained stable disease for 10 weeks.

In the second trial, 30 patients have been treated with intravenous VEGF-Trap every 2 weeks at one of five dose levels (0.3, 1.0, 2.0, 3.0, and 4.0 mg/kg).[32,33] Drug-related grade 3 adverse events included arthralgia and fatigue. One patient with metastatic RCC has maintained stable disease for more than 11 months (at the 1.0 mg/kg dose level). Vascular imaging with dynamic contrast-enhanced magnetic resonance imaging performed at baseline and after 24 hours indicated effects on tumor perfusion at higher dose levels ($\geq 2.0$ mg/kg). Complete binding of circulating VEGF was documented at higher dose levels ($\geq 2.0$ mg/kg). Further investigation is ongoing via a cooperative group trial that randomizes metastatic patients with RCC who have failed one prior tyrosine kinase inhibitor (eg, sunitinib,

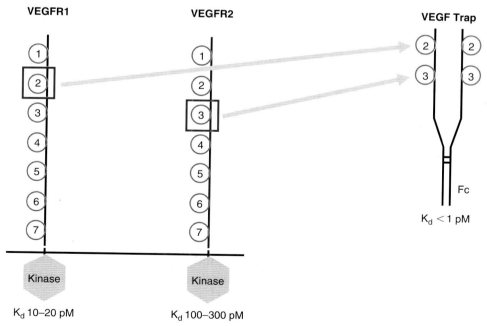

**Figure 3.** Vascular endothelial growth factor (VEGF)-Trap structure. VEGF-Trap is a fusion protein comprised of the human VEGF receptor VEGFR-1 (Flt-1), extracellular immunoglobulin (Ig) domain 2, and the VEGFR-2 (KDR) extracellular Ig domain 3 fused to human IgG1 Fc molecule.

| Table 1.  DATA FROM KEY TRIALS OF BEVACIZUMAB IN METASTATIC RENAL CELL CARCINOMA | | | | |
| --- | --- | --- | --- | --- |
| Agent/Study | Study Design/Patient Population | Number of Patients | PFS (months)* | ORR |
| Bevacizumab (VEGF ligand-binding antibody) | | | | |
| Bevacizumab vs placebo[18] | Randomized phase II in cytokine-refractory | 116 | 4.8 vs 2.5 | 10 vs 0% |
| Bevacizumab vs bevacizumab + erlotinib[35] | Randomized phase II in previously untreated | 104 | 8.5 vs 9.9 | 13 vs 14% |
| Bevacizumab + IFNA vs IFNA[24] | Randomized phase III in previously untreated | 638 | 10.2 vs 5.4 | 31 vs 13% |
| Bevacizumab + IFNA vs IFNA[23] | Randomized phase III in previously untreated | 732 | 8.5 vs 5.2 | 26 vs 13% |

IFN = interferon; ORR = ; VEGF = vascular endothelial growth factor; PFS = progression-free survival; RCC = renal cell carcinoma.

sorafenib) to 1 mg/kg or 4 mg/kg IV every 2 weeks. There is cross over at progression for the low-dose group to high-dose therapy with the primary end point of PFS at 8 weeks.

## VEGF Antisense

Although not a VEGF ligand-binding approach, VEGF antisense aims to reduce VEGF levels and has been tested in RCC. This molecule is a 21-mer antisense oligonucleotide that targets the coding region of VEGF mRNA and thus reduces VEGF-A (and some VEGF-C, VEGF-D) levels. A phase I trial of 51 patients (including 7 patients with RCC) of VEGF antisense IV every day × 5, repeated every other week from 15 mg/m² to 250 mg/m² was conducted.[34] VEGF levels decreased by a median of 33% and VEGF-C levels by 11%. There was a greater decline at higher doses and in patients with RCC. No obvious clinical activity in RCC was reported. Further investigation is ongoing.

## FUTURE DIRECTIONS

Several ongoing clinical trials with VEGF binding strategies have been described above, which will further define the activity of this approach as monotherapy and combination therapy in metastatic RCC. As the clinical development of these active agents has far outpaced the ability to study them in preclinical models and/or with correlative studies, the understanding of the exact antitumor mechanism(s) is imprecise. It is believed that inhibition of

VEGF results in decreased angiogenesis, ie, reducing the growth of new blood vessels to prevent tumor growth, yet the sometimes dramatic tumor shrinkage observed may imply an additional effect on the tumor cell itself. In addition, the effect of these agents on existing blood vessel function and mechanism(s) of toxicity are not well characterized. Additional translational studies involving blood and tissue-based correlates, along with functional imaging of tumor blood flow, is needed.

## CONCLUSIONS

*VHL* gene inactivation is a frequent event in clear cell RCC, leading indirectly to overexpression of VEGF. Strategies to bind or neutralize the VEGF protein have undergone investigation in metastatic RCC. These strategies target the secreted ligand itself, removing the source of receptor activation to effectively inhibit this pathway of angiogenesis signal transduction (Figure 4). These approaches differ substantially from the therapeutic approaches, which target the activation of specific cell surface receptors and although the drugs function as a class of agents, the molecular signature of upstream versus downstream signaling strategies will be distinct. These differences will be of further clinical importance as the sequential and combination treatment strategies move to the forefront in RCC. Bevacizumab has demonstrated prolongation of time to progression versus placebo and continues to be investigated in multiple RCC settings. VEGF-Trap is a distinct VEGF-binding molecule with evidence of effects on vasculature leading to tumor regression.

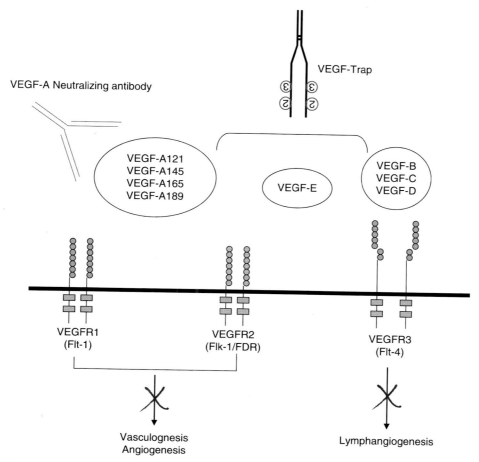

**Figure 4.** Activities of vascular endothelial growth factor (VEGF) ligand-binding agents on VEGF receptor activation. VEGF neutralizing antibody therapy is targeted to the VEGF-A isoforms and effectively removes these ligands from interacting with their cognate receptors, interfering with VEGF receptor (VEGFR) signaling to promote angiogenesis. VEGF-Trap differs by acting as a dual-specificity mimic of VEGFR-1 and VEGFR-2, which together have affinity for all classes of VEGF-secreted ligands.

Results from ongoing and future trials will more precisely define the role of VEGF binding strategies in RCC.

## REFERENCES

1. Ross R. Angiogenesis. Successful growth of tumours. Nature 1989;339:16–7.

2. Tsuzuki Y, Fukumura D, Oosthuyse B, et al. Vascular endothelial growth factor (VEGF) modulation by targeting hypoxia-inducible factor-1α—hypoxia response element—VEGF cascade differentially regulates vascular response and growth rate in tumors. Cancer Res 2000;60:6248–52.

3. Li VW, Folkerth RD, Watanabe H, et al. Microvessel count and cerebrospinal fluid basic fibroblast growth factor in children with brain tumours. Lancet 1994;344:82–6.

4. Brattstrom D, Bergqvist M, Larsson A, et al. Basic fibroblast growth factor and vascular endothelial growth factor in sera from non-small cell lung cancer patients. Anticancer Res 1998;18:1123–7.

5. Yamamoto Y, Toi M, Kondo S, et al. Concentrations of vascular endothelial growth factor in the sera of normal controls and cancer patients. Clin Cancer Res 1996; 2:821–6.

6. Salven P, Ruotsalainen T, Mattson K, Joensuu H. High pre-treatment serum level of vascular endothelial growth factor (VEGF) is associated with poor outcome in small-cell lung cancer. Int J Cancer 1998;79:144–6.

7. Gasparini G, Toi M, Gion M, Verder, et al. Prognostic significance of vascular endothelial growth factor protein in node-negative breast carcinoma. J Natl Cancer Inst 1997;89:139–47.

8. Guidi AJ, Abu-Jawdeh G, Berse B, et al. Vascular permeability factor (vascular endothelial growth factor) expression and angiogenesis in cervical neoplasia. J Natl Cancer Inst 1995;87:1237–45.

9. Shweiki D, Itin A, Soffer D, Keshet E. Vascular endothelial growth factor induced by hypoxia may mediate hypoxia-initiated angiogenesis. Nature 1992;359:843–45.

10. Iliopoulos O, Levy AP, Jiang C, et al. Negative regulation of hypoxia-inducible genes by the von Hippel-Lindau protein. Proc Natl Acad Sci USA 1996;93:10595–99.

11. Presta LG, Chen H, O'Connor SJ, et al. Humanization of an anti-vascular endothelial growth factor monoclonal antibody for the therapy of solid tumors and other disorders. Cancer Res 1997;57:4593–9.

12. Gordon MS, Margolin K, Talpaz M, et al. Phase I safety and pharmacokinetic study of recombinant human anti-vascular endothelial growth factor in patients with advanced cancer. J Clin Oncol 2001;19:843–50.

13. Hsei V, Deguzman GG, Nixon A, Gaudreault J. Complexation of VEGF with bevaczumab decreases VEGF clearance in rats. Pharm Res 2002;19:1753–6.

14. Wang Y, Fei D, Vanderlaan M, Song A. Biological activity of bevacizumab, a humanized anti-VEGF antibody in vitro. Angiogenesis 2004;7:335–45.

15. Gerber HP, Ferrara N. Pharmacology and pharmacodynamics of bevacizumab as monotherapy or in combination with cytotoxic therapy in preclinical studies. Cancer Res 2005;65:671–80.

16. Rowe DH, Huang J, Kayton ML, et al. Anti-VEGF antibody suppresses primary tumor growth and metastasis in an experimental model of Wilms' tumor [discussion]. J Pediatr Surg 2000;35:30–3.

17. Willett CG, Boucher Y, di Tomaso E, et al. Direct evidence that the VEGF-specific antibody bevacizumab has antivascular effects in human rectal cancer. Nat Med 2004;10:145–7.

18. Yang JC, Haworth L, Sherry RM, et al. A randomized trial of bevacizumab, an anti-vascular endothelial growth factor antibody, for metastatic renal cancer. N Engl J Med 2003;349:427–34.

19. Yang JC. Bevacizumab for patients with metastatic renal cancer: an update. Clin Cancer Res 2004;10:6367S-70S.

20. Yuan F, Chen Y, Dellian M, et al. Time-dependent vascular regression and permeability changes in established human tumor xenografts induced by an anti-vascular endothelial growth factor/vascular permeability factor antibody. Proc Natl Acad Sci USA 1996;93:14765–770.

21. Viloria-Petit A, Crombet T, Jothy S, et al. Acquired resistance to the antitumor effect of epidermal growth factor receptor-blocking antibodies in vivo: a role for altered tumor angiogenesis. Cancer Res 2001;61:5090–101.

22. Spigel DR, Hainsworth JD, Sosman JA, et al. Bevacizumab and erlotinib in the treatment of patients with metastatic renal carcinoma (RCC): update of a phase II multicenter trial. Proc Am Soc Clin Oncol 2005;23:4540.

23. Rini BI, Halabi S, Rosenberg J, et al. Bevacizumab plus interferon-$\alpha$ vs interferon-$\alpha$ Monotherapy in patients with metastatic RCC: Results of CALGB 90206. J Clin Onc (in press).

24. Escudier B, Pluzanska A, Koralewski P, et al. Bevacizumab plus interferon alpha-2a for treatment of metastatic renal cell carcinoma: a randomized, double-blind Phase III trial. Lancet 2007;320:2103–2111.

25. Gabrilovich DI, Cunningham HT, Carbone DP. IL-12 and mutant P53 peptide-pulsed dendritic cells for the specific immunotherapy of cancer. J Immunother Emphasis Tumor Immunol 1996;19:414–8.

26. Gabrilovich DI, Ishida T, Nadaf S, Ohm JE, et al. Antibodies to vascular endothelial growth factor enhance the efficacy of cancer immunotherapy by improving endogenous dendritic cell function. Clin Cancer Res 1999;5:2963–70.

27. Posadas E, Kwitkowski V, Liel M. Clinical synergism from combinatorial VEGF signal transduction inhibition in patients with advanced solid tumors—early results from a phase I study of sorafenib (BAY 43-9006) and bevacizumab. Eur J of Cancer Suppl 2005;3:419.

28. Holash J, Davis S, Papadopoulos N, et al. VEGF-trap: a VEGF blocker with potent antitumor effects. Proc Natl Acad Sci USA 2002;99:11393–8.

29. Konner J, Dupont J. Use of soluble recombinant decoy receptor vascular endothelial growth factor trap (VEGF trap) to inhibit vascular endothelial growth factor activity. Clin Colorectal Cancer 2004;4 Suppl 2:S81–5.

30. Frischer JS, Huang J, Serur A, et al. Effects of potent VEGF blockade on experimental Wilms tumor and its persisting vasculature. Int J Oncol 2004;25:549–53.

31. Dupont J, Koutcher J. Phase I and pharmacakinetic study of VEGF trap administered subcutaneously (sc) to patients with advanced solid malignancies. Proc Am Soc Clin Oncol 2004;23.

32. Dupont JR, Spriggs D. Safety and pharmacokinetic of intravenous VEGF Trap in a phase I clinical trial of patients with advanced solid tumors. Proc Am Soc Clin Oncol 2005;23.

33. Lockhart A, Muruganandham M, Schwartz L. Pharmacodynamic indicators of VEGF trap activity in patients with advanced solid tumors. Clin Cancer Res 2005;11.

34. Levine AM, Tulpule A, Quinn DI, et al. Phase I study of antisense oligonucleotide against vascular endothelial growth factor: decrease in plasma vascular endothelial growth factor with potential clinical efficacy. J Clin Oncol 2006;24:1712–9.

35. Bukowski RM, Kabbinavar F, Figlin RA, et al. Bevacizumab with or without erlotinib in metastatic renal cell carcinoma (RCC). J Clin Oncol, 2006 ASCO Annual Meeting Proceedings (Post-Meeting Edition) Part I. 2006;24:4523.

36. Kashmiri SV, De Pascalis R, Gonzales NR, Schlom J. SDR grafting-a new approach to antibody humanization. Methods 2005;36:25–34.

# Antivascular Endothelial Growth Factor Therapy In Metastatic Renal Cell Carcinoma

## Therapeutic Inhibition of Vascular Endothelial Growth Factor Receptors

OLIVIER RIXE, MD, PHD
BERTRAND BILLEMONT, MD
FREDERIC THIBAULT, MD
HASSAN IZZEDINE, MD, PHD

The identification of the von Hippel-Lindau (*VHL*) tumor suppressor gene, whose loss of function results both in the predisposition to cancer in the von Hippel-Lindau disease and in sporadic renal cell carcinoma (RCC), has played an important role in our understanding of the human renal carcinogenesis.[1] A chromosome arm 3p loss has been observed in most clear cell RCC, and somatic alterations of the *VHL* gene have been found in this subtype and consisted of point mutations in 42 to 57% and promoter methylation in 5 to 19% of these tumors.[2] The VHL protein (pVHL) plays an important role in angiogenesis by binding to the α subunit of the hypoxia-inducible factor (HIF), a key transcription factor for hypoxia-dependent gene expression. Disruption of *VHL* results in an abnormal accumulation of HIF, leading to the upregulation of downstream genes such as vascular endothelial growth factor (VEGF), platelet-derived growth factor (PDGF), erythropoietin (EPO), and transforming growth factor α (TGF-α).[3] These factors can bind to their receptors, members of the tyrosine kinase transmembrane protein family, containing extracellular ligand-binding domains and intracellular catalytic domains, inducing tumor growth, survival, and angiogenesis.[4] Inhibiting these targets in concert might be expected to result in broad antitumor efficacy and particularly with the use of antiangiogenic therapy.[5] Despite progress accomplished in other tumor types, metastatic RCC (mRCC) remains one of the most therapy-resistant cancers. The modest benefit of biologic therapy with interferon-α (IFN-α) and/or interleukin-2 could be demonstrated only in good-prognosis patients.[6]

Alternative strategies have been developed to inhibit angiogenesis in metastatic RCC. From the historical studies of the 1970s conducted by Folkman,[5] the first major advance in the inhibition of angiogenesis in humans has been reached with the development of humanized monoclonal antibodies against VEGF (Bevacizumab, Avastin).[7] One of the key steps toward a deeper understanding of the biology of angiogenis was the discovery and the characterization of the tyrosine kinase VEGF receptors by

Ferrara's and Williams's group in 1992.[8–9] After the identification of the crucial role of both receptors (and additional kinases involved in angiogenesis and cell proliferation including PDGF receptors), several small molecules targeting the VEGF receptors (VEGFRs) were further developed beyond anti-VEGF monoclonal antibodies (Figure 1). Synthetic small (low molecular weight) compounds have been specifically designed to target and inhibit the VEGFRs and have shown outstanding activity in mRCC in the early phase of their development. Sorafenib and sunitinib are the leading molecules, registered by the North American and European agencies in 2006 and early 2007, whereas several additional molecules are curently under clinical development including axitinib and pazopanib.

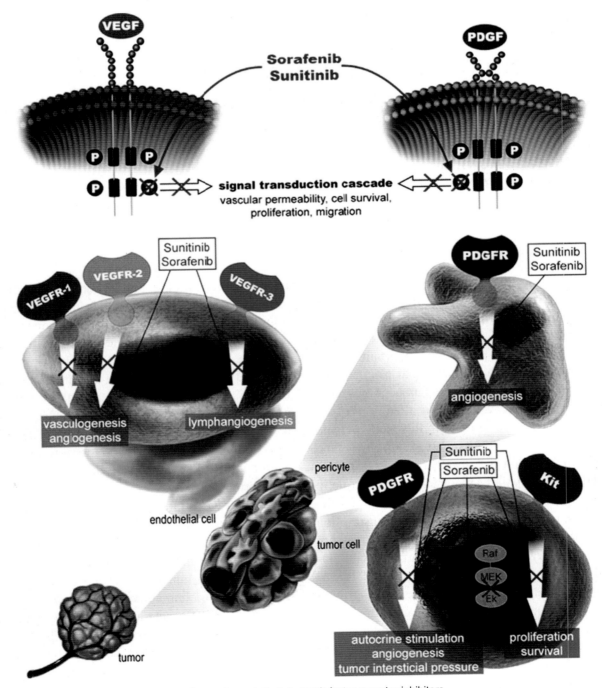

**Figure 1.** Mechanisms of action of vascular endothelial growth factor receptor inhibitors.

In this chapter, we will review the characteristics of the molecules directed against the VEGFRs, the radical modifications in the standard care of mRCC, and the potential unlimited perspectives opened by those new tools. However, the limits reached with those strategies including the development of acquired drug resistance and the potential severe drug toxicities will also be evaluated in this article.

## VEGFR INHIBITORS: SUNITINIB AND SORAFENIB

### Sunitinib

Sunitinib (Sunitinib malate; SU11248; SUTENT; Pfizer Inc, New York, NY) is an orally bioavailable, oxindole, (Figure 2) multitargeted tyrosine kinase inhibitor with antitumor and antiangiogenic activities. Sunitinib is a multitargeted agent and has been identified as a potent inhibitor of VEGFRs (types 1 to 3), PDGFR (α and β), as well as FLT3, Kit (stem-cell factor [SCF] receptor) colony-stimulating factor type 1 and glial cell-line derived neurotrophic factor receptor (RET), in both biochemical and cellular assays.[10]

### Mechanism of Action

Mechanisms of action of antiangiogenic inhibitors including VEGFR inhibitors remain controversial.

Both cytotoxicity and cytostasis have been reported.[11] This activity is related to the structure of the molecule and the spectrum of kinase inhibition, restricted to the VEGF receptors or enlarged to additional targets (ie, PDGF receptors (PDGFRs), c-Kit).

Direct antitumor effects on tumor cells has been suggested with sunitinib, such as wild type and activated mutants of FLT3, expressed by acute myeloid leukemia-derived cell lines[12] and small cell lung cancer-derived cell lines expressed c-Kit. Indirect antitumour activity of sunitinib by inhibition of VEGFR expressed on endothelial cells and PDGFR-β on pericytes or stromal cells has also been demonstrated, and its full antitumour efficacy was associated with prolonged (at least 12 to 24 hours), but not continuous, inhibition of VEGFR-2 and PDGFR-β.[13]

### Clinical Pharmacology

In vitro metabolism studies have demonstrated that sunitinib was primarily metabolized by cytochrome CYP3A4, resulting in the formation of a major, pharmacologically active *N*-desethyl metabolite, SU012662. This metabolite has been shown to be equipotent to the parent compound in biochemical tyrosine kinase and cellular proliferation assays, acting toward VEGFR, PDGFR, and c-Kit.[14] Pharmacokinetic (PK) data indicate good oral absorption,

| Compound | Structure | VEGFR | PDGFR | c-Kit | CSF1R | Flt-3 | FGFR | Other kinases |
|----------|-----------|-------|-------|-------|-------|-------|------|---------------|
| Sorafenib | 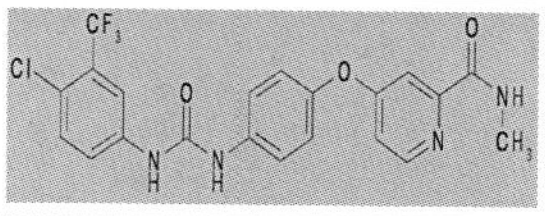 | ■ | ■ | ■ | ■ | ■ | ■ | Yes (Raf kinase) |
| Sunitinib | 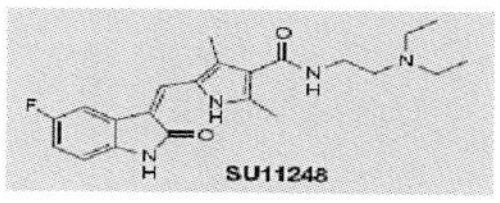 | ■ | ■ | ■ | ■ | ■ | ■ | yes (Lck,PhK,CK1) |
| Axitinib | 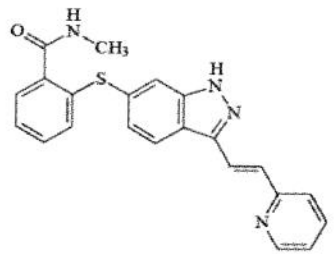 | ■ | ■ | ■ | ■ | ■ | ■ | ? |
| Pazopanib | 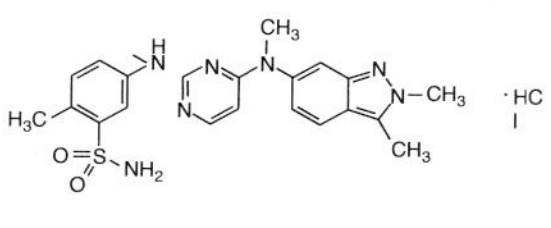 | ■ | ■ | ■ | ■ | ■ | ■ | ? |

■ : high affinity;   ■ : low affinity;   ■ : absence of affinity.

**Figure 2.** Structure and spectrum of activity of vascular endothelial growth factor receptor inhibitors.

a prolonged half-life for sunitinib (~40 hours) and its active metabolite, SU12662 (~80 hours) and linear kinetics at the doses that are administered. PK/pharmacodynamic data from animal studies showed that target plasma concentrations of sunitinib plus SU012662 capable of inhibiting PDGFR-β and VEGFR-2 phosphorylation were established in the range of 50 to 100 ng/mL. From 2 phase II mRCC trials including 169 patients, a population PK analysis was performed to assess the exposure-response relationship between PK and tumor volume changes, clinical response, and time to tumor progression (TTP). Plasma clearance decreased by an average of 28% in mRCC patients relative to healthy volunteers. Improved clinical response and longer time to progression were associated with greater AUCs. Within 12 weeks of treatment, mean tumor volume decreased by 24 to 32% in each trial. The authors concluded that over the first 12 weeks of treatment at 50 mg daily on schedule 4/2, increased exposure was associated with improved clinical response and decreased tumor volumes.[15] However, at higher doses (≥ 75 mg/d), tumor responses were often associated with reduced intratumoral vascularization and central tumor necrosis, eventually resulting in organ perforation or fistula (Table 1).[16]

## Clinical Experience in Renal Cell Carcinoma

Objective responses have been observed in the phase I study conducted in Gustave-Roussy Institute.[16] In this early phase of development including 22 patients, objective responses have been documented in 3 out of 6 mRCC. On the basis of both this report and a solid biological background, 2 single arm consecutive phase II studies involving patients with advanced RCC who had experienced failure of prior cytokine-based therapy have been conducted. Patients received the Gustave-Roussy schedule (50 mg/d continuously for 4 weeks followed by 2 weeks off) until they met withdrawal criteria or had progressive disease.

In the first study,[17] 63 patients with advanced RCC were enrolled. The majority of patients had clear cell carcinoma (87%). An outstanding response rate of 40% (using RECIST criteria) was reported with a duration of response of 8.7 months. Median duration of treatment was 9 months, and median time to progression was 8.7 months. To confirm the antitumor activity and safety observed in the first phase II trial, a second larger study[18] involving 106 patients with clear cell mRCC was conducted. The objective response rate was 39%. Of

| Features | Sunitinib | Sorafenib |
|---|---|---|
| Mechanism of action | Multitargeted tyrosine kinase inhibitor, including VEGFR (types 1 to 3), and PDGFR, (α and β). | Multitargeted tyrosine kinase inhibitor, including VEGFR (types 1 to 3), and PDGFR, (α and β) and Raf kinase. |
| Route of administration | Oral | Oral |
| Metabolization | CYP3A4 | CYP3A4 |
| Glucuronidation | — | UGT1A9 |
| Metabolite | Predominent active metabolite:SU12662 | Non-modified active sorafenib (70%) and 8 different metabolites |
| Elimination | Fecal (> 60%) | Fecal (> 75%) |
| Half-life | 40 to 60 h | 25 to 28 h |
| Protein binding | 90% (metabolite) | 99% (sorafenib) |
| Principal toxicities | Asthenia, diarrhea, nausea, mucositis, hypertension. | Rash, hand-foot skin reaction, diarrhea, asthenia. |
| Dosing in organ dysfunction | Absence of recommendations | Absence of recommendations |

Table 1. SUNITINIB AND SORAFENIB: PRINCIPAL CHARACTERISTICS

PDGFR = platelet-derived growth factor receptor; VEGFR = vascular endothelial growth factor receptor.

the 106 patients who were evaluable for efficacy analyses, 36 patients achieved partial response (34%; 95% CI; 25 to 44%), and a median progression-free survival of 8.3 months as evaluated by an independant third-party assessment. No complete responses were reported in these 2 studies.

An international randomized phase III trial[19] compared the efficacy and safety of sunitinib to IFN-α in first-line treatment of patients with advanced RCC. In all, 690 untreated patients with clear cell advanced RCC were randomized 1:1 to receive sunitinib (375 patients) (6-week cycles: 50 mg orally once daily for 4 weeks followed by 2 weeks off) or IFN-α (375 patients) (6-week cycles: subcutaneous injection 9 MU given 3 times weekly). Ninety percent of the patients had prior nephrectomy. Median progression-free survival was 47.3 weeks (95% CI: 40.9) for sunitinib versus 24.9 weeks (95% CI: 21.9, 37.1) for IFN-α [hazard ratio = 0.394 (95% CI: 0.297, 0.521) ($p < .000001$)]. The objective response rate by a third-party independent review was 37% for sunitinib versus 9% for IFN-α ($p < .000001$). The objective response rate by investigator assessment was 31 % (95% CI: 30.9, 40.8) for sunitinib versus 6% (95% CI: 6.1, 12.1) for IFN-α ($p < .000001$). Eight percent withdrew from

the study due to adverse event on sunitinib arm versus 13% on IFN-α arm. The toxicity profile was similar to that reported in second-line trials. On the basis of this large phase III study, sunitinib is one of the standard therapies for first-line treatment of mRCC (Table 2).

## Sorafenib

Although sorafenib was initially developed as a Raf kinase inhibitor, the lack of activity in the clinic against tumors with mutant Raf and the demonstration of activity against renal cell carcinoma led to an emphasis on its ability to target VEGFR-1, -2, -3, and PDGFR-β[20] (see Figure 2). In vivo studies with the murine renal adenocarcinoma (Renca) model and a VHL knockout model have demonstrated a cytostatic effect for sorafenib, albeit a very modest growth delay.[21] In these preclinical models documenting a mechanism of cytostasis proved to be difficult. For example, when colon xenografts treated with sorafenib were examined, no significant inhibition of ERK 1/2 phosphorylation was detected indicating that the MAPK pathway was not blocked, and therefore, could not be correlated with tumor stasis.[22] An effect on angiogenesis was considered because

| Compound | Trial | Characteristics of the Trial | Control Arm | Number of Patients | Objective Response: Number of Patients* | Disease Free Survival (mo) | Reference |
|---|---|---|---|---|---|---|---|
| Sunitinib | Phase II | Single arm, second-line therapy, Any RCC histology | — | 63 | CR = 0, PR = 25 (40%) | 8.7 | Motzer et al[17] |
| Sunitinib | Phase II | Single arm, second-line therapy | — | 106 | CR = 0, PR = 36 (34%) | 8.3 | Motzer et al[18] |
| Sunitinib | Phase III | Randomized study, First-line therapy | Interferon | 335 | CR = 0, PR = 103 (31%) | 11 (vs 5.1), $p < .001$ | Motzer et al[19] |
| Sorafenib | Phase II | Randomized study, first-line therapy | Interferon | 189 | CR/PR = 5% | 5.7 (vs 5.6), N.S. | Szczylik et al[68] |
| Sorafenib | Phase II | Randomized study, second-line therapy | Placebo | 202 | CR = 0, PR² = 73 | 6 (vs 1.5), $p = .0087$ | Ratain et al[28] |
| Sorafenib | Phase III | Randomized study, second-line therapy | Placebo | 451 | CR = 1, PR = 43 (10%) | 5.5 (vs 2.8), $p < 0.001$ | Escudier etal[29] |

Table 2. CLINICAL ACTIVITY OF SUNITINIB AND SORAFENIB

*Objective responses by independent review.

†Tumor shrinkage of > or = 25%.

sorafenib, as discussed above, exhibits significant activity against receptor tyrosine kinases that are known to promote angiogenesis. In some models, inhibition of angiogenensis was inferred from data showing reduced MVA and MVD in the treated tumors compared with controls.[23] However, sorafenib has also demonstrated significant tumor regression in the human breast carcinoma MDA-MB-231 xenografts. Significant necrosis in sorafenib treated mice was visualized by hematoxylin staining at day 5 after initiation of drug treatment associated with a significant reduction of pERK 1/2 and Ki-67, and 50% to 80% inhibition of MVA and MVD, but despite extensive studies, a convincing mechanistic explanation for tumor stasis remains elusive.[24] A recent report suggests a potential unexpected role of the peroxisome proliferation-activated receptor-β (PPARβ) implicated in tumorigenesis, in constraining tumor endothelial cell proliferation and blocking tumor growth, via the *Cdkn1c* gene encoding the cell cycle inhibitor *p57* (Kip2).[25] A recent study[26] reported that transcriptional induction of the tumor suppressors TGF-β and Notch contribute to *p21* induction and epithelial cytostasis.

### Clinical Experience in Renal Cell Carcinoma

In 4 phase I studies that enrolled 163 patients, low objective antitumor activity as defined by RECIST criteria was documented (2 partial responses in kidney cancer and hepatocellular carcinoma), but disease stabilization associated with clinical benefit encouraged investigators to continue drug development.[27] A multicentre phase II randomized discontinuation study (RDT) was conducted to distinguish cytostatic antitumor activity from spontaneous indolent tumor growth in metastatic clear cell carcinoma.[28] In this trial, all patients were initially treated with sorafenib. Using modified WHO criteria, a total of 73 patients (36%) had tumor shrinkage after 12 weeks, which was ≥ 25% of their baseline, whereas 51 patients (25%) showed either tumor growth ≥ 25% or other evidence of progression. Sixty-nine patients (34%) had tumor measurements that remained within 25% of baseline levels (stable disease). Sixty-five out of these 69 patients were randomized to continue either therapy or begin placebo.

A significant improvement in progression-free survival was reported for the patients who continued on sorafenib compared with those who received the placebo (24 vs 6 weeks, $p = .0087$). In a subsequent phase III study, 903 patients with metastatic clear cell carcinoma whose disease had progressed following 1 prior systemic treatment were randomized to receive either sorafenib 400 mg bid ($n = 451$) or placebo ($n = 452$). Treatment with sorafenib prolonged progression-free survival (5.5 months for sorafenib vs 2.8 months for placebo, $p < .01$): a result interpreted by many as an evidence of cytostasis. As in the RDT, objective responses were recorded with partial responses reported as the best objective response in 10% of patients receiving sorafenib and in 2% of those receiving placebo ($p < .001$). However, tumor shrinkage was observed in 76% of the patients in the sorafenib treated cohort, suggesting cytotoxic properties for sorafenib.[29] Finally, patients in the sorafenib group had a significantly better quality of life than patients receiving IFN. The primary end point was overall survival (OS), but the first interim analysis of OS did not reach the prespecified O'Brien-Fleming boundaries for statistical significance. Furthermore, additional evidence of a cytotoxic effect may be found when higher doses are used. A recent abstract reported significant tumor shrinkage associated with a high response rate (52% objective response with 16% complete response) in metastatic clear cell carcinoma treated with sorafenib of 600 or 800 mg bid (see Table 2).[30]

## SECOND GENERATION VEGFR INHIBITORS: AXITINIB, PAZOPANIB AND OTHER MOLECULES

### Axitinib (AG-013736)

Axitinib is an orally available imidazole derivative that acts as a potent inhibitor of angiogenesis mediated by the multitarget receptor tyrosine kinase inhibition including VEGFRs 1 and 2, PDGFR-β, and c-Kit[31] (see Figure 2).

In the phase I study, 36 patients received doses ranging from 5 to 30 mg bid.[32] The dose-limiting toxicities were hypertension and stomatitis with other toxicities, including diarrhea, fatigue, nausea, and vomiting. The recommended dose for phase II study was 5 mg bid, administered in the fasti state. Two objective responses were reported in patients with RCC. The activity and safety of axitinib was evaluated in mRCC patients after failure of a prior cytokine-based regimen (interleukin-2 and/or IFN-α).[33] Fifty-two patients were enrolled in a multicenter phase II study. In the final analysis completed in January 2007, two complete and 21 partial responses were reported for an ORR of 44.2% (95% CI: 30.5 to 58.7). Median response duration was 23 months (95% CI: 20.9, not estimable). Additionally, 22 patients (42.3%) demonstrated stable disease > 8 weeks, including 13 (25%) with stable disease for ≥ 24 weeks. Median TTP was 15.7 months (95% CI: 8.4 to 23.4), and median OS was 29.9 months (95% CI: 20.3, not estimable).

### Pazopanib (GW786034)

Pazopanib (see Figure 2) is another multitargeted, oral inhibitor of VEGFR, PDGFR-α and β, and c-Kit. Objective responses have been documented in the phase I study for patients with metastastic RCC.[34] In a randomized phase II study conducted by Hutson and colleagues in patients with mRCC (in first line or after immunotherapy failure), a high response rate was reported in the preliminary results reported on the first 60 patients.[35] The high response rate, the profile of toxicity, and the spectrum of kinase inhibition show similar characteristics with axitinib. Phase III studies are planned in mRCC.

### Other Molecules

Several other VEGFR inhibitors are currently under development. Most of these compounds are evaluated in phase I studies and have not yet reached the phase II evaluation. Several reports already suggest activity in mRCC in this early phase of development. BMS-582664, ZK261991 are multitargeted inhibitors of VEGF receptors.[36,37] LY2401401 is inhibiting VEGFreceptors, PDGF receptors, kit, and flt-3.[38] BMS690514 and ZD 6474 are potent dual inhibitors of VEGF and EGF receptors.[39,40] By contrast, the spectrum of activity of Ki23057 and CT-322 are limited to VEGFR-2.[41,42]

AZD2171, a potent orally available inhibitor of VEGFR, PDGF-β, and c-KIT, is currently evaluated in refractory, mRCC patients.[43] PTK787/ZK222584 (valatinib) is an oral, potent inhibitor of VEGFR, PDGFR-β, and c-Kit. A phase I study of PTK787 demonstrated that a dose of 1200mg/d was well tolerated with activity in patients with mRCC.[44] XL880 is an oral, small molecule inhibitor of several kinases including VEGFRs.[45] A recent phase I trial including 25 patients demonstrated a confirmed PR in 1 patient with papillary renal carcinoma. A phase II study of XL880 is currently enrolling patients with hereditary or sporadic papillary renal carcinoma.

## TOXICITY

Side effects of VEGFR inhibitors are moderate compared with other therapies. They are usually manageable and regressive upon drug withdrawal. Since the preclinical studies and the early phases of clinical development, class side effects have been extensively reported, including hypertension, gastrointestinal, and skin toxicities. However, the mechanisms related to those toxicities are often poorly understood.

### Sunitinib

In the 2 phase II RCC trials,[17,18] the most common side effects that were noted were fatigue (74%), diarrhea (55%), nausea (54%), and mucositis and stomatitis (53%). In most instances, symptoms improved with dose modification. Similar observations were reported in the phase III study.

The exact mechanisms of sunitinib toxicities are not well understood. Several additional toxicities have also been reported as skin and/or hair depigmentation or discoloration.[46]

Concomitant treatment with potent CYP3A4 inducers or inhibitors should be avoided when sunitinib is used in patients with cancer to limit treatment failure and risk of side effects. Otherwise, dose reductions (to a minimum of 25 mg/d) or increase doses (to a maximum of 87.5 mg/d) are more likely to be considered when sunitinib is administered concomitantly with strong CYP3A4 inhibitors or inducers, respectively.[15,47]

## Sorafenib

In the phase III study, drug-related toxicities for sorafenib versus placebo were rash (34%), diarrhea (33%), hand-foot skin reactions (27%), and fatigue (26% versus 23% in the placebo arm). Thirty percent of the patients experienced a grade 3 or 4 toxicity compared with 22% on placebo. Of note, in the randomized phase II study versus IFN, the patients treated with sorafenib had a significantly better quality of life.

## HYPERTENSION AND PROTEINURIA

Hypertension and proteinuria have been experienced in patients treated with VEGFRs inhibitors. This class effect toxicity is frequent, potentially severe, and has been extensively reported and studied since the phase I studies.[48]

## Incidence of Hypertension and Proteinuria With Sunitinib, Sorafenib, and Axitinib (Table 3)

### Sunitinib

In the phase I dose ranging study of sunitinib in 28 patients, hypertension was seen in 5 patients and required antihypertensive treatment for grade ¾ hypertension in 2 patients treated at doses ≥ 75 mg/d.[16] Hypertension usually occurred after 3 to 4 weeks of treatment. In the phase 2 study, hypertension was only seen in 3 out of 163 patients (5%) treated with 50 mg daily for advanced RCC, and only 1 patient experienced grade 3 or 4 hypertension.[19] Information regarding incidence of proteinuria was not available in those studies.

### Sorafenib

In a phase II study, hypertension was seen in 86 out of 202 patients (43%) and was the most common grade ¾ adverse event noted in 62 patients (31%). Antihypertensive therapy was needed in 46% of patients. No patients died from toxicity.[28] In the Veronese study,[48] an increase of > 10 mm Hg or > 20 mm Hg in systolic blood pressure (SBP) was reported in 75% (15/20) and 60% (12/20) of treated patients, respectively, compared with their baseline value (mean = 130.6 mm Hg) after 3 weeks of therapy. The mean diastolic blood pressure (DBP) showed a corresponding significant increase (mean = +9.3 mm Hg). One patient required antihypertensive medication after 6 weeks of treatment (BP increased to 200/100 mm Hg). In the phase III evaluation of sorafenib versus placebo in mRCC, drug-related adverse events hypertension of any grade was noted in 8 versus < 1%.[29] Information regarding proteinuria was not available in those studies.

### Axitinib

A phase I dose-escalating study in 36 patients with advanced cancers revealed that hypertension was the primary dose limiting toxicity, which is occurring in 22 patients (61%). The majority of cases (18 patients)

| Compound | Trial | Number of Patients | Hypertension | | Proteinuria | | Kidney Biopsy | Reference |
|---|---|---|---|---|---|---|---|---|
| | | | All Grade (%) | Grade ¾ (%) | All Grade (%) | Grade ¾ % | | |
| Sunitinib | Phase I | 28 | 18 | 7 | NA | NA | ND | Faivre et al[16] |
| Sunitinib | Phase II (RCC) | 63 | 5 | 2 | NA | NA | ND | Motzer et al[17] |
| Sunitinib | Phase III | 375 | 24 | 8 | NA | NA | ND | Motzer et al[19] |
| Sorafenib | Phase II (RCC) | 202 | 43 | 31 | NA | NA | ND | Ratain et al[28] |
| Sorafenib | Phase III (RCC) | 384 | 8 | 1 | NA | NA | ND | Escudier et al[29] |
| Axitinib | Phase I | 36 | 61 | 30 | 8 | 3 | ND | Rugo et al[33] |
| Axitinib | Phase II (RCC) | 52 | 33 | 12 | NA | NA | ND | Rixe et al[34] |
| Vatalanib | Phase I | 43 | 16 | 9 | NA | NA | ND | Morgan et al[45] |

Table 3. INCIDENCE OF HYPERTENSION AND PROTEINURIA IN SELECTED TRIALS WITH VASCULAR ENDOTHELIAL GROWTH FACTOR RECEPTOR INHIBITORS.

NA = not available; ND = not done; RCC = renal cell carcinoma.

were controlled easily with antihypertensive medications. The incidence and severity of hypertension was dose dependent. In the first 2 cohorts in which doses ranged from 10 mg qd to 30 mg bid, hypertension was observed in all 10 patients and was grade 3 or 4 in severity in 5 patients. Asymptomatic proteinuria was observed in 7 out of 10 patients enrolled in the first 2 cohorts, including 2 patients with grade 3 proteinuria by dipstick. The protocol was subsequently amended to exclude patients with proteinuria > 500 mg over 24 hours; dose adjustment or suspension of AG-013736 dosing was required for patients with proteinuria ≥ 1 g over 24 hours. In subsequent cohorts treated at lower doses of AG-013736, proteinuria was less frequent and less severe. Of these 26 patients, only 6 developed grade 1 or 2 proteinuria after starting the treatment.[32]

In the phase II study, hypertension was the most common grade ¾ adverse event affecting 6 patients (12%), with 1 patient discontinuing treatment due to worsening hypertension.[33]

## General Considerations on Hypertension and Proteinuria

Veronese and colleagues[49] and Sane and colleagues[50] have contributed to the understanding of the mechanisms underlying anti-VEGF–induced hypertension. A drop in BP with angiogenic growth factor administration in animal and human studies has been observed. VEGF exerts a stimulatory effect on endothelial nitric oxide (NO) production by upregulating endothelial nitric oxide synthase expression. NO in turn has a vasodilatory effect. A possible explanation for the occurrence of hypertension associated with anti-VEGF may be related to the inhibition of NO. Preclinical data support this hypothesis; in vitro evaluation of axitinib in human umbilical vein endothelial cells revealed inhibition of endothelial nitric oxide synthase activity.[51] Sane and colleagues also hypothesized that VEGF may have effects on the renin-angiotensin system, particularly on receptors associated with angiotensin I and angiotensin II. However, Veronese and colleagues find no statistically significant changes in humoral factors (catecholamines, endothelin I, urotensin II, renin, and aldosterone) in patients treated with sorafenib, although there was a statistically significant inverse

relationship between decreases in catecholamines and increases in SBP, suggesting a secondary response to BP elevation.

Another important factor contributing to hypertension and independently predicting cardiovascular risk is aortic stiffness as measured from aortic pulse wave velocity and central aortic augmentation index.[52] This was demonstrated in Veronese study. However, increased vascular stiffness can be demonstrated in any group of hypertensive patients, and it is not possible to determine whether increase in vascular stiffness is the direct result of sorafenib or whether it is the consequence of hypertension and only indirectly caused by the drug. Further study of this area is necessary to understand the mechanism of hypertension-related angiogenesis inhibitors.

Proteinuria is also a class effect of VEGF antagonists, but its mechanism is not as well understood as that of hypertension. Dose-response effects of AG-013736 observed in Kamba and colleagues study indicates the involvement of a VEGF-related mechanism.[53] Proteinuria is reversible by stopping the VEGF antagonist, and with BP control, suggesting a possible hemodynamic effect. In clinical trials, patients developed proteinuria or experienced worsening of preexisting proteinuria. Only 2 kidney biopsies are reported in patients treated with Tyrosine Kinase Inhibitors (TKIs) and who experienced proteinuria. One patient showed thrombotic microangiopathy under sunitinib treatment.[54] The other patient revealed acute interstitial nephritis related to sorafenib treatment in the setting of facial erythema.[55] However, as renal biopsies were not largely performed in those patients who developed proteinuria during antiangiogenic therapy, these hypotheses still need to be confirmed.

Podocytes, which are the specialized cells that make up the support structures of the functional glomerulus, normally express VEGF at high levels. A dual effect of VEGF can be spoken of in the sense that too little or too much VEGF expression induces proteinuria. Eremina and colleagues demonstrated that podocyte specific heterozygosity for VEGF resulted in renal disease by 2.5 weeks of age in mice.[56] The renal disease was characterized by nephrotic range proteinuria, endotheliosis, and hyaline deposits that resemble the pathologic lesions seen in renal biopsies from patients with preeclampsia[57] whose subsequent development can be predicted by increased levels of soluble VEGF receptor 1 protein (sFlt-1) and reduced levels of PlGF.[58] Mesangial cell contribution to glomeruli was also abnormal in mice that is specifically lacking PDGFB in endothelial cells. Together, these results suggest that endothelial cells, which are recruited, matured, and maintained by VEGF from podocytes, promote further maturation of podocytes and mesangial cells and formation of a functional glomerulus. Endothelial cell maintenance through regulated VEGF levels is crucial for continued glomerular function in adults.

## FURTHER DEVELOPMENTS

VEGFR inhibitors have clearly revolutionized the treatment of mRCC and were approved based on robust phase II and III studies. However, several major questions need to be addressed in prospective trials. To enhance efficacy, combination studies with conventional agents (ie, IFN) or agents that target non-VEGF pathways, such as mTOR inhibitors, are currently under development (Table 4). Combination of VEGFR inhibitors (such as sorafenib) and bevacizumab appears to provide preliminary high antitumour

### Table 4.  DRUG-COMBINATION TRIALS WITH VEGFRS INHIBITORS

| Compounds and Design | Phase | Status | Site/Sponsor | Number of Patients | Characteristics |
|---|---|---|---|---|---|
| Sunitinib (4 weeks on/2 weeks off), + Bevacizumab (J1 = J14)l | I | Active | USA/pfizer | 36 | Metastatic cell rena carcinoma |
| Sunitinib (J1 to J14), + Gemcitabine (J1, J8, and J21) | II | Not yet active | USA | 36 | Sarcomatoid and/or poor-risk patients with metastatic renal cell carcinoma |
| Sunitinib (4 weeks on/2 weeks off), + Bevacizumab (J1 = J14), vs sunitinib vs bevacizumab | II | Not yet active | USA/pfizer/ genetech | 81 | Sunitinib-refractory patients with metastatic renal cell carcinoma |
| Sunitinib (4 weeks on/2 weeks off), + Rad001 weekly schedule | I | Active | USA/novartis | 28 | Metastatic renal cell carcinoma |
| Sunitinib (4 weeks on/2 weeks off), + Iressa | I and II | Not yet active | USA/pfizer | 69 | Metastatic renal cell carcinoma |
| Sunitinib (4 weeks on/2 weeks off), + cG250 | I | Not yet active | USA/pfizer/wilex | 14 | Metastatic renal cell carcinoma |
| Sunitinib (4 weeks on/2 weeks off), + Temsirolimus | I and II | Closed | USA/wyeth | 124 | Metastatic renal cell carcinoma |
| Sunitinib (4 weeks on/2 weeks off), + Erlotinib | II | active | USA/NCI | 49 | Metastatic renal cell carcinoma |
| Sorafenib (400 mg bid), + Rad001 (2.5 mg/d) | I and II | active | USA/novartis | 55 | Metastatic renal cell carcinoma |
| Sorafenib (400 mg bid) with or without interferon α-2b | II | Not yet active | USA/NCI | 80 | Metastatic renal cell carcinoma |
| Sorafenib (400 mg bid), + Rad001 (2.5mg/d) | II | active | USA/novartis | 73 | Metastatic renal cell carcinoma |
| Sorafenib (400 mg bid), + gemcitabine, + capecitabine | II | active | Spain/Spanish Oncology Genito-Urinary Group | 40 | Metastatic renal cell carcinoma |

activity, with manageable toxicities with respect to the schedule recommended in the phase I study.

Quest for identification of predictive factors of VEGFR inhibitors activity is currently explored including clinical or biologic parameters (erytropoietin level, proteomic, or genomic analysis). For example, a preliminary report has demonstrated a potential relationship between the occurence of hypertension and sunitinib activity.[59]

Cross-resistance between antiangiogenic compounds needs to be adressed. Preliminary preclinical studies tried to demonstrate the putative mechanisms involved in acquired resistance to antiangiogenic compounds.[60] They underline the heterogeneity of endothelial cell, angiogenic factors and tumor cells, the role of the microenvironment, the potential angiogeno-independence, or the implication of PK parameters (Table 5). In the clinical setting, 2 major studies have evaluated the cross-resistance between VEGFR inhibitors (Table 6) and offer some perspectives for the management of second- and third-line therapy. In the study conducted by Rini and colleagues,[61] mRCC patients with sorafenib-refractory disease were treated by axitinib in a multicenter, open-label, phase II trial. Partial response was observed in 6 of 42 evaluable patients (14%; 95% CI: 5 to 29%), stable disease was observed in 15 patients (36%), progressive disease was experienced by 12 patients (29%); and 9 patients (21%) withdrew due to adverse events. Overall, 57% of patients experienced some degree of tumor regression. Similar observations have been reported by Sablin and colleagues when sunitinib activity has been evaluated after sorafenib failure or sorafenib after sunitinib progression.[62] In the limit of the small number of evaluated patients, those preliminary data are demonstrating a different spectrum of activity from those VEGFR inhibitor agents and putative different mechanisms of acquired resistance in a subset population.

**Table 5. DRUG RESISTANCE AND VASCULAR ENDOTHELIAL GROWTH FACTOR RECEPTOR INHIBITORS**

| Mechanism | Example |
|---|---|
| Endothelial cell heterogeneity | Cytogenetic endothelial cell alterations (endothelial cells with tumor DNA) |
| Angiogenic factors heterogeneity | Secretion of alternative angiogenic growth factors |
| Tumor cells heterogeneity | Vascular mimicry from tumor cells |
| Role of microenvironment | Pericytes and stroma cells interactions |
| Angiogeno-independance | Vascular cooptation, Tumor cell tubulisation, Vasculogenesis, Intussusception |
| Pharmacokinetic parameters | Drug interactions, Decreased biodisponibility (necrosis) |

**Table 6. CROSS-RESISTANCE TRIALS WITH VASCULAR GROWTH FACTOR RECEPTOR INHIBITORS. IN METASTATIC RENAL CELL CARCINOMA**

| Compound | Trial | Previous Treatment | Number of Patients | Objective Response Rate (%) | Reference |
|---|---|---|---|---|---|
| Axitinib | Phase II | Sorafenib failure | 42 | 14 | Rini et al[62] |
| Sorafenib | Retrospective study | Sunitinib failure | 22 | 17, 6 | Sablin et al[63] |
| Sunitinib | Retrospective study | Sorafenib failure | 68 | 22, 7 | Sablin et al[63] |

Methodological issues have been addressed with the development of this new class of compounds. Objective response using RECIST criteria may not be appropriate for evaluation.[63] Possible new end points might include changes in tumor markers, measures of target inhibition, time to tumor progression, or proportion of patients with evidence of tumor progression at a defined time point after the initiation of the treatment. Additional dynamic imaging can improve the determination of the activity of the compound, using positron emission tomography scanning, DCI-magnetic resonance imaging, dynamic-computed tomography scan, and ultrasonography.[64,65] Novel trial designs, such as the RDT, represent innovative new approaches that have been successfully tested with sorafenib. Any trial design should also focus on identifying clinical side effects that may be associated with drug activity. Finally, the activity of VEGFRs inhibitors in nonclear cell RCC is warranted, and specific trials are underway in histology subtype based on specific genetic modifications (ie, *c-Met* alterations in papillary carcinoma).[67]

## CONCLUSION

On the basis of robust biological rationale, the rapid clinical development of VEGFR inhibitors over the past few years has radically modified the natural course of patients with mRCC. Sunitinib is a treatment of choice (in addition to bevacizumab-IFN) for most good and intermediate-risk patients. After cytokine failure, sorafenib is a treatment of choice, although data with sunitinib in this setting are convincing but not randomized. Data with sorafenib and sunitinib in the poor-risk group are still anecdotal and remain to be extended. However, radical cure of the metastatic disease has not been achieved with this new class of agents. We must continue offering to our patients to be treated in the framework of clinical trials (combined with translational studies) to find the answers of unaddressed questions.

## ACKNOWLEDGMENT

We thank the Fondation Martine Midy, Paris, France for technical assistance in preparation of this manuscript.

## REFERENCES

1. Richard S, Graff J, Lindau J, Resche F. Von Hippel-Lindau disease. Lancet 2004;363:1231–4.
2. Cohen HT, McGovern FJ. Renal-cell carcinoma. N Engl J Med 2005;353:2477–90.
3. Kim WY, Kaelin WG. Role of VHL gene mutation in human cancer. J Clin Oncol 2004;22:4991–5004.
4. Schlessinger J. Cell signaling by receptor tyrosine kinases. Cell 2000;103:211–25.
5. Folkman J. Tumor angiogenesis: therapeutic implications. N Engl J Med 1971;285:1182–6.
6. Motzer RJ, Bacik J, Schwartz LH, et al. Prognostic factors for survival in previously treated patients with metastatic renal cell carcinoma. J Clin Oncol 2004;22:454–463.
7. Yang C, Haworth L, Sherry RM, et al. A randomized trial of bevacizumab, an anti-vascular endothelial growth factor antibody, for metastatic renal cancer. N Engl J Med 2003;349:427–34.
8. de Vries C, Escobedo JA, Ueno H, et al. The fms-like tyrosine kinase, a receptor for vascular endothelial growth factor. Science 1992;255:989–91.
9. Rini BI, Small EJ. Biology and clinical development of vascular endothelial growth factor-targeted therapy in renal cell carcinoma. J Clin Oncol 2005;23:1028–43.
10. Mendel DB, Laird AD, Xin X, et al. In vivo antitumor activity of SU11248, a novel tyrosine kinase inhibitor targeting VEGF and PDGF receptors: determination of a pharmacokinetic/pharmacodynamic relationship. Clin Cancer Res 2003;9:327–37.
11. Abrams TJ, Murray LJ, Pesenti E, et al. Preclinical evaluation of the tyrosine kinase inhibitor SU11248 as a single agent and in combination with "standard of care" therapeutic agents for the treatment of breast cancer. Mol Cancer Ther 2003;2:1011–21.
12. Gilliland DG, Griffin JD. Role of FLT3 in leukemia. Curr Opin Hematol 2002;9:274–81.
13. Gale NW, Yancopoulos GD. Growth factors acting via endothelial cell-specific receptor tyrosine kinases: VEGFs, angiopoietins, and ephrins in vascular development. Genes Dev 1999;13:1055–66.
14. Baratte S, Sarati S, Frigerio E, et al. Quantitation of SU11248, an oral multi-target tyrosine kinase inhibitor, and its metabolite in monkey tissues by liquid chromatograph with tandem mass spectrometry following semi-automated liquid-liquid extraction. J Chromatogr A 2004;1024:87–94.
15. Houk BE, Amantea M, Motzer RJ, et al. Pharmacokinetics (PK) and efficacy of sunitinib in patients with metastatic renal cell carcinoma (mRCC). Journal of Clinical Oncology, 2006 ASCO Annual Meeting Proceedings Part I. Vol 24, No. 18S.
16. Faivre S, Delbaldo C, Vera K, et al. Safety, pharmacokinetic, and antitumor activity of SU11248, a novel oral multitarget tyrosine kinase inhibitor, in patients with cancer. J Clin Oncol 2006;24:25–35.
17. Motzer RJ, Michaelson MD, Redman BG, et al. Activity of SU11248, a multitargeted inhibitor of vascular endothelial growth factor receptor and platelet derived growth factor receptor, in patients with metastatic renal cell carcinoma. J Clin Oncol 2006;24:16–24.

18. Motzer RJ, Rini BI, Bukowski RM, et al. Sunitinib in patients with metastatic renal cell carcinoma. JAMA 2006;295:2516–24.

19. Motzer RJ, Hutson TE, Tomczak P, et al. Sunitinib versus interferon α in metastatic renal-cell carcinoma. N Engl J Med 2007;356:115–24.

20. Flaherty KT. Sorafenib in renal cell carcinoma. Clin Cancer Res 2007;13(2 Pt 2):747S–752S.

21. Chang YS, Adnane J, Trail PA, et al. Sorafenib (BAY 43-9006) inhibits tumor growth and vascularization and induces tumor apoptosis and hypoxia in RCC xenograft models. Cancer Chemother Pharmacol 2007;59:561–74.

22. Wilhelm SM, Carter C, Tang L, et al. BAY 43-9006 exhibits broad spectrum oral antitumor activity and targets the RAF/MEK/ERK pathway and receptor tyrosine kinases involved in tumor progression and angiogenesis. Cancer Res 2004;64:7099–109.

23. Liu L, Cao Y, Chen C, et al. Sorafenib blocks the RAF/MEK/ERK pathway, inhibits tumor angiogenesis, and induces tumor cell apoptosis in hepatocellular carcinoma model PLC/PRF/5. Cancer Res 2006;66:11851–8.

24. Carter CA, Chen C, Brink C, et al. Sorafenib is efficacious and tolerated in combination with cytotoxic or cytostatic agents in preclinical models of human non-small cell lung carcinoma. Cancer Chemother Pharmacol 2007;59:183–95.

25. Muller-Brusselbach S, Komhoff M, Rieck M, et al. Deregulation of tumor angiogenesis and blockade of tumor growth in PPARβ-deficient mice. EMBO J 2007;26:3686–98.

26. Campos AH, Wang W, Pollman MJ, Gibbons GH. Determinants of Notch-3 receptor expression and signaling in vascular smooth muscle cells: implications in cell-cycle regulation. Circ Res 2002;91:999–1006.

27. Kane RC, Farrell AT, Saber H, et al. Sorafenib for the treatment of advanced renal cell carcinoma. Clin Cancer Res 2006;12:7271–8.

28. Ratain MJ, Eisen T, Stadler WM, et al. Phase II placebo-controlled randomized discontinuation trial of sorafenib in patients with metastatic renal cell carcinoma. J Clin Oncol 2006;24:2505–12.

29. Escudier B, Eisen T, Stadler WM, et al. TARGET Study Group. Sorafenib in advanced clear-cell renal-cell carcinoma. N Engl J Med 2007;356:125–34.

30. Amato RJ, Harris P, Dalton M, et al. A phase II trial of intrapatient dose-escalated sorafenib in patients (pts) with metastatic renal cell cancer (MRCC). J Clin Oncol 2007 ASCO Annual Meeting Proceedings Part I. Vol 25, No. 18S, 5026.

31. Wickman G, Hallin M, Salansky KA, et al. Further characterization of the potent VEGF/PDGF receptor tyrosine kinase inhibitor AG-013736 in preclinical tumor models for its antiangiogenesis and antitumor activity [abstract 3780]. Proc Am Assoc Cancer Res 2003;44:865.

32. Rugo HS, Herbst RS, Liu G, et al. Phase I trial of the oral antiangiogenesis agent AG-013736 in patients with advanced solid tumors: pharmacokinetic and clinical results. J Clin Oncol 2005;23:5474–83.

33. Rixe O, Bukowski RM, Michaelson MD, et al. Axitinib treatment in patients with cytokine-refractory metastatic renal-cell cancer: a phase II study. Lancet Oncol 2007;8:975–84.

34. Kumar R, Knick VB, Rudolph SK, et al. Pharmacokinetic-pharmacodynamic correlation from mouse to human with pazopanib, a multikinase angiogenesis inhibitor with potent antitumor and antiangiogenic activity. Mol Cancer Ther 2007;6:2012–21.

35. Sonpavde G, Hutson TE. Pazopanib: a novel multitargeted tyrosine kinase inhibitor. Curr Oncol Rep 2007;9:115–9.

36. Ayers M, Fargnoli J, Lewin A, et al. Discovery and validation of biomarkers that respond to treatment with brivanib alaninate, a small-molecule VEGFR-2/FGFR-1 antagonist. Cancer Res 2007;67:6899–906.

37. Thierauch K, Haberey M, Hess-Stumpp H, et al. ZK 261991, a Novel VEGFR Inhibitor for Tumour Therapy. [abstract 2135]. Proceedings of the American Association for Cancer Research Annual Meeting; 2007 Apr 14–18; Los Angeles, CA. Philadelphia: AACR; 2007.

38. Considine EL, Bloem LJ, Burkholder TP, et al. A novel and orally bioavailable inhibitor of angiogenesis can be distinguished from other multi-targeted kinase inhibitors by its unique target selectivity profile and preclinical efficacy [abstract 1623]. Proceedings of the American Association for Cancer Research Annual Meeting; 2007 Apr 14–18; Los Angeles, CA. Philadelphia: AACR; 2007.

39. Wong TW, Ayers M, Emanuel S, et al. Inhibition of EGFR/HER2 signaling in tumor cells and VEGFR2 activity in tumor endothelium contribute to the preclinical antitumor activity of BMS-690514 [abstract 4007]. Proceedings of the American Association for Cancer Research Annual Meeting; 2007 Apr 14-18; Los Angeles, CA. Philadelphia: AACR; 2007.

40. Tamura T, Minami H, Yamada Y, et al. A phase I dose-escalation study of ZD6474 in Japanese patients with solid,malignant tumors. J Thorac Oncol 2006;1:1002–9.

41. Sakurai K, Yamada N, Yashiro M, et al. A novel angiogenesis inhibitor, Ki23057, is useful for preventing the progression of colon cancer and the spreading of cancer cells to the liver. Eur J Cancer 2007.

42. Carvajal IM, Short S, Zhou Y, et al. CT-322: A specific VEGFR-2-blocking protein therapeutic agent with activity in pre-clinical tumor models comparable to pan-specific tyrosine kinase receptor inhibitors sutent and sorafenib [abstract 4189]. Proceedings of the American Association for Cancer Research Annual Meeting; 2007 Apr 14–18; Los Angeles, CA. Philadelphia: AACR; 2007.

43. Wedge SR, Kendrew J, Hennequin LF, et al. AZD2171: a highly potent, orally bioavailable, vascular endothelial growth factor receptor-2 tyrosine kinase inhibitor for the treatment of cancer. Cancer Res 2005;65:4389–400.

44. Morgan B, Thomas AL, Drevs J, et al. Dynamic contrast-enhanced magnetic resonance imaging as a biomarker for the pharmacological response of PTK787/ZK 222584, an inhibitor of the vascular endothelial growth factor receptor tyrosine kinases, in patients with advanced colorectal cancer and liver metastases: results from two phase I studies. J Clin Oncol 2003;21:3955–64.

45. Eder J, Appleman L, Heath E, et al. A phase I study of a novel spectrum selective kinase inhibitor (SSKI), XL880, administered orally in patients (pts) with advanced solid tumors (STs). Proc Am Soc Clin Oncol 2006;24:3041.

46. Robert C, Soria JC, Spatz A, et al. Cutaneous side-effects of kinase inhibitors and blocking antibodies. Lancet Oncol 2005;6:491–500.

47. Bello C, Houk B, Sherman L, et al. Effect of rifampin on the pharmacokinetics of SU11248 in healthy volunteers [abstract 3078]. J Clin Oncol, ASCO Annual Meeting Proceedings Vol 23, No. 16S, Part I of II (June 1 Supplement), 2005.

48. Izzedine H, Rixe O, Billemont B, et al. Angiogenesis inhibitor therapies: focus on kidney toxicity and hypertension. Am J Kidney Dis 2007;50:203–18.

49. Veronese ML, Mosenkis A, Flaherty KT, et al. Mechanisms of hypertension associated with BAY 43-9006. J Clin Oncol 2006;24:1363–9.

50. Sane DC, Anton L, Brosnihan KB. Angiogenic growth factors and hypertension. Angiogenesis 2004;7:193–201.

51. Tang JR, Markham NE, Lin YJ, et al. Inhaled nitric oxide attenuates pulmonary hypertension and improves lung growth in infant rats after neonatal treatment with a VEGF receptor inhibitor. Am J Physiol Lung Cell Mol Physiol 2004;287:L344–51.

52. Safar ME, Levy BI, Struijker-Boudier H. Current perspectives on arterial stiffness and pulse pressure in hypertension and cardiovascular diseases. Circulation 2003;107:2864–9.

53. Kamba T, Tam BY, Hashizume H, et al. VEGF-dependent plasticity of fenestrated capillaries in the normal adult microvasculature. Am J Physiol Heart Circ Physiol 2006;290:H560–76.

54. Kapiteijn E, Brand A, Kroep J, Gelderblom H. Sunitinib induced hypertension, thrombotic microangiopathy and reversible posterior leukencephalopathy syndrome. Ann Oncol 2007;18:1745–7.

55. Izzedine H, Brocheriou I, Rixe O, Deray G. Interstitial nephritis in a patient taking sorafenib. Nephrol Dial Transplant 2007;22:2411.

56. Eremina V, Sood M, Haigh J, et al. Glomerular-specific alterations of VEGF-A expression lead to distinct congenital and acquired renal diseases. J Clin Invest 2003r;111:707–16.

57. Kincaid-Smith, P. The renal lesion of preeclampsia revisited. Am J Kidney Dis 1991;17:144–8.

58. Levine RJ, Maynard SE, Qian C, et al. Circulating angiogenic factors and the risk of preeclampsia. N Engl J Med 2004;350:672–83.

59. Rixe O, Billemont B, Izzedine H. Hypertension as a predictive factor of Sunitinib activity. Ann Oncol 2007;18:1117.

60. Glade Bender J, Cooney EM, Kandel JJ, Yamashiro DJ. Vascular remodeling and clinical resistance to antiangiogenic cancer therapy. Drug Resist Updat 2004;7:289–300.

61. Rini BI, Wilding GT, Hudes G, et al. Axitinib (AG-013736; AG) in patients (pts) with metastatic renal cell cancer (RCC) refractory to sorafenib. Journal of Clinical Oncology, ASCO Annual Meeting Proceedings. 2007;25:No 18S, 5032.

62. Sablin MP, Bouaita L, Balleyguier C, et al. Sequential use of sorafenib and sunitinib in renal cancer: Retrospective analysis in 90 patients. Journal of Clinical Oncology, 2007 ASCO Annual Meeting Proceedings Part I 2007;25:No. 18S (June 20 Supplement), 5038.

63. Korn EL, Arbuck SG, Pluda JM, et al. Clinical trial designs for cytostatic agents: are new approaches needed? J Clin Oncol 2001;19:265–72.

64. Hylton N. Dynamic contrast-enhanced magnetic resonance imaging as an imaging biomarker. J Clin Oncol 2006;24:3293–8.

65. Rixe, J. Meric, J. Bloch, et al. Surrogate markers of activity of AG-013736, a multi-target tyrosine kinase receptor inhibitor, in metastatic renal cell cancer (RCC). Journal of Clinical Oncology, 2005 ASCO Annual Meeting Proceedings 2005;23:No. 16S, Part I of II (June 1 Supplement), 3003.

66. Pouessel D, Culine S. Targeted therapies in metastatic renal cell carcinoma: the light at the end of the tunnel. Expert Rev Anticancer Ther 2006;6:1761–7.

67. Zbar B, Tory K, Merino M, et al. Hereditary papillary renal cell carcinoma. J Urol 1994;151:561–6.

68. Szczylik C, Demkow T, Staehler M, et al. Randomized phase II trial of first-line treatment with sorafenib versus interferon in patients with advanced renal cell carcinoma: Final results. Journal of Clinical Oncology, 2007 ASCO Annual Meeting Proceedings Part I. Vol 25, No. 18S (June 20 Supplement), 2007: 5025.

# mTOR Pathway Biology in Renal Cell Carcinoma

WILLIAM Y. KIM
ANDREW J. ARMSTRONG
DANIEL J. GEORGE, MD

The biology of renal cell carcinoma (RCC) has been elucidated recently, resulting in a greater understanding of cellular pathways that lead to disease growth and progression. One of these pathways, that involving mammalian target of rapamycin (mTOR) and related signaling proteins, has been identified as a key component of RCC pathophysiology.

## The *PTEN* Tumor Suppressor Gene

The *PTEN* tumor suppressor gene (also called *MMAC1*, mutated in multiple advanced cancers 1, or *TEP1*, TGFβ-regulated and epithelial cell enriched phosphatase) is one of the most frequently deleted genes in human cancer with somatic deletions or mutations identified in a high percentage of glioblastomas, endometrial, and prostate tumors.[1] Inherited germline mutations of *PTEN* have been described in several autosomal dominantly inherited hamartomatous syndromes including Cowden Syndrome and Bannayan-Riley-Ruvalcaba syndrome.[2] The *PTEN* gene product encodes a dual specificity phosphatase active against the lipid substrate phosphoinositide-3,4,5 triphosphate (PIP3), a product of the phosphoinositide-3 kinase (PI3K).[3] PTEN thus serves as a direct antagonist to PI3K activity.

PI3K exists as a heterodimer consisting of a p85 regulatory subunit and a p110 catalytic subunit and regulates growth and proliferation downstream of growth factor receptor tyrosine kinases (RTKs) and G-protein-coupled receptors.[4] PI3K activity is tightly regulated in normal cells and ordinarily exists within the cytoplasm as a preformed, inactive complex of p85 and p110. PI3K can be activated by several different mechanisms including direct mutation, loss of PTEN, and activation of RTKs. Additionally, however, direct binding of PI3K by mutated, membrane bound Ras can induce activation of PI3K.[5,6] In the canonical pathway, activation of RTKs by extracellular ligands or oncogenic mutation results in their autophophorylation and the subsequent recruitment of PI3K to the cytoplasmic domain of the receptor (Figure 1). This recruitment leads to increased PI3K activity not only by increasing its physical proximity to its substrates but also by inducing a conformation change in its structure.

Studies examining *PTEN* knockout mice have reported that *PTEN* expression is necessary for embryonic development. Mice deficient in both alleles of *PTEN* are early embryonic lethal and die before embryonic day 7.5.[7] Additionally, although classic models of oncogenic transformation require that both alleles of a tumor suppressor gene to be lost to gain the selective proliferation and survival advantage necessary for overt malignant transformation, contrary to this paradigm, inactivation of a single *PTEN* allele can result in both a growth advantage and defects in apoptosis.[8] Thus, *PTEN* haploinsufficiency results in functional consequences and its role in the early pathogenesis of human tumors may have been underestimated. On the basis of these studies in murine models and the detection of inactivating mutations and deletions in human cancers, PTEN appears to have a clear well-established role in tumorigenesis.

## Akt/Protein Kinase B (PKB)

The crucial downstream target of PI3K is the Akt serine-threonine kinase family, members of which include Akt1, 2, 3 (also known as PKB).[9] Generation of PIP3 at the inner leaflet of the plasma membrane following PI3K activation results in the recruitment of phosphoinositol 3-dependent kinase 1 (PDK1),

2 (PDK2), and Akt. PDK1 then phosphorylates and partially activates Akt. However, secondary phosphorylation of Akt by PDK2 is required for its maximal activation. Akt is itself a serine, threonine kinase, and phosphorylation and subsequent inactivation of downstream target genes (including GSK3, NF-kB, BCL-2, FOXO proteins, hDM2, and TSC2) result in the promotion of cell proliferation (cell number), cell growth (cell size), and cell survival. Thus, cells lacking *PTEN* have elevated levels of PI3K activity resulting in increased Akt activity (Figure 1).

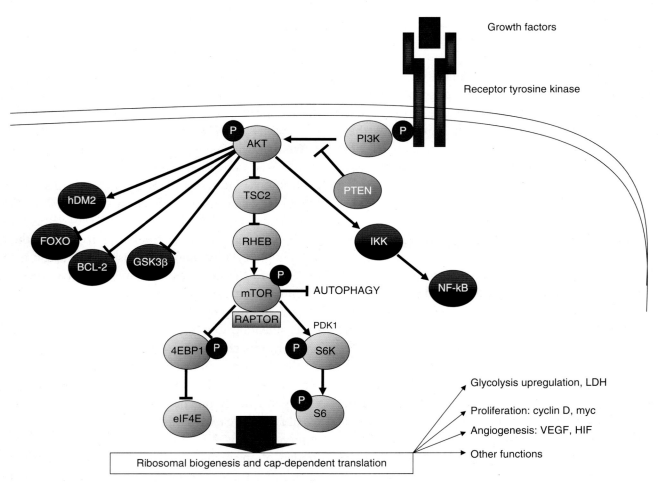

**Figure 1.    The PI3K/Akt/mammalian target of rapamycin (mTOR) Pathway.** The mTOR/Raptor complex integrates signals from a diverse set of stimuli. In the canonical pathway, activation of receptor tyrosine kinases (RTKs) by extracellular ligands or oncogenic mutation results in RTK autophosphorylation and the subsequent recruitment of PI3K to the cytoplasmic domain of the receptor. PI3K phosphorylates and activates Akt, which in turn phosphorylates and negatively regulates the TSC2. The TSC complex acts as a GAP for Rheb, therefore negatively restraining mTOR. mTOR's kinase activity is directed towards two substrates involved in translational initiation and protein synthesis. First, mTOR directly phosphorylates ribosomal subunit S6 kinase (S6K), which in turn phosphorylates a number of proteins including the ribosomal S6 protein and the translational regulators eIF2 kinase and eIF-4B. In total, activation of S6K results in the increased translation of mRNAs, which contain TOP (terminal oligopyrimidine tracts). Second, mTOR indirectly regulates the eukaryotic initiation factor 4E (eIF-4E), which is released from its inhibitory binding partner 4E-BP1 through phosphorylation by mTOR. eIF4E is the mRNA cap binding subunit of the eIF4F complex, which is responsible for the initiation of protein translation of mRNAs with regulatory elements in the 5′ untranslated terminal regions, so called CAP-dependent mRNAs, such as cyclin D1, c-MYC, LDH, HIF, and VEGF.

Although Akt is widely believed to be the critical oncogenic downstream mediator of PI3K activity, and thus the mediator of oncogenesis in the setting of *PTEN* loss, there is genetic evidence to suggest that *PTEN* has other targets as well. For example, in mouse models, complementary gain or loss of function mutations in *PTEN* and *Akt* have incompletely overlapping phenotypes.[9] Importantly, although various transgenic mice expressing activated forms of *Akt* in differing tissues results in increases in cell size or cell number, activation of the *Akt* pathway is not sufficient to cause cancer unless combined with mutation or activation of a second pathway. On the contrary, *PTEN*-deficient mice readily develop a high incidence of T-cell lymphomas, gonadostromal and germ-line tumors, and cancers of the endometrium, thyroid, prostate, breast, liver, and intestine.

## mTOR

mTOR is a serine/threonine kinase that functions as a gatekeeper of cell growth, metabolism, and proliferation, receiving signals from a diverse set of growth factor receptors and sensors of cellular nutrient levels such as *STK11/LKB1*. TOR is evolutionarily conserved from yeast to mammals and is necessary for development because mTOR knockout mice are embryonic lethal.[10] Additionally, studies in *Drosophila* using tissue-specific knockout technology have shown that dTOR, and specifically its kinase activity, regulate cell size.[11,12]

mTOR was originally identified and cloned from a screen in the budding yeast *Saccharomyces cerevisiae* looking for resistance to the immunosuppressant drug rapamycin.[13–17] mTOR exists in two distinct multiprotein complexes, one which is sensitive to rapamycin and the other which is not. The rapamycin sensitive complex contains mTOR and GβL and raptor (regulatory associated protein of mTOR) proteins, whereas the rapamycin insensitive complex contains mTOR and GβL but instead of raptor binds to the rictor (rapamycin-insensitive companion of mTOR) protein (Figure 2).[18–22] Although the rictor/mTOR complex has recently been shown to activate the Akt pathway and regulate the actin cytoskeleton through mechanisms that are PKCα and Rho dependent,[22,23] the discussions below are

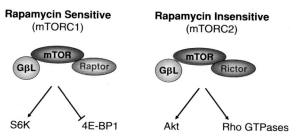

**Figure 2. Mammalian target of rapamycin mTORC1 and mTORC2.** mTOR exists in two biochemically distinct complexes, one which is sensitive to rapamycin and the other which is not. The rapamycin sensitive complex contains mTOR and GβL and raptor (regulatory associated protein of mTOR) proteins, whereas the rapamycin insensitive complex contains mTOR and GβL but instead of raptor binds to the rictor (rapamycin-insensitive companion of mTOR) protein. The rictor/mTOR complex has recently been shown to activate the Akt pathway and regulate the actin cytoskeleton through mechanisms that are Rho dependent.

restricted to those pertaining to the rapamycin sensitive mTOR complex. Interestingly, recent data suggest that long-term therapy with mTOR inhibitors may reduce mTOR/rictor complex activity in addition to mTOR/raptor activity, thus leading to some degree of Akt inhibition.[24] It remains to be determined if the antitumor activity of mTOR inhibitors correlates with their ability over time to inhibit Akt indirectly.

mTOR's kinase activity is directed towards two substrates involved in translational initiation and protein synthesis. First, mTOR directly phosphorylates ribosomal subunit S6 kinase (S6K),[25–27] which in turn phosphorylates a number of proteins including the ribosomal S6 protein and the translational regulators eIF2 kinase and eIF-4B.[28] In total, activation of S6K results in the increased translation of mRNAs, which contain conserved sequences within their 5′ untranslated regions, so called, TOP (terminal oligopyrimidine tracts). These mRNAs encode many components of the translational machinery including ribosomal proteins, elongation factors, and poly (A)-binding protein.[29] Second, mTOR indirectly regulates the eukaryotic initiation factor 4E (eIF-4E), which is released from its inhibitory binding partner 4E-BP1 through phosphorylation by mTOR (Figure 1).[30] eIF4E is the mRNA cap binding subunit of the eIF4F complex, which is responsible for the initiation of protein translation of mRNAs with regulatory elements in the 5′ untranslated terminal regions, so called CAP-dependent mRNAs, such as cyclin D1 and c-MYC.[31,32]

Although mTOR may integrate some signals directly, such as the ability to sense amino acid levels, it normally integrates a diverse set of signaling pathways including growth factors, intracellular nutrient levels, and hypoxia via its negative regulation by the tuberous sclerosis complex (TSC). TSC is composed of TSC1 (tuberin) and TSC2 (hamartin) both of which are necessary for TSC's functions and both have been characterized as tumor suppressor genes. TSC2 acts as a GTPase activating protein (GAP) for the kinase, Rheb, resulting in Rheb being in its GDP-bound (and inactive) state. Rheb when bound to GTP (Rheb-GTP) is active and phosphorylates and activates mTOR. Thus, TSC through its GAP activity towards Rheb works to restrain mTOR activity.

Growth factors bind to their RTK receptors on the cell surface and activate mTOR via the PI3K/Akt pathway (Figure 3). Intracellular nutrient levels are sensed by the AMP Kinase (AMPK), which phosphorylates and negatively regulates TSC2. In this same regard, hypoxia has been shown to downregulate mTOR activity in a manner dependent upon the REDD1 kinase, which phosphorylates TSC2 in response to hypoxia (Figure 3).[33,34] Although all these physiologic signals impact mTOR function, oncogenic activation of mTOR occurs through these very same pathways as well. However, which protein or set of proteins, downstream of mTOR, is responsible for its transforming potential has yet to be defined.

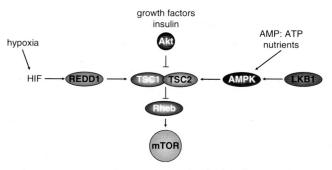

**Figure 3. Physiologic regulation of mammalian target of rapamycin (mTOR).** Growth factors bind to their receptor tyrosine kinases receptors on the cell surface and activate mTOR via the PI3K/Akt pathway. Intracellular nutrient levels are sensed by the AMPK, which phosphorylates and negatively regulates TSC2. In this same regard, hypoxia has been shown to downregulate mTOR activity in a manner dependent upon the REDD1 kinase, which phosphorylates TSC2 in response to hypoxia. Although all these physiologic signals impact physiologic mTOR function, oncogenic activation of mTOR occurs through these very same pathways as well.

## PI3K/Akt/mTOR Activation Results in Hypoxia-inducible Factor (HIF) Upregulation

Loss of the von Hippel-Lindau tumor suppressor gene results in the stabilization of the α subunits of the HIF, events thought to be critical in the development of clear cell renal carcinoma. HIF is a heterodimeric transcription factor composed of a labile α-subunit and a stable β-subunit. Humans possess three α-subunit genes (*HIF1α*, *HIF2α*, and *HIF3α*) and three *HIFβ* genes.[35] HIF acts not only as a key regulator of the cellular response to hypoxia but also plays a critical role in the adaptation of cancer cells to the unfavorable environment that develops as they outgrow their blood supply. HIF is polyubiquitinated within a region termed the oxygen-dependent degradation domain by the *VHL* (von Hippel-Lindau) gene product, pVHL. The binding of pVHL to HIF is governed by an oxygen-dependent, posttranslational prolyl hydroxylation of HIFα subunits.[36,37] Thus, HIFα subunits are normally degraded in the presence of oxygen but are stabilized under hypoxic conditions or in the setting of pVHL loss, leading to transactivation of HIF target genes.

HIF can be upregulated at the transcriptional level as well. Mutations in *Ras* family members or of *BRaf* result in activation of the Ras/Raf/Erk pathway with resultant increases in HIF mRNA levels[38–40]. Additionally, translation of HIF mRNA is dependent upon mTOR activity because treatment with mTOR inhibitors results in a decrease in both normoxic and hypoxic accumulation of HIF protein.[41–43] This effect is at least partially mediated by the presence of TOP tracts located in the 5′ UTR of both HIF1 and HIF2[43] as protein levels of variants of HIF lacking their native 5′ UTRs (and thus their TOP tracts) are insensitive to mTOR inhibitors and their growth inhibitory effects.[43]

## Activation of the PI3K/Akt Pathway in RCC

Analysis of human tumors by tissue microarray has shown that RCCs stain highly for markers of PI3K/mTOR pathway activation.[44] In this study, 85% of RCCs were noted to have increased staining for phosphorylated S6 (pS6) with significantly higher expression observed in tumors with higher

T classification, higher Fuhrman grade, and metastatic disease. There are several possible mechanisms of PI3K/mTOR activation in RCC discussed below.

### PTEN Loss

Activation of the PI3K/Akt pathway in RCC may occur through distinct mechanisms. *PTEN* loss of heterozygosity (LOH) and homozygous deletion has been documented in both renal carcinoma cell lines and primary human tumors, although at a low frequency (< 10%).[45,46] On the contrary, its expression at the protein level has been shown to be decreased in up to 30% of primary RCC specimens relative to adjacent normal kidney and its absence has been associated in multivariate analyses as a negative prognostic factor in disease-specific survival,[47–50] suggesting alternative mechanisms of PTEN silencing other than at the level of the genome. As expected, Akt activation appears to be concordant with PTEN loss[49] and interestingly was noted in over 80% of metastatic tumor biopsies in one series.[51] Although mutations in PI3K or Akt have been described in other solid tumors such as breast, ovarian, and colorectal cancer, none have been reported in RCC to date.

PTEN loss or Akt activation in RCC may play a role in immune escape and response to immunotherapy. Loss of PTEN and Akt activation in glioma cells, for example, led to the overexpression of the immunosuppressive protein B7-H1 and loss of T-cell-mediated killing of tumor cells.[52] Whether this same paradigm exists in RCC remains to be validated.

### Ras

Mutations of one of the three Ras family members (*K-Ras*, *H-Ras*, or *N-Ras*) activate PI3K in a PTEN independent manner. However, the Ras family of oncogenes has been thoroughly studied and appears to be rarely mutated in RCC.[53–56] Of note, however, is that the majority of these studies were performed before the advent of more sensitive sequencing techniques such as single nucleotide polymorphism. Frequent homozygous deletion and LOH of 3p21 in both RCC and other tumor types has led to the search for a putative tumor suppressor gene in this region. In this regard, silencing of the Ras association domain family 1A (*RASSF1A*) gene by hypermethylation has been documented and occurs in up to 56% of primary RCCs[57] irregardless of *VHL* status.[58] Although the exact biochemical understanding of RASSF1A remains to be understood, preliminary evidence points to a role in opposing Ras function.[59] Whether or not silencing of *RASSF1A* in RCC has true functional effects has yet to be proven.

### Growth Factor Receptors

Activation of the PI3K/Akt pathway by stimulation of growth factor RTKs is likely the most common event resulting in elevated levels in Akt signaling. There are several well-known growth factors that are dysregulated in RCC. Many of these are HIF target genes and thus implicated in the pathogenesis of *VHL* –/– RCC. Specifically, these include the activation of EGFR via autocrine or paracrine secretion of TGFα, stimulation of VEGFR via secretion of VEGF and PDGF.

### Cooperation Between VHL Loss and Akt Activation

Cooperation between *VHL* loss and Akt activation may lead to higher HIF levels through a cooperative effect on increased translation and protein stabilization, thus leading to hypoxia-independent growth and survival in RCC. Although *VHL* loss leads to stabilization of the HIFα subunits despite normoxic conditions, Akt activation increases the mTOR-mediated, CAP-dependent translation of HIF. In addition, the PI3K/Akt pathway may lead to heat shock protein expression and stabilization of the HIF complex to facilitate this signaling program.[60] These findings suggest that agents that inhibit the PI3K/Akt pathway may reverse several of the oncogenic molecular lesions associated with *VHL* loss and HIF deregulation.

### Nonclear Cell RCC and the PI3K/Akt/m TOR Pathway

Nonclear cell RCC is composed of several pathologic subgroups, including papillary, chromophobe, collecting duct, oncocytoma, and rarer pathologies such as small cell variants and medullary carcinoma.

The underlying molecular events implicated in several of these pathologic subtypes have now been identified and appear to activate the PI3K/Akt/mTOR pathway or result in hypoxia-independent stabilization of HIFα subunits, resulting in a pseudo-hypoxic state. These alterations may represent shared molecular pathways similar to clear cell RCC.[61]

In papillary RCC, c-met on chromosome 7 is amplified, mutated, or overexpressed in the majority of tumors and likely contributes to the pathogenesis of both familial and sporadic tumors.[61] Activation of the met pathway can occur in response to hypoxia as well leading to a genetic program of invasive growth and metastasis.[62] Although the mechanisms underlying met transformation, motility and metastasis, and survival are imperfectly understood, the PI3K pathway is likely essential for the lethal metastatic phenotype in these tumors.[62] Thus, in addition to selective c-met inhibitors, HIF inhibitors and PI3K/Akt/mTOR pathway inhibitors may reduce c-met levels or activity in papillary RCC and confer clinical benefit. A recent caveat to this finding is the discovery of c-myc amplification and expression signatures in the subset of aggressive papillary carcinomas, indicative of a secondary transformative event in these tumors that is associated with poor survival and therapeutic resistance.[63]

In lieu of c-met activation, hereditary papillary RCC patients may have mutations in the gene for fumarate hydratase (FH), located on chromosome 1q42. These patients typically have hereditary leiomyoma and renal cell cancer, and extremely aggressive papillary or collecting duct histology.[64] This gene product is involved in the Krebs cycle of oxidative phosphorylation, and loss of function of FH leads to accumulation of fumarate and succinate, which competitively inhibits HIF prolyl hydroxylase.[65] This results in increased HIF levels and activity, not due to VHL loss, but due to reduced hydroxylation and degradation by VHL, thus mimicking hypoxia. This dependence on HIF signaling may thus be amenable to therapeutic intervention with mTOR inhibition.

Finally, in chromophobe RCC, mutations and LOH occur in the Birt-Hogg-Dube (BHD) gene on chromosome 17p, and have been identified in familial cases.[66,67] The gene BHD gene product, folliculin, is a putative tumor suppressor protein, the exact function of which remains unknown. Recent data, however, suggest that folliculin is phosphorylated by and downstream of the AMPK/mTOR pathway, although its exact role in nutrient sensing remains to be clarified.[68] Its interaction with the mTOR pathway is intriguing and leaves open the possibility that mTOR inhibitors may have clinical utility in BHD defective RCCs.

## Inhibitors of the PI3K/Akt/mTOR Pathway

Inhibitors of PI3K and Akt are available. In vitro, inhibition of PI3K with LY294002 results in the downregulation of Ras induced increases of HIF and interestingly inhibits the growth of both VHL wild type and VHL deficient cells.[38] In vivo, treatment of mice with VHL deficient renal carcinoma xenografts produces not only inhibition of tumor growth but also regression, thought to be secondary to increased apoptosis of the tumor cells.[69]

The prototypical mTOR inhibitor, rapamycin (sirolimus), was isolated from the soil of Easter Island (Rapa Nui) in the 1970s, found to be produced by the bacterium Streptomyces hygroscopicus, and had potent antifungal properties.[70] It was soon noted, however, to have immunosuppressive effects, inhibiting both the production of and T-cell response to IL-2 and other cytokines, which led to its approval by the FDA in 1999 for the prevention of acute graft rejection in combination with cyclosporine and steroids in renal transplant patients.[71] Around the same time, the development of CCI-779 (cell cycle inhibitor-779, Wyeth) rejuvenated interest in this class of compounds as a cancer therapeutic. There are now four mTOR inhibitors available for clinical trials: the prototype rapamycin and three rapamycin derivatives, CCI-779 (temsirolimus, Wyeth), AP23573 (Ariad), and RAD001 (everolimus, Novartis). Inhibitors of mTOR mediate their effect by complexing with the FK506 binding protein 12 (FKBP12). The resulting complex inhibits mTOR and subsequent translation (Figure 4).

Preclinical models of RCC have reported significant sensitivity of renal carcinoma cells to mTOR inhibition not only in vitro but also in vivo. Growth of VHL deficient renal carcinoma xenografts was

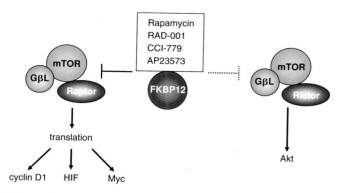

**Figure 4.** Mammalian target of rapamycin (mTOR) Inhibitors. There are now four mTOR inhibitors available for clinical trials: the prototype rapamycin and three rapamycin derivatives, CCI-779 (temseirolimus, Wyeth), AP23573 (Ariad), and RAD001 (everolimus, Novartis). Inhibitors of mTOR mediate their effect by complexing with the FK6 binding protein 12 (FKBP12). The resulting complex inhibits mTOR and subsequent translation of several genes thought to be critical to renal cell carcinogenesis such as cyclin D1, HIF, and Myc. Recent data suggest that long-term therapy with mTOR inhibitors may reduce mTOR/rictor complex activity and mTOR/raptor activity, thus leading to some degree of Akt inhibition.

inhibited by treatment with the mTOR inhibitor CCI-779, whereas the same cells expressing stabilized HIF variants lacking their 5′ TOP tracts were insensitive to the growth inhibitory effects of CCI-779. Thus, although loss of function mutations of *PTEN* result in an Akt-dependent increase in mTOR-dependent translation of many genes, HIF has been reported to be the downstream oncogenic mediator of mTOR in RCC.[41,43]

## Clinical Experience with PI3K/Akt/mTOR Inhibitors in RCC

PI3K inhibitors have not been studied specifically in the context of RCC. However, a phase I trial of the Akt inhibitor perifosine (NSC 639966) showed 1 partial response (in a patient with sarcoma) and stable disease in two of six patients with metastatic RCC (6 and 14 weeks each),[72] suggesting that Akt inhibitors may have activity *in vivo* in patients with RCC.

mTOR inhibitors have shown encouraging results in the treatment of RCC leading to the recent FDA approval of temsirolimus (CCI-779, Wyeth) for the treatment of advanced RCC. Despite high expectations for this class of compounds and other inhibitors of the PI3K pathway, their success in the

clinic as monotherapies other than in RCC has been limited. One potential explanation for the somewhat disappointing results of these compounds in clinical trials to date is that pharmacologic inhibition of mTOR can result in the feedback activation of PI3K.[73,74] In this regard, recent reports show that the combined inhibition of mTOR and the p110 subunit of PI3K result in significant proliferative arrest in glioma cells, whereas inhibition of either alone did not.[74] These results suggest that PI3K activation, as a consequence of mTOR inhibition, results in stimulation of mTOR independent effector pathways. The promising clinical trial results in RCC suggest that these mTOR independent functions of PI3K may not be relevant in RCC. This may reflect the fact that the majority of RCCs harbor inactivating mutations or silencing by hypermethylation of the *VHL* tumor suppressor gene, resulting in upregulation of HIF and rendering them sensitive to its inhibition. This hypothesis is consistent with preclinical data that has established that HIF as both necessary and sufficient for renal carcinogenesis as well as the fact that ectopic expression of HIF variants that are insensitive to mTOR inhibition are sufficient to overcome the growth inhibitory properties of mTOR inhibitors.[43,75–78] An equally plausible hypothesis is that feedback activation of PI3K upon mTOR inhibition does not occur in renal carcinoma cells. These questions will hopefully be addressed with preclinical and correlative studies in the near future.

## SUMMARY

Activation of the PI3K/Akt/mTOR pathway through its effects on HIF translation appears to play a fundamental role in the pathogenesis of RCC. Although alternative effector pathways of Akt possibly play a role in renal carcinogenesis, studies to this effect are lacking. The mTOR inhibitor, temsirolimus, has recently been FDA approved for the treatment of metastatic RCC as monotherapy and is the first compound to show an overall survival advantage in this difficult to treat disease. Further studies to determine the exact effects of mTOR inhibitors on the immune system of cancer patients are warranted. Finally, information on predictors of clinical response to inhibitors of the mTOR pathway is needed.

# REFERENCES

1. Ali IU, Schriml LM, et al. Mutational spectra of PTEN/MMAC1 gene: a tumor suppressor with lipid phosphatase activity. J Natl Cancer Inst 1999; 91:1922–32.

2. Eng C. PTEN: one gene, many syndromes. Hum Mutat 2003; 22:183–98.

3. Maehama T, Dixon JE. The tumor suppressor, PTEN/MMAC1, dephosphorylates the lipid second messenger, phosphatidylinositol 3,4,5-trisphosphate. J Biol Chem 1998; 273:13375–8.

4. Engelman JA, Luo J, et al. The evolution of phosphatidylinositol 3-kinases as regulators of growth and metabolism. Nat Rev Genet 2006; 7:606–19.

5. Kodaki T, Woscholski R, et al. The activation of phosphatidylinositol 3-kinase by Ras. Curr Biol 1994; 4:798–806.

6. Rodriguez-Viciana P, Warne PH, et al. Phosphatidylinositol-3-OH kinase as a direct target of Ras. Nature 1994; 370:527–32.

7. Di Cristofano A, Pesce B, et al. Pten is essential for embryonic development and tumour suppression. Nat Genet 1998; 19:348–55.

8. Di Cristofano A, Kotsi P, et al. Impaired fas response and autoimmunity in PTEN+/– mice. Science 1999; 285: 2122–5.

9. Vivanco I, Sawyers CL. The phosphatidylinositol 3-kinase AKT pathway in human cancer. Nat Rev Cancer 2002; 2:489–501.

10. Murakami M, Ichisaka T, et al. mTOR is essential for growth and proliferation in early mouse embryos and embryonic stem cells. Mol Cell Biol 2004; 24:6710–8.

11. Oldham S, Montagne J, et al. Genetic and biochemical characterization of dTOR the Drosophila homolog of the target of rapamycin. Genes Dev 2000; 14:2689–94.

12. Zhang H, Stallock JP, et al. Regulation of cellular growth by the Drosophila target of rapamycin dTOR. Genes Dev 2000; 14:2712–24.

13. Brown EJ, Albers MW, et al. A mammalian protein targeted by G1-arresting rapamycin-receptor complex. Nature 1994; 369:756–8.

14. Chiu MI, Katz H, et al. RAPT1, a mammalian homolog of yeast Tor, interacts with the FKBP12/rapamycin complex. Proc Natl Acad Sci U S A 1994; 91:12574–8.

15. Sabatini DM, Erdjument-Bromage H, et al. RAFT1: a mammalian protein that binds to FKBP12 in a rapamycin-dependent fashion and is homologous to yeast TORs. Cell 1994; 78:35–43.

16. Kunz J, Henriquez R, et al. Target of rapamycin in yeast, TOR2, is an essential phosphatidylinositol kinase homolog required for G1 progression. Cell 1993; 73:585–96.

17. Helliwell SB, Wagner P, et al. TOR1 and TOR2 are structurally and functionally similar but not identical phosphatidylinositol kinase homologues in yeast. Mol Biol Cell 1994; 5:105–18.

18. Hara K, Maruki Y, et al. Raptor, a binding partner of target of rapamycin (TOR), mediates TOR action. Cell 2002; 110:177–89.

19. Kim DH, Sarbassov DD, et al. mTOR interacts with raptor to form a nutrient-sensitive complex that signals to the cell growth machinery. Cell 2002; 110:163–75.

20. Loewith R, Jacinto E, et al. Two TOR complexes, only one of which is rapamycin sensitive, have distinct roles in cell growth control. Mol Cell 2002; 10:457–68.

21. Kim DH, Sarbassov DD, et al. GβL, a positive regulator of the rapamycin-sensitive pathway required for the nutrient-sensitive interaction between raptor and mTOR. Mol Cell 2003; 11:895–904.

22. Sarbassov DD, Ali SM, et al. Rictor, a novel binding partner of mTOR, defines a rapamycin-insensitive and raptor-independent pathway that regulates the cytoskeleton. Curr Biol 2004; 14:1296–302.

23. Jacinto E, Loewith R, et al. Mammalian TOR complex 2 controls the actin cytoskeleton and is rapamycin insensitive. Nat Cell Biol 2004; 6:1122–8.

24. Sarbassov DD, Ali SM, et al. Prolonged rapamycin treatment inhibits mTORC2 assembly and Akt/PKB. Mol Cell 2006; 22:159–68.

25. Chung J, Kuo CJ, et al. Rapamycin-FKBP specifically blocks growth-dependent activation of and signaling by the 70 kd S6 protein kinases. Cell 1992; 69:1227–36.

26. Kuo CJ, Chung J, et al. Rapamycin selectively inhibits interleukin-2 activation of p70 S6 kinase. Nature 1992; 358:70–3.

27. Price DJ, Grove JR, et al. Rapamycin-induced inhibition of the 70-kilodalton S6 protein kinase. Science 1992; 257:973–7.

28. Sarbassov DD, Ali SM, et al. Growing roles for the mTOR pathway. Curr Opin Cell Biol 2005; 17:596–603.

29. Meyuhas O. Synthesis of the translational apparatus is regulated at the translational level. Eur J Biochem 2000; 267:6321–30.

30. Thomas GV. mTOR and cancer: reason for dancing at the crossroads? Curr Opin Genet Dev 2006; 16:78–84.

31. Rosenwald IB, Kaspar R, et al. Eukaryotic translation initiation factor 4E regulates expression of cyclin D1 at transcriptional and post-transcriptional levels. J Biol Chem 1995; 270:21176–80.

32. Mendez R, Myers MG Jr, et al. Stimulation of protein synthesis, eukaryotic translation initiation factor 4E phosphorylation, and PHAS-I phosphorylation by insulin requires insulin receptor substrate 1 and phosphatidylinositol 3-kinase. Mol Cell Biol 1996; 16:2857–64.

33. Brugarolas J, Lei K, et al. Regulation of mTOR function in response to hypoxia by REDD1 and the TSC1/TSC2 tumor suppressor complex. Genes Dev 2004; 18:2893–904.

34. Reiling JH, Hafen E. The hypoxia-induced paralogs Scylla and Charybdis inhibit growth by down-regulating S6K activity upstream of TSC in Drosophila. Genes Dev 2004; 18:2879–92.

35. Semenza GL. HIF-1 and mechanisms of hypoxia sensing. Curr Opin Cell Biol 2001; 13:167–71.

36. Ivan M, Kondo K, et al. HIFα targeted for VHL-mediated destruction by proline hydroxylation: implications for $O_2$ sensing. Science 2001; 292:464–8.

37. Jaakkola P, Mole DR, et al. Targeting of HIF-α to the von Hippel-Lindau ubiquitylation complex by $O_2$-regulated prolyl hydroxylation. Science 2001; 292:468–72.

38. Blancher C, Moore JW, et al. Effects of Ras and von Hippel-Lindau (VHL) gene mutations on hypoxia-inducible factor (HIF)-1α, HIF-2α, and vascular endothelial growth factor expression and their regulation by the phosphatidylinositol 3′-kinase/Akt signaling pathway. Cancer Res 2001; 61:7349–55.

39. Sodhi A, Montaner S, et al. MAPK and Akt act cooperatively but independently on hypoxia inducible factor-1α in RasV12 upregulation of VEGF. Biochem Biophys Res Commun 2001; 287:292–300.

40. Kumar SM, Yu H, et al. Mutant V600E BRAF increases hypoxia inducible factor-1α expression in melanoma. Cancer Res 2007; 67:3177–84.

41. Hudson CC, Liu M, et al. Regulation of hypoxia-inducible factor 1α expression and function by the mammalian target of rapamycin. Mol Cell Biol 2002; 22:7004–14.

42. Treins C, Giorgetti-Peraldi S, et al. Insulin stimulates hypoxia-inducible factor 1 through a phosphatidylinositol 3-kinase/target of rapamycin-dependent signaling pathway. J Biol Chem 2002; 277:27975–81.

43. Thomas GV, Tran C, et al. Hypoxia-inducible factor determines sensitivity to inhibitors of mTOR in kidney cancer. Nat Med 2006; 12:122–7.

44. Pantuck AJ, Seligson DB, et al. Prognostic relevance of the mTOR pathway in renal cell carcinoma: implications for molecular patient selection for targeted therapy. Cancer 2007; 109:2257–67.

45. Alimov A, Li C, et al. Somatic mutation and homozygous deletion of PTEN/MMAC1 gene of 10q23 in renal cell carcinoma. Anticancer Res 1999; 19:3841–6.

46. Kondo K, Yao M, et al. PTEN/MMAC1/TEP1 mutations in human primary renal-cell carcinomas and renal carcinoma cell lines. Int J Cancer 2001; 91:219–24.

47. Brenner W, Farber G, et al. Loss of tumor suppressor protein PTEN during renal carcinogenesis. Int J Cancer 2002; 99:53–7.

48. Shin Lee J, Seok Kim H, et al. Expression of PTEN in renal cell carcinoma and its relation to tumor behavior and growth. J Surg Oncol 2003; 84:166–72.

49. Hara S, Oya M, et al. Akt activation in renal cell carcinoma: contribution of a decreased PTEN expression and the induction of apoptosis by an Akt inhibitor. Ann Oncol 2005; 16:928–33.

50. Kim HL, Seligson D, et al. Using tumor markers to predict the survival of patients with metastatic renal cell carcinoma. J Urol 2005; 173:1496–501.

51. Horiguchi A, Oya M, et al. Elevated Akt activation and its impact on clinicopathological features of renal cell carcinoma. J Urol 2003; 169:710–3.

52. Parsa AT, Waldron JS, et al. Loss of tumor suppressor PTEN function increases B7-H1 expression and immunoresistance in glioma. Nat Med 2007; 13:84–8.

53. Fujita J, Kraus MH, et al. Activated H-Ras oncogenes in human kidney tumors. Cancer Res 1988; 48: 5251–5.

54. Nanus DM, Mentle IR, et al. Infrequent Ras oncogene point mutations in renal cell carcinoma. J Urol 1990; 143:175–8.

55. Rochlitz CF, Peter S, et al. Mutations in the Ras protooncogenes are rare events in renal cell cancer. Eur J Cancer 1992; 28:333–6.

56. Uchida T, Wada C, et al. Genomic instability of microsatellite repeats and mutations of H-, K-, and N-Ras, and p53 genes in renal cell carcinoma. Cancer Res 1994; 54:3682–5.

57. Yoon JH, Dammann R, et al. Hypermethylation of the CpG island of the RASSF1A gene in ovarian and renal cell carcinomas. Int J Cancer 2001; 94:212–7.

58. Dreijerink K, Braga E, et al. The candidate tumor suppressor gene, RASSF1A, from human chromosome 3p21.3 is involved in kidney tumorigenesis. Proc Natl Acad Sci U S A 2001; 98:7504–9.

59. Agathanggelou A, Cooper WN, et al. Role of the Ras-association domain family 1 tumor suppressor gene in human cancers. Cancer Res 2005; 65:3497–508.

60. Zhou J, Schmid T, et al. PI3K/Akt is required for heat shock proteins to protect hypoxia-inducible factor 1α from pVHL-independent degradation. J Biol Chem 2004; 279:13506–13.

61. Linehan WM, Pinto PA, et al. Identification of the genes for kidney cancer: opportunity for disease-specific targeted therapeutics. Clin Cancer Res 2007; 13(2 Pt 2): 671s–9s.

62. Boccaccio C, Comoglio PM. Invasive growth: a MET-driven genetic programme for cancer and stem cells. Nat Rev Cancer 2006; 6:637–45.

63. Furge KA, Tan MH, et al. Identification of deregulated oncogenic pathways in renal cell carcinoma: an integrated oncogenomic approach based on gene expression profiling. Oncogene 2007; 26:1346–50.

64. Toro JR, Nickerson ML, et al. Mutations in the fumarate hydratase gene cause hereditary leiomyomatosis and renal cell cancer in families in North America. Am J Hum Genet 2003; 73:95–106.

65. Pollard PJ, Spencer-Dene B, et al. Targeted inactivation of fh1 causes proliferative renal cyst development and activation of the hypoxia pathway. Cancer Cell 2007; 11:311–9.

66. Nickerson ML, Warren MB, et al. Mutations in a novel gene lead to kidney tumors, lung wall defects, and benign tumors of the hair follicle in patients with the Birt-Hogg-Dube syndrome. Cancer Cell 2002; 2:157–64.

67. Gad S, Lefevre SH, et al. Mutations in BHD and TP53 genes, but not in HNF1β gene, in a large series of sporadic chromophobe renal cell carcinoma. Br J Cancer 2007; 96:336–40.

68. Baba M, Hong SB, et al. Folliculin encoded by the BHD gene interacts with a binding protein, FNIP1, and AMPK, and is involved in AMPK and mTOR signaling. Proc Natl Acad Sci U S A 2006; 103:5552–7.

69. Sourbier C, Lindner V, et al. The phosphoinositide 3-kinase/Akt pathway: a new target in human renal cell carcinoma therapy. Cancer Res 2006; 66:5130–42.

70. Vezina C, Kudelski A, et al. Rapamycin (AY-22,989), a new antifungal antibiotic. I. Taxonomy of the producing streptomycete and isolation of the active principle. J Antibiot (Tokyo) 1975; 28:721–6.

71. Law BK. Rapamycin: an anti-cancer immunosuppressant? Crit Rev Oncol Hematol 2005; 56:47–60.

72. Van Ummersen L, Binger K, et al. A phase I trial of perifosine (NSC 639966) on a loading dose/maintenance dose schedule in patients with advanced cancer. Clin Cancer Res 2004; 10:7450–6.

73. Sun SY, Rosenberg LM, et al. Activation of Akt and eIF4E survival pathways by rapamycin-mediated mammalian target of rapamycin inhibition. Cancer Res 2005; 65:7052–8.

74. Fan QW, Knight ZA, et al. A dual PI3 kinase/mTOR inhibitor reveals emergent efficacy in glioma. Cancer Cell 2006; 9:341–9.

75. Kondo K, Klco J, et al. Inhibition of HIF is necessary for tumor suppression by the von Hippel-Lindau protein. Cancer Cell 2002; 1:237–46.

76. Maranchie JK, Vasselli JR, et al. The contribution of VHL substrate binding and HIF1-α to the phenotype of VHL loss in renal cell carcinoma. Cancer Cell 2002; 1:247–55.

77. Kondo K, Kim WY, et al. Inhibition of HIF2α is sufficient to suppress pVHL-defective tumor growth. PLoS Biol 2003; 1:E83.

78. Zimmer M, Doucette D, et al. Inhibition of hypoxia-inducible factor is sufficient for growth suppression of VHL –/– tumors. Mol Cancer Res 2004; 2:89–95.

79. Atkins MB, Hidalgo M, et al. Randomized phase II study of multiple dose levels of CCI-779, a novel mammalian target of rapamycin kinase inhibitor, in patients with advanced refractory renal cell carcinoma. J Clin Oncol 2004; 22:909–18.

80. Hudes G, Carducci M, et al. Temsirolimus, interferon alfa, or both for advanced renal-cell carcinoma. N Engl J Med 2007; 356:2271–81.

# 17

# Clinical Results of Mammalian Target of Rapamycin Inhibition in Renal Cell Carcinoma

GARY R. HUDES, MD

## THE MAMMALIAN TARGET OF RAPAMYCIN

Mammalian target of rapamycin (mTOR) is a member of the phosophoinositol-3-kinase (PI3K)-like kinase family, a group of structurally similar protein kinases (Figure 1) that includes the ataxia-telangiectasia mutated (ATM), ATMR (ATM and rad3) kinase, and DNA protein kinase.[1] Members of this family have a domain structure that includes FAT, FATC, and HEAT sequences, the latter which mediate protein-protein interaction. This structure underlies the numerous protein interactions of mTOR and its key role as a regulator of cellular homeostasis.[2] A rapamycin binding domain(RBD) is centrally located, whereas the kinase domain is located near the carboxyl terminus. Inhibition of mTOR kinase by rapamycin first requires that the drug form a complex with FKBP-12, an abundant intracellular protein. This requirement also holds for temsirolimus and likely for other rapamycin analogs.[3,4] The drug-FKBP-12 complex binds mTOR at the RBD to inhibit kinase function by an allosteric mechanism. This mechanism confers remarkable selectivity, and there are no other known molecular targets of rapamycin and its analogs.

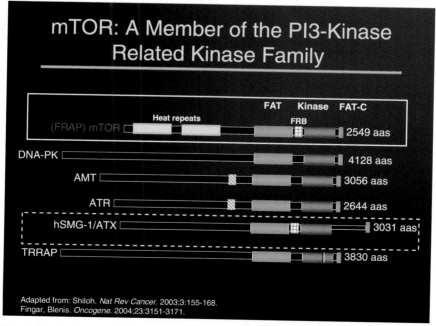

**Figure 1.** Structures of mammalian target of rapamycin and related proteins.

## mTOR ACTIVATION AND SIGNALING

mTOR integrates numerous signals including cellular growth stimuli, nutrition and energy status, and stress. Early biochemical studies positioned mTOR in the growth factor-activated phosphatidylinositol-3-kinase (PI3K), Akt (protein kinase B) signaling pathway, and downstream from Akt.[5] mTOR kinase is also activated by genetic alterations that reduce function of the PTEN tumor suppressor protein[6] or increase function of the catalytic subunit of PI3K,[7] both of which cause abnormal activation of Akt. A parallel pathway through which mTOR is activated involves cellular levels of cyclic AMP (cAMP), the cAMP-dependent protein kinase (AMPK), and the tuberous sclerosis complex 1 and 2 proteins (Figure 2). This upstream branch of the mTOR pathway is sensitive to cellular energy balance and nutritional status.[2]

mTOR functions in 2 main multiprotein complexes, target of rapamycin complex (TORC) 1 and TORC2.[8] TORC2 is implicated in the regulation of protein kinase Cα and consequently in the control of cell morphology and adhesion. TORC2 has also been shown to phosphorylate and activate Akt.[9]

Through phosphorylation of 2 downstream effectors, S6 kinase (S6K) and the binding protein for eukaryotic initiation factor 4E (4E-BP1), TORC1 controls the translation of cyclin D, c-Myc, and other key proteins involved in cell proliferation.[10] TORC1 also regulates expression and stability of HIF-1α.[11,12] These mTOR functions are relevant to renal cell carcinoma (RCC), which is characterized by alterations of the von Hippel-Lindau gene (*VHL*), leading to the upregulation of HIFα subunits, vascular endothelial growth factor (VEGF), and other molecules that increase angiogenesis.[13] Loss of VHL function in RCC also results in deregulation of Cyclin D1, a cyclin-dependent kinase cofactor required for cell cycle progression.[14,15] Thus, mechanisms underlying the antitumor activity of temsirolimus in renal carcinoma probably include inhibition of both angiogenesis and tumor cell proliferation. Importantly, mTOR kinase associated with TORC2 is relatively resistant to inhibition by rapamycin in vitro, suggesting that temsirolimus and other rapamycin analogs may effectively inhibit the activities TORC1 but not those of TORC2, a potential mechanism of resistance.[16]

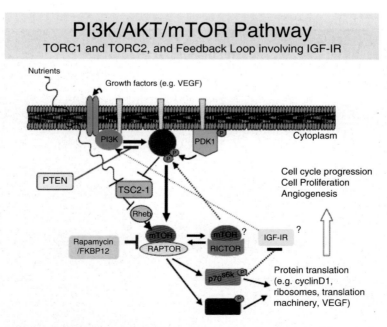

**Figure 2.** Phosphatidylinositol-3-kinase/Akt/mammalian target of rapamycin pathway, TORC1 and TORC2, and feedback loop involving insulin receptor substrate (IGF-IR) phosphorylation by p70[S6 kinase].

## THE PI3K/Akt/mTOR PATHWAY IN RENAL CARCINOMA

Using immunohistochemical methods, Robb and colleagues found evidence of mTOR activation in approximately 60% of 25 primary clear cell RCC.[17] Pantuck and colleagues found that activation of the mTOR pathway affects prognosis for patients with localized and metastatic kidney cancer. In their tissue microarray-based immunohistochemical study, mTOR pathway activation occurred most significantly in clear cell carcinomas, high grade tumors, and tumors with poor-prognostic features.[18] The frequency of mTOR pathway activation in RCC metastases and how this correlates with activation in the primary tumor has not yet been reported.

Laboratory investigations indicate that PI3K/Akt activation could be an important predictor of sensitivity to mTOR inhibitor therapy in the clinic,[19] and the preliminary report of a small correlative study supports this possibility.[20] A large clinical trial of mTOR inhibitor therapy that correlates treatment outcomes with tissue biomarkers of mTOR pathway activation would provide a more definitive answer to this important question.

## CLINICAL TRIALS OF mTOR INHIBITORS

Three inhibitors of mTOR have undergone clinical evaluation (Table 1). Each of these agents is analogs of rapamycin differing only at the C43 position, which is modified to increase solubility and bioavailability by the addition of an ester, ether or phosphonate group for temsirolimus, everolimus (RAD001), and deferolimus (AP23573) (Figure 3). Temsirolimus, the first mTOR inhibitor to enter the clinic, was approved in 2007 for patients with advanced or metastatic renal carcinoma. Temsirolimus will also be tested as second-line therapy following progression on sunitinib and as first-line therapy of patients with nonclear cell renal carcinoma. Everolimus is being evaluated as second-line therapy for patients with metastatic RCC who have progressed after treatment with sunitinib or sorafenib, ie, after VEGFR tyrosine kinase inhibitor therapy. Deferolimus has not yet been evaluated in RCC. Combination studies of temsirolimus and other mTOR inhibitors will be discussed below.

## TEMSIROLIMUS

The potential role for temsirolimus as a therapeutic agent in renal cancer and other tumors was first observed in phase I evaluation. Two schedules were evaluated, a 5 consecutive day, every 2 week schedule,[21] and a weekly schedule.[22] A conventional maximal tolerated dose was not defined for either of these schedules in minimally pretreated patients, but

| Table 1. SUMMARY OF PHASE I STUDIES OF TEMSIROLIMUS | | | |
|---|---|---|---|
| | Temsirolimus | RAD001 | AP-23573 |
| Sirolimus Analog | Yes | Yes | Yes |
| Metabolized to sirolimus | Yes | No | No |
| Schedules and phase II doses | Daily IV × 5: 15 (19.2) mg/d, weekly IV: 25 to 250 mg | Daily PO: 10 mg/d, weekly PO: 50 to 70 mg | Daily IV × 5: 12.5 mg, weekly 50 to 75 mg, daily PO: ? |
| Main AEs and DLTs | Anemia, rash, stomatitis, hyperlipidemia, hyperglycemia neutropenia, thrombocytopenia | Rash, anorexia, fatigue, stomatitis, hyperlipidemia, headache | Stomatitis, fatigue, anemia, rash, diarrhea thrombocytopenia, neutropenia (daily) |
| Activity (incl SD > 3 mo) | RCC, sarcoma, endometrial, cervical NSCLCa | Sarcoma, RCC, hepatoma, NSCLCa | Sarcoma, RCC, bladder, mesothelioma, bile duct, CRC |

AE = ; CRC = ; DLT = ; IV = intravenous; NSCLCa = ; PO = ; RCC = renal cell carcinoma.

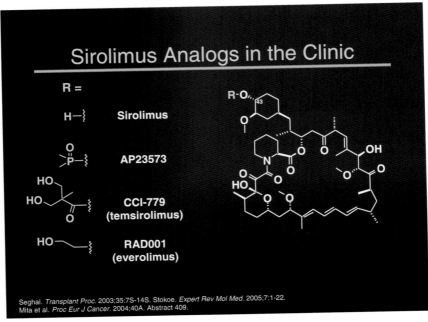

**Figure 3.**   Structures of rapamycin and analogs.

adverse events were more common at higher doses levels in each study. Two unconfirmed partial responses (PRs) were observed in 16 patients with RCC enrolled on the 5-day q 2 week phase I trial of temsirolimus, and 1 confirmed PR was seen in the weekly schedule phase I study. Several other patients had prolonged stable disease on the weekly schedule over a broad range of doses.

The pharmacologic parameters for temsirolimus are summarized in Table 2. Also, summarized are the key pharmacokinetic and pharmacodynamic findings for everolimus and deferolimus. Temsirolimus is metabolized to sirolimus (rapamycin), which has a longer terminal half-life than the parent molecule. Because temsirolimus and sirolimus bind similarly to FK-BP12, and exert similar antiproliferative effects in vitro,[4] both the parent drug and metabolite are likely responsible for inhibition of mTOR and antitumor effects after administration of temsirolimus.

The weekly dosing schedule was chosen for clinical development of temsirolimus, and the question of optimal dose was further evaluated in a randomized phase II study of weekly temsirolimus in patients with cytokine-refractory metastatic RCC.[23] A total of 111 patients were enrolled in this trial and treated with temsirolimus at a dose of 25, 75, or 250 mg as a weekly 30 minute intravenous infusion. The study subjects had received a median of 2 prior therapies for metastatic disease, and 91% subjects had received prior interleukin-2 or interferon (IFN). The median time to progression was 5.8 months, and median overall survival (OS) was 15 months. The objective response rate was only 7%, but 51% of patients had clinical benefit defined as either objective response or stable disease for at least 6 months. The lowest dose of temsirolimus in this study (25 mg) seemed to be as effective as the higher doses and was better tolerated over multiple cycles. Accordingly, the 25 mg weekly dose was selected for future studies in RCC.

In an exploratory subgroup analysis of OS using the MSKCC prognostic factor model,[24] 8, 46, and 47% of patients were classified as good, intermediate, or poor prognosis (ie, having ≥ 3 of 5 predictors of shorter survival). The median OS times for these groups were 23.8, 22.5, and 8.2 months (Table 3). Although short, the OS of the poor-prognosis subgroup receiving temsirolimus was better than expected compared with a group of patients with 3 or more of the MSKCC risk factors treated with IFN as first-line therapy.[24] Based on these results, a larger randomized trial was conducted to determine whether mTOR inhibition with temsirolimus could improve the OS of patients with poor-prognosis RCC.

| Table 2. mTOR INHIBITORS COMPARED PK AND PD | | | | |
|---|---|---|---|---|
| | Sirolimus | Temsirolimus | Everolimus | AP23573 |
| PK<br>Median half-life (h)<br>Clearance AUC | 40–50 | 12–15<br>↑ with dose<br>↑ less than proportional | 26–38<br>↑ with dose | 49<br>↑ with dose<br>↑ less than proportional |
| PD<br>Peripheral blood<br>mononuclear cell | | ↓ S6K1 activity, variable duration (n = 9) | ↓ pS6K1 at 20–30 mg/week | ↓ p4E-BP1, 7–10 day duration* ≥ 50% |
| Tumor Specimens | | ↓ pS6 (greater with low/absent PTEN) in prostate cancer; ↓ pS6K1, ↑ pAkt in paired neuroendocrine tumor biopsies (n = 13) | ↓ pS6K1 ↓ p4E-BP1* ↑ p-Akt* (n = 33) | ↓ pS6K1 in brain tumors after 12.5 to 15 mg × 4 days (n = 8) |

*Dose-related change

Desai et al. *J Clin Oncol.* 2004;22(14s):3150. Mita et al. *J Clin Oncol.* 2004;22(14s):3076. Raymond et al. *J Clin Oncol.* 2004;22:2336–2347.

| Table 3. RANDOMIZED PHASE II STUDY OF TEMSIROLIMUS IN CYTOKINE-REFRACTORY RENAL CELL CARCINOMA: OVERALL SURVIVAL BY PROGNOSTIC GROUP | | | |
|---|---|---|---|
| Risk Group | No. (%) Patients | Median Survival, Mo | Survival, 95% CI, Mo |
| Good | 8 (7) | 23.8 | 17.7 to 27.1 |
| Intermediate | 48 (43) | 22.5 | 16.9 to 25.7 |
| Poor | 49 (44) | 8.2 | 7.0 to 10.1 |

Data from Atkins MB.[23]

*Does not include 6 patients (5%) with unknown risk category.

## Phase III Trial of Temsirolimus, IFN, or Temsirolimus Plus IFN in RCC

The global Advanced Renal Cell Carcinoma (ARCC) trial was designed to determine whether temsirolimus as a single agent or in combination with IFNα improves the OS of patients with advanced (unresectable) or metastatic poor-prognosis RCC.[25] Several aspects of the Global ARCC trial design distinguish it from other contemporary phase III trials of new agents in RCC. First, the primary study endpoint was OS, targeting a 40% improvement in median OS for each of 2 comparisons: temsirolimus versus IFN and the combination of temsirolimus and IFN versus IFN. Second, the study enrolled patients with all RCC histologies and did not exclude those with predominantly nonclear cell tumors. Third,

patients were not required to undergo cytoreductive or adjuvant nephrectomy prior to enrollment. Finally, the study enrolled a predominantly poor-prognosis population defined by requiring subjects to have at least 3 of 6 factors known to be associated with short survival. This prognostic factor model was adapted from the 5 prognostic factor MSKCC model[24] by adding a sixth factor (multiple organ sites of metastases) as initially described by Mekhail and colleagues from the Cleveland Clinic.[26]

A total of 626 patients with ≥ 3 factors predicting short survival were randomized to 1 of 3 treatment groups: temsirolimus 25 mg intravenously (IV) each week; IFNα 3 million units (MU) subcutaneously (SC) 3 times weekly (escalating to 18 MU SC 3 times weekly or maximum tolerated dose); and the combination of temsirolimus 15 mg IV weekly and IFNα 6 MU SC 3 times weekly. The schedule and doses of temsirolimus and IFNα for the combination treatment were established in a preceding phase I and II study[27] (Figure 4).

The study was conducted in 23 countries between July 2003 and April 2005. The majority of patients (80%) had clear cell histology, and 67% of patients had undergone nephrectomy to remove the primary tumor. Patients with Karnofsky performance score < 80 comprised 82% of the population. By the MSKCC prognostic model,[28] 74% of patients were in the poor-prognosis category.

The common adverse events by treatment are summarized in Table 4. Asthenia was more frequent in the groups receiving IFN, whereas rash, peripheral edema, and stomatitis affected more patients who received temsirolimus alone or in the combination treatment. Myelosuppression was more common in patients treated with the combination of temsirolimus and IFNα. Compared with IFN monotherapy, temsirolimus was associated with a higher incidence of hyperlipidemia, hyperglycemia, and hypercholesterolemia

(see Table 4). These metabolic effects of temsirolimus are consistent with inhibition of insulin signaling through the PI3K/Akt/mTOR signaling pathway and are generally manageable with diet control or standard medical therapies. Compared with IFN and combination therapy, fewer patients receiving single-agent temsirolimus had grade 3 or 4 adverse events.

The efficacy endpoints for this trial are summarized in Table 5, and the Kaplan–Meier estimates of OS and PFS are shown in Figure 5. OS was greater for patients who received temsirolimus than for patients who received IFN (hazard ratio for death, 0.73; 95% CI 0.58 to 0.92; $p = .008$). Progression-free survival was also greater for patients receiving temsirolimus ($p < .001$). By contrast, OS for the group receiving combination therapy was not significantly different from that of the group treated with IFN (hazard ratio, 0.96; 95% CI, 0.76 to 1.20; $p = .70$) although PFS was significantly longer for the combination group. The median survival times for the groups receiving temsirolimus, IFN, and combination were 7.3, 10.9, and 8.4 months, respectively. The ORR was

| Table 4.  PHASE III STUDY OF TEMSIROLIMUS AND IFNα: SELECTED TREATMENT RELATED ADVERSE EVENTS (% OF PATIENTS) | | | | | | |
|---|---|---|---|---|---|---|
| | IFN ($n = 200$) | | Temsirolimus ($n = 208$) | | Temsirolimus + IFN ($n = 208$) | |
| Adverse event | All Grades | Grade 3 or 4 | All Grades | Grade 3 or 4 | All Grades | Grade 3 or 4 |
| Asthenia | 64 | 26 | 51 | 11 | 62 | 28 |
| Nausea | 41 | 4 | 37 | 2 | 40 | 3 |
| Rash | 6 | 0 | 47 | 4 | 21 | 1 |
| Dyspnea | 24 | 6 | 28 | 9 | 26 | 10 |
| Diarrhea | 20 | 2 | 27 | 1 | 27 | 5 |
| Peripheral edema | 8 | 0 | 27 | 2 | 16 | 0 |
| Vomiting | 28 | 2 | 19 | 2 | 30 | 2 |
| Stomatitis | 4 | 0 | 20 | 1 | 21 | 5 |
| Anemia | 42 | 22 | 45 | 20 | 61 | 38 |
| Hyperlipidemia | 14 | 1 | 27 | 3 | 38 | 8 |
| Hyperglycemia | 11 | 2 | 26 | 11 | 17 | 6 |
| Hypercholesteremia | 4 | 0 | 24 | 1 | 26 | 2 |
| Thrombocytopenia | 8 | 0 | 14 | 1 | 38 | 9 |
| Neutropenia | 12 | 7 | 7 | 3 | 27 | 15 |

Hudes G et al.[25]

## Phase 3 Study of TEMSR and IFN in Advanced RCC

- 626 patients with advanced metastatic RCC with poor-risk features
- 209 sites (26 countries)

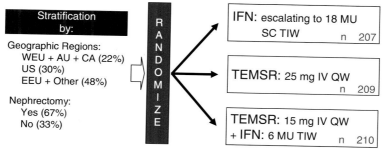

**Figure 4.**   Design of the global Advanced Renal Cell Carcinoma trial.

**Table 5. SUMMARY OF EFFICACY MEASURES FROM GLOBAL ADVANCED RENAL CELL CARCINOMA TRIAL**

| Endpoint | Interferon | Temsirolimus | Temsirolimus + Interferon |
|---|---|---|---|
| Overall survival, mo (95% CI) | 7.3 (6.1 to 8.8) | 10.9 (8.6 to 12.7) | 8.4 (6.6 to 10.3) |
| Progression-free survival in months (95% CI) | | | |
| Investigator assessment | 1.9 (1.9 to 2.2) | 3.8 (3.6 to 5.2) | 3.7 (2.9 to 4.4) |
| Independent assessment* | 3.1 (2.2 to 3.8) | 5.5 (3.9 to 7.0) | 4.7 (3.9 to 5.8) |
| Objective response rate (95% CI) | 4.8% (1.9 to 7.8) | 8.6% (4.8 to 12.4) | 8.1% (4.4 to 11.8) |
| Clinical benefit (complete and partial response, and stable disease ≥ 24 weeks) (95% CI) | 15.5% (10.5 to 20.4) | 32.1% (25.7 to 38.4) | 28.1% (22.0 to 34.2) |

Hudes G et al[25].

*This category includes only patients who had at least one tumor assessment after the baseline assessment: 153 patients in the interferon group (74%), 192 patients in the temsirolimus group (92%), and 168 patients in the combination group (80%).

not significantly different, 8.6, 4.8, and 8.1%, for the temsirolimus, IFN, and combination groups. Clinical benefit, defined as objective response or stable disease for ≥ 24 weeks, was observed in 32.1, 15.5, and 28.1% of the temsirolimus, combination, and IFN groups, respectively.

A prespecified subgroup analysis revealed that the OS advantage for temsirolimus was consistent across most of the subgroups examined, including sex, time from initial diagnosis to randomization (< 1 vs ≥ 1 year), KPS (≤ 70 vs > 70), prior nephrectomy (yes vs no), tumor histology (clear cell vs other), hemoglobin level (normal vs < normal value), corrected serum calcium level (≤ 10 mg/dL vs > 10 mg/dL), and geographic area. By contrast, the survival benefit of temsirolimus was greater for patients less than 65 years old than for older patients ($p = .02$) and for patients with serum LDH levels > 1.5 × ULN than for those with LDH values ≤ 1.5 × ULN, ($p = .008$).

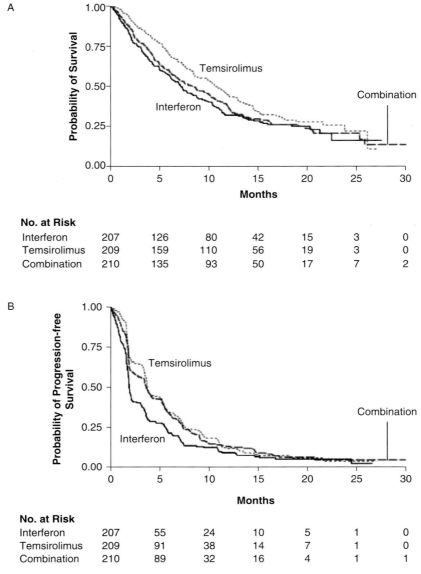

**Figure 5.**   Kaplan–Meier estimates of overall survival (panel A) and progression-free survival (panel B).

## EVEROLIMUS

Everolimus (RAD001) is an orally administered rapamycin analog and the second mTOR inhibitor in clinical development (see Figure 1). Phase I studies defined tolerable doses for daily and weekly administration. Continuous daily administration of 10 mg was selected for a phase II study in patients with metastatic, progressive, predominantly clear cell RCC and up to 1 prior therapy. In a preliminary report,[29] 37 of 41 patients enrolled were evaluated for response and toxicity. Adverse events related to everolimus treatment were stomatitis, skin rash, hypophosphatemia,

hypertriglyceridemia, hyperglycemia, anemia, thrombocytopenia, and pneumonitis—a toxicity profile similar to that of temsirolimus. Objective PR was observed in 12 patients, and 19 patients had stable disease for ≥ 3 months. The median duration of therapy exceeded 8 months, and median OS exceeded 11.5 months. These encouraging results formed the basis for a phase III study comparing daily everolimus with placebo "in 410 patients with disease progression after sunitinib, sorafenib, or both treatments. Progression free survival was the primary efficacy indicator for this double-blind randomized trial. Patients receiving everolimus had significantly

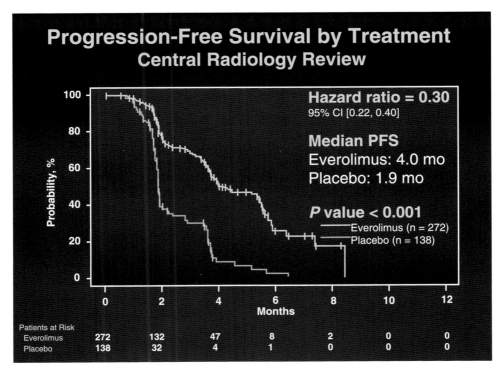

**Figure 6.** Progression-free survival of patients receiving RAD001 (everolimus) or placebo in the RECORD-1 Trial. Adapted from Motzer RJ, Escudier B, Oudard S, et al. RAD001 vs placebo in patients with metastatic renal cell carcinoma after progression on VEGFr-TKI therapy: Results from a randomized, double blind, multicenter phase III study. Presented at the 2008 annual meeting of the American Society of Clinical Oncology.

longer PFS than those receiving placebo (hazard ratio 0.30; 95% confidence interval 0.22–0.40; $p < .001$). The median PFS for everolimus and placebo groups were 4.0 and 1.9 months, respectively (Figure 6). The OS analysis will include patients assigned to placebo who received everolimus at the time of disease progression."

## COMBINATION STUDIES

Ideally, combination therapies should employ effective agents with differing mechanisms of action and adverse effect profiles. Accordingly, the possibility of achieving greater efficacy in metastatic RCC with the combination of mTOR inhibitor and a VEGF or VEGFR inhibitor seems appealing. Preliminary results of a phase I study of temsirolimus and bevacizumab have been the most encouraging. Each agent was delivered at the standard single-agent dose for multiple cycles, and eight PRs were observed in 14 patients.[31] By contrast, the combination of temsirolimus with sorafenib, a Raf kinase and VEGF receptor tyrosine kinase inhibitor, required a 50%

reduction of the single-agent dose of sorafenib. The recommended doses for phase II evaluation were sorafenib 200 mg bid and temsirolimus 25 mg IV weekly.[32] As noted above, the combination of temsirolimus and IFN was feasible only at reduced doses of each agent and was not more effective than single-agent temsirolimus in metastatic RCC.[25]

Temsirolimus combinations will be more rigorously assessed in the BEST trial sponsored by the Eastern Cooperative Oncology Group and National Cancer Institute. This randomized phase II study will compare 3 2-drug combinations, including the aforementioned temsirolimus/bevacizumab and temsirolimus/sorafenib doublets, with single-agent bevacizumab as first-line treatment for metastatic RCC.

## POTENTIAL RESISTANCE MECHANISMS

As referenced above, TORC2 can signal back to Akt phosphorylating the protein at Ser 473.[9] This positive feedback loop may limit the therapeutic effects of rapamycin analog mTOR inhibitors, which mainly inhibit mTOR associated with TORC1.[16] A second potential resistance mechanism involves inhibition of S6K as a downstream consequence of mTOR (TORC1) inhibition. Through interactions with the insulin receptor and insulin-like growth factor (IGF) receptors, and with PI3K, insulin receptor substrates 1 and 2 (IRS-1 and IRS-2) couple insulin and IGF-1 signaling to PI3K and the subsequent activation of Akt and mTOR. S6K phosphorylates IRS-1 and IRS-2, a modification that destabilizes these proteins and uncouples IGF/insulin signaling to PI3K. Thus, mTOR/S6K signaling constitutes a negative feedback mechanism for insulin and IGF-1 signaling. Loss of this negative feedback mechanism has been shown to occur in cells and tumors exposed to rapamycin,[33–35] everolimus,[36] and temsirolimus,[37] and in certain contexts could limit the antitumor effects of mTOR inhibition with these agents. This specific mechanism of resistance—increased IGF/PI3K/Akt signaling with mTOR inhibition—could be counteracted by simultaneous inhibition of IGF-1R signaling.[35–37]

Finally, evidence for a rapamycin-insensitive, mTOR-independent mechanism of protein translation that requires PI3K signaling, but not S6K or phosphorylation of the S6 ribosomal protein, is another potential barrier to effective therapy with mTOR inhibitors.[38] Depending on the expression of the alternate pathway in tumor cells, inhibition of TORC1 and its downstream effectors (S6 kinase, 4E-BP1) may not be sufficient to reduce the translation of HIFs and cell cycle regulators such as cyclin D.

## SUMMARY AND FUTURE CONSIDERATIONS

Although the mechanisms that lead to increased mTOR activation in RCC are incompletely defined, it is clear that mTOR kinase is an important therapeutic target for RCC.

All 3 mTOR inhibitors in clinical development are analogs of the bacterial product rapamycin, and they likely share a common mechanism of action with the natural product inhibitor. Compared with IFNα, temsirolimus administered as a weekly infusion improved the survival of a poor-prognosis

population with RCC and was subsequently approved for treatment of RCC. Everolimus, an orally administered mTOR inhibitor with activity in RCC, is being investigated as second-line treatment after sunitinib and sorafenib treatment. The third mTOR inhibitor, deferolimus (AP23573), has not been evaluated in RCC. These agents are generally well tolerated with metabolic abnormalities noted to be the most common dose-limiting toxic effects.

How to use mTOR inhibitors most effectively in RCC and other tumors is an active area of clinical research. Current investigations include comparison of mTOR inhibition with VEGF/PDGF tyrosine kinase inhibition, both as first- and second-line therapy, and as treatment for patients with nonclear cell histology. Additional studies have been initiated to assess the feasibility and efficacy of mTOR inhibitors in combination with targeted agents and cytotoxic drugs. Many of these studies will include correlations of tumor biomarkers with treatment outcomes toward the important goal of establishing who will benefit the most from therapeutic mTOR inhibition. The complexity of mTOR biology suggests that many new insights await basic and clinical investigators working in this field.

## REFERENCES

1. Shiloh Y. ATM and related protein kinases: safeguarding genome integrity. Nature Rev Cancer 2003;3:155–68.
2. Fingar DC, Blenis J. Target of rapamycin (TOR): an integrator of nutrient and growth factor signals and coordinator of cell growth and cell cycle progression. Oncogene 2004;23:3151–71.
3. Harding MW. Immunophilins, mTOR, and pharmacodynamic strategies for a targeted cancer therapy. Clin Cancer Res 2003;9:2882–86.
4. Skotnicki JS, Leone CL, Smith AL, et al. Design, synthesis and biological evaluation of C-42 hydroxyesters of rapamycin: the identification of CCI-779. Clin Cancer Res 2001;7:3749S–50S.
5. Schmelzle T, Hall MN. TOR, a central controller of cell growth. Cell 2000;103:253–62.
6. Neshat MS, Mellinghoff IK, Tran C, et al. Enhanced sensitivity of PTEN-deficient tumors to inhibition of FRAP/mTOR. PNAS 2001;98:10314–19.
7. Kang S, Bader AG, Vogt PK. Phosphatidylinositol 3-kinase mutations identified in human cancer are oncogenic. PNAS 2005;102:802–7.

8. Inoki K, Guan K-L. Complexity of the TOR signaling network. Trends in Cell Biol 2006;16:206–12.

9. Sarbassov DD, Guertin DA, Ali SM, et al. Phosphorylation and regulation of Akt/PKB by the rictor-mTOR complex. Science 2005;307:1098–1101.

10. Fingar DC, Richardson CJ, Tee AR, et al. mTOR controls cell cycle progression through its cell growth effectors S6K1 and 4EBP1/Eukaryotic Translation Factor 4E. Mol Cell Biol 2004;24:200–16.

11. Hudson CC, Liu M, Chiang GG, et al. Regulation of hypoxia-inducible factor 1α expression and function by the mammalian target of rapamycin. Mol Cell Biol 2002;22:7004–14.

12. Thomas GV, Tran C, Mellinghoff IK, et al. Hypoxia-inducible factor determines sensitivity to inhibitors of mTOR in kidney cancer. Nature Medicine 2005;12:122–7.

13. Pantuck AJ, Zeng G, Belldegrun AS, Figlin RA. Pathobiology, prognosis, and targeted therapy for renal cell carcinoma: exploiting the hypoxia-induced pathway. Clin Cancer Res 2003;9:4641–52.

14. Baba M, Hirai S, Yamada-Okabe H, et al. Loss of von-Hippel-Lindau protein causes cell density dependent deregulation of Cyclin D1 expression through Hypoxia-inducible factor. Oncogene 2003;22:2728–38.

15. Zatyka M, da Silva NF, Clifford SC, et al. Identification of Cyclin D1 and other novel targets for the von Hippel-Lindau tumor suppressor gene by expression array analysis and investigation of cyclin D1 genotype as a modifier in von Hippel-Lindau disease. Cancer Research 2002;62:3803–11.

16. Sarbassov DD, Ali SM, Sengupta S, et al. Prolonged rapamycin treatment inhibits mTORC2 assembly and Akt/PKB.

17. Robb VA, Karbowniczek M, Klein-Szanto AJ, et al. Activation of the mTOR signaling pathway in renal clear cell carcinoma. J Urol 2007;177:346–52.

18. Pantuck AJ, Seligson DB, Klatte T, et al. Prognostic relevance of the mTOR pathway in renal cell carcinoma. Cancer 2007;109:2257–67.

19. Neshat MS, Mellinghoff IK, Tran C, et al. Enhanced sensitivity of PTEN-deficient tumors to inhibition of FRAP/mTOR. PNAS 2001;98:10314–19.

20. Cho D, Signoretti S, Regan M, et al. Low expression of surrogates for mTOR pathway activation predicts resistance to CCI-779 in patients with advanced renal cell carcinoma [abstract C137]. Proc of the AACR-NCI-EORTC International Conference on Molecular Therapeutics, 2005.

21. Raymond E, Alexandre J, Faivre S, et al. Safety and pharmacokinetics of weekly intravenous infusion of CCI-779, a novel mTOR inhibitor, in patients with cancer. J Clin Oncol 2004;22:2336–47.

22. Hidalgo M, Buckner JC, Erlichman C, et al. A phase I and pharmacokinetic study of temsirolimus (CCI-779) administered intravenously daily for 5 days every 2 weeks to patients with advanced cancer. Clinical Cancer Res 2006. [In press].

23. Atkins M. Randomized phase II study of multiple dose levels of CCI-779, a novel mammalian target of rapamycin kinase inhibitor, in patients with advanced refractory renal cell carcinoma. J Clin Oncol 2004;22:909–18.

24. Motzer RJ, Murphy BA, Bacik J, et al. Interferon-α as a comparative treatment for clinical trials of new therapies against advanced renal cell carcinoma. J Clin Oncol 2002;20:289–96.

25. Hudes G, Carducci M, Tomczak P, et al. Temsirolimus, interferon-α, or both in advanced renal-cell carcinoma. N Engl J Med 2007;356:2271–81.

26. Mekhail TM, Abou-Jawde RM, BouMerhi G, et al. Validation and extension of the Memorial Sloan-Kettering prognostic factors model for survival in patients with previously untreated metastatic renal cell carcinoma. J Clin Oncol 2005;23:832–41.

27. Motzer RJ, Hudes GR, Curti BD, et al. Temsirolimus plus interferon α phase I trial in patients with advanced renal cell carcinoma. J Clin Oncol 2007;25:3958–64.

28. Motzer RJ, Mazumdar M, Bacik J, et al. Survival and prognostic stratification of 670 patients with advanced renal cell carcinoma. J Clin Oncol 1999;17:2530–40.

29. Jac J, Giessinger S, Khan M, et al. A phase II trial of RAD001 in patients with metastatic renal cell carcinoma [abstract 5107]. Proc Am Soc Clin Oncol 2007;25.

30. Motzer RJ, Escudier B, Oudard S, et al. Efficacy of everolimus in advanced renal cell carcinoma: a double-blind, randomized, placebo-controlled phase III trial. Lancet 2008;372:449–456.

31. Merchan, JR. Phase I/II trial of CCI-779 and bevacizumab in stage IV renal cell carcinoma: phase I safety and.

32. Patnaik A. Phase I, pharmacokinetic and pharmacodynamic study of sorafenib, a multitargeted kinase inhibitor, in combination with temsirolimus, an mTOR inhibitor, in patients with advanced solid malignancies.

33. Shah O, Wang Z, Hunter T. Inappropriate activation of the TSC/Rheb/mTOR/S6k cassette induces IRS1/2 depletion, insulin resistance, and cell survival deficiencies. Current Biol 2004;14:1650–56.

34. Sun S-Y, Rosenberg LM, Wang X, et al. Activation of Akt and eIF4E survival pathways by rapamycin-mediated mammalian target of rapamycin inhibition. Cancer Res 2005;65:7052–58.

35. Wan X, Harkavy B, Shen N, et al. Rapamycin induces feedback activation of Akt signaling through an IGF-1R-dependent mechanism. Oncogene 2007;26:1932–40.

36. O'Reilly KE, Rojo F, She Q, et al. mTOR inhibition induces upstream receptor tyrosine kinase signaling and activates Akt. Cancer Res 2006;6:1500–8.

37. Shi Y, Yan H, Frost P, et al. Mammalian target of rapamycin inhibitors activate the AKT kinase in multiple myeloma cells by up-regulating the insulin-like growth factor receptor/insulin receptor substrate-1/phosphatidylinositol 3-kinase cascade. Mol Cancer Ther 2005;4:1533–40.

38. Stolovich M, Tang H, Hornstein E, et al. Transduction of growth or mitogenic signals into translational activation of TOP mRNAs is fully reliant on the phosphatidylinositol 3-kinase-mediated pathway but requires neither S6K1 nor rpS6 phosphorylation. Mol Cell Biol 2002;22:8101–13.

# 18

# Response, Resistance and Future Therapeutics in Metastatic Renal Cell Carcinoma

**KEITH T. FLAHERTY, MD**

Despite the successful development of new therapies for metastatic renal cell carcinoma (RCC) in the past five years, nearly all patients with metastatic disease will succumb to their disease. Cleary, there is a need for continued exploration for more effective agents or regimens. Progress has been most clearly documented in the treatment of clear cell RCC, but there is evidence that the currently FDA approved therapies also benefit some patients with papillary and chromophobe RCC. Given that the molecular pathophysiology of each of those entities is distinct, a separate discussion of each RCC subtype is appropriate when considering signal transduction inhibitors. This chapter will focus on the broad area of optimizing current application of tumor-targeted therapies and future directions.

Two essential questions remain unanswered in the field of systemic therapy for metastatic RCC: what tumor or host factors predict long-term benefit from the currently available agents and what mechanisms underlie resistance to therapy. This second issue can be further dissected into the mechanisms that mediate resistance for those patients who progress early in the course of therapy and the mechanisms that mediate disease progression for those patients who remain progression-free for many months or years. Consideration of these areas is necessary as a first step in the rational development of the next generation of therapies for metastatic RCC.

## MECHANISM OF ACTION AND PREDICTIVE BIOMARKERS FOR CURRENT THERAPIES

A thorough understanding of the mechanism of action is lacking for the agents that have been shown to definitively alter the natural history of metastatic RCC: bevacizumab, sorafenib, sunitinib, and temsirolimus. Bevacizumab is, perhaps, the agent for which the mechanism of action is best described, although critical questions regarding the limits of its effects remain to be elucidated. Vascular endothelial growth factor (VEGF) signaling is clearly critical for endothelial cell proliferation and recruitment into the tumor microenvironment.[1] Yet, the cellular and macroscopic consequences of pure VEGF antagonism are more far-reaching than just inhibition of new tumor blood vessel formation. Reductions in tumor volume and induction of new areas of necrosis within tumors point to additional functions of VEGF within the tumor microenvironment.[2] If the endothelial cell is the primary or sole "target" of VEGF deprivation, then it may be that tumor blood vessels other than those that lack the support of pericytes may also be susceptible to VEGF depletion. Experimental evidence does not suggest this, but it is likely that preclinical models of tumor angiogenesis do not capture the complexity of endothelial cell homeostasis in human tumors as has been elucidated by some recent reports.[3] VEGF receptor expression on tumor cells has recently been described for a significant subset of clear cell RCCs.[4] For this subset of tumors, VEGF-targeted therapy with VEGF ligand or VEGF receptor inhibitors may mediate direct tumor-cell effects, independent of effects on tumor vessels.[5] However, this cannot entirely explain the regression of established metastases, which occurs more frequently than VEGF receptor overexpression.

Defining the factors that accurately predict which patients experience prolonged benefit from single-agent therapy would provide a rational basis for improving treatment outcomes for the latter group. There are no reports of predictive markers for any of the four proven targeted therapies, and this area of investigation remains largely exploratory. Under consideration are tumor factors, such as von Hippel-Lindau (VHL) gene status, hypoxia inducible factor (HIF) expression, and expression of HIF responsive genes (VEGF, platelet-derived growth factor (PDGF), and basic fibroblast growth factor (bFGF), amongst others). (Figure 1) Endothelial cell factors such as expression of receptors for these same growth factors and down-stream activation of signal transduction pathways are also plausible distinguishing features of responsive versus refractory tumors. Lastly, host factors that may influence outcome in the setting of these therapies include functional polymorphisms in the genes encoding the direct targets of each agent or

the downstream signaling mediators of drug effect. Even differences in drug exposure among a population of treated patients may explain differences in outcome as data from phase II trials with sunitinib suggest.[6] It is likely that multiple factors influence outcome and unraveling their respective contribution of each factor will require building statistical models incorporating apparently predictive markers for large cohorts of patients.

The exploration of predictive markers of outcome in the setting of therapy with bevacizumab, sorafenib, sunitinib, and temsirolimus in clear cell RCC is in its infancy. The only published report regarding predictive marker in the setting of therapy investigated the predictive value of VHL function or loss of function in patients with clear cell RCC treated with either bevacizumab, sunitinib, or axitinib (another potent inhibitor of VEGF and PDGF receptors).[7] In this relatively small cohort, the presence of mutations in VHL or hypermethylation of the VHL promotor, which would be expected to result in silencing of gene expression, were weakly predictive of better progression-free survival (PFS). When only those mutations that would result in complete loss of functional VHL protein were considered, along with those tumors with promoter hypermethylation, a stronger association was seen between VHL status and PFS but still not statistically

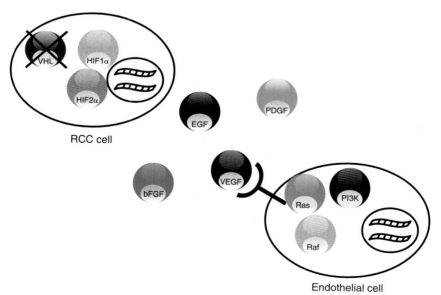

**Figure 1.** The central genetic event in clear cell renal cell carcinoma is the loss of VHL function through allelic deletion, inactivating mutation or gene expression silencing. This results in the unregulated activity of HIF1 and HIF2 which are responsible for increased expression of the pro-angiogenic growth factors: VEGF, PDGF, EGF, bFGF, amongst others.

significant. The implication of these findings is that VEGF-targeted therapy may be most beneficial for those patients whose tumors lack functional VHL and therefore have unique dependence on HIF activity and subsequent VEGF expression. This categorization of patients is supported by the preclinical data describing the central role of VHL loss of function in the pathophysiology of clear cell RCC. If tumors with VHL intact are uniquely unresponsive to VEGF-targeted therapy, then that population merits a focused search for better therapeutic targets than VEGF or VEGF receptors. Even among the patients whose tumors have VHL loss of function, there is a great range in disease control, indicating that further characterization is required to define the factors that predict outcome in this subgroup, which represents at least two-thirds of the clear cell RCC population.

The characteristics of each of the proven targeted agents must be considered to create testable hypotheses pertaining to improvements in therapy. Bevacizumab specifically binds VEGF-A, the isoform of VEGF that has been described as the ligand for VEGF receptors 1 and 2.[8] At doses of 0.3 mg/kg and higher, bevacizumab ligates all detectable serum VEGF.[9] It is not clear whether this effect also reflects complete binding of VEGF in the interstitial space between tumor cells and tumor vessel endothelial cells. The half-life of bevacizumab is approximately two weeks. Thus, repeated doses given every two to three week intervals result in drug accumulation. Although the dose that has been most thoroughly evaluated in RCC is 10 mg/kg given every 2 weeks,[2,10,11] on the basis of pharmacokinetic and pharmacodynamic data, one would anticipate that even lower doses and less-frequent administration would achieve complete or near complete VEGF binding.

Sorafenib and sunitinib are both kinase inhibitors with potency against VEGF receptors −1, −2, and −3.[12,13] Although these may be the most relevant targets in clear cell RCC, the additional activity against PDGF receptor β (PDGFRβ) associated with both the agents is likely a valuable property when targeting tumor angiogenesis given the role of PDGF in recruiting pericytes to sprouting tumor vessels.[14] Each drug inhibits additional kinases, and the spectrum of kinases beyond VEGF and PDGF receptors differs significantly.[15] Having demonstrated clear benefit in clear cell RCC, the possibility remains that many of the kinases inhibited by each agent may contribute to toxicity and not to efficacy. In that sense, the therapeutic index of more narrow spectrum VEGF receptor inhibitors may be greater. The phase II trial experience with axitinib lends some support to this hypothesis, however, comparative trials will be needed with careful attention to impact on biomarkers to resolve this issue.[16] It is also possible that the extended spectrum of sorafenib and sunitinib offer some therapeutic advantages in RCC. Sorafenib, for example, is a potent inhibitor of Raf kinases. These constituents of the mitogen activated protein (MAP) kinase pathway have been shown to be essential for VEGF-stimulated proliferation of endothelial cells. In preclinical models, Raf antagonism results in endothelial cell apoptosis and inhibition of angiogenesis.[17,18] Thus, Raf inhibition could complement VEGF receptor inhibition by blocking serial steps in endothelial cell signaling.

## MECHANISMS OF RESISTANCE TO TARGETED THERAPY IN RCC

Mechanisms of resistance to VEGF-targeted therapy in clear cell RCC are not defined. To the same degree that responsiveness to VEGF-targeted therapy is highly variable, resistance may be mediated by different factors for patients whose tumors progress early or late in the course of therapy. In the setting of VEGF receptor inhibition in clear cell RCC patients, serum VEGF levels increase significantly within the first few weeks of treatment.[19,20] Of note, this phenomenon is observed with bevacizumab as well.[9] However, it has been shown that the amount of available unbound bevacizumab is sufficient to adsorb this excess VEGF. It has been hypothesized that this increase reflects effective VEGF receptor blockade and that an intracellular or intercellular feedback loop leads to greater HIF activity and more VEGF production. If this increase reflects the degree to which VEGF receptors are inhibited, as opposed to a macroscopic effect on tumor vasculature architecture leading to increased tumor hypoxia and HIF activation, then one might expect that greater increases in VEGF would associate with improved clinical outcome.[21] A very strong association would only be expected if all tumors were equally dependent on VEGF signaling for progression. Based on variable loss of VHL, amongst other factors, this is likely not the case. Additional hypotheses regarding the significance of rising VEGF levels following VEGF receptor inhibition are that tumor progression might ultimately be mediated by overcoming incomplete receptor inhibition or stimulation of lower affinity VEGF receptors. Experimental evidence regarding this phenomenon is lacking. There are, however, ample data from animal models of tumor angiogenesis (not RCC) that VEGF or VEGF receptor inhibition leads to increased production of PDGF and bFGF by tumors.[22] PDGF upregulation may be addressed by the cross reactivity to PDGFRβ inherent with sorafenib and sunitinib, but pro-angiogenesis growth factors, including bFGF, transforming growth factor β (TGFβ), hepatocyte growth factor (HGF) angiopoetin, and ephrins, may mediate tumor escape in the face of VEGF and VEGF receptor inhibition.

mTOR inhibition was added to the list of successful molecular interventions in RCC with the phase IV trial comparing temsirolimus to interferon.[23] This agent was taken into phase III testing based on clinical activity observed in a large phase II trial, but a robust understanding of mTOR in RCC pathophysiology was lacking.[24] It had been observed that tumor angiogenesis is inhibited with mTOR inhibition in preclinical models.[25] It has since been described that mTOR regulates HIF expression and activity in several tumor models.[26,27] This provides a plausible mechanistic link between mTOR and the known role of VHL and HIF in clear cell RCC. However, it also known that the phosphoinositol-3-phosphate kinase pathway (PI3 kinase pathway), in which mTOR plays a critical role, is responsible for a significant element of VEGF receptor and other growth factor receptor signaling in endothelial cells.[28,29] Thus, it remains possible that temsirolimus exerts a significant effect on both the tumor cell and endothelial cell that would result in inhibition of angiogenesis. These points aside, the role of the PI3 kinase pathway in tumor cell survival, independent of HIF, cannot be ignored as a possible contributor to efficacy with mTOR inhibition. The potential mechanisms of resistance to mTOR inhibited may be quite distinct compared to that observed with VEGF-targeted therapy. One observation that deserves closer attention is that rapamycin analogs, including temsirolimus, inhibit only one of two signaling complexes of which mTOR is a part. The TORC1 complex is potently inhibited by the temsirolimus and other rapamycin analog mTOR inhibitors, whereas the TORC2 complex is not.[30] As a consequence, one downstream consequence of mTOR activation is unopposed. It has been demonstrated in preclinical studies that mTOR inhibition with rapamycin analogs results in feedback upregulation of the PI3 kinase pathway, assessed by activation of Akt, which is more proximal in the PI3 kinase pathway than mTOR.[31] This is analogous to VEGF upregulation in the setting of VEGF receptor blockade. Because Akt can activate the TORC2 complex, which is not inhibited by rapamycin analogs, it is possible that the upregulation of this pathway compensates for TORC1 inhibition in tumors that are refractory to temsirolimus. This question requires further preclinical and clinical evaluation.

The cell signaling consequences of VEGF- or mTOR-targeted therapies are currently being studied in several ongoing clinical trials. These *neoadjuvant* studies share the feature that therapy is administered prior to cytoreductive nephrectomy for patients with metastatic RCC at presentation. Provided that an adequate baseline biopsy is obtained to allow baseline assessment of the expression and activity of HIF, VEGF, VEGF receptors, the MAP kinase, and PI3 kinase pathways, the impact of therapy can be assessed in the nephrectomy specimen. By the same token, the upregulation of pro-angiogenic growth factors that may mediate resistance to therapy can be investigated in the nephrectomy specimen. For studies that administer therapy for a relatively short time prior to nephrectomy, these putative mechanisms of resistance may reflect only be relevant for RCC that is refractory early in the course of therapy. (Figure 2) Mechanisms of delayed resistance would only manifest with more prolonged exposure, which would require delaying the performance of nephrectomy until months have passed. This poses a challenge in study

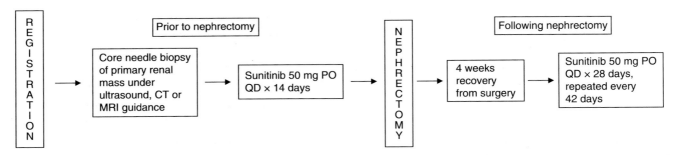

**Figure 2.** Design of UPCC 01807, a neoadjuvant trial of sunitinib for patients with metastastic clear cell renal cell carcinoma at the time of initial diagnosis. As cytoreductive remains the standard-of-care for initial management, there is an opportunity to study the pharmacodynamic effects of novel agents in this patient population. Numerous studies of similar design are underway, exploring the mechanism of action for sunitinib, sorafenib, temsirolimus, and bevacizumab.

design as planning the scientifically appropriate interval prior to surgery may not align with the most clinically appropriate time. As all angiogenesis inhibitors have the potential risk of delaying wound healing, a fine line must be drawn between having enough drug exposure in the tumor at the time of nephrectomy to be informative of mechanism of action while not having so much systemic exposure that postoperative healing is significantly impaired. This can be accomplished with sorafenib, sunitinib, and temsirolimus, which are cleared relatively quickly, but not with bevacizumab with a two week half-life.[32,33,34]

## DEVELOPMENT OF NOVEL TARGETED AGENTS IN CLEAR CELL RCC

Sorafenib and sunitinib are members of the largest class of cancer therapeutics in development, with 15 other VEGF receptor inhibitors in clinical trials. To the same extent that differences between the mechanism of action of sorafenib and sunitinib in RCC are difficult to discern, it is unclear what advantages may come from VEGF receptor inhibitors that have greater or less potency against members of the VEGF receptor family. Sorafenib and sunitinib both exert relatively greater effect on VEGFR-2, compared with VEGFR-1 or VEGFR-3. Given that VEGFR-1 is a receptor for VEGF-A, and preclinical evidence supports it unique contribution to tumor angiogenesis,[35] it may be that having VEGFR-1 inhibiting is beneficial for complete VEGF-A signaling inhibition. Axitinib and AMG-706 are examples of agents that offer potent inhibition of VEGFR-1, in addition to VEGFR-2.[36,37] Unlike

sorafenib and sunitinib, these agents are associated with proteinuria in a minority of patients enrolled on phase I trials.[38,39] Bevacizumab frequently induces proteinuria and had been the only VEGF signaling inhibitor to cause this toxicity.[9] Because bevacizumab only impacts VEGF-A signaling, it may be that the observation of proteinuria with the newer VEGF receptor inhibitors reflects more complete suppression of VEGF-A signaling with these agents. VEGFR-3 mediates lymphangiogenesis,[40] which is clearly a component of tumor pathophysiology, but the therapeutic value of blocking lymphangiogenesis, as opposed to angiogenesis, in RCC is unknown. Many of the VEGF receptor inhibitors currently in development have nearly equal potency against VEGFR-1, -2, and -3, with far less potency against other kinases. Axitinib, which potently inhibits all VEGF receptors, has demonstrated the highest objective response rate and longest median PFS of any agents evaluated in RCC to date.[16] However, comparative trials against sorafenib or sunitinib will be required to determine if efficacy is truly greater. And if so, further preclinical evaluation will be needed to understand what unique aspects of the drug underlie greater efficacy.

Novel VEGF ligand inhibitors are also in clinical development. VEGF trap is the best characterized of this class, but phase II data in RCC have not been reported.[41] The theoretical advantages of VEGF trap over bevacizumab are that the affinity for VEGF is higher and other isoforms of VEGF, beyond VEGF-A, are bound. Analogous to the potential advantage of agents that potently inhibit all VEGF receptors, VEGF trap and other related agents. The affinity of bevacizumab for VEGF-A is very high, with no detectable free VEGF remaining in patients treated at the doses used currently in clinical trials. So, it is not clear that whether there is benefit in developing agents whose sole feature is higher affinity for VEGF.

VEGF and VEGF receptor activation are downstream consequences of HIF activity in RCCs. However, there are other consequences of HIF activity that contribute to carcinogenesis. For example, HIF2α controls the expression of c-*myc*, which is critical cell cycle regulator.[42] Selective inhibition of VEGF signaling clearly alters the natural history of metastatic RCC, but concomitant inhibition of other HIF regulated signaling is a clear direction for novel therapy development. Amongst other potential advantages, antagonism of HIF would potentially downregulate angiogenesis promoting growth factors other than VEGF. There are unique challenges to develop HIF-targeted therapies, in that HIF is a transcription factor, which lacks an enzymatic domain that can be blocked with a competitive inhibitor.[43] It is possible that non-competitive inhibitors that block the protein-protein interactions that are essential for HIF function can be developed, but large peptides and proteins have very limited bioavailability and cellular penetration.

A promising new direction for RCC therapeutics is agents that modulate HIF stability and expression. As discussed previously, mTOR appears to serve this function, and the mechanism of action of temsirolimus may, in part, derive from this effect. Other constituents of the PI3 kinase pathway have been independently demonstrated to regulate HIF protein stability, including Akt and glycogen synthase kinase (GSK3)β.[44,45] Inhibitors of Akt are in preclinical development, and GSK3β inhibitors are in clinical trials for neurodegenerative diseases and, more recently, cancer. Given the large number of factors that have been associated with regulation of HIF expression and stability, it is not surprising that many different classes of novel cancer therapies have been observed to alter HIF levels in preclinical models. These include class II HDAC inhibitors, c-kit inhibitors, STAT3 inhibitors, and HSP90 inhibitors.[46,47,48,49] Although the ability of these inhibitors to downregulate HIF in vitro has been demonstrated, the clinical effects of these agents in RCC has not been thoroughly evaluated. Any one of these HIF regulators may offer incomplete inhibition of HIF activity and thus minimal single-agent activity

in RCC patients. However, these agents may be ideally suited to be used in combination with VEGF-targeted therapies that appear to upregulate HIF activity.

Dysregulated HIF activity results in the upregulation of numerous growth factors that stimulate angiogenesis. Although VEGF may be the single most potent endothelial cell mitogen, angiopoetin, bFGF, HGF, and TGFβ each have the ability to stimulate tumor angiogenesis.[50,51,52,53] Thus, any of these are plausible partners for VEGF-targeted therapies as a strategy for broadening the coverage of angiogenesis mediators. Inhibition of epidermal growth factor receptor (EGFR), the receptor for TGFβ, has been explored in phase II trials with single-agent EGFR inhibitors and in combination with bevacizumab or sunitinib.[54,55] In single-agent EGFR inhibitor trials, objective response rates were observed among patients with clear cell RCC in 5 to 10% of cases, and similarly, a small percentage of patients had disease stabilization for more than 6 months.[56,57] The most definitive test of EGFR inhibition was a randomized phase II trial in which bevacizumab was administered with or without erlotinib among 100 patients with clear cell RCC.[10] Although a trial of this size does not reliably rule out a small added clinical benefit, there was no difference detected in either PFS or objective response rate. Thus, among unselected RCC patients, this approach does not appear to warrant further testing. Phase I trials are being conducted with inhibitors of the receptors for angiopoetin, bFGF, and HGF: Tie-2, FGF receptor, and c-met. The latter two targets are genetically related to other receptor tyrosine kinases. Thus, it is not surprising that small molecule kinase inhibitors have been identified that have potency against either FGF receptor or c-met in addition to VEGF receptor and PDGF receptor β.[58,59] Such broad-spectrum inhibitors are, therefore, similar to sorafenib and sunitinib in some respects, but their spectrum is somewhat more tailored to the high priority angiogenesis targets.

## COMBINATIONS OF TARGETED AGENTS FOR CLEAR CELL RCC

The mechanistic overlap of sorafenib, sunitinib, temsirolimus, and bevacizumab has prompted investigators to hypothesize that combinations of these agents may synergistically inhibit angiogenesis. Of the possible combinations of these agents, sorafenib and sunitinib have not been paired together given their shared effects at the level of receptor tyrosine kinases. Each of the other combinations has been explored in phase I trials among RCC patients and are currently entering phase II and phase III trials.

As noted previously, sorafenib, sunitinib, and bevacizumab treatment are associated with significant increases in VEGF above baseline levels. To the extent that this effect may reflect further HIF activation in tumor cells and may underlie eventual resistance to these agents, antagonizing this response is a rational strategy for improving the duration of disease control. (Figure 3)

Sorafenib has been combined with bevacizumab in a phase I trial restricted to patients with metastatic RCC.[60] Forty-eight patients were enrolled, 85% of them had clear cell RCC. The doses of bevacizumab ranged from 3 mg/kg to 10 mg/kg every 2 weeks, and the dose of sorafenib were varied between 200 mg once daily to 400 mg twice daily. Doses of sorafenib at 200 mg twice daily or 400 mg twice daily combined

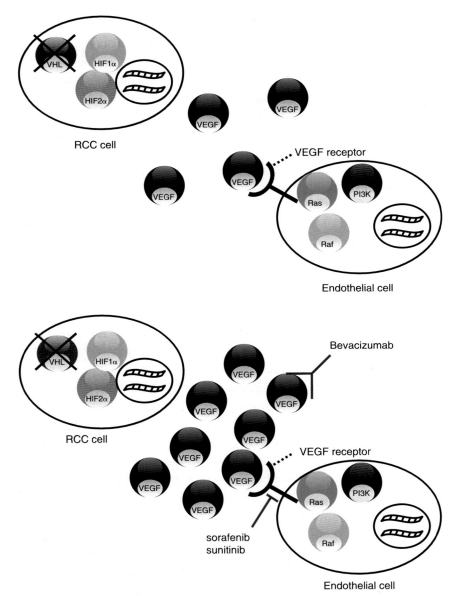

**Figure 3.** In the setting of treatment with either the VEGF receptor inhibitors, sorafenib and sunitinib, VEGF levels increase. While this increase has been weakly correlated with improved response to therapy, it is unknown whether this increase eventually mediates resistance to therapy. It is this possibility that have led to the hypothesis that the addition of bevacizumab to sorafenib or sunitinib therapy might enhance the blockade of VEGF signaling and delay the emergence of refractory disease.

with any dose of bevacizumab resulted in severe rash, hand-foot syndrome, and declines in performance status. Thus, the dose-limiting toxicities were those typically observed with sorafenib, but more severe than would be expected with sorafenib alone at 400 mg twice daily. Conversely, any dose of sorafenib combined with bevacizumab at 10 mg/kg every 2 weeks resulted in dose limiting hypertension and proteinuria. These are typically associated with bevacizumab single-agent therapy but were more prevalent and severe for the patients receiving combination therapy. Bevacizumab appears to enhance the severity of hand-foot syndrome in this combination despite the lack of hand-foot syndrome with bevacizumab single-agent therapy. Likewise, sorafenib appears to enhance the severity of proteinuria, even though it does not cause proteinuria when given alone. In the absence of a pharmacokinetic interaction, it is most likely that this interaction is at the level of target inhibition. The maximum tolerated dose in this trial was determined to be sorafenib 200 mg once daily (25% of the standard single-agent dose) combined with 5 mg/kg of bevacizumab every 2 weeks (50% of the standard single-agent dose). In a separate phase I trial among patients with advanced solid tumors, interrupted schedules of sorafenib administration were explored as a means to limit the severity of hand-foot syndrome. By administering sorafenib for 5 days out of every seven, a dose of 200 mg twice daily could be tolerably combined with 5 mg/kg of bevacizumab every 2 weeks.[61] This more dose-intense regimen was selected for further development in RCC.

Sunitinib has been combined with bevacizumab in two phase I trials, one exclusively among patients with RCC and the other among patients with advanced solid tumors.[62,63] In both the cases, a standard 50 mg daily dose of sunitinib for 28 days out of every 42 days was tolerable in combination with bevacizumab 10 mg/kg every 2 weeks. Although the severe toxicity rate was sufficiently low to allow these doses to be declared to recommended phase II doses, there was one case of fatal myocardial infarction in the second cycle and a case of severe subcutaneous hemorrhage in the first cycle. Although infrequent, these toxicities raise the concern that severe vascular toxicity could be a unique concern with this combination. More recently, updated results from one of these two trials revealed several cases of microangiopathic hemolytic

anemia. Vascular homeostasis is clearly regulated, in part, by VEGF, and it may be that near complete antagonism of VEGF signaling will disrupt even mature vasculature. A randomized phase II trial administering sunitinib with or without bevacizumab in patients with metastatic clear cell RCC was intiated, but now halted in the face of these events.

Combining temsirolimus with either sorafenib or sunitinib provides another strategy for countering the apparent HIF activation following administration of the VEGF receptor inhibitors. The combination of sunitinib and temsirolimus proved to be intolerable at doses that were 50% lower than the standard single-agent doses for each agent.[64] Therefore, this regimen was declared unsuitable for further testing. Sorafenib and temsirolimus could be safely combined, but a reduction in the dose of sorafenib to 200 mg twice daily was required to administer temsirolimus at its standard single-agent dose (25 mg weekly).[65] In this phase I trial among patients with advanced solid tumors, the dose-limiting toxicities were rash, hand-foot syndrome, mucositis, elevated creatinine and thrombocytopenia each being commonly observed with less severity for single-agent sorafenib or temsirolimus. The rate of severe toxicity was higher when the dose of sorafenib was maximized (400 mg twice daily) with any dose of temsirolimus as opposed to combinations with 25 mg of temsirolimus and any dose of sorafenib.

The combination of bevacizumab and temsirolimus has been evaluated in a phase I trial among patients with metastatic RCC.[66] The standard single-agent doses of both the agents could be combined with an acceptable toxicity profile (bevacizumab 10 mg/kg every 2 weeks and temsirolimus 25 mg every week). There was one case of dose-limiting stomatitis, which can be observed with temsirolimus, although infrequently so severe. Thus, this combination appears to be perhaps the least problematic regarding enhancement of known toxicities. This could relate to the high degree of specificity of these agents for VEGF and mTOR, whereas the broad-spectrum kinase inhibitors have been more problematic to combine with these agents.

Definitive conclusions regarding the efficacy of these various combinations cannot be made because the only available data are from phase I trials, and several of these trials were not conducted exclusively in patients with RCC. In the case of the three trials that were restricted to patients with RCC, the objective response rates reported for the combinations of sorafenib with bevacizumab and temsirolimus with bevacizumab were notably higher than one would expect for any of those agents given alone.[60,66] These initial observations will need to be validated in phase II trials, but observing response rates of 40 to 60% when combining agents with single-agent response rates of 10 to 15% certainly supports the notion that these agents could act synergistically in RCC.

Several randomized trials, phase II and phase III, have been undertaken to determine which combinations are most promising. Several pharmaceutical industry-sponsored trials have been initiated comparing an individual doublet with one of the single agents. These trials will provide important information regarding the magnitude of clinical benefit associated with the various combinations. However, it will not be possible to compare the results of these trials to determine which doublet is most worthy of subsequent evaluation in a definitive phase III trial. To address this need, a randomized phase II trial has been initiated in the cooperative groups (E2804). (Figure 4) This trial is simultaneously evaluating the combinations of bevacizumab/temsirolimus, bevacizumab/sorafenib, and sorafenib/temsirolimus. The only doublet missing, for which a phase II dose has been established, is sunitinib/bevacizumab. A benchmark, single-agent bevacizumab arm is included, making this a four-arm trial. The purpose of this trial is to select the combination with the most promising PFS. This regimen would be suited for a definitive phase III trial comparing doublet therapy with sequential single-agent therapy with each of the drugs in the doublet. Currently, sequential single-agent therapy has evolved as the clinical standard, and thus, combination therapy must be proven superior to this approach to warrant declaring a new standard of care.

## NONCLEAR CELL RCC

The progress made in the treatment of metastatic RCC has largely been confined to clear cell RCC. By design, most phase III trials, and many phase II trials, excluded patients with histologic subtypes other than clear cell. Although it is true that the molecular underpinning of papillary and chromophobe RCC appears to be independent of VHL, it is not clear that HIF and downstream upregulation of VEGF is not a viable therapeutic target in either subtype. Yet, the evidence for benefit with the four proven clear cell RCC therapies in papillary or chromophobe RCC is scant.

Fifteen patients with papillary RCC and fewer with chromophobe RCC were included in the the randomized discontinuation, phase II trial of sorafenib.[67] Minor and partial responses were observed in that small group, suggesting that there may be activity. In the phase III trial comparing tem-

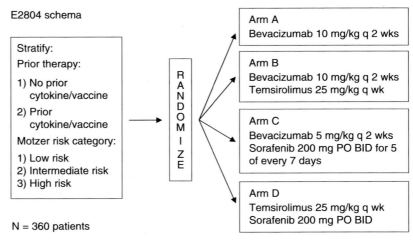

**Figure 4.** Design of E2804, a randomized phase II trial evaluating doublet combinations of bevacizumab, sorafenib and temsirolimus. The goal of this trial is to understand the safety and efficacy of this approach. Provided that at least one of the combination arms provides a median progression-free survival of 14 months or greater, a phase III trial would be considered comparing the best combination therapy to the best available single-agent therapy.

sirolimus to interferon, the vast majority of the patients enrolled on had clear cell RCC, but a notable subset of patients (20%) had papillary RCC.[23] In a subset analysis of overall survival between the two arms, patients with papillary RCC appeared to obtain an even greater benefit from temsirolimus compared to interferon than those with clear cell RCC.[68] This result indicates that further investigation with mTOR inhibitors in papillary RCC is warranted.

Although papillary RCC has intact VHL, genetic amplification of c-met has been identified in the majority of sporadic Type I papillary RCC cases and activating mutations in c-met in nearly all cases of familial Type I papillary RCC.[69] This receptor tyrosine kinase represents a unique target and one that is not inhibited by temsirolimus, bevacizumab, sorafenib, or sunitinib. Broad-spectrum kinase inhibitors with potency against c-met are currently in clinical development and one, XL880, has entered phase II testing in papillary RCC. Specific c-met inhibitors are also in development, but only one has progressed into a phase I trial (ARQ197).[70]

The molecular pathophysiology of chromophobe RCC is not well understood. The only commonly observed defect is mutation or deletion of the Burt-Hogg-Dube gene.[71] The function of this tumor suppressor is under investigation, and no upregulated pathway has been identified for which an inhibitor can be tested. Thus, this subtype remains without a rational therapeutic target.

## CONCLUSION

Although significant progress has been made in the treatment of RCC with the emergence of VEGF and mTOR signaling inhibitors, the most fruitful future direction for improved therapy remains obscure. In clear cell RCC, three strategies are being pursued in parallel: (1) more potent and specific inhibitors of HIF or VEGF signaling, (2) inhibitors of angiogenesis mediators other than VEGF and PDGF, and (3) combinations of individually active agents that act at distinct points in the HIF to endothelial cell axis. Certainly, there are additional avenues that must be pursued, particularly for clear RCCs for which VHL is intact. The aberrant signaling pathways in that important

subgroup require focused preclinical investigation. Arguably, the greatest strides will come when a molecular classification can be defined that explains the heterogeneity of response to current therapy for RCC and identifies the best subgroup-specific therapeutic targets.

## REFERFENCES

1. Ferrara N. VEGF as a therapeutic target in cancer. Oncology 2005; 69(Suppl 3):11–16.
2. Yang JC, Haworth L, Sherry RM, Hwu P, et al. A randomized trial of bevacizumab, an anti-vascular endothelial growth factor antibody, for metastatic renal cancer. N Engl J Med 2003; 349:427–34.
3. Gee MS, Procopio WN, Makonnen S, et al. Tumor vessel development and maturation impose limits on the effectiveness of anti-vascular therapy. Am J Pathol 2003; 162: 183–93.
4. Badalian G, Derecskei K, Szendroi A, et al. EGFR and VEGFR2 protein expressions in bone metastases of clear cell renal cancer. Anticancer Res 2007; 27:889–94.
5. Yu C, Friday BB, Lai JP, et al. Cytotoxic synergy between the multikinase inhibitor sorafenib and the proteasome inhibitor bortezomib in vitro: induction of apoptosis through Akt and c-Jun NH2-terminal kinase pathways. Mol Cancer Ther 2006; 5:2378–87.
6. Houk BE, Bello CL, Michaelson MD, et al. Exposure-response of sunitinib in metastatic renal cell carcinoma: A population pharmacokinetic/pharmacodynamic approach. J Clin Oncol 2007. ASCO Annual Meeting ProceedingsPart I Vol 25, No. 18S (June 20 Supplement)2007. 5027.
7. Rini BI, Jaeger E, Weinberg V, et al. Clinical response to therapy targeted at vascular endothelial growth factor in metastatic renal cell carcinoma: impact of patient characteristics and Von Hippel-Lindau gene status. BJU Int 2006.
8. Ferrara N, Hillan KJ, Gerber HP, Novotny W. Discovery and development of bevacizumab, an anti-VEGF antibody for treating cancer. Nat Rev Drug Discov 2004; 3:391–400.
9. Gordon MS, Margolin K, Talpaz M, et al. Phase I safety and pharmacokinetic study of recombinant human anti-vascular endothelial growth factor in patients with advanced cancer. J Clin Oncol 2001; 19:843–50.
10. Bukowski RM, Kabbinavar FF, Figlin RA, et al. Randomized phase II study of Erlotinib Combined With Bevacizumab Compared With Bevacizumab Alone in Metastatic Renal Cell Cancer. J Clin Oncol 2007 [Epub ahead of print].
11. Escudier B, Koralewski P, Pluzanska A, et al. A randomized, controlled, double-blind phase III study (AVOREN) of bevacizumab/interferon-α2a vs placebo/interferon-α2a as first-line therapy in metastatic renal cell carcinoma. J Clin Oncol 2007. ASCO Annual Meeting Proceedings Part IVol 25, No. 18S (June 20 Supplement) 20073.
12. Wilhelm SM, Carter C, Tang L, et al. BAY 43-9006 43-9006 exhibits broad spectrum oral antitumor activity and targets the RAF/MEK/ERK pathway and receptor tyrosine kinases involved in tumor progression and angiogenesis. Cancer Res 2004; 64:7099–109.

13. Mendel DB, Laird AD, Xin X, et al. In vivo antitumor activity of SU11248, a novel tyrosine kinase inhibitor targeting vascular endothelial growth factor and platelet-derived growth factor receptors: determination of a pharmacokinetic/pharmacodynamic relationship. Clin Cancer Res 2003; 9:327–37.

14. Benjamin LE, Hemo I, Keshet E. A plasticity window for blood vessel remodelling is defined by pericyte coverage of the preformed endothelial network and is regulated by PDGF-B and VEGF. Development 1998; 125:1591–8.

15. Fabian MA, Biggs WH III, Treiber DK, et al. A small molecule-kinase interaction map for clinical kinase inhibitors. Nat Biotechnol 2005; 23:329–36. [Epub 2005 Feb 13]

16. Rini BI. SU11248 and AG013736: current data and future trials in renal cell carcinoma. Clin Genitourin Cancer 2005; 4:175–80.

17. Hood JD, Bednarski M, Frausto R, et al. Tumor regression by targeted gene delivery to the neovasculature. Science 2002; 296:2404–7.

18. Alavi A, Hood JD, Frausto R,. Role of Raf in vascular protection from distinct apoptotic stimuli. Science 2003; 301:94–6.

19. Veronese ML, Mosenkis A, Flaherty KT, et al. Mechanisms of hypertension associated with BAY 43-9006. J Clin Oncol 2006; 24:1363–9.

20. Deprimo SE, Bello CL, Smeraglia J, et al. Circulating protein biomarkers of pharmacodynamic activity of sunitinib in patients with metastatic renal cell carcinoma: modulation of VEGF and VEGF-related proteins. J Transl Med 2007; 5:32.

21. Flaherty KT. Sorafenib in renal cell carcinoma. Clin Cancer Res 2007; 13(2 Pt 2):747S–752S.

22. Jubb AM, Oates AJ, Holden S, Koeppen H. Predicting benefit from anti-angiogenic agents in malignancy. Nat Rev Cancer 2006; 6:626–35. [Epub 2006 Jul 13]

23. Hudes G, Carducci M, Tomczak P, et al. Temsirolimus, interferon alfa, or both for advanced renal-cell carcinoma. N Engl J Med 2007; 356:2271–81.

24. Atkins MB, Hidalgo M, Stadler WM, et al. Randomized phase II study of multiple dose levels of CCI-779, a novel mammalian target of rapamycin kinase inhibitor, in patients with advanced refractory renal cell carcinoma. J Clin Oncol 2004; 22:909–18.

25. Humar R, Kiefer FN, Berns H, et al. Hypoxia enhances vascular cell proliferation and angiogenesis in vitro via rapamycin (mTOR)-dependent signaling. FASEB J 2002; 16:771–80.

26. Land SC, Tee AR. Hypoxia-inducible factor $1\alpha$ is regulated by the mammalian target of rapamycin (mTOR) via an mTOR signaling motif. J Biol Chem 2007; 282:20534–43. [Epub 2007 May 14]

27. Pore N, Jiang Z, Shu HK, et al. Akt1 activation can augment hypoxia-inducible factor-$1\alpha$ expression by increasing protein translation through a mammalian target of rapamycin-independent pathway. Mol Cancer Res 2006; 4:471–9.

28. Hamada K, Sasaki T, Koni PA, et al. The PTEN/PI3K pathway governs normal vascular development and tumor angiogenesis. Genes Dev 2005; 19:2054–65.

29. Riesterer O, Zingg D, Hummerjohann J, et al. Degradation of PKB/Akt protein by inhibition of the VEGF receptor/mTOR pathway in endothelial cells. Oncogene 2004 ; 23:4624–35.

30. Inoki K, Guan KL. Complexity of the TOR signaling network. Trends Cell Biol 2006; 16:206–12.

31. O'Reilly KE, Rojo F, She QB, et al. mTOR inhibition induces upstream receptor tyrosine kinase signaling and activates Akt. Cancer Res 2006; 66:1500–8.

32. Strumberg D, Richly H, Hilger RA, et al. Phase I clinical and pharmacokinetic study of the novel raf kinase and vascular endothelial growth factor receptor inhibitor BAY 43-9006 in patients with advanced refractory solid tumors. J Clin Oncol 2005; 23:965–72.

33. Faivre S, Delbaldo C, Vera K, et al. Safety, pharmacokinetic, and antitumor activity of SU11248, a novel oral multitarget tyrosine kinase inhibitor, in patients with cancer. J Clin Oncol 2006; 24:25–35.

34. Hidalgo M, Buckner JC, Erlichman C, et al. A phase I and pharmacokinetic study of temsirolimus (CCI-779) administered intravenously daily for 5 days every 2 weeks to patients with advanced cancer. Clin Cancer Res 2006; 12:5755–63.

35. Fong GH, Rossant J, Gertsenstein M, Breitman ML. Role of the Flt-1 receptor tyrosine kinase in regulating the assembly of vascular endothelium. Nature 1995; 376:66–70.

36. Inai T, Mancuso M, Hashizume H, et al. Inhibition of vascular endothelial growth factor (VEGF) signaling in cancer causes loss of endothelial fenestrations, regression of tumor vessels, and appearance of basement membrane ghosts. Am J Pathol 2004; 165:35–52.

37. Polverino A, Coxon A, Starnes C, et al. AMG 706, an oral, multikinase inhibitor that selectively targets vascular endothelial growth factor, platelet-derived growth factor, and kit receptors, potently inhibits angiogenesis and induces regression in tumor xenografts. Cancer Res 2006; 66:8715–21.

38. Rugo HS, Herbst RS, Liu G, et al. Phase I trial of the oral antiangiogenesis agent AG-013736 in patients with advanced solid tumors: pharmacokinetic and clinical results. J Clin Oncol 2005; 23:5474–83. [Epub 2005 Jul 18]

39. Rosen LS, Kurzrock R, Mulay M, et al. Safety, pharmacokinetics, and efficacy of AMG 706, an oral multikinase inhibitor, in patients with advanced solid tumors. J Clin Oncol 2007; 25:2369–76.

40. Karpanen T, Egeblad M, Karkkainen MJ, et al. Vascular endothelial growth factor C promotes tumor lymphangiogenesis and intralymphatic tumor growth. Cancer Res 2001; 61:1786–90.

41. Holash J, Davis S, Papadopoulos N, et al. VEGF-Trap: a VEGF blocker with potent antitumor effects. Proc Natl Acad Sci USA 2002; 99:11393–8.

42. Gordan JD, Bertout JA, Hu CJ, et al. HIF-$2\alpha$ promotes hypoxic cell proliferation by enhancing c-myc transcriptional activity. Cancer Cell 2007; 11:335–47.

43. Park EJ, Kong D, Fisher R, et al. Targeting the PAS-A domain of HIF-$1\alpha$ for development of small molecule inhibitors of HIF-1. Cell Cycle 2006; 5:1847–53.

44. Majumder PK, Febbo PG, Bikoff R, et al. mTOR inhibition reverses Akt-dependent prostate intraepithelial neoplasia through regulation of apoptotic and HIF-1-dependent pathways. Nat Med 2004; 10:594–601.

45. Flugel D, Gorlach A, Michiels C, Kietzmann T. Glycogen synthase kinase 3 phosphorylates hypoxia-inducible factor.

46. Qian DZ, Kachhap SK, Collis SJ, et al. Class II Histone Deacetylases are associated with VHL-independent regulation of hypoxia-inducible factor 1α. Cancer Res 2006; 66:8814–21.

47. Litz J, Krystal GW. Imatinib inhibits c-Kit-induced hypoxia-inducible factor-1α activity and vascular endothelial growth factor expression in small cell lung cancer cells. Mol Cancer Ther 2006; 5:1415–22.

48. Jung JE, Lee HG, Cho IH, et al. STAT3 is a potential modulator of HIF-1-mediated VEGF expression in human renal carcinoma cells. FASEB J 2005; 19:1296–8.

49. Isaacs JS, Jung YJ, Mimnaugh EG, et al. Hsp90 regulates a von Hippel Lindau-independent hypoxia-inducible factor-1α-degradative pathway. J Biol Chem 2002; 277:29936–44.

50. Lin P, Buxton JA, Acheson A, et al. Antiangiogenic gene therapy targeting the endothelium-specific receptor tyrosine kinase Tie2. Proc Natl Acad Sci USA 1998; 95:8829–34.

51. Jouanneau J, Plouet J, Moens G, Thiery JP. FGF-2 and FGF-1 expressed in rat bladder carcinoma cells have similar angiogenic potential but different tumorigenic properties in vivo. Oncogene 1997; 14:671–6.

52. Kuba K, Matsumoto K, Date K, et al. HGF/NK4, a four-kringle antagonist of hepatocyte growth factor, is an angiogenesis inhibitor that suppresses tumor growth and metastasis in mice. Cancer Res 2000; 60:6737–43.

53. Ananth S, Knebelmann B, Gruning W, et al. Transforming growth factor beta1 is a target for the von Hippel-Lindau tumor suppressor and a critical growth factor for clear cell renal carcinoma. Cancer Res 1999; 59:2210–6.

54. Hainsworth JD, Sosman JA, Spigel DR, et al. Treatment of metastatic renal cell carcinoma with a combination of bevacizumab and erlotinib. J Clin Oncol 2005; 23:7889–96.

55. Patel PH, Kondagunta GV, Redman BG, et al. Phase I/II study of sunitinib malate in combination with gefitinib in patients (pts) with metastatic renal cell carcinoma. Journal of Clinical Oncology, 2007 ASCO Annual Meeting Proceedings Part I. Vol 25, No. 18S (June 20 Supplement), 2007: 5097.

56. Schwartz G, Dutcher JP, Vogelzang NJ, et al. Phase 2 clinical trial evaluating the safety and effectiveness of ABX-EGF in renal cell cancer (RCC) [Abstract 91]. Proc Am Soc Clin Oncol 2002; 21.

57. Jermann M, Joerger M, Pless M, et al. An open-label phase II trial to evaluate the efficacy and safety of gefitinib in patients with locally advanced, relapsed or metastatic renal cell cancer [abstract 1681]. Proc Am Soc Clin Oncol 2003; 22.

58. Ayers M, Fargnoli J, Lewin A, et al. Discovery and validation of biomarkers that respond to treatment with brivanib alaninate, a small-molecule VEGFR-2/FGFR-1 antagonist. Cancer Res 2007; 67:6899–906.

59. Zou HY, Li Q, Lee JH, et al. An orally available small-molecule inhibitor of c-Met, PF-2341066, exhibits cytoreductive antitumor efficacy through antiproliferative and antiangiogenic mechanisms. Cancer Res 2007; 67: 4408–17.

60. Sosman JA, Flaherty K, Atkins MB, et al. A phase I/II trial of sorafenib with bevacizumab in metastatic renal cell cancer patients. J Clin Oncol, 2006 ASCO Annual Meeting Proceedings Part I. Vol 24, No. 18S (June 20 Supplement), 2006: 3031.

61. Azad NS, Annunziata C, Barrett T, et al. Dual targeting of vascular endothelial growth factor (VEGF) with sorafenib and bevacizumab: Clinical and translational results. J Clin Oncol 2007 ASCO Annual Meeting Proceedings Part I. Vol 25, No. 18S (June 20 Supplement), 2007: 3542.

62. Feldman DR, Kondagunta GV, Ronnen EA, et al. Phase I trial of bevacizumab plus sunitinib in patients (pts) with metastatic renal cell carcinoma (mRCC). J Clin Oncol 2007 ASCO Annual Meeting Proceedings Part I. Vol 25, No. 18S (June 20 Supplement), 2007: 5099.

63. Cooney MM, Garcia J, Brell J, et al. A phase I study of bevacizumab in combination with sunitinib in advanced solid tumors. J Clin Oncol 2007 ASCO Annual Meeting Proceedings Part I. Vol 25, No. 18S (June 20 Supplement), 2007: 15532.

64. Feldman DR, Gnsberg MS, Baum M, et al. Phase I trial of beracizumab plus sunitinib in patients with metastatic renal cell carcinoma. J Clin Oncol 26:2008 (may 20 suppl, abstr 5100).

65. Patnaik A, Ricart A, Cooper J, et al. A phase I, pharmacokinetic and pharmacodynamic study of sorafenib (S), a multi-targeted kinase inhibitor in combination with temsirolimus (T), an mTOR inhibitor in patients with advanced solid malignancies. J Clin Oncol 2007 ASCO Annual Meeting Proceedings Part I. Vol 25, No. 18S (June 20 Supplement), 2007: 3512.

66. Merchan JR, Liu G, Fitch T, et al. Phase I/II trial of CCI-779 and bevacizumab in stage IV renal cell carcinoma: Phase I safety and activity results. J of Clin Oncol 2007 ASCO Annual Meeting Proceedings Part I. Vol 25, No. 18S (June 20 Supplement), 2007: 5034.

67. Ratain MJ, Eisen T, Stadler WM, et al. Phase II placebo-controlled randomized discontinuation trial of sorafenib in patients with metastatic renal cell carcinoma. J Clin Oncol 2006; 24:2505–12.

68. Dutcher JP, Szczylik C, Tannir N, et al. Correlation of survival with tumor histology, age, and prognostic risk group for previously untreated patients with advanced renal cell carcinoma (adv RCC) receiving temsirolimus (TEMSR) or interferon-α (IFN). J Clin Oncol 2007 ASCO Annual Meeting Proceedings Part I. Vol 25, No. 18S (June 20 Supplement), 2007: 5033.

69. Lubensky IA, Schmidt L, Zhuang Z, et al. Hereditary and sporadic papillary renal carcinomas with c-Met mutations share a distinct morphological phenotype. Am J Path 1999; 155:517–26.

70. Garcia A, Rosen L, Cunningham CC, et al. Phase 1 study of ARQ 197, a selective inhibitor of the c-Met RTK in patients with metastatic solid tumors reaches recommended phase 2 dose. J Clin Oncol 2007; ASCO Annual Meeting Proceedings Part I. Vol 25, No. 18S (June 20 Supplement), 2007. 3525.

71. Nickerson ML, Warren MB, Toro JR, et al. Mutations in a novel gene lead to kidney tumors, lung wall defects, and benign tumors of the hair follicle in patients with the Birt-Hogg-Dube syndrome. Cancer Cell 2002:157–64.

# 19

# The Role of Surgery in Advanced Renal Cell Carcinoma

**ERIC C. NELSON, MD**
**BRIAN I. RINI, MD**
**STEVEN C. CAMPBELL, MD, PHD**
**CHRISTOPHER P. EVANS, MD, FACS**

Despite improvements in renal imaging, surgical techniques, and development of novel biologic agents for metastatic renal cell carcinoma (mRCC), curative therapy for is still lacking for the majority of these patients. Nevertheless, the current literature shows that a multimodal approach that integrates surgery and systemic therapies can improve outcomes for this challenging patient population. However, this approach should not be applied indiscriminately. Careful patient selection that takes into account performance status, sites and burden of disease, and other established prognostic factors is paramount and must be combined with a well-planned and judicious surgical approach to optimize results.

Historically, the role of surgery in mRCC was limited to palliation of symptoms such as intractable pain, hemorrhage, hematuria, or paraneoplastic syndromes. Improvements in symptomatic care and angioinfarction further limited the use of nephrectomy in this patient population.[1,2] The rare patient presenting with resectable metastatic disease was offered complete surgical extirpation largely because of a lack of effective systemic therapies.[3]

With the development of effective immunotherapy regimens, interest in the surgical treatment of mRCC was reawakened. Cumulative results from retrospective studies led some centers to advocate cytoreductive nephrectomy before systemic treatment.[4–6] Other institutions, citing the morbidity of nephrectomy in this patient population, recommended consolidative nephrectomy following immunotherapy in responding patients.[7,8] In 2001, results from two prospective, randomized studies further substantiated the role of cytoreductive surgery in the era of immunotherapy, and this has become standard of care for appropriately selected patients.[9,10] Cytoreductive nephrectomy is still being performed routinely in the era of targeted molecular agents because this paradigm is now ingrained in the urologic mindset. However, a careful reassessment of the optimal ways to integrate systemic therapies and surgery is now in progress with consideration of neoadjuvant and adjuvant approaches for various target populations.

This chapter will be divided into three main sections based on extent of disease. First, the role of metastasectomy in patients with mRCC that is potentially amenable to complete resection will be discussed. Second, those with unresectable disease who respond to systemic therapy and are candidates for subsequent consolidative resection will be considered. Finally, the role of cytoreductive surgery will be reviewed.

## METASTASECTOMY

### Synchronous Metastases

The metastatic progression of RCC is unpredictable. Although any area of the body may be affected, the most common organs involved by metastases are (in order of incidence) lung, bone, liver, and brain.[11] Overall, only 1 to 3% of patients with mRCC have solitary metastases, although additional patients may have limited and potentially resectable disease.[12–14] Despite recent advances in targeted biologic agents, complete surgical resection, when possible, still forms the basis of treatment for this small subset of patients.

The rationale for attempting what is sometimes an extensive operation is based on several factors. First, up to 30% of carefully selected patients amenable to metastasectomy will experience significant progression-free survival. Second, survival may be improved even for those patients who do not experience cure—the "biological clock" of their disease process is potentially reset by removing the identifiable metastases. In addition, some patients require resection for palliation or prevention of local symptoms.[15,16]

### Patient Selection

Clearly, estimating prognosis is important not only for individual counseling but also for determining how extensive a surgical resection should be attempted. As discussed below, several algorithms have been developed that can stratify patients into various prognostic categories. Factors specifically affecting patients with potentially resectable metastases include the number, location and size of metastatic lesions, status of regional lymphatics, and ability to perform a second resection if recurrent disease develops. The primary tumor stage, grade, and lymph node status, as discussed later, also affect prognosis and should be considered.

In relation to the number of metastatic sites, cumulative data from retrospective analysis indicates a favorable effect associated with lower disease burden.[15,17] Han and colleagues retrospectively analyzed patients with N0M1 disease and found disease in one organ system versus multiple organ systems was a statistically significant independent predictor of improved survival (27 months versus 11 months median survival, respectively).[18] Within an organ system, fewer metastatic lesions also portends an improved prognosis. The number of pulmonary metastases serves as the primary example, with multiple studies showing improved survival with fewer metastases.[19,20] Patients with more radiographically identifiable metastases are more likely to have occult metastases—the surgery is only addressing the "tip of the iceberg".

The impact of different metastatic locations on prognosis has been controversial. Traditionally, pulmonary lesions were thought to have a better prognosis than most other sites.[18,21–23] However, some studies have not reported a survival advantage for lung metastases when compared with bone metastases.[15,18,24] Most data suggests that liver and central nervous system involvement carry a worse prognosis than pulmonary metastases.[17,25] However, two multivariate analyses of all common metastatic sites for RCC found no independent predictive status for any metastatic site.[26,27] Although robust statistical analysis of very rare sites of mRCC is impossible, lesions such as true metastasis to the adrenal gland or pancreas seem to carry a relatively good prognosis with up to 50% 10-year survival rates.[25,28] Although this literature is not conclusive, the general consensus is that lung metastases tend to carry a more favorable prognosis with liver and brain metastases at the other end of the spectrum, and with bone metastases likely somewhere in between.

The decision to attempt a complete resection of mRCC should involve careful consultation between the surgical subspecialties involved and extensive patient counseling regarding appropriate expectations. Criteria for attempting such a resection include: 1) the patient is at good operative risk; 2) the primary RCC is controlled or can be readily controlled; 3) complete resection of the metastatic site is possible; and 4) no other metastatic sites exist, or if they exist, they can also be completely resected.

### Metachronous Metastases

Compared with synchronous metastases, metastasectomy plays a greater role in the treatment of metachronous metastases because these are more common and less likely to be rapidly progressive. Increasing disease-free interval (DFI) from initial nephrectomy to the development of metastases indicates a better prognosis, likely reflecting a more indolent disease course.[19] Isolated renal fossa recurrence will also be discussed here because it may be considered a special case of metachronous metastasis.

The rationale for resecting metachronous metastases or local recurrence of RCC is similar to that for synchronous disease, including the attempt to cure some patients and perhaps extend survival in those who are not rendered disease-free. As DFI increases, greater consideration should be given to metastasectomy—these patients have had more time to declare themselves and may actually be free of occult metastatic disease.[15] For patients with isolated locally recurrent RCC, retrospective data suggest that disease-specific survival may be improved by surgical intervention, although the morbidity of this procedure can be prohibitive in some cases and patient selection is thus critically important.

## Prognostic Factors

Prognostic factors for metachronous metastases are similar to those discussed above, with the addition of DFI. In one retrospective study of patients undergoing metastasectomy, those with a DFI of less than 12 months had only a 9% overall 5-year survival compared with 55% for patients with a longer DFI.[15] A similar study limited to pulmonary metastasectomy showed 5-year survivals of 25 and 47% for patients with DFI less than or greater than 23 months, respectively.[19] Both studies also showed that selected patients may undergo sequential resections for recurrent mRCC with surgical morbidity and overall prognoses similar to the initial or previous resections.

Isolated renal fossa recurrence following nephrectomy for RCC is an uncommon event and prognostic factors are difficult to ascertain. Two retrospective analyses suggest that shorter DFI may be a significant predictor of poor outcomes in these patients as well.[30,31] Symptoms caused by the tumor recurrence occur in less than 30% of patients, emphasizing the need for close surveillance.[30–33] Patient selection for surgical intervention must include careful preoperative imaging, remembering

that isolated renal fossa recurrence is much less common than local recurrence associated with disseminated metastases.[34]

## Operative Factors

As the lung is the most common site for mRCC, pulmonary metastasectomy is one of the most commonly performed. Initial thoracotomy or wedge resection of these lesions resulted in a high rate of recurrence. This led to the use of sternotomy with direct examination or palpation of both lungs, which showed that up to half of the patients with apparently unilateral disease may show contralateral lesions intraoperatively.[35] One disadvantage of median sternotomy is the difficulty accessing the lower lobes, especially the left lower lobe, and this approach is also associated with increased morbidity compared with minimally invasive approaches. Lesions difficult to access may require bilateral staged thoracotomies or the use of video-assisted thoracic surgery.[36] Despite the increased accuracy provided by modern computed tomography scanning modalities, Parsons and colleagues suggest that palpation of the lung may still be necessary for complete resection of metastatic disease. However, this must be counterbalanced by careful consideration of the morbidity that each approach may entail.[37]

Surgical approaches to osseous metastases are largely a function of location because this affects the feasibility of enucleation or partial bone resection before osteosynthesis. Spinal lesions may require treatment even when curative resection is impossible to prevent compression fractures and resulting morbidity (Figure 1).[38] For such lesions, the combination of surgery and radiation is superior compared with radiation alone.[39] Metastatic deposits in bone are rarely solitary, but complete resection of such lesions may result in long-term survival.[22] Preoperative embolization can reduce the blood loss that often accompanies these procedures and thus may serve as an useful adjunct.

Liver metastases are felt to have a particularly poor prognosis and are less amenable to metastasectomy. Nevertheless, some patients experience long-term disease control and complete resection may be attempted in selected cases. Right hepatectomy is

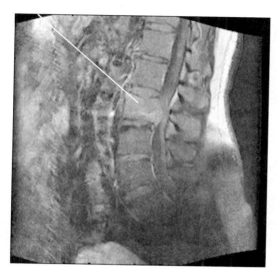

**Figure 1.** This 70-year-old man with a history of RCC, status post left radical nephrectomy 9 years prior, presented with progressive low back pain radiating to the left knee. MRI demonstrates bone metastases to the L3 vertebrae, which required treatment for prevention of compression fracture.

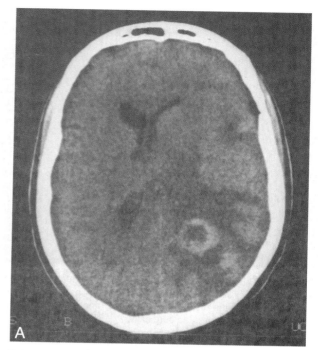

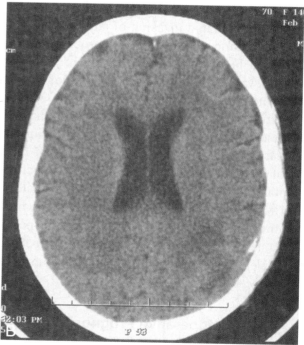

**Figure 2.** *A*, One year following a left nephrectomy for RCC, this 69-year-old woman presented with expressive aphasia, right hemiparesis and visual field deficits. Note midline shift because of left parietal mRCC. *B*, CT of the same patient 6 weeks later following palliative excision of brain metastasis and whole brain radiotherapy.

most often performed, sometimes extending the resection to segment 4. Intraoperative ultrasonography may be helpful to ensure complete resection of all disease. Alves and colleagues' series of 10 patients undergoing hepatic metastasectomy for mRCC yielded 4 survivors at 6, 18, 26, and 96 months follow-up.[25,40] In contrast, to earlier series reporting over 30% perioperative mortality, no perioperative deaths occurred in this series, probably because of careful patient selection. Most operations use either Pringle's maneuver to occlude the portal vein or total vascular exclusion of the liver. Nevertheless, this is a formidable surgical challenge and most patients require intraoperative blood transfusions.[25,40]

Metastatic RCC affects the brain in 5 to 15% of cases, carries a poor prognosis and is frequently symptomatic. Operative interventions in this setting are usually palliative in intent.[41] Very rarely is total excision of all lesions possible and other options for local control of symptomatic disease include whole-brain radiation, stereotactic radiosurgery, or a combination of these with surgery (Figure 2A,B).[42] The minimally invasive nature of stereotactic radiosurgery and the ability to treat multiple lesions in the same setting makes it a particularly attractive option. In one series of 69 patients with intracranial mRCC, local control was possible in over 90% of cases with

minimal morbidity and a treatment-related mortality rate of 1.4%.[43]

The surgical excision of isolated locally recurrent RCC is often difficult—tissue planes have

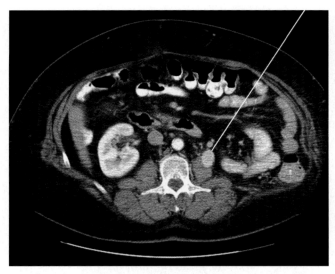

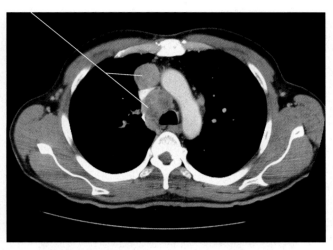

**Figure 3.** This patient is a 63-year-old male status post left nephrectomy for T3b RCC. Despite negative margins, three sequential recurrences of the diaphragm, renal bed, and the shown psoas recurrence have been treated surgically.

**Figure 4.** This 48-year-old male initially presented with fatigue and hematuria. CT showed a right renal tumor, stage T3b, associated with this extensive mediastinal lymphadenopathy and lung metastases (not shown).

been obliterated and invasion of adjacent organs is not uncommon. Hence, these procedures may require en bloc removal of the spleen, tail of the pancreas, various segments of bowel, part of the liver, or surrounding muscle/body wall (Figure 3).[29,31,32] In addition, venous thrombosis or invasion may also be present and may require vascular isolation and reconstruction. Reflecting this, most series of resection of local recurrence of RCC report perioperative complication rates of 30–50% and mortality rates of 5–10%.[29–31] Preoperative counseling and intraoperative decision-making must weigh the performance status of the patient and the possible benefits of complete resection against the potential morbidity of the procedure.

## Postoperative Prognosis

Surgical pathology from the metastasectomy specimen gives prognostic information that may guide further therapy. Up to 30% of patients are at increased risk for recurrence because of unsuspected positive surgical margins, grossly incomplete resection, or nodal disease and should be strongly considered for adjuvant systemic therapy trials.[11] Studies of pulmonary metastases confirm that complete resection is an independent prognostic factor for

improved survival.[19,20] Although small patient numbers limit analysis of similar data in hepatic metastasectomy, complete versus incomplete resection appears to be a significant predictor of postoperative prognosis.[25]

Locally positive lymph nodes associated with metastatic disease sites also represents a poor prognostic feature. Again, the primary example is pulmonary metastasectomy with 10 to 30% of patients showing lymphatic involvement at the time of surgery (Figure 4).[19,36] Pfannschmidt and colleagues found a 24 vs 42% 5-year survival for positive and negative pulmonary or mediastinal lymph nodes, respectively, with node status being an independent prognostic factor on multivariate analysis.[19]

Another pathologic factor showing possible prognostic significance is the size of the largest metastatic deposit. For example, Piltz and colleagues reported that increasing size of the largest pulmonary metastasis correlated strongly with a shorter survival, with divisions at 2, 3, and 4 cm, and this remained significant on multivariate analysis.[44] Although limited by small patient numbers, one study suggests that larger hepatic metastases also correspond with a compromised prognosis.[25]

In patients with isolated renal fossa recurrence, long-term prognosis may be similar to patients with metachronous metastases, with 5-year survival following complete excision ranging from 18 to 51%.[29,33] Examination of the pathology specimen adds prognostic data in that smaller size of the recurrence may correlate with improved survival.[30] In addition, the presence of positive surgical margins correlates with both local and distant failure and shorter survival.[34,45]

## Summary

Patients with mRCC only occasionally presents with resectable metastatic disease. However, for those who do, surgery offers the chance of long-term survival and might extend survival and maximize quality of life in those who eventually relapse. Careful patient selection is the key to success with these procedures. Different sites of metastatic spread may indicate unique biological characteristics and can be associated with divergent prognoses. In addition, each site requires special consideration of the relevant anatomy, surgical options, and potential morbidities, and this should be conveyed during individualized patient counseling. In general, patients with metachronous lesions have a better prognosis, which improves with increasing DFI. Repeat excisions of recurrent mRCC, if possible, can carry a prognosis similar to initial resection. The special case of isolated renal fossa recurrence is similar in many respects to metachronous mRCC, but en bloc excision of adjacent organs may be required and can be associated with substantial morbidity.

## CONSOLIDATIVE NEPHRECTOMY

Current treatment of mRCC emphasizes multimodal therapy to optimize response rates and survival. Systemic treatment using biologic or targeted agents, combined with surgical intervention, appears to be superior to either alone. As discussed below, results from prospective, randomized trials suggest that initial cytoreductive nephrectomy may be superior to initial cytokine therapy. However, the role of consolidative nephrectomy may need to be re-examined as systemic therapy improves.

The rationale for initial systemic therapy followed by consolidative nephrectomy is multidimensional. If the goal is curative, patients with mRCC will need to respond to systemic therapy. Identification of these patients by initial systemic therapy could spare nonresponding patients the morbidity of surgery. In addition, some patients may be unable to receive systemic therapy following nephrectomy because of progressive deterioration in performance status. Multiple retrospective studies listed in Table 1 show that this group typically represents 10 to 30% of patients after cytoreductive nephrectomy but has been as high as 77%, probably

### TABLE 1. REPRESENTATIVE RETROSPECTIVE CASE SERIES OF CYTOREDUCTIVE NEPHRECTOMY

| Series | Number of Patients | Surgical Mortality Number (%) | Unable to Receive Systemic tx (%) | Total Response Rate (%) | Median Survival (months) | Year of Publication | Reference |
|---|---|---|---|---|---|---|---|
| Cleveland Clinic | 37 | 1 (2.7%) | 22% | 8% | 12 | 1994 | 52 |
| Albert Einstein College | 30 | 5 (17%) | 77% | 13% | NR | 1995 | 95 |
| Tufts | 28 | 1 (3.6%) | 7% | 39% | 20.5 | 1997 | 4 |
| National Cancer Institute | 195 | 2 (1%) | 38% | 18% | NR | 1997 | 5 |
| UCLA | 62 | 0 (0%) | 11% | 35% | 22 | 1997 | 96 |
| MD Anderson | 66 | 2 (3%) | 18% | NR | NR | 1998 | 97 |
| UCSF | 63 | 2 (3.6%) | 27% | NR | 17.8 | 2000 | 6 |
| UCLA | 89 | NR | NR | NR | 16.7 | 2001 | 71 |
| Indiana | 32 | 1 (3%) | 25% | NR | NR | 2003 | 66 |

because of variable patient selection criteria.[46] Finally, delay in administration of systemic therapy because of surgical trauma and recovery may be associated with disease progression, perhaps because of the effects of surgery on immunologic parameters.[47,48]

Despite this strong rationale, the largest study of initial systemic immunotherapy followed by consolidative nephrectomy reported by Wagner and colleagues reported somewhat disappointing results. This group reported a response rate to initial cytokine therapy of only 6% with the primary tumor in place, and responses in the primary tumor were particularly uncommon.[7] Only a minority of patients were thus candidates for nephrectomy. These results appear to be substantially inferior to those following cytoreductive nephrectomy.[49] However, comparison is difficult because of potential selection bias—patients with more advanced disease or poor performance status may have been channeled toward initial systemic therapy rather than surgery. Surgical consolidation for responders to systemic immunotherapy has reported persistence of viable cancer in many metastatic lesions and up to 90% of primary tumors.[7] Similar studies for surgical consolidation after targeted molecular therapy have not yet been reported.

## Prognostic Factors

Predicting response to systemic therapies might allow identification of those patients most likely to benefit from this approach. Perhaps, the most widely used prognostic model stratifies patients with mRCC into three categories predicting survival while undergoing immunotherapy. Low Karnofsky performance score, high serum lactate, low hemoglobin, high serum calcium, and time from initial RCC diagnosis to start of immunotherapy of less than 1 year were all predictive of shorter survival.[50] Other factors that might influence the response to immunotherapy include histologic type, CAIX expression, or other molecular factors, but their use for predicting response to systemic therapy for any individual patient is rather limited, and this is particularly true as we move into the era of targeted molecular therapeutics.[51]

## Postoperative Prognosis

Patients who respond to systemic therapy and subsequently undergo consolidation resection represent a highly selected population with widely differing prognoses. Reported median survival following consolidation nephrectomy varies from 12 to 26 months, but some studies find up to one-third of patients are long-term survivors.[7,8,47,49,52]

## Summary

In light of the prospective, randomized studies in favor of cytoreduction discussed below, consolidative nephrectomy following initial systemic treatment is not widely used in this era. Occasional patients who are poor surgical candidates will respond to systemic therapy with a subsequent improvement in performance status, and can then be considered for consolidative nephrectomy and/or metastasectomy.[53] This is now one of the few undisputed indications for consolidative surgery for patients with mRCC. However, given the increased response rates reported for targeted molecular agents and the current trend to use these agents earlier in the treatment paradigm, consolidative surgery will likely play an increasingly important role in the future. Identification of clinical or molecular parameters that can predict response to these agents would greatly facilitate progress in this field.

## CYTOREDUCTIVE NEPHRECTOMY

Some early reports suggested that spontaneous regression of mRCC may be promoted by cytoreductive or "debulking" nephrectomy.[54–56] Although later analysis established that this is an extremely rare phenomenon, the development of modestly effective immunotherapy treatments also reawakened the debate about the impact of cytoreductive nephrectomy on patient outcomes.[46,57] For lack of better data, the discussion at that time focused on multiple retrospective case series analyzing survival following cytoreductive nephrectomy (Table 1).

**Table 2**

**Rationale for Cytoreductive Nephrectomy**

Immunologic/Biologic
  Remove immunologic "sink" trapping circulating
    lymphocytes and antibodies
  Remove source of cytokines/growth factors
  Primary tumor will probably not respond to systemic
    therapy
  Remove source of additional metastasis

Palliative
  Reduce tumor burden, decreasing local symptoms
  Prevent future complications
  Prevent future metastases
  Possible improvement in performance status
  Patient psychological factors

Experimental Therapies
  Adoptive immunotherapy strategies require isolation of
    tumor infiltrative lymphocytes or other tumor related
    factors from nephrectomy specimen
  Future individually targeted biologic agents may require
    pathology specimen to guide therapy

## Rationale

Multiple factors comprise the rationale for cytoreductive nephrectomy before systemic therapy. These may be conceptually grouped into the three categories listed below and summarized in Table 2.

First, removal of the primary tumor may improve the body's immunologic function through a variety of biologic mechanisms.[58–60] For instance, cytokines produced by the tumor may be responsible for both local and systemic immune dysfunction.[53,61] The presence of the primary tumor may also act as an immunologic "sink" trapping lymphocytes and antibodies, thereby further decreasing the systemic immune response.[53,62–64] Biologic agents target growth factor pathways upregulated by RCC and the primary tumor is usually the most important source of these growth factors.[65] Cytoreductive nephrectomy may maximize the effect of such therapies, but this has yet to be reported.

Second, removal of the primary tumor may provide effective palliation and improve quality of life. Palliation is rarely a sole indication for nephrectomy because medical management and embolization are usually sufficient.[16] However, cytoreductive nephrectomy will prevent future hematuria, anemia, or pain, and it can ameliorate some paraneoplastic

symptoms. In addition, some patients experience a postoperative improvement in performance status, possibly increasing tolerance of subsequent systemic therapy.[66] Finally, psychological factors and patient attitudes regarding removal of the primary tumor may also play a role in decision-making.[67]

Third, certain experimental treatments depend upon examination of the nephrectomy specimen. Some tumor vaccine strategies require sizeable pathologic specimens to purify tumor infiltrating lymphocytes or tumor tissue.[68,69] Future targeted biologic therapies may also depend upon pathologic information, such as histologic subtype or other related analyses, to guide treatment.

## Current Status

Current best evidence on the role of surgery in mRCC comes from two prospective, randomized controlled trials examining the efficacy of cytoreductive nephrectomy.[9,10] These studies were designed to detect a 50% improvement in median survival and 15% improvement in response rate with 0.85 power. Accrual randomized 331 total patients, 246 by Southwestern Oncology Group (SWOG) and an additional 85 by the European Organization for the Research and Treatment of Cancer (EORTC) in two nearly identical and parallel study designs. Enrollment criteria included biopsy-proven mRCC with a resectable primary tumor, Eastern Cooperative Oncology Group (ECOG) performance status of 0 or 1, and no previous systemic or radiation therapy. Patients were stratified by ECOG performance status, measurable disease, and metastatic site, and then randomized to receive cytoreductive nephrectomy followed by interferon $\alpha$-2b, or interferon $\alpha$-2b alone. All analyses were by intent-to-treat criteria. Survival was measured from date of surgery or date of first immunotherapy treatment. Primary and secondary outcomes were survival and response, respectively.

The conclusions of these studies are strengthened by the fact that they independently arrived at similar results supporting cytoreductive nephrectomy. Combined analysis shows a survival advantage for the cytoreductive nephrectomy group of 5.8 months (13.6 vs 7.8 months, $p = 0.002$; Figure 5). No significant difference in response

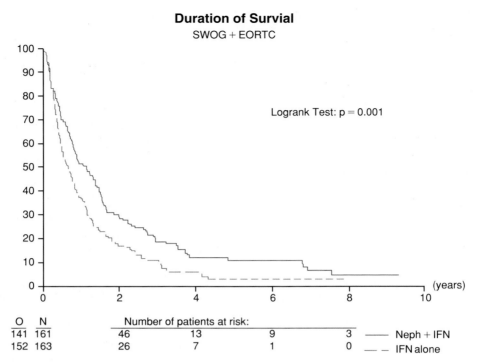

**Figure 5.**   Kaplan–Meier survival curves showing duration of survival in combined SWOG and EORTC trials. *O*, observation; *N*, nephrectomy. Reproduced with permission from Flanigan and colleagues.[70]

to immunotherapy was observed (6.9 vs 5.7%, $p = 0.60$). Surgical complications were much lower in this series compared with the historical series listed in Table 1. Only 23% of patients experienced operative complications and perioperative mortality was only 1.4%. Importantly, only 5.6% of patients did not receive postoperative immunotherapy for reasons related to surgery, which is also lower than historical series.[70]

Also strengthening the conclusions of these studies is the fact that the survival advantage for the cytoreductive nephrectomy group remained significant across all stratified subgroups. However, patients with ECOG performance status of 0 had a significantly greater survival benefit compared with those with a performance status of 1 (5.7 vs 2.1 months).[9]

In light of this data, most authors agree that for appropriately selected patients, cytoreductive nephrectomy followed by systemic therapy is superior to primary immunotherapy followed by consolidation nephrectomy.[2,16,46,53,67,71–73] Future studies will examine methods for maximizing the efficacy of cytoreductive nephrectomy. Phase II data suggest that perioperative immunomodulation may prevent the immune dysfunction caused by major surgery.

Low-dose cytokines before cytoreductive nephrectomy led to a small but significant survival advantage along with significant improvements in serum parameters for cellular and humoral immunity.[74]

## Prognostic Factors

Cytoreductive nephrectomy is only of benefit as part of multimodal therapy. Therefore, identifying those most likely to undergo and respond to systemic therapy following surgery is an important goal. Patient education regarding treatment options and associated prognoses will clarify expectations. Finally, patients should be encouraged to participate in clinical trials whenever possible.

Criteria discussed above predict overall patient survival with immunotherapy and give general prognostic information helpful for patients undergoing cytoreductive nephrectomy. The current consensus is that the most important factors when considering cytoreductive nephrectomy are performance status and sites and overall burden of disease. Other relevant factors include the tumor stage, particularly locally invasive disease, and clinical node status. Locally invasive tumor requiring en

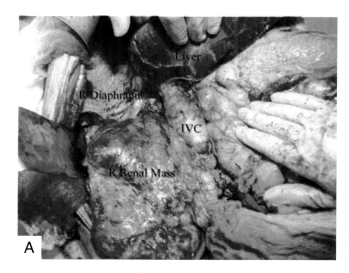

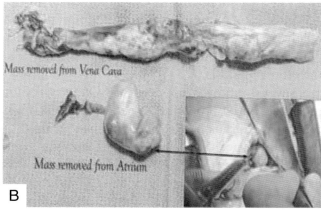

**Figure 6.** *A,* Intraoperative photograph of debulking right radical nephrectomy for stage T3c tumor. Note liver is mobilized and rotated to left upper quadrant. Short hepatic veins are ligated to facilitate infra-hepatic vena caval occlusion and thrombectomy. *B,* Photograph of thrombus removed from vena cava and atria.

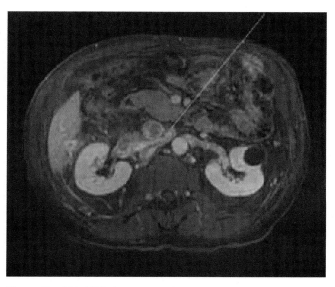

**Figure 7.** This MRI shows extensive lymphadenopathy because of a right renal tumor (not shown). Line indicates 1.5 × 2.5 cm interaortocaval node.

bloc resection of adjacent organs, bulky lymphadenopathy that encases the renal hilum, or large tumor in proximity to vital structures such as the mesenteric vasculature may substantially increase the morbidity of surgery and thereby alter the risk or benefit analysis in an unfavorable direction. Tumor thrombus alone is not an absolute contraindication to cytoreductive nephrectomy, although surgical morbidity and mortality increase significantly with level III/IV tumor thrombi (Figure 6A,B).[75]

Bulky retroperitoneal lymph nodes (see Figure 7) are almost always malignant and represent a poor prognostic indicator. For instance, Vasselli and colleagues retrospectively reported that absence of preoperative lymphadenopathy (hazard ratio 1.82,

$p = 0.002$) was a stronger predictor of survival than performance status (hazard ratio 1.42, $p = 0.0139$).[76] Preoperative estimation of the volume of lymphadenopathy also correlated with survival in this series. In addition, response to postoperative cytokine therapy may be superior in patients without lymph node disease.[77]

Inclusion criteria for cytoreductive nephrectomy have been proposed by Fallick and colleagues[4] and include the following: 1) tumor debulking greater than 75% possible, 2) no central nervous system, bone, or liver metastases, 3) adequate cardiopulmonary function, 4) ECOG performance status of 0 or 1, and 5) no nonclear cell histology on biopsy, if performed. Some authors recommend relaxing one or more of these criteria to allow more patients the potential benefits of cytoreductive nephrectomy.[66] In particular, although some sites of disease, namely CNS or liver, will usually preclude a benefit from cytoreductive nephrectomy, there is still room for individualized decision making, and some such patients with limited burden of disease may still benefit. The rationale for uniformly excluding patients with nonclear cell histology is also not strong. This subgroup of patients has not been adequately studied and definitive conclusions about the potential utility of cytoreductive nephrectomy are not possible.

## Operative Considerations

Operative factors affecting cytoreductive nephrectomy outcomes are generally similar to standard nephrectomy. Locally advanced disease is more likely in patients with metastatic disease compared with those without, although all tumor stages are represented.[78] Stage for stage, no difference in surgical complications is noted for cytoreductive nephrectomy compared with curative nephrectomy.[79]

Retrospective analyses show that patients with mRCC experience significantly improved survival if lymph node dissection is included as part of surgical debulking before immunotherapy.[77] As lymphadenectomy did not add significantly to surgery time, blood loss, or complication rate, it should be considered a standard part of cytoreductive nephrectomy. Although having a poor prognosis in general, one study showed that survival rates for patients receiving complete resection of the primary tumor and associated lymphadenopathy were not significantly different than patients with no clinically positive nodes. Unfortunately, complete resection of lymph nodes was possible in less than 25% of patients with gross nodal involvement, and small patient numbers may not allow sufficient power to accurately calculate survival differences.[76]

These data regarding cytoreductive nephrectomy and the benefit of cytoreductive lymphadenectomy cumulatively suggest a survival benefit associated with maximal debulking before systemic therapy. This has lead some institutions to advocate a possible role for cytoreductive metastasectomy.[20,22,80] However, most patients in these retrospective series have metachronous lesions and there is likely a strong selection bias—most patients have excellent performance status and disease that appears to be completely resectable. Therefore, the role of cytoreductive metastasectomy for unresectable synchronous metastases remains undefined. Cytoreduction in these patients should be limited to the primary tumor, any local extension, and regional lymph nodes. Metastases easily accessible through the same incision may be considered for resection if the potential added morbidity is minimal.

## Postoperative Prognosis

Pathologic confirmation of the stage and nodal status of the nephrectomy specimen predicted by preoperative imaging gives little new information with significant upstaging or downstaging occurring very rarely.[81–83] However, histologic features of the specimen may give important data. For example, higher tumor grade and sarcomatoid features are associated with worsening prognosis, even when adjusted for stage.[84] Uncommon histologic subtypes such as type 2 papillary, collecting duct, and renal medullary carcinomas also carry a poor prognosis.[85–87]

A retrospective analysis of the SWOG trial discussed above suggests a role for postoperative azotemia and acidosis in determining prognosis.[53] Patients with greater postoperative rise in urea nitrogen and creatinine experienced significantly longer survival. Computer modeling suggests that the relative acidity of the peritumoral environment may play a role in determining invasive behavior and therefore prognosis.[88]

Several algorithms predicting postoperative prognosis based on pathologic stage and histologic features are discussed elsewhere in this volume. Two algorithms specifically relevant to patients with mRCC were developed by Leibovich and colleagues[78,89] In both, a numeric score is assigned based on symptoms, characteristics of the primary tumor and metastatic sites, and histologic features. The numeric score can then used to predict cancer-specific survival at 0.5, 1, 2, and 3 years.

## Laparoscopic Cytoreductive Nephrectomy

Four retrospective patient series suggest that laparoscopy may play a role in cytoreduction, even in patients with bulky disease.[46,90–92] These series show at least an equal number of patients who subsequently enter systemic therapy compared with open surgery, and the shorter recovery time from laparoscopic surgery enabled earlier therapy. It should be emphasized that the complexity of laparoscopic cytoreductive nephrectomy necessitates a high level of expertise, and applications of this procedure should therefore be limited to specialized institutions.

## SUMMARY

Current best evidence indicates cytoreductive nephrectomy to be the treatment of choice for carefully selected patients in combination with immunotherapy. However, the optimal timing of surgery will need to be reevaluated by prospective studies in the era of targeted biologic agents. Meanwhile, further study into the mechanism of improved survival with cytoreductive nephrectomy will help inform current treatment decisions and patient selection. Perioperative immunomodulation and laparoscopic techniques may extend the efficacy of cytoreductive nephrectomy.

## CONCLUSIONS

The historical lack of effective systemic therapy for mRCC led to radical surgical attempts at cure with occasional successes. Immunotherapy offered the first hope of effective systemic treatment, although response rates were generally modest and accompanied by extensive side effects. Attempts to maximize outcomes of systemic therapy led to examination of cytoreductive nephrectomy and a beneficial effect on survival was confirmed by subsequent prospective studies.

The current standard of care for patients with mRCC involves complete surgical resection for patients amenable to nephrectomy and metastasectomy, and cytoreductive nephrectomy for selected patients with more extensive metastases. Laparoscopic surgery, when possible, may benefit patients by enabling earlier entry into systemic therapy.

The treatment of mRCC is undergoing rapid change with new, targeted biologic agents offering treatment options in addition to immunotherapy. The concept of combination therapy for mRCC is firmly established, but will need to be redefined as systemic therapy improves. However, surgical resection of disease is likely to remain an integral component of therapy for patients with mRCC in the future.

## REFERENCES

1. Yonover PM, Flanigan RC. Should radical nephrectomy be performed in the face of surgically incurable disease? Curr Opin Urol 2000;10:429–34.
2. Wood CG. The role of cytoreductive nephrectomy in the management of metastatic renal cell carcinoma. Urol Clin North Am 2003;30:581–8.
3. Flanigan RC. Role of surgery in patients with metastatic renal cell carcinoma. Semin Urol Oncol 1996;14:227–9.
4. Fallick ML, McDermott DF, LaRock D, et al. Nephrectomy before interleukin-2 therapy for patients with metastatic renal cell cancer. J Urol 1997;158:1691–5.
5. Walther MM, Yang JC, Pass HI, et al. Cytoreductive surgery before high dose interleukin-2 based therapy in patients with metastatic renal cell carcinoma. J Urol 1997;158:1675–8.
6. Tigrani VS, Reese DM, Small EJ, et al. Potential role of nephrectomy in the treatment of metastatic renal cell carcinoma: a retrospective analysis. Urology 2000;55:36–40.
7. Sella A, Swanson DA, Ro JY, et al. Surgery following response to interferon-alpha-based therapy for residual renal cell carcinoma. J Urol 1993;149:19–21; discussion 21–2.
8. Krishnamurthi V, Novick AC, Bukowski RM. Efficacy of multimodality therapy in advanced renal cell carcinoma. Urology 1998;51:933–7.
9. Flanigan RC, Salmon SE, Blumenstein BA, et al. Nephrectomy followed by interferon alfa-2b compared with interferon alfa-2b alone for metastatic renal-cell cancer. N Engl J Med 2001;345:1655–9.
10. Mickisch GH, Garin A, van Poppel H, et al. Radical nephrectomy plus interferon-alfa-based immunotherapy compared with interferon alfa alone in metastatic renal-cell carcinoma: a randomised trial. Lancet 2001;358:966–70.
11. Vogl UM, Zehetgruber H, Dominkus M, et al. Prognostic factors in metastatic renal cell carcinoma: metastasectomy as independent prognostic variable. Br J Cancer 2006;95:691–8.
12. Middleton RG. Surgery for metastatic renal cell carcinoma. J Urol 1967;97:973–7.
13. Tolia BM, Whitmore WF Jr. Solitary metastasis from renal cell carcinoma. J Urol 1975;114:836–8.
14. O'Dea MJ, Zincke H, Utz DC, et al. The treatment of renal cell carcinoma with solitary metastasis. J Urol 1978;120:540–2.
15. Kavolius JP, Mastorakos DP, Pavlovich C, et al. Resection of metastatic renal cell carcinoma. J Clin Oncol 1998;16:2261–6.
16. Sengupta S, Leibovich BC, Blute ML, et al. Surgery for metastatic renal cell cancer. World J Urol 2005;23:155–60.
17. Atzpodien J, Royston P, Wandert T, et al. Metastatic renal carcinoma comprehensive prognostic system. Br J Cancer 2003;88:348–53.
18. Han KR, Pantuck AJ, Bui MH, et al. Number of metastatic sites rather than location dictates overall survival of patients with node-negative metastatic renal cell carcinoma. Urology 2003;61:314–9.
19. Pfannschmidt J, Hoffmann H, Muley T, et al. Prognostic factors for survival after pulmonary resection of metastatic renal cell carcinoma. Ann Thorac Surg 2002;74:1653–7.
20. Hofmann HS, Neef H, Krohe K, et al. Prognostic factors and survival after pulmonary resection of metastatic renal cell carcinoma. Eur Urol 2005;48:77–81; discussion 81–2.
21. Mani S, Todd MB, Katz K, et al. Prognostic factors for survival in patients with metastatic renal cancer treated with biological response modifiers. J Urol 1995;154:35–40.
22. van der Poel HG, Roukema JA, Horenblas S, et al. Metastasectomy in renal cell carcinoma: A multicenter retrospective analysis. Eur Urol 1999;35:197–203.
23. Kankuri M, Pelliniemi TT, Pyrhonen S, et al. Feasibility of prolonged use of interferon-alpha in metastatic kidney carcinoma: a phase II study. Cancer 2001;92:761–7.
24. Tsuda S, Koga S, Nishikido M, et al. Evaluation of bone metastases from renal cell carcinoma. Hinyokika Kiyo 2001;47:155–8.

25. Alves A, Adam R, Majno P, et al. Hepatic resection for metastatic renal tumors: is it worthwhile? Ann Surg Oncol 2003;10:705–10.

26. Citterio G, Bertuzzi A, Tresoldi M, et al. Prognostic factors for survival in metastatic renal cell carcinoma: retrospective analysis from 109 consecutive patients. Eur Urol 1997;31:286–91.

27. Ljungberg B, Landberg G, Alamdari FI. Factors of importance for prediction of survival in patients with metastatic renal cell carcinoma, treated with or without nephrectomy. Scand J Urol Nephrol 2000;34:246–51.

28. Kuczyk MA, Bokemeyer C, Kohn G, et al. Prognostic relevance of intracaval neoplastic extension for patients with renal cell cancer. Br J Urol 1997;80:18–24.

29. Itano NB, Blute ML, Spotts B, et al. Outcome of isolated renal cell carcinoma fossa recurrence after nephrectomy. J Urol 2000;164:322–5.

30. Schrodter S, Hakenberg OW, Manseck A, et al. Outcome of surgical treatment of isolated local recurrence after radical nephrectomy for renal cell carcinoma. J Urol 2002;167:1630–3.

31. Master VA, Gottschalk AR, Kane C, et al. Management of isolated renal fossa recurrence following radical nephrectomy. J Urol 2005;174:473–7; discussion 477.

32. Gogus C, Baltaci S, Beduk Y, et al. Isolated local recurrence of renal cell carcinoma after radical nephrectomy: experience with 10 cases. Urology 2003;61:926–9.

33. Bruno JJ 2nd, Snyder ME, Motzer RJ, et al. Renal cell carcinoma local recurrences: impact of surgical treatment and concomitant metastasis on survival. BJU Int 2006;97:933–8.

34. Sandhu SS, Symes A, A'Hern R, et al. Surgical excision of isolated renal-bed recurrence after radical nephrectomy for renal cell carcinoma. BJU Int 2005;95:522–5.

35. Dowling RD, Landreneau RJ, Miller DL. Video-assisted thoracoscopic surgery for resection of lung metastases. Chest 1998;113:2S–5S.

36. Cerfolio RJ, Allen MS, Deschamps C, et al. Pulmonary resection of metastatic renal cell carcinoma. Ann Thorac Surg 1994;57:339–44.

37. Parsons AM, Detterbeck FC, Parker LA. Accuracy of helical CT in the detection of pulmonary metastases: is intraoperative palpation still necessary? Ann Thorac Surg 2004;78:1910–6; discussion 1916–8.

38. Vrionis FD, Small J. Surgical management of metastatic spinal neoplasms. Neurosurg Focus 2003;15:E12.

39. Patchell RA, Tibbs PA, Regine WF, et al. Direct decompressive surgical resection in the treatment of spinal cord compression caused by metastatic cancer: a randomised trial. Lancet 2005;366:643–8.

40. Stief CG, Jahne J, Hagemann JH, et al. Surgery for metachronous solitary liver metastases of renal cell carcinoma. J Urol 1997;158:375–7.

41. Harada Y, Nonomura N, Kondo M, et al. Clinical study of brain metastasis of renal cell carcinoma. Eur Urol 1999;36:230–5.

42. Doh LS, Amato RJ, Paulino AC, et al. Radiation therapy in the management of brain metastases from renal cell carcinoma. Oncology (Williston Park) 2006;20:603–13; discussion 613, 616, 619–20 passsim.

43. Sheehan JP, Sun MH, Kondziolka D, et al. Radiosurgery in patients with renal cell carcinoma metastasis to the brain: long-term outcomes and prognostic factors influencing survival and local tumor control. J Neurosurg 2003;98:342–9.

44. Piltz S, Meimarakis G, Wichmann MW, et al. Long-term results after pulmonary resection of renal cell carcinoma metastases. Ann Thorac Surg 2002;73:1082–7.

45. Tanguay S, Pisters LL, Lawrence DD, et al. Therapy of locally recurrent renal cell carcinoma after nephrectomy. J Urol 1996;155:26–9.

46. Healy KA, Marshall FF, Ogan K. Cytoreductive nephrectomy in metastatic renal cell carcinoma. Expert Rev Anticancer Ther 2006;6:1295–304.

47. Bex A, Horenblas S, Meinhardt W, et al. The role of initial immunotherapy as selection for nephrectomy in patients with metastatic renal cell carcinoma and the primary tumor in situ. Eur Urol 2002;42:570–4; discussion 575–6.

48. Bohm M, Ittenson A, Schierbaum KF, et al. Pretreatment with interleukin-2 modulates peri-operative immuno-dysfunction in patients with renal cell carcinoma. Eur Urol 2002;41:458–67; discussion 467–8.

49. Wagner JR, Walther MM, Linehan WM, et al. Interleukin-2 based immunotherapy for metastatic renal cell carcinoma with the kidney in place. J Urol 1999;162:43–5.

50. Motzer RJ, Bacik J, Murphy BA, et al. Interferon-alfa as a comparative treatment for clinical trials of new therapies against advanced renal cell carcinoma. J Clin Oncol 2002;20:289–96.

51. Lam JS, Shvarts O, Leppert JT, et al. Renal cell carcinoma 2005: new frontiers in staging, prognostication and targeted molecular therapy. J Urol 2005;173:1853–62.

52. Rackley R, Novick A, Klein E, et al. The impact of adjuvant nephrectomy on multimodality treatment of metastatic renal cell carcinoma. J Urol 1994;152:1399–403.

53. Flanigan RC. Debulking nephrectomy in metastatic renal cancer. Clin Cancer Res 2004;10:6335S–41S.

54. Freed SZ, Halperin JP, Gordon M. Idiopathic regression of metastases from renal cell carcinoma. J Urol 1977;118:538–42.

55. de Riese W, Goldenberg K, Allhoff E, et al. Metastatic renal cell carcinoma (RCC): spontaneous regression, long-term survival and late recurrence. Int Urol Nephrol 1991;23:13–25.

56. Marcus SG, Choyke PL, Reiter R, et al. Regression of metastatic renal cell carcinoma after cytoreductive nephrectomy. J Urol 1993;150:463–6.

57. Lokich J. Spontaneous regression of metastatic renal cancer. Case report and literature review. Am J Clin Oncol 1997;20:416–8.

58. Montie JE, Straffon RA, Deodhar SD, et al. In vitro assessment of cell-mediated immunity in patients with renal cell carcinoma. J Urol 1976;115:239–42.

59. Dadian G, Riches PG, Henderson DC, et al. Immunological parameters in peripheral blood of patients with renal cell carcinoma before and after nephrectomy. Br J Urol 1994;74:15–22.

60. Fujikawa K, Matsui Y, Miura K, et al. Serum immunosuppressive acidic protein and natural killer cell activity in

patients with metastatic renal cell carcinoma before and after nephrectomy. J Urol 2000;164:673–5.

61. Lahn M, Fisch P, Kohler G, et al. Pro-inflammatory and T cell inhibitory cytokines are secreted at high levels in tumor cell cultures of human renal cell carcinoma. Eur Urol 1999;35:70–80.

62. Ng CS, Novick AC, Tannenbaum CS, et al. Mechanisms of immune evasion by renal cell carcinoma: tumor-induced T-lymphocyte apoptosis and NFkappaB suppression. Urology 2002;59:9–14.

63. Tatsumi T, Herrem CJ, Olson WC, et al. Disease stage variation in CD4+ and CD8+ T-cell reactivity to the receptor tyrosine kinase EphA2 in patients with renal cell carcinoma. Cancer Res 2003;63:4481–9.

64. Biswas K, Richmond A, Rayman P, et al. GM2 expression in renal cell carcinoma: potential role in tumor-induced T-cell dysfunction. Cancer Res 2006;66:6816–25.

65. Rini BI, Campbell SC, Rathmell WK. Renal cell carcinoma. Curr Opin Oncol 2006 May;18:289–96.

66. Mosharafa A, Koch M, Shalhav A, et al. Nephrectomy for metastatic renal cell carcinoma: Indiana University experience. Urology 2003;62:636–40.

67. Mickisch GH, Mattes RH. Combination of surgery and immunotherapy in metastatic renal cell carcinoma. World J Urol 2005;23:191–5.

68. Figlin RA, Thompson JA, Bukowski RM, et al. Multicenter, randomized, phase III trial of CD8(+) tumor-infiltrating lymphocytes in combination with recombinant interleukin-2 in metastatic renal cell carcinoma. J Clin Oncol 1999;17:2521–9.

69. Jocham D, Richter A, Hoffmann L, et al. Adjuvant autologous renal tumour cell vaccine and risk of tumour progression in patients with renal-cell carcinoma after radical nephrectomy: phase III, randomised controlled trial. Lancet 2004;363:594–9.

70. Flanigan RC, Mickisch G, Sylvester R, et al. Cytoreductive nephrectomy in patients with metastatic renal cancer: a combined analysis. J Urol 2004;171:1071–6.

71. Pantuck AJ, Belldegrun AS, Figlin RA. Nephrectomy and interleukin-2 for metastatic renal-cell carcinoma. N Engl J Med 2001;345:1711–2.

72. Russo P. Surgical intervention in patients with metastatic renal cancer: current status of metastasectomy and cytoreductive nephrectomy. Nat Clin Pract Urol 2004;1:26–30.

73. Klotz L. Back to nephrectomy for patients with metastatic renal cancer. Lancet 2001;358:948–9.

74. Klatte T, Ittenson A, Rohl FW, et al. Perioperative immunomodulation with interleukin-2 in patients with renal cell carcinoma: results of a controlled phase II trial. Br J Cancer 2006;95:1167–73.

75. Sweeney P, Wood CG, Pisters LL, et al. Surgical management of renal cell carcinoma associated with complex inferior vena caval thrombi. Urol Oncol 2003;21:327–33.

76. Vasselli JR, Yang JC, Linehan WM, et al. Lack of retroperitoneal lymphadenopathy predicts survival of patients with metastatic renal cell carcinoma. J Urol 2001;166:68–72.

77. Pantuck AJ, Zisman A, Dorey F, et al. Renal cell carcinoma with retroperitoneal lymph nodes. Impact on survival and benefits of immunotherapy. Cancer 2003;97:2995–3002.

78. Leibovich BC, Cheville JC, Lohse CM, et al. A scoring algorithm to predict survival for patients with metastatic clear cell renal cell carcinoma: a stratification tool for prospective clinical trials. J Urol 2005;174:1759–63; discussion 1763.

79. Zisman A, Pantuck AJ, Chao DH, et al. Renal cell carcinoma with tumor thrombus: is cytoreductive nephrectomy for advanced disease associated with an increased complication rate? J Urol 2002;168:962–7.

80. Lee SE, Kwak C, Byun SS, et al. Metastatectomy prior to immunochemotherapy for metastatic renal cell carcinoma. Urol Int 2006;76:256–63.

81. Schlomer B, Figenshau RS, Yan Y, et al. How does the radiographic size of a renal mass compare with the pathologic size? Urology 2006;68:292–5.

82. Herr HW, Lee CT, Sharma S, et al. Radiographic versus pathologic size of renal tumors: implications for partial nephrectomy. Urology 2001;58:157–60.

83. Yaycioglu O, Rutman MP, Balasubramaniam M, et al. Clinical and pathologic tumor size in renal cell carcinoma; difference, correlation, and analysis of the influencing factors. Urology 2002;60:33–8.

84. Tsui KH, Shvarts O, Smith RB, et al. Prognostic indicators for renal cell carcinoma: a multivariate analysis of 643 patients using the revised 1997 TNM staging criteria. J Urol 2000;163:1090–5; quiz 1295.

85. Amin MB, Amin MB, Tamboli P, et al. Prognostic impact of histologic subtyping of adult renal epithelial neoplasms: an experience of 405 cases. Am J Surg Pathol 2002;26:281–91.

86. Frank I, Blute ML, Cheville JC, et al. An outcome prediction model for patients with clear cell renal cell carcinoma treated with radical nephrectomy based on tumor stage, size, grade and necrosis: the SSIGN score. J Urol 2002;168:2395–400.

87. de Peralta-Venturina M, Moch H, Amin M, et al. Sarcomatoid differentiation in renal cell carcinoma: a study of 101 cases. Am J Surg Pathol 2001;25:275–84.

88. Gatenby RA, Gawlinski ET, Tangen CM, et al. The possible role of postoperative azotemia in enhanced survival of patients with metastatic renal cancer after cytoreductive nephrectomy. Cancer Res 2002;62:5218–22.

89. Leibovich BC, Han KR, Bui MH, et al. Scoring algorithm to predict survival after nephrectomy and immunotherapy in patients with metastatic renal cell carcinoma: a stratification tool for prospective clinical trials. Cancer 2003; 98:2566–75.

90. Walther MM, Lyne JC, Libutti SK, et al. Laparoscopic cytoreductive nephrectomy as preparation for administration of systemic interleukin-2 in the treatment of metastatic renal cell carcinoma: a pilot study. Urology 1999;53:496–501.

91. Rabets JC, Kaouk J, Fergany A, et al. Laparoscopic versus open cytoreductive nephrectomy for metastatic renal cell carcinoma. Urology 2004;64:930–4.

92. Matin SF, Madsen LT, Wood CG. Laparoscopic cytoreductive nephrectomy: the M. D. Anderson Cancer Center experience. Urology 2006;68:528–32.

93. Virgo KS, Naunheim KS, Johnson FE. Preoperative workup and postoperative surveillance for patients undergoing pulmonary metastasectomy. Thorac Surg Clin 2006; 16:125–31, v.

94. Evans CP. Follow-up surveillance strategies for genitourinary malignancies. Cancer 2002;94:2892–905.

95. Bennett RT, Lerner SE, Taub HC, et al. Cytoreductive surgery for stage IV renal cell carcinoma. J Urol 1995;154:32–4.

96. Figlin RA, Pierce WC, Kaboo R, et al. Treatment of metastatic renal cell carcinoma with nephrectomy, interleukin-2 and cytokine-primed or CD8(+) selected tumor infiltrating lymphocytes from primary tumor. J Urol 1997;158:740–5.

97. Levy DA, Swanson DA, Slaton JW, et al. Timely delivery of biological therapy after cytoreductive nephrectomy in carefully selected patients with metastatic renal cell carcinoma. J Urol 1998;159:1168–73.

# SUPPORTIVE CARE IN METASTATIC RENAL CELL CARCINOMA

## Bisphosphonates

ABRAHAM B. SCHWARZBERG, MD
M. DROR MICHAELSON, MD, PHD

Bone is a dynamic tissue that undergoes continuous remodeling through a balance of bone formation and resorption. Bone homeostasis is perturbed in the setting of skeletal metastasis from solid tumors. Skeletal complications related to metastatic disease to the bone occur in approximately 30% of patients with advanced renal cell carcinoma (RCC).[1] The morbidity that results from skeletal metastasis is often challenging to manage, and historically, treatments have focused on temporizing interventions with the goal of stabilizing local lesions. With the introduction of bisphosphonates into the armamentarium, the focus of therapy has shifted toward delaying or preventing skeletal complications. Bisphosphonates have reduced the morbidity experienced by patients with metastatic RCC and other solid tumors.

## BONE BIOLOGY

Bone remodeling involves the continual breakdown of mature bone and subsequent replacement by new bone. Approximately 10% of the total bone mass turns over each year because of the remodeling process. Physiologic bone resorption is directed by osteoclast activity. These tissue-specific macrophages are giant multinucleated cells, which are formed by the fusion of several precursor cells derived from hematopoietic stem cells. Osteoclasts attach to the endosteal and periosteal surfaces and tunnel their way through the mineralized bone to dissolve the bone matrix and resorb the bone mass. This process is closely regulated and is balanced by osteoblast activity. The osteoblasts are mesenchymal in origin and are responsible for bone formation. Alkaline phosphatase is an enzyme essential to the process of bone formation, and serum levels of alkaline phosphatase can reflect osteoblast activity. Bone formation by osteoblasts is stimulated by factors including transforming growth factor-$\beta$, insulin-like growth factor, and platelet-derived growth factor. Bone resorption via osteoclasts is activated by interleukin-1, interleukin-6, tumor necrosis factor $\alpha$ and $\beta$, and cortisol. Under normal circumstances, these factors allow for balanced bone remodeling but become deranged in the presence of metastatic cancer to the bone. Tumors alter directly and/or indirectly the homeostasis of bone remodeling and can lead to excess bone formation or breakdown. This imbalance causes significant morbidity, which often requires immediate attention and intervention.

## CLINICAL MANIFESTATIONS OF BONY METASTASIS

Bony metastases from RCC are the second most common organ site of distant spread, occurring approximately 30% of the time.[1] In 2001, Zekri and colleagues reviewed 103 cases of metastatic RCC and reported that the most commonly affected bony sites are the pelvis (48%), ribs (48%), and spine (42%). Pain is the most common symptom of bony metastasis. Additional skeletal-related events (SRE) observed include pathologic fractures, hypercalcemia, spinal cord compression, cauda equine syndrome, and nerve root compression. Zekri and colleagues reported that 81% of patients with skeletal metastasis required radiation treatment, 42% of patients experienced long bone fractures, and 29% of patients underwent orthopedic surgery. Lipton and colleagues observed that 74% of bony metastasis from RCC resulted in at least one skeletal complication during a 9-month period in patients receiving placebo as part of a randomized double-blind trial.[2] Patients with RCC experienced a higher rate of SREs (74%) compared with other cancer subsets (44%), indicating the higher risk of skeletal complications as a result of bony metastases from RCC.

Tumor mediated osteoclast activity, as commonly observed in metastatic RCC, causes extensive bone resorption and subsequent osteolytic bone lesions. These lesions result in SREs as described previously. Unfortunately, bony metastases historically respond poorly to systemic treatment for RCC and are a major cause of morbidity. An important advance in the supportive management of patients with bony metastases has been the addition of bisphosphonates in routine oncology care.

## BISPHOSPHONATE THERAPY

Bisphosphonates are synthetic analogs of inorganic pyrophosphate with a backbone of two phosphonate groups linked by nonhydrolyzable phosphoether bonds to a central carbon atom (Figure 1). The potency of bisphosphonates is enhanced when a nitrogen moiety is included in the side chain of the middle carbon, and the most potent in this class of drugs is zoledronic acid.[3] Bisphosphonates have skeletal half-lives measured in years because of their nonbiodegradable properties and strong adherence to mineralized surfaces.[4]

Bisphosphonates are ingested selectively by normal and pathologically activated osteoclasts and result in inhibition of bone resorption through multiple mechanisms including inhibition of recruitment to bone surface, inhibition of activity on the bony surface, reduced life span of osteoclasts, and alteration of the bone or bone mineral to reduce the rate of dissolution.[5]

Two bisphosphonates are approved for use in the treatment of bony metastasis from solid tumors, zoledronic acid, and pamidronate. Their characteristics and dosing recommendations are detailed in Table 1. Bisphosphonates have been extensively investigated and used to treat SRE (which include pathologic fracture, spinal cord compression, hypercalcemia of malignancy (HCM), need for radiation treatment, or surgery to bone) caused by bone

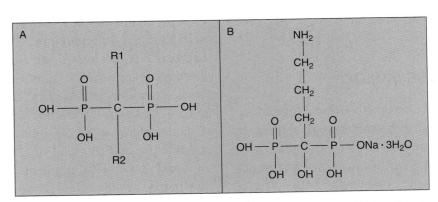

**Figure 1.** Structure of bisphosphonates. Structure of a generic bisphosphonate (A) and a nitrogen-containing bisphosphonate. B, Reproduced with permission from Bilezikian JP.[17]

Supportive Care in Metastatic Renal Cell Carcinoma    275

| Table 1. BISPHOSPHONATE CHARACTERISTICS | | |
|---|---|---|
| Bisphos-phonate | Recommended Dosing and Administration | Indications for Cancer Patients |
| Pamidronate* | 90 mg intravenously infused over at least 2 hours administered every 3 to 4 weeks | HCM—less effective than zoledronate[11] |
| | Duration of treatment not defined | Prevention and delay of SREs in patients with bony lesions from breast cancer or multiple myeloma[6,9] |
| Zoledronic acid* | 4 mg intravenously infused over at least 15 minutes administered every 3 to 4 weeks | HCM—superior to pamidronate[11] |
| | Duration of treatment not defined | Prevention and delay with of SREs in patients bony lesions from multiple myeloma and all solid tumors[9,10,12,19] (especially RCC patients[2]) |

*Check creatinine prior to each dose and supplement with vitamin D and calcium.

HCM = hypercalcemia of malignancy; SRE = Skeletal-related events.

metastases in patients with breast cancer or multiple myeloma. In multiple placebo-controlled trials, pamidronate showed significant delays in the onset and reduced incidences of SREs in patients with breast cancer or myeloma.[6–8] These studies led to the approval of pamidronate and its routine use in the management of patients with breast cancer and myeloma with bony metastases. Subsequently, zoledronic acid was proven to be at least as effective as pamidronate in preventing SRE in patients with multiple myeloma and breast cancer.[9] A large randomized phase III study showed its efficacy as the first bisphosphonate to reduce significantly the incidence of SRE in patients with advanced prostate cancer from 44% in the placebo arm to 33% in the 4 mg zoledronic acid group ($p = .021$).[10] In addition, zoledronic acid has been shown to be superior in the treatment of HCM and in reducing the risk of developing skeletal complications from breast cancer (Table 2).[9,11]

A pivotal study evaluated the efficacy of zoledronic acid in the treatment of skeletal metastases

from other solid tumors.[12] This randomized phase III trial compared zoledronic acid (4 or 8 mg dosing as a 15-minute infusion) every 3 weeks for 9 months with placebo in 773 patients with a variety of solid tumors including 74 patients with RCC (Table 2). Because of the concerns about safety, the 8 mg dosing was decreased to 4 mg. The primary end point was the percentage of patients with ≥ 1 SRE, not including HCM. Results showed no significant difference in SRE in comparing 4 mg of zoledronic acid with placebo (38 vs 44%; $p = .127$). When analysis of SREs included HCM, the 4 mg zoledronic acid dosing significantly reduced the rate of skeletal events compared with placebo (38% vs 47%; $p = .039$).

Another statistically significant finding was the delay in time to first SRE by more than 2 months when treated with zoledronic acid (230 days to first event for the 4 mg dosing group compared with 163 days for placebo [$p = .023$]). There were no statistically significant differences between zoledronic acid and placebo with respect to quality of life, bone lesion response, disease progression, or overall survival, although the study was not powered for these end points. Multiple-event analysis showed that zoledronic acid provides a 31% risk reduction of developing skeletal complications (including HCM) compared with placebo and is a well-tolerated intervention.

## EFFICACY OF ZOLEDRONIC ACID IN RCC

In an attempt to establish the efficacy of zoledronic acid in the treatment of bony metastases from RCC, Lipton and colleagues analyzed the subset of patients with RCC who were included in the phase III trial by Rosen and colleagues.[12] Of the 773 patients in the original trial, 74 (10%) were identified to have RCC.[2] Patients were randomized to treatment with zoledronic acid (4 or 8 mg as a 15-minute infusion) every 3 weeks for 9 months or placebo. Baseline characteristics for RCC patients were well balanced between the 4 mg zoledronic acid group and the placebo group. Zoledronic acid reduced the percent of patients with SREs by 50% (37 vs 74% with placebo, $p = .015$). In addition, zoledronic acid prolonged the time to first SRE from 72 days for placebo to median not reached at

**Table 2. SELECTED RANDOMIZED CONTROLLED TRIALS OF IV BISPHOSPHONATES IN CANCER**

| Trial | Study Population | Treatment | Major Outcome |
|---|---|---|---|
| Major and colleagues (275 patients)[11] | All cancer types | Zoledronic acid vs pamidronate | Complete resolution of HCM at 10 days: 88% for the zoledronic acid arm vs 70% for the placebo arm+ |
| Rosen and colleagues (1648 patients)[9] | Breast cancer or multiple myeloma | Zoledronic acid vs pamidronate | No significant difference in SRE. Multiple-event analysis demonstrated 16% risk reduction with use of zoledronate* |
| Saad and colleagues (643 patients)[10] | Androgen independent prostate cancer | Zoledronic acid vs placebo | Significant decrease in SREs* from 44% in the placebo arm to 33% in the zoledronic acid arm |
| Rosen and colleagues (773 patients)[12] | Solid tumors (excluding breast and prostate cancer) | Zoledronic acid vs placebo | No significant difference in SRE. Zoledronic acid provided > 2 month delay in time to first SRE. Multiple-event analysis demonstrated 31% risk reduction with use of zoledronate |
| Lipton and colleagues (74 patients)[2] | Renal cell carcinoma | Zoledronic acid vs placebo | Significant reduction in SRE by 50% (74% vs 37%), prolongation of time to first SRE, and 21% reduction in skeletal morbidity rate* |

All zoledronic acid dosing is 4 mg and pamidronate dosing is 90 mg.

HCM = hypercalcemia of malignancy; SRE = Skeletal-related events.

*p value ≤ .05.

9 months ($p$ = .006) and reduced the skeletal morbidity rate by approximately 21% ($p$ = .014).

Patients receiving zoledronic acid also experienced notable responses in bony lesions as measured by increased median time to bone lesion progression and number of patients with partial responses or stable disease in their bone lesions. These additional clinical benefits may support the preclinical models, which have shown antiangiogenic activity of zoledronic acid. In addition, there is a suggestion that for the patients with RCC, treatment with zoledronic acid might provide direct antitumor effects or prevent bone metastasis. Despite these observations, there was no significant change to overall survival and further investigation is needed to confirm these hypotheses.

In summary, multiple-event analysis showed that zoledronic acid provides a 61% risk reduction of developing skeletal complications and delays time to first SRE by almost 1 year compared with placebo.[2,13] This reduction is more profound than that observed in the overall cancer patient population (31%), suggesting that RCC patients may receive greater benefit from treatment with zoledronic acid than other subsets of solid tumor patients.

## TOXICITY

The most common adverse effects reported in solid tumor patients (all grades) receiving bisphosphonates are bone pain, nausea, anemia, vomiting, constipation, dyspnea, and fatigue (Table 3 and 4).[12] Acute-phase reactions during infusions have been well documented and include nausea, emesis, dyspnea, headache, and flu-like symptoms. These symptoms are self-limited and often mild to moderate in severity.[14] These reactions are more common after the first few infusions of bisphosphonates and are less frequent with subsequent treatments. Despite good tolerability, bisphosphonates present rare but potentially serious complications, including renal failure, hypocalcemia, and jaw osteonecrosis.

Significant renal toxicity from bisphosphonate use is a serious but uncommon complication of treatment. Pamidronate has been associated with renal

**Table 3. ALL GRADE TOXICITY IN SOLID TUMOR PATIENTS (N = 773)**

| Adverse Event | Zoledronic Acid 4 mg Number of Patients (%) | Placebo Number of Patients (%) |
|---|---|---|
| Bone pain | 130 (51.2) | 150 (60.7) |
| Nausea | 124 (48.8) | 90 (36.4) |
| Emesis | 96 (37.8) | 75 (30.4) |
| Dyspnea | 90 (35.4) | 74 (30) |
| Fever | 69 (27.2) | 58 (23.5) |
| Headache | 43 (16.9) | 27 (10.9) |

Adverse events in patients with solid tumors adapted from Rosen and colleagues.[14]

**Table 4. ALL GRADE TOXICITY IN RENAL CELL CARCINOMA PATIENTS (n = 74)**

| Adverse Event | Zoledronic Acid 4 mg Number of Patients (%) | Placebo Number of Patients (%) |
|---|---|---|
| Rigors | 6 (22) | 2 (11) |
| Lower extremity edema | 6 (22) | 2 (11) |
| Hypocalcemia | 5 (19) | 0 (0) |
| Abdominal pain | 4 (15) | 0 (0) |
| Dyspepsia | 3 (11) | 0 (0) |
| Total renal-related events | 2 (11) | 3 (20) |
|    Hyperuricemia | 1 (5.6) | 0 (0) |
|    Blood creatinine increase | 0 (0) | 0 (0) |
|    Renal failure | 1 (5.6) | 0 (0) |

Adverse events in subgroup of patients with RCC only adapted from Lipton and colleagues.[2]

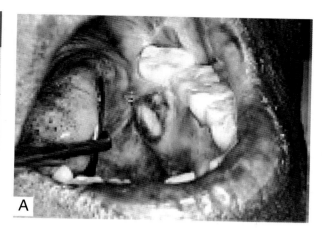

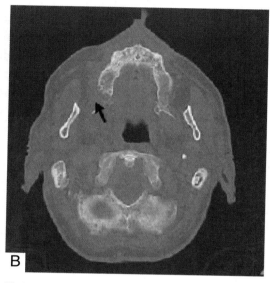

**Figure 2.** Osteonecrosis of the jaw. *A,* Patient with bisphosphonate-associated ONJ. (Reproduced with permission from Treister N and Woo S-B).[20] *B,* Computed tomographic scan showing ONJ of the right maxilla — black arrow. Reproduced with permission from S-B Woo.

insufficiency and nephrotic syndrome in multiple myeloma patients but these complications are rarely seen in solid malignancies. Administration of pamidronate for less than 2 hours appears to increase the risk of renal toxicity and should be avoided. Zoledronic acid is associated with renal insufficiency predominantly with higher doses (8 mg) or rapid infusions (less than 15 minutes) of the drug.[9] Many studies have shown the safety and absence of clinically significant renal toxicity when bisphosphonates are given at currently approved schedules for prolonged courses in patients with RCC and other solid tumors.[2,15,16] Due to the potential for renal toxicity, general recommendations are to check creatinine prior to each bisphosphonate dose, and any unexplained elevation ≥ 0.5 mg/dL in serum creatinine should warrant temporary discontinuation of the drug until renal function returns to baseline. If renal function does not return to normal, either indefinite discontinuation of the drug or resumption of therapy with prolonged infusion time and close observation are reasonable.

Hypocalcemia is an uncommon but potentially serious complication of bisphosphonate therapy (Table 4). Due to compensatory mechanisms, this complication is rarely observed. General recommendations include periodic monitoring of serum calcium, magnesium, and phosphate while patients are on therapy.

Osteonecrosis of the jaw (ONJ) is a recently described complication of long-term use of bisphosphonate, typically occurring in patients receiving treatment for 1.5 to 3 years.[17] This process involves avascular necrosis of the jaw with subsequent exposed bone in the mandible, maxilla, and/or palate that heals poorly over a prolonged period (Figure 2). The rate of occurrence is estimated to be between 4 and 7%.[18] Predisposing factors include dental disease or surgery, oral trauma, poor dental hygiene, and periodontitis.[17] Prior to initiation of bisphosphonate therapy, patients should optimize their dental hygiene and while on therapy should follow routine oral health maintenance. After developing ONJ, management includes minimal local debridement of dead bone, rinses with cyclohexidine or hydrogen peroxide, antibiotics and analgesics. There is no clear evidence to guide the timing and duration of discontinuing bisphosphonates in patients who develop ONJ but cessation of treatment should be strongly considered.[18]

## CONCLUSIONS

Skeletal-related events cause significant morbidity for patients with metastatic RCC. Bone lesions from RCC are particularly destructive, likely due to their predominantly osteolytic nature, and usually result in skeletal-related complications including pain and fractures. Zoledronic acid is proven to reduce SRE from bony metastasis in patients with RCC. Potential toxicities include mild acute phase reaction, renal dysfunction, and jaw osteonecrosis. Additional studies are needed to determine the optimal time to initiate therapy, to establish the necessary duration of treatment, and to investigate the possible antineoplastic effects of bisphosphonates. Answers to these questions will help to define further the role of bisphosphonates in the systemic management of metastatic RCC.

## REFERENCES

1. Zekri J, Ahmed N, Coleman RE, Hancock BW. The skeletal metastatic complications of renal cell carcinoma. Int J Oncol 2001; 19:379–82.
2. Lipton A, Zheng M, Seaman J. Zoledronic acid delays the onset of skeletal-related events and progression of skeletal disease in patients with advanced renal cell carcinoma. Cancer 2003; 98:962–9.
3. Fleisch H. Bisphosphonates: mechanisms of action. Endocr Rev 1998; 19:80–100.
4. Licata AA. Discovery, clinical development, and therapeutic uses of bisphosphonates. Ann Pharmacother 2005; 39:668–77.
5. Rodan GA, Fleisch HA. Bisphosphonates: mechanisms of Action. J Clin Invest 1996; 97:2692–6.
6. Lipton A, Theriault RL, Hortobagyi GN, et al. Pamidronate prevents skeletal complications and is effective palliative treatment in women with breast carcinoma and osteolytic bone metastases: long term follow-up of two randomized, placebo-controlled trials. Cancer 2000; 88:1082–90.
7. Theriault RL, Lipton A, Hortobagyi GN, et al. Pamidronate reduces skeletal morbidity in women with advanced breast cancer and lytic bone lesions: a randomized, placebo-controlled trial. Protocol 18 Aredia Breast Cancer Study Group. J Clin Oncol 1999; 17:846–54.
8. Berenson JR, Lichtenstein A, Porter L, et al. Efficacy of pamidronate in reducing skeletal events in patients with advanced multiple myeloma. Myeloma Aredia Study Group. N Engl J Med 1996; 334:488–93.
9. Rosen LS, Gordon D, Kaminski M, et al. Long-term efficacy and safety of zoledronic acid compared with pamidronate disodium in the treatment of skeletal complications in patients with advanced multiple myeloma or breast carcinoma. Cancer 2003; 98:1735–44.
10. Saad F, Gleason DM, Murray R, et al. A randomized, placebo-controlled trial of zoledronic acid in patients with hormone-refractory metastatic prostate carcinoma. J Natl Cancer Inst 2002;94:1458–68.
11. Major P, Lortholary A, Hon J, et al. Zoledronic acid is superior to pamidronate in the treatment of hypercalcemia of malignancy: a pooled analysis of two randomized, controlled clinical trials. J Clin Oncol 2001; 19:558–67.
12. Rosen LS, Gordon D, Tchekmedyian S, et al. Zoledronic Acid Versus Placebo in the Treatment of Skeletal Metastases in Patients With Lung Cancer and Other Solid Tumors: A Phase III, Double-Blind, Randomized Trial—The Zoledronic Acid Lung Cancer and Other Solid Tumors Study Group. J Clin Oncol 2003; 21:3150–7.
13. Lipton A, Seaman J, Zheng M. Efficacy and safety of zoledronic acid in patients with bone metastases from renal cell carcinoma. In: What Is New in Bisphosphonates? Seventh Workshop on Bisphosphonates—From the Laboratory to the Patients; 2004 March 24–26; Davos, Switzerland. Poster 28; 2004.

14. Rosen LS, Gordon D, Tchekmedyian NS, et al. Long-term efficacy and safety of zoledronic acid in the treatment of skeletal metastases in patients with nonsmall cell lung carcinoma and other solid tumors. Cancer 2004; 100: 2613–21.

15. Kohno N, Aogi K, Minami H, et al. Zoledronic Acid Significantly Reduces Skeletal Complications Compared With Placebo in Japanese Women With Bone Metastases From Breast Cancer: A Randomized, Placebo-Controlled Trial. J Clin Oncol 2005; 23:3314–21.

16. Guarneri V, Donati S, Nicolini M, et al. Renal safety and efficacy of i.v. bisphosphonates in patients with skeletal metastases treated for up to 10 Years. Oncologist 2005; 10:842–8.

17. Bilezikian JP. Osteonecrosis of the Jaw—Do Bisphosphonates Pose a Risk? N Engl J Med 2006; 355:2278–81.

18. Woo S-B, Hellstein JW, Kalmar JR. Systematic review: bisphosphonates and osteonecrosis of the jaws. Ann Intern Med 2006; 144:753–61.

19. Saad F, Lipton A. Zoledronic acid is effective in preventing and delaying skeletal events in patients with bone metastases secondary to genitourinary cancers. BJU International 2005; 96:964–9.

20. Treister N, Woo S-B. Bisphosphonate-associated osteonecrosis of the jaw. N Engl J Med 2006; 355:2348.

# SUPPORTIVE CARE IN METASTATIC RENAL CELL CARCINOMA

## Management of Central Nervous System Metastasis from Renal Carcinoma

**GURU SONPAVDE, MD**

**BIN S. TEH, MD**

**THOMAS E. HUTSON, DO, PHARMD**

Central nervous system metastasis is a significant cause of morbidity and early mortality from renal cell carcinoma. Whole brain radiotherapy has typically been offered in the past. Surgical resection followed by conventional radiotherapy appears to improve outcomes when feasible. Although renal cell carcinoma has historically been felt to be radioresistant, stereotactic radiosurgery appears promising with minimal morbidity. Future investigation and integration of radiation and/or surgery with novel multitargeted tyrosine kinase inhibitors is of paramount importance and may further improve outcomes.

In the United States, 38,890 new cases of renal cell carcinoma (RCC) are expected in 2006, with the majority being clear cell RCC.[1] One-third of the patients with RCC have evidence of metastases at the time of the diagnosis, whereas up to 50% of the patients who are treated for localized disease eventually develop a recurrence.[2] The widely used Memorial Sloan-Kettering Cancer Center risk group categorization in mostly untreated metastatic patients defines the 5 poor-risk features: Karnofsky performance status (KPS) < 80, a serum calcium > 10 (corrected for albumin), a hemoglobin below normal, absence of prior nephrectomy, and a lactate dehydrogenase > 1.5 times the upper limit of normal.[3,4] The median survivals were 20, 10, and 4 months for good (no risk factors), intermediate (1 to 2 risk factors), and poor-risk patients (≥ 3 risk factors), respectively. The novel multitargeted tyrosine kinase inhibitors sunitinib, malate, and sorafenib have supplanted cytokines for the therapy of good- and intermediate-risk metastatic clear cell RCC.[5,6] High-dose interleukin-2 may be appropriate for good performance status in patients with clear cell RCC and favorable risk status.[7,8] Temsirolimus, an mammalian target of rapamycin (mTOR) inhibitor, has been proven to improve survival in poor-risk RCC.[9]

Patients with untreated brain metastasis from RCC have a poor prognosis with a median survival of 17 weeks to 7 months.[10,11] This has led to pessimism about the prognosis of patients with RCC brain metastasis. Therefore, most clinical trials have either excluded or not included patients with RCC who had central nervous system (CNS) metastasis. A special focus and innovative strategies are necessary for this population. We will review recent data and approaches to manage patients with clear cell RCC and CNS metastasis.

## BIOLOGY OF CNS METASTASIS FROM RCC

RCC has traditionally been considered radioresistant.[11] DNA double strand breakage is considered to be the most important lesion related to cell death induced by ionizing radiation. Radioresistant cells have lower initial DNA double-strand break frequencies and a faster rate at which DNA double-strand breaks are repaired.[12] In the linear-quadratic model, a low $\alpha$-$\beta$ ratio implies radioresistance.[13] Recent experiments with human cell lines of RCC have revealed a low $\alpha$-$\beta$ ratio ranging from 2.6 to 6.92.[14,15] The exact cellular mechanisms of radioresistance in RCC remain elusive, but various molecular markers (*TP53*, BRCA1, BRCA2, Bcl-2, PI3k, IFG-1, EGFR, *HER2*, vascular endothelial growth factor [VEGF]) have been demonstrated to influence radiation sensitivity for other tumor types. Several of these pathways (notably VEGF, vascular endothelial growth factor) are upregulated in clear cell RCC[16,17]

## CLINICAL FEATURES AND DIAGNOSTIC EVALUATION OF CNS METASTASIS FROM RCC

Common metastatic sites of advanced RCC include the lung (75%), soft tissues (36%), bone (20%), liver (18%), cutaneous (8%), and CNS (8%).[18] Four to 17% of all RCC patients will eventually develop brain metastases with 50% of these suffering from multiple lesions.[19] The incidence of brain metastasis following a diagnosis of RCC is 10 to 20% in autopsy studies.[20–22] The brain as the sole site of metastasis has been occasionally described.[23,24] Spinal cord compression has been observed less commonly, and in 1 study, 13% of patients are with bone metastases from RCC.[25] The kidney was reported to be the site of primary tumor in 5 to 10% of all patients presenting with initial brain metastasis.[26–29]

The most frequent complaints of brain metastasis include headaches, cognitive changes, focal weakness, and seizures.[30,31] Other symptoms include gait difficulty, visual loss, speech abnormalities, and sensory loss. Physical examination may reveal hemiparesis, cognitive changes, speech abnormalities, papilledema, gait disturbance, and hemianopsia.

Brain metastases of RCC may be hemorrhagic, and occasionally bleed, and cause acute neurological symptoms because they are hypervascular.[32,33] Multifocal abnormalities at multiple sites in the CNS are suggestive of leptomeningeal disease which can be proven by the demonstration of malignant cells in the CSF or by a high quality magnetic resonance imaging (MRI) of the brain and spinal cord. Spinal cord compression is characterized by lower extremity motor and sensory symptoms.

## MANAGEMENT OF CNS METASTASIS FROM RCC

Conventional treatment for cerebral metastases includes initial glucocorticoids.[34,35] The routine use of prophylactic antiepileptic drugs for patients with brain metastases without seizures is currently not recommended.[36,37] Definitive therapeutic options for brain metastasis include whole brain radiotherapy (WBRT), stereotactic radiosurgery (SRS), and surgical resection. Spinal cord compression from epidural metastasis is generally managed by conventional radiation with or without surgery.

### Whole Brain Radiotherapy

#### WBRT for Brain Metastasis: General Concepts

WBRT is considered to be the traditional treatment for patients with brain metastases. It can delay/prevent neurological deficits, restore neurological function, decrease steroid dependency, and result in symptomatic improvement in up to 80% of patients within 3 weeks of treatment in more radiosensitive malignancies.[38–41] WBRT is the treatment of choice for patients with single brain metastasis not amenable to surgery or SRS, for patients with poorly controlled systemic disease, and thus, relatively short life expectancy, and for patients with multiple brain metastases that are too numerous for SRS or surgery. A dose of 30 Gy in 10 fractions is the most commonly reported dose for WBRT in RCC.

WBRT alone results in a median survival, which is 7.1, 4.2, and 2.3 months for Radiation Therapy Oncology Group (RTOG) recursive partitioning analysis (RPA) class I, II, and III, respectively, for patients with brain metastases from historically nonradioresistant tumors.[42] The 3 RPA classes were defined as follows: Class 1, patients with KPS $\geq$ 70, < 65 years of age with controlled primary, and no extracranial metastases; Class 3, KPS < 70; Class 2, all others. The most common treatment schedule used is 30 Gy in 10 fractions over 2 weeks. However, for patients with a good prognosis who are likely to survive longer than 1 year, more prolonged fractionated schedules may reduce long-term morbidity from radiation. For patients with a solitary brain metastasis, surgical resection followed by WBRT has been advocated and is discussed in detail in another section in this chapter.[43,44] However, many patients suffer from unresectable brain metastases because of the presence of multiple sites of intracranial disease or critical tumor location.[45] Autopsy studies indicate that 60 to 85% of all patients with brain metastases have multiple lesions.[46]

### WBRT for RCC Brain Metastasis

In retrospective studies, patients with brain metastases from RCC treated with WBRT displayed a median survival of 3 to 7 months (Table 1).[10,32,47]

| Table 2. SURVIVAL FOR DIFFERENT RADIATION THERAPY ONCOLOGY GROUP RECURSIVE PARTITIONING ANALYSIS CLASSES WITH WHOLE BRAIN RADIOTHERAPY (NON–RANDOMIZED COMPARISONS ACROSS DIFFERENT STUDIES) | | | |
|---|---|---|---|
| RTOG RPA | Description | Non-RCC Median Survival (mo) | RCC Median Survival (mo) |
| I | KPS $\geq$ 70, age < 65, controlled primary, and no extracranial disease | 7.1 | 8.5 |
| II | All others | 4.2 | 3 |
| III | KPS < 70 | 2.3 | 0.6 |

KPS = Karnofsky Performance Status; RCC = renal cell carcinoma; RTOG = radiation therapy oncology group.

Moreover, WBRT provided up to 60% local control (LC, control at the sites of radiographically apparent disease) with only 8% distant brain failure rate (incidence of new brain lesions away from initial sites of disease).[32] The median survivals for metastatic RCC by RTOG RPA classes (8.5, 3, and 0.6 months for RPA classes I, II, and III, respectively) further support the efficacy of WBRT because outcomes appear similar to patients with other malignancies (Table 2).[42,47]

### Dose Response and Hyperfractionation of WBRT

The role of dose escalation and/or hyperfractionation in WBRT for non-RCC brain metastases is controversial. In practice, the dose and fraction size of WBRT should be individualized to take into consideration the status of systemic or extracranial disease as well as performance status. The RTOG has conducted 2 randomized studies, which demonstrated that different fractionation schedules of 40 Gy in 15 or 20 fractions, 30 Gy in 10 or 15 fractions, and 20 Gy in 5 fraction yield comparable results.[38,48] In these randomized trials, there was no difference in neurological function, duration of improvement, time to progression, and survival. This was recently challenged by Epstein and colleagues[49] who reported superior survival times and improved neurologic function in patients with solitary brain metastases with doses of 32 Gy administered in 1.6 Gy fractions twice daily followed by boost doses to 48, 54, 64, and 70 Gy.

| Table 1. RETROSPECTIVE REPORTS OF RENAL CELL CARCINOMA PATIENTS TREATED WITH WHOLE BRAIN RADIATION THERAPY ALONE | | | |
|---|---|---|---|
| Series | Wronski et al, 1997 | Cannady et al, 2004* | Culine et al, 1998 |
| No. of patients | 119 | 46 | 50 |
| Patients with multiple brain metastses | 70 | 30 | NR |
| Dose (Gy) | 30 | 30 | 18–36 |
| CR% | NR | 2 | NR |
| LC% | NR | 61 | NR |
| DBF% | NR | 8 | NR |
| median OS | 4.4 | 3.0 | 7 |

CR = Complete response; DBF = distant brain failure; LC = local control, OS = overall survival.

Fifty patients were available for SRS alone arm and 39 patients were available for SRS + WBRT arm. The local control rates were 100% and 92% for SRS with WBRT and for SRS alone respectively. The DBF rates were 31% and 21% for SRS with WBRT and for SRS alone respectively. A trend towards improved local and distant control rates are seen with the addition of WBRT with p–values of 0.05 and 0.14. However, the results must be viewed with caution as patient or institutional selection biases may be present and have not been accounted for.

Survivals increased with increasing dose from 4.9 months with 48 Gy to 8.2 months with 70 Gy. Nieder and colleagues[50] found patients who received WBRT with 30 Gy in 10 fractions had 50% the response rate of the group receiving 40 to 60 Gy in 20 to 30 fractions without survival benefit. These retrospective studies suggest that there may be a dose response at higher doses, which is not evident at lower doses such as the ones used in the randomized trials by RTOG.

Data supporting a dose response for WBRT in RCC patients are scant. The retrospective study of RCC patients by Cannady and colleagues[47] has found that patients who receive greater than 30 Gy had significantly longer survival than patients who received 30 Gy or less. However, the result was confounded by the fact that patients who received higher doses also had better prognostic factors such as KPS and RPA class. Thus, it is unclear if dose or fractionation has an impact in RCC patients with brain metastases.

## Surgery Followed by Adjuvant WBRT

### Non–RCC Metastasis

Surgical resection of a metastatic brain tumor has several advantages including confirmation of pathology, rapid reversal of neurological symptoms, no risk of radionecrosis, and durable LC. In non-RCC patients, randomized trials has evaluated the benefits of surgery in patients with good performance status or limited or controlled systemic disease.[43,51,52] Three randomized trials (American, Dutch, and Canadian) have evaluated surgery and WBRT versus WBRT alone. The American and the Dutch study have included mainly patients with controlled or limited systemic disease, and both have reported 9 to 10 months of median survival with surgery + WBRT versus 3 to 6 months with WBRT alone.[43,51] In contrast, the Canadian study that included a higher proportion of patients with an active systemic disease and lower performance status failed to show any advantage of surgery + WBRT over WBRT alone.[52] In addition, it has been shown for patients with brain metastasis from non-RCC that with accessible lesions in patients with good performance status complete surgical resections of up to 3 lesions yielded similar results

to those with single lesions.[53,54] The benefits of postoperative WBRT, including a 52% reduction of in brain recurrences, have been validated in a phase III randomized trial of patients with solitary brain metastases.[55] A trial that randomized patients with spinal cord compression caused by metastatic cancer to either surgery followed by radiotherapy (*n* = 50) or radiotherapy alone (*n* = 51) demonstrated a similar benefit for surgery in these patients.[56] Radiotherapy for both treatment groups was given in ten 3 Gy fractions. More patients in the surgery group (84%) than in the radiotherapy group (57%) were able to walk after treatment (*p* = .001). The need for corticosteroids and opioid analgesics was significantly reduced in the surgical group.

### RCC Brain Metastasis

Surgical resection of brain metastasis from RCC has been investigated in retrospective studies.[57–59] Wronski, O'Dea, and Salvati have reported a median survival of 14.5 to 27.5 months (Table 3). Patients in the surgical series for RCC had a much lower burden of disease (80% had only solitary brain metastasis) and higher performance status than in the nonsurgical series. Therefore, it is difficult to assess the true impact of surgery in RCC patients with brain metastasis in the absence of a dedicated randomized study. However, given the weight of data from the non-RCC randomized trials, as well as retrospective studies from RCC series, current data support surgery for patients with good performance status, limited systemic disease, and single brain metastasis. Furthermore, on the basis of non-RCC data, the benefits of surgery may extend to patients with up to 3 brain metastases from RCC. The role of adjuvant WBRT following surgery for RCC is controversial. The RCC surgical reports by Wronski and Salvati did not suggest a benefit to postoperative WBRT both in terms of brain recurrences or overall survival.[57,59] Notably, the radiation doses used by Wronski and Salvati were lower than in the randomized trial by Patchell.[55] The average dose in Wronski's series was 30 Gy in 10 to 15 fractions, whereas Salvati used various doses and fractions of 30 Gy in 10 fractions, 40 Gy in 20 fractions, 45 Gy in 25 fractions, or SRS. No significant differences

| | Table 3. SURGERY FOR RENAL CELL CARCINOMA BRAIN METASTASIS | | | | | | |
|---|---|---|---|---|---|---|---|
| | Median Survival (mo) | | Brain Relapse | | | Died of Widely | |
| Series | Surgery Alone | Surgery + XRT | Surgery Alone | Surgery + XRT | Solitary Brain Met | Metastatic Disease | No. of patients |
| Salvati et al,[59] | 23 | 28.1 | 33.9% | 32.8% | 100% | n/a | 28 |
| Wronski et al,[57] | 14.5 | 13.3 | 44% | 64% | 82% | 51% | 40 |
| O'Dea et al,[58] | 27.5 | NA | NA | NA | 100% | n/a | 8 |

The Wronski and colleagues series with the lowest median survival had more patients with multiple brain metastases and widely metastatic disease. In a highly selected group of patients with single brain metastasis and controlled primary, Salvati and colleagues reported higher median survival for patients who received postoperative radiotherapy.

NA = not available.

of survival time were noted in the various radiotherapy groups. Whether patients with RCC would benefit from higher WBRT doses remain a subject for investigation.

## Toxicities of WBRT

Data specific for RCC do not exist. Acute side effects occurring during or soon after radiotherapy include hair loss, otitis media, skin irritations, and brain edema. These symptoms with the possible exception of hair loss are generally transient and can be managed conservatively. The long-term side effects of radiotherapy are usually not a significant issue in the treatment of brain metastases because of the relatively short survival of these patients. Long-term survivors (> 12 months) will frequently develop radiographic changes on CT or MRI including hypodense areas in the white matter, cerebral atrophy, and an increase in the sulcal width and/or enlargement of the ventricles. However, only some long-term survivors (up to 11%) will develop clinical symptoms such as dementia, ataxia, and urinary incontinence.[60,61] Although the pathogenesis of these alterations is unknown, leukoencephalopathy is implicated. Leukoencephalopathy or white matter necrosis is generally associated with combination treatment of brain radiotherapy and intravenous or intrathecal methotrexate with the greatest injury occurring when all 3 modalities are used.[62] High-fractional dose (> 2 Gy per fraction) and high-dose

schedules may also be a factor.[59] Consequently, patients with favorable prognostic factors are probably optimally treated with conventional fractions of 1.8 to 2 Gy to a total dose of 40 to 50 Gy instead of the conventional fractions of 3 Gy to a total dose of 30 Gy.

Radiation necrosis refers to changes noted on imaging that are felt to represent radiation effect rather than recurrent tumor.[63] This potential complication is associated with SRS as well as WBRT. Radiation necrosis can produce symptoms that are as disabling as tumor recurrence and can be progressive and fatal. Surgical debulking should be performed if corticosteroids do not provide relief. Although biopsy proven rates as high as 24% have been reported, the true incidence of radiation necrosis is difficult to assess as chemotherapy, fraction size, total dose, and diagnostic modalities may all contribute.[64] In a report by Sheline and colleagues,[65] the brain could tolerate a total dose of 50 to 54 Gy if given in 2 Gy once daily with the estimated cerebral necrosis at 0.04% to 0.4%.

Radcliffe published a prospective study of 19 children treated for brain tumors with WBRT, of whom 19 also received adjuvant chemotherapy.[66] Children younger than 7 years at diagnosis had a mean intelligence quotient (IQ) loss of 27 points, whereas children over 7 years at diagnosis showed no significant decrease in IQ. Decline in IQ occurred between baseline and year 2 of follow-up; none could be documented between years 2 and 4.

In adults, many studies have shown decreases in mental function after brain radiation, but most of these fail to include pretreatment mental function assessment. Decline in cognitive function has been associated with radionecrosis.[67,68] In a prospective study of patient with small cell lung cancer, prophylactic cranial irradiation was not associated with decline in mental function for the duration of the follow-up (6 to 20 months).[69] NCCTG protocol 86-72-51 conducted a 2-arm prospective trial with 203 eligible adult patients with supratentorial, low-grade gliomas randomized to 50.4 Gy versus 64.8 Gy localized radiation therapy.[70] Patients were evaluated with an extensive battery of psychometric tests at baseline (before radiation therapy) and at approximate 18-month intervals up to 5 years after completing radiation therapy. Formal cognitive testing did not document significant detrimental effects. Deterioration from baseline occurred at years 1, 2, and 5 in 8.2%, 4.6%, and 5.3% of patients, respectively.[71] Thus, in contrast to children, adults have exhibited little decline in mental function following WBRT.

## Stereotactic Radiosurgery

### Stereotactic Radiosurgery for Non–RCC

Stereotactic radiosurgery provides, in a single session, a high dose of radiation to a localized brain tumor volume while minimizing the dose to the surrounding normal tissues.[72–74] For patients with brain metastases from non-RCC, SRS can produce results equivalent to surgery. Bindal and colleagues[53] have reported improved survival and LC in a small retrospective analysis of patients undergoing surgery compared to SRS. However, most studies support the notion that SRS, alone or in conjunction with WBRT, yields results that are comparable to those reported for surgery followed by WBRT for brain lesions < 3 cm and for up to 2 metastases.[54,75,76] In general, SRS provides a local tumor response rate of 80 to 90% with a median survival of 7 to 12 months.[77]

### Stereotactic Radiosurgery for RCC

Many retrospective studies have investigated the role of SRS in brain metastases from RCC (Table 4).

When SRS is one of the major components of the treatment of brain metastases from RCC, the results are encouraging.[19,78–87] The aggregate LC rate was 94% (ranging from 85 to 100%), with a distant brain failure (DBF) rate of 37% (ranging from 17.2 to 50%) and a median survival of 11 months (ranging from 6.7 to 17.8 months).[88] Other recent reports corroborate the value of SRS.[45,89] Several patients on these reports had multiple metastases and received repeated SRS.

### Stereotactic Radiosurgery Dose–Response

The optimal dose of SRS for brain metastasis is unclear. Hemibrain irradiation of normal beagle dogs in a single fraction suggests that there may be a sigmoid shaped dose-effect curve with a sharp increase in the brain changes from radiation occurring around 14 to 15 Gy.[90] Breneman and colleagues[91] have reported a significant improvement in LC with radiation dose > 18 Gy (median time to failure 52 weeks with high dose versus 25 weeks with low dose; $p = .008$). An analysis by Shiau and colleagues[92] found that a minimum dose ≥ 18 Gy yields greater failure-free survival at 1 year of 90% versus 77% for those who were treated with < 18 Gy. On the other hand, Alexander, Flickinger, and Shirato did not detect an impact of dose on LC or survival.[93–95] In general, larger tumors have been treated with lower dose, which are confounding the presently available retrospective data. Currently, the dose is generally guided by toxicities and not the minimum effective dose. Maximum tolerable dose of 24, 18, and 15 Gy for lesions < 2 cm, 2 to 3 cm, and 3 to 4 cm, respectively, has been recommended by RTOG 90 to 05, a prospective dose-escalation trial of SRS in patients with recurrent or previously irradiated primary brain tumors and brain metastases.[96]

SRS has been used multiple times to treat multiple lesions. Approximately, 50% of the patients treated with SRS in RCC series had multiple brain metastases. However, the maximum number of lesions that can be safely and efficaciously treated with SRS has not been identified for either RCC or other types of metastases. Some have suggested that patients with 10 or more metastases can be safely treated with good quality of life outcomes.[97,98]

Although multiple lesions can safely be treated with SRS, there is no evidence for superiority compared with WBRT. Other retrospective studies suggest that WBRT may be equivalent to SRS alone for patients with ≥ 3 brain metastases.[93,99]

## SRS Plus WBRT

### SRS Plus WBRT for Non–RCC

In non-RCC patients, a retrospective study by Sanghavi and colleagues[100] have reported an improved median survival ($p < .05$) for patient treated with SRS boost, in addition to WBRT, when compared with RPA-stratified patients from earlier RTOG studies of WBRT alone for non–RCC patients. Three randomized studies have shown LC benefit of adding SRS to WBRT.[101–103] The largest of the three studies by RTOG 95–08 (333 patients) demonstrated a median survival benefit of 1.5 months (6.5 vs 4.9 months) when SRS was added to WBRT in the pre-planned subset analysis of patients with a solitary metastasis.[103] In a post hoc analysis, subsets with 1 to 3 metastases and age < 50 years, RPA class I or non-small cell lung cancer also demonstrated improved survival. However, overall survival for all patients did not improve for the combination, although functional outcomes improved. A randomized study published by Brown University in abstract form only compared SRS versus WBRT versus SRS + WBRT in patients with 1 to 3 metastases.[102] No improvement in survival was observed with combination therapy, although 53% of the patients had undergone prior surgery, and there may have been an uneven distribution among the arms. In a recent Japanese randomized trial of 132 patients with 1 to 4 brain metastases, each less than 3 cm in diameter, patients were randomly assigned to receive WBRT + SRS (65 patients) or SRS alone (67 patients).[104] The median survival time and the 1-year actuarial survival rate were 7.5 months and 38.5% in the WBRT + SRS group and 8.0 months and 28.4% for SRS alone ($p = .42$). The 12-month brain tumor recurrence rate was 46.8% in the WBRT + SRS group and 76.4% for SRS alone group ($p < .001$). Salvage brain treatment was less frequently required in the WBRT + SRS group ($n = 10$) than with SRS alone ($n = 29$) ($p < .001$). Consequently, salvage treatment

| Table 4. STEREOTACTIC RADIO SURGERY AS ONE MAJOR COMPONENT FOR RENAL CELL CARCINOMA BRAIN METASTASIS | | | | |
|---|---|---|---|---|
| Series | No. of patients | LC (%) | DBF (%) | median OS |
| Mori et al,[83] 1998 | 35 | 90 | 46 | 11 |
| Schoggl et al,[84] 1998 | 23 | 96 | 30 | 11 |
| Goyal et al,[85] 2000 | 29 | 91 | 39 | 6.7 |
| Payne et al,[86] 2000 | 21 | 100 | 50 | 10 |
| Brown et al,[78] 2002 | 16 | 85 | 44 | 17.8 |
| Hoshi et al,[79] 2002 | 42 | 93 | 34 | 12.5 |
| Amendola et al,[80] 2000 | 22 | 91 | 36 | 8.4 |
| Wowra et al,[81] 2002 | 75 | 95 | 36 | 11.1 |
| Hernandez et al,[87] 2002 | 29 | 100 | 17.2 | 7 |
| Sheehan et al,[19] 2003 | 69 | 96 | 39 | 15 |
| Noel et al,[82] 2004 | 28 | 97 | 36 | 15 |
| **Total** | 389 | 94 | 37 | 11 |

DBF = distant brain failure; LC = local control; OS = overall survival.

was more frequently required when up–front WBRT was not used.

### SRS Plus WBRT for RCC

To investigate the role of combination of SRS and WBRT in patients with brain metastases from RCC, we performed a subgroup analysis on patients who were treated initially with SRS and WBRT or SRS alone and had local and distant failure rate published. The analysis was performed on the 11 small retrospective RCC series that included SRS as one of the main treatment modalities (see Table 4). Thirty-nine patients were eligible for analysis in the SRS + WBRT arm, and 50 patients were eligible in the SRS arm alone. SRS + WBRT resulted in a local failure rate of 0% and a distant brain failure rate of 21% in this selected group.[84–87] In comparison, SRS alone resulted in a mean LC rate of 8% with

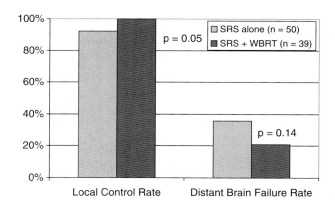

**Figure 1.**   Retrospective analysis of local control rates (LCR) and distant brain failure rates (DBF) for stereotactic radiosurgery (SRS) with and without whole brain radiotherapy (WBRT) for RCC.

distant brain failure rate of 36% (Figure 1). Therefore, SRS alone compared with SRS + WBRT may result in higher rates of distant brain failure and may have high risk of local failures. Some suggest that salvage WBRT is effective for both recurrences and new metastasis after SRS, and this approach would spare majority of patients the toxicities of up-front WBRT.[94,95,105] To date, the retrospective series of RCC patients as well and prospective studies from non-RCC patients suggest that the addition of SRS to WBRT improves control of brain metastases without undue toxicities. The benefits of reserving WBRT for salvage therapy over up-front SRS and WBRT remain to be proven.

## Hypofractionated Stereotactic Radiotherapy (FSRT)

Ikushima and colleagues have reported a series of 35 patients with brain metastases from RCC who were treated with FSRT (10 patients), surgery and conventional radiation (11 patients) versus conventional radiation only (14 patients).[106] The FSRT group was treated to 42 Gy in 7 fractions over 2.3 weeks. Median survival rates were 25.6 months for the FSRT group, 18.7 months for the surgery and conventional radiation group, and 4.3 months for the conventional radiation group. FSRT had 88% and 55.2% 1- and 2-year LC rates, respectively. None of the FSRT patients suffered from acute or late complications during and following FSRT with median follow-up of 17.5 months. This LC rate for the FSRT group does not appear to be

better than the historically reported values for SRS in RCC. Although the idea that FSRT could limit toxicities is intriguing, it remains to be established.

## Toxicities of SRS

Specific data reporting acute toxicity for SRS are scarce and limited to small numbers of retrospective studies.[107,108] Acute toxicities are similar to that of WBRT and for the most part can be medically managed. They include edema, headaches, nausea and vomiting, worsening of preexisting neurological deficits, and seizures. Chronic complications consist mainly of radionecrosis, cranial nerve palsies, and chronic steroid dependence. Treatment volume is the most consistent risk factor for long-term toxicity from SRS.[95,108] RTOG 90-05 prospectively determined that the risk of complications from SRS increases with tumor size.[95] Varlotto and colleagues[109] published a long-term toxicity data for 137 patients treated with $\gamma$ knife at the University of Pittsburgh Medical Center. The mean peripheral dose was 16 Gy (ranging from 12 to 25 Gy). They reported 1- and 5-year incidence of late complication as 2.8% and 11.4%, respectively. Treatment volume was the only significant factor associated with complications. For tumors $\leq 2$ cm$^3$, the 1- and 5-year incidence of complications was 2.3% and 3.7% respectively. For tumors $> 2$ cm$^3$, the 1- and 5-year incidence of complications were 3.4% and 16%, respectively. Reducing long-term toxicities will be more important in the future when systemic control of RCC improves.

## Systemic Therapy Plus Radiation for Radiosensitization

Although radiation sensitizers and chemotherapeutic agents have been used concurrently with radiation for brain metastases in other malignancies, no data exist for RCC.[110–123] Motexafin Gadolinium (Gd-Tex) is a paramagnetic compound which has been demonstrated to be taken up by tumor may sensitize cells to ionizing radiation by increasing oxidative stress as a consequence of futile redox cycling.[116–118] A Phase III study of brain metastases comparing WBRT alone (30 Gy in 10 fractions) to WBRT with Gd-Tex given before each fraction has demonstrated improved time to neurologic progression in all patients with greatest benefit in lung cancer, which made up approximately 60% of the patients in the study.[123] Currently, this agent is being investigated in patients with metastatic RCC. The role of novel agents including tyrosine kinase inhibitors (sunitinib and sorafenib) and mTOR inhibitors (temsirolimus) in combination with radiation needs to be investigated.

## Systemic Therapy Alone for RCC CNS Metastasis

Traditionally, chemotherapy has played a limited role in the management of brain metastases. The blood brain barrier appears to be disrupted near tumor vasculature.[124] In support, a prospective study that assessed the activity of a cisplatin/etoposide without radiation in patients with brain metastases reported overall response rate of 38%, 30%, and 0% for the breast cancer, nonsmall cell lung cancer, and melanoma patients, respectively; these results were similar to those in patients with systemic disease who did not have brain metastases.[125] Temozolomide has shown promise in gliomas and brain metastases alone and in combination with WBRT but has no defined role in RCC.[126–138] The activity of novel tyrosine kinase inhibitors in RCC brain metastasis is unknown. However, given their low molecular weight (associated with penetration of the blood brain barrier), they need to be evaluated, and significant activity can be expected. A recent case report describes a patient with spinal cord compression from RCC who was progressing following recent radiotherapy and responded dramatically to sunitinib malate.[139] Zole dronic acid administered prophylactically to patients with bone metastasis may diminish the risk of skeletal morbidity including spinal cord compression.[140]

## CONCLUSION

Radiotherapy has played an important role in the management of brain metastases from renal cell carcinoma despite its radioresistance. WBRT alone appears to be as beneficial for patients with multiple brain metastases from RCC as it is for other tumor types. More recently, SRS with or without WBRT have resulted in encouraging short-term LC rates of greater than 90%. Surgical resection followed by WBRT should be considered in patients with limited systemic and brain disease and good performance status, although SRS may be substituted for surgery in this population too. Systemic agents have not been shown to be effective either alone or with radiation in the treatment of brain metastasis from RCC. Opportunities in the management of brain metastases from renal cell carcinoma are expanding rapidly with the emergence of novel tyrosine kinase inhibitors. The biotechnology of gene expression profiling may help us to identify the radioresistance gene in renal cell carcinoma and enable targeted approaches.[141–144] It is important to integrate radiotherapy (SRS, WBRT) optimally with surgery and systemic treatment to maximize tumor control and, hopefully, prolong the survival of patients with this disease.

## REFERENCES

1. Jemal A, Siegel R, Ward E, et al. Cancer statistics, 2006. CA Cancer J Clin 2006;56:106–130.
2. Flanigan RC, Campbell SC, Clark JI, et al. Metastatic renal cell carcinoma. Curr Treat Options Oncol 2003;4:385–90.
3. Motzer RJ, Mazumdar M, Bacik J, et al. Survival and prognostic stratification of 670 patients with advanced renal cell carcinoma. J Clin Oncol 1999;17:2530–40.
4. Mekhail TM, Abou-Jawde RM, Boumerhi G, et al. Validation and extension of the memorial sloan-kettering prognostic factors model for survival in patients with previously untreated metastatic renal cell carcinoma. J Clin Oncol 2005;23:832–41.
5. Motzer RJ, Hutson TE, Tomczak P, et al. Phase III randomized trial of sunitinib malate (SU11248) versus interferon-α as first-line systemic therapy for patients with metastatic renal cell carcinoma [abstract LBA3]. Proc Am Soc Clin Oncol 2006;24:2S.

6. Eisen T, Bukowski RM, Staehler M, et al. Randomized phase III trial of sorafenib in advanced renal cell carcinoma (RCC): impact of crossover on survival. J Clin Oncol 2006;24(18S):4524.

7. Yang JC, Sherry RM, Steinberg SM, et al. Randomized study of high-dose and low-dose interleukin-2 in patients with metastatic renal cancer. J Clin Oncol 2003;21:3127–132.

8. McDermott DF, Regan MM, Clark JI, et al. Randomized phase III trial of high-dose interleukin-2 versus subcutaneous interleukin-2 and interferon in patients with metastatic renal cell carcinoma. J Clin Oncol 2005;23:133–41.

9. Hudes G, Carducci M, Tomczak P, et al. A phase III, randomized, 3-arm study of temsirolimus (TEMSR) or interferon-α (IFN) or the combination of TEMSR + IFN in the treatment of first-line poor-prognosis patients with advanced renal cell carcinoma [Abstract LBA4]. J Clin Oncol 2006;24:2S.

10. Culine S, Bekradda M, Kramar A, et al. Prognostic factors for survival in patients with brain metastases from renal cell carcinoma. Cancer 1998;83:2548–53.

11. Maor MH, Frias AE, Oswald MJ. Palliative radiotherapy for brain metastases in renal carcinoma. Cancer 1988;62:1912–17.

12. Wei K, Wandl E, Karcher KH. X-ray induced DNA double-strand breakage and rejoining in a radiosensitive human renal carcinoma cell line estimated by CHEF electrophoresis. Strahlenther Onkol 1993;169:740–4.

13. Hall EJ. Radiobiology for the radiobiologist. 3rd ed. Philadelphia: J. B. Lippincott;1988:116–25.

14. Ning S, Trisler K, Wessels BW, et al. Radiobiologic studies of radioimmunotherapy and external beam radiotherapy in vitro and in vivo in human renal cell carcinoma xenografts. Cancer 1997;80(12 Suppl):2519–28.

15. Syljuasen RG, Belldegrun A, Tso CL, et al. Sensitization of renal carcinoma to radiation using alpha interferon (IFNA) gene transfection. Radiat Res 1997;148:443–8.

16. Cohen HT, McGovern FJ. Medical progress: renal-cell carcinoma. N Engl J Med 2005;353:2477–90.

17. Hicklin DJ, Ellis LM. Role of the vascular endothelial growth factor pathway in tumor growth and angiogenesis. J Clin Oncol 2005;23:1011–27.

18. Maldazys JD, deKernion JB. Prognostic factors in metastatic renal carcinoma. J Urol 1985;136:376–9.

19. Sheehan JP, Sun MH, Kondziolka D, et al. Radiosurgery in patients with renal cell carcinoma metastasis to the brain: long-term outcomes and prognostic factors influencing survival and local tumor control. J Neurosurg 2003;98:342–9.

20. Decker DA, Decker VL, Herskovic A, et al. Brain metastases in patients with renal cell carcinoma: prognosis and treatment. J Clin Oncol 1984;2:169–73.

21. Gay PC, Litchy WJ, Cascino TL. Brain metastasis in hypernephroma. J Neurooncol 1987;5:51–6.

22. Saitoh H. Distant metastasis of renal adenocarcinoma. Cancer 1981;48:1487–91.

23. Taxy JB. Renal adenocarcinoma presenting as a solitary metastasis: contribution of electron microscopy to diagnosis. Cancer 1981;48:2056–62.

24. Ammirati M, Samii M, Skaf G, Sephernia A. Solitary brain metastasis 13 years after removal of renal adenocarcinoma. J Neurooncol 1993;15:87–90.

25. Zekri J, Ahmed N, Coleman RE, Hancock BW. The skeletal metastatic complications of renal cell carcinoma. Int J Oncol 2001;19:379–82.

26. Ebels EJ, Van Der Meulen JD. Cerebral metastases without known primary tumour: a retrospective study. Clin Neurol Neurosurg 1978;80:195–7.

27. Le Chevalier T, Smith FP, Caile P, et al. Sites of primary malignancies in patients presenting with cerebral metastases. Cancer 1985;56:880–2.

28. Merchut MP. Brain metastases from undiagnosed systemic neoplasms. Arch Intern Med 1989;149:1076–80.

29. Posner JB, Chernick NL. Intracranial metastases from systemic cancer. Adv Neurol 1978;19:579–91.

30. Patchell RA. The management of brain metastases. Cancer Treat Rev 2003;29:533–40.

31. Chidel MA, Suh JH, Barnett GH. Brain metastases: presentation, evaluation, and management. Cleve Clin J Med 2000;67:120–7.

32. Wronski M, Maor MH, Davis BJ, et al. External radiation of brain metastases from renal carcinoma: a retrospective study of 119 patients from the M.D. Anderson Cancer Center. Int J Radiat Oncol Biol Phys 1997;37:753–9.

33. Wowra B, Siebels M, Muacevic A, et al. Repeated gamma knife surgery for multiple brain metastases from renal cell carcinoma. J Neurosurg 2002;97:785–793.

34. Ruderman NB, Hall TC. Use of glucocorticoides in the palliative treatment of metastatic brain tumors. Cancer 1965;18:298–306.

35. Bruce JN, Criscuols GR, Merrill MJ, et al. Vascular permeability induced by protein product of malignant brain tumors: inhibition of dexamethasone. J Neurosurg 1987;67:880–4.

36. Glantz MJ, Cole BF, Forsyth PA, et al. Practice parameter: anticonvulsant prophylaxis in patients with newly diagnosed brain tumors. Report of the quality standards subcommittee of the American Academy of neurology. Neurology 2000;54:1886–1893.

37. Cohen N, Strauss G, Lew R, et al. Should prophylactic anticonvulsants be administered to patients with newly-diagnosed cerebral metastases? a retrospective analysis. J Clin Oncol 1998;6:1621–4.

38. Hoskin PJ, Crow J, Ford HT. The influence of extent and local management on the outcome of radiotherapy for brain metastases. Int J Radiat Oncol Biol Phys 1990;19:111–5.

39. Borgelt B, Gelber R, Kramer S, et al. The palliation of brain metastases: final results of the first two studies by the radiation therapy oncology group. Int J Radiat Oncol Biol Phys 1980;6:1–9.

40. Kurtz JM, Gelber R, Brady LW, et al. The palliation of brain metastases in a favorable patient population: a randomized clinical trial by the radiation therapy oncology group. Int J Radiat Oncol Biol Phys 1981;7:891–5.

41. West J, Maor M. Intracranial metastases: behavioral patterns related to primary site and results of treatment by whole brain irradiation. Int J Radiat Oncol Biol Phys 1980;6:11–5.

42. Gaspar L, Scott C, Rotman M, et al. Recursive partitioning analysis (RPA) of prognostic factors in three radiation therapy oncology group (RTOG) brain metastases trials. Int J Radiat Oncol Biol Phys 1997;37:745–51.

43. Patchell RA, Tibbs PA, Walsh JW, et al. A randomized trial of surgery in the treatment of single metastases to the brain. N Engl J Med 1990;322:494–500.

44. Patchell RA, Tibbs PA, Regine WF, et al. Postoperative radiotherapy in the treatment of single metastases to the brain. JAMA 1998;280:1485–9.

45. Muacevic A, Kreth FW, Mack A, et al. Stereotactic radiosurgery without radiation therapy providing high local tumor control of multiple brain metastases from renal cell carcinoma. Minim Invasive Neurosurg 2004;47:203–8.

46. Posner JB. Management of brain metastases. Rev Neurol (Paris) 1992;148:477–487.

47. Cannady SB, Cavanaugh KA, Lee SY, et al. Results of whole brain radiotherapy and recursive partitioning analysis in patients with brain metastases from renal cell carcinoma: a retrospective study. Int J Radiat Oncol Biol Phys 2004;58:253–8.

48. Gelber RD, Larson M, Borgelt BB, et al. Equivalence of radiation schedules for the palliative treatment of brain metastases in patients with favorable prognosis. Cancer 1981;48:1749–53.

49. Epstein BE, Scott CB, Sause WT, et al. Improved survival duration in patients with unresected solitary brain metastasis using accelerated hyperfractionated radiation therapy at total doses of 54.4 gray and greater results of radiation therapy oncology group 85–28. Cancer 1993;71:1362–7.

50. Nieder C, Berberich W, Nestle U, et al. Relation between local result and total dose of radiotherapy for brain metastases. Int J Radiat Oncol Biol Phys 1995;33:349–55.

51. Vecht CJ, Haaxma–Reiche H, Noordijk EM, et al. Treatment of single brain metastasis: radiotherapy alone or combined with neurosurgery? Ann Neurol 1993;33:583–90.

52. Mintz AH, Kestle J, Rathbone MP, et al. A randomized trial to assess the efficacy of surgery in addition to radiotherapy in patients with a single cerebral metastasis. Cancer 1996;78:1470–6.

53. Bindal AK, Bindal RK, Hess KR, et al. Surgery versus radiosurgery in the treatment of brain metastasis. J Neurosurg 1996;84:748–754.

54. Nussbaum ES, Djalilian HR, Cho KH, et al. Brain metastases. histology, multiplicity, surgery, and survival. Cancer 1996;78:1781–8.

55. Patchell RA, Tibbs PA, Regine WF, et al. Postoperative radiotherapy in the treatment of single metastases to the brain: a randomized trial. JAMA 1998;280:1485–9.

56. Patchell RA, Tibbs PA, Regine WF, et al. Direct decompressive surgical resection in the treatment of spinal cord compression caused by metastatic cancer: a randomised trial. Lancet 2005;366:643–8.

57. Wronski M, Arbit E, Russo P, et al. Surgical resection of brain metastases from renal cell carcinoma in 50 patients. Urology 1996;47:187–93.

58. O'Dea MJ, Zincke H, Utz DC, et al. The treatment of renal cell carcinoma with solitary metastasis. J Urol 1978;120:540–2.

59. Salvati M, Scarpinati M, Orlando ER, et al. Single brain metastases from kidney tumors. clinico-pathologic considerations on a series of 29 cases. Tumori 1992;78:392–4.

60. DeAngelis LM, Delattre JY, Posner JB. Radiation–induced dementia in patients cured of brain metastases. Neurology 1989;39:789–96.

61. Nieder C, Schwerdtfeger K, Steudel WI, et al. Patterns of relapse and late toxicity after resection and whole-brain radiotherapy for solitary brain metastases. Strahlenther Onkol 1998;174:275–8.

62. Griffin T. White matter necrosis, microangiopathy and intellectual abilities in survivors of childhood leukemia. Association with central nervous system irradiation and methotrexate therapy. In: Gilbert H, Kagan A. editors. Radiation damage to the nervous system. New York: Raven Press;1980.

63. Giglio P, Gilbert M. Cerebral radiation necrosis. Neurologist 2003;9:180–8.

64. Kumar AJ, Leeds NE, Fuller GN, et al. Malignant gliomas: MR imaging spectrum of radiation therapy-and chemotherapy-induced necrosis of the brain after treatment. Radiology 2000;217:377–84.

65. Sheline GE, Wara WM, Smith V. Therapeutic irradiation and brain injury. Int J Radiat Oncol Biol Phys 1980;6:1215–28.

66. Radcliffe J, Packer RJ, Atkins TE, et al. Three-and four-year cognitive outcome in children with noncortical brain tumors treated with whole-brain radiotherapy. Ann Neurol 1992;32:551–4.

67. Cheung MC, Chan AS, Law SC, et al. Impact of radionecrosis on cognitive dysfunction in patients after radiotherapy for nasopharyngeal carcinoma. Cancer 2003;97:2019–26.

68. Cheung M, Chan AS, Law SC, et al. Cognitive function of patients with nasopharyngeal carcinoma with and without temporal lobe radionecrosis. Arch Neurol 2000;57:1347–52.

69. Komaki R, Meyers CA, Shin DM, et al. Evaluation of cognitive function in patients with limited small cell lung cancer prior to and shortly following prophylactic cranial irradiation. Int J Radiat Oncol Biol Phys 1995;33:179–82.

70. Laack N, Brown P, Furth A. Neurocognitive function after radiotherapy (RT) for supratentorial low-grade gliomas (LGG): results of a north central cancer treatment group (NCCTG) prospective study. Int J Radiat Oncol Biol Phys 2003;57(2 Suppl):S134.

71. Brown PD, Buckner JC, O'Fallon JR, et al. Effects of radiotherapy on cognitive function in patients with low-grade glioma measured by the folstein mini-mental state examination. J Clin Oncol 2003;21:2519–24.

72. Lutz W, Winston KR, Maleki N. A system for stereotactic radiosurgery with a linear accelerator. Int J Radiat Oncol Biol Phys 1988;14:373–81.

73. Yeung D, Palta J, Fontanesi J, et al. Systematic analysis of errors in target localization and treatment delivery in stereotactic radiosurgery (SRS). Int J Radiat Oncol Biol Phys 1994;28:493–8.

74. Chang SD, Main W, Martin DP, et al. An analysis of the accuracy of the CyberKnife: a robotic frameless stereotactic radiosurgical system. Neurosurgery 2003;52:140–6; discussion 146–7.

75. Auchter RM, Lamond JP, Alexander E, et al. A multiinstitutional outcome and prognostic factor analysis of radiosurgery for resectable single brain metastasis. Int J Radiat Oncol Biol Phys 1996;35:27–35.

76. Muacevic A, Kreth FW, Horstmann GA, et al. Surgery and radiotherapy compared with gamma knife radiosurgery in the treatment of solitary cerebral metastases of small diameter. J Neurosurg 1999;91:35–43.

77. Soffietti R, Ruda R, Mutani R. Management of brain metastases. J Neurol 2002;249:1357–69.

78. Brown PD, Brown CA, Pollock BE, et al. Stereotactic radiosurgery for patients with "radioresistant" brain metastases. Neurosurgery 2002;51:656–65;discussion 665–7.

79. Hoshi S, Jokura H, Nakamura H, et al. Gamma-knife radiosurgery for brain metastasis of renal cell carcinoma: results in 42 patients. Int J Urol 2002;9:618–25;discussion 626;author reply 627.

80. Amendola BE, Wolf AL, Coy SR, et al. Brain metastases in renal cell carcinoma: management with gamma knife radiosurgery. Cancer J 2000;6:372–6.

81. Wowra B, Siebels M, Muacevic A, et al. Repeated gamma knife surgery for multiple brain metastases from renal cell carcinoma. J Neurosurg 2002;97:785–93.

82. Noel G, Valery CA, Boisserie G, et al. LINAC radiosurgery for brain metastasis of renal cell carcinoma. Urol Oncol 2004;22:25–31.

83. Mori Y, Kondziolka D, Flickinger JC, et al. Stereotactic radiosurgery for brain metastasis from renal cell carcinoma. Cancer 1998;83:344–53.

84. Schoggl A, Kitz K, Ertl A, et al. Gamma-knife radiosurgery for brain metastases of renal cell carcinoma: results in 23 patients. Acta Neurochir (Wien) 1998;140:549–55.

85. Goyal LK, Suh JH, Reddy CA, et al. The role of whole brain radiotherapy and stereotactic radiosurgery on brain metastases from renal cell carcinoma. Int J Radiat Oncol Biol Phys 2000;47:1007–12.

86. Payne BR, Prasad D, Szeifert G, et al. Gamma surgery for intracranial metastases from renal cell carcinoma. J Neurosurg 2000;92:760–5.

87. Hernandez L, Zamorano L, Sloan A, et al. Gamma knife radiosurgery for renal cell carcinoma brain metastases. J Neurosurg 2002;97(5 Suppl):489–93.

88. Doh LS, Amato RJ, Paulino AC, Teh BS. Radiation therapy in the management of brain metastases from renal cell carcinoma. Oncology (Williston Park) 2006;20:603–13.

89. Shuto T, Inomori S, Fujino H, Nagano H. Gamma knife surgery for metastatic brain tumors from renal cell carcinoma. J Neurosurg 2006;105:555–60.

90. Fike JR, Cann CE, Turowski K, et al. Radiation dose response of normal brain. Int J Radiat Oncol Biol Phys 1988;14:63–70.

91. Breneman JC, Warnick RE, Albright RE Jr, et al. Stereotactic radiosurgery for the treatment of brain metastases. Results of a single institution series. Cancer 1997;79:551–7.

92. Shiau CY, Sneed PK, Shu HK, et al. Radiosurgery for brain metastases: relationship of dose and pattern of enhancement to local control. Int J Radiat Oncol Biol Phys 1997;37:375–83.

93. Alexander E III, Moriarty TM, Davis RB, et al. Stereotactic radiosurgery for the definitive, noninvasive treatment of brain metastases. J Natl Cancer Inst 1995;87:34–40.

94. Flickinger JC, Kondziolka D, Lunsford LD, et al. A multi-institutional experience with stereotactic radiosurgery for solitary brain metastasis. Int J Radiat Oncol Biol Phys 1994;28:797–802.

95. Shirato H, Takamura A, Tomita M, et al. Stereotactic irradiation without whole-brain irradiation for single brain metastasis. Int J Radiat Oncol Biol Phys 1997;37:385–91.

96. Shaw E, Scott C, Souhami L, et al. Single dose radiosurgical treatment of recurrent previously irradiated primary brain tumors and brain metastases: final report of RTOG protocol 90–05. Int J Radiat Oncol Biol Phys 2000;47:291–8.

97. Suzuki S, Omagari J, Nishio S, et al. Gamma knife radiosurgery for simultaneous multiple metastatic brain tumors. J Neurosurg 2000;(93 Suppl 3):30–1.

98. Serizawa T, Iuchi T, Ono J, et al. Gamma knife treatment for multiple metastatic brain tumors compared with whole-brain radiation therapy. J Neurosurg 2000;(93 Suppl 3):32–6.

99. Joseph J, Adler JR, Cox RS, et al. Linear accelerator-based stereotactic radiosurgery for brain metastases:the influence of number of lesions on survival. J Clin Oncol 1996;14:1085–92.

100. Sanghavi SN, Miranpuri SS, Chappell R, et al. Radiosurgery for patients with brain metastases: a multi–institutional analysis, stratified by the RTOG recursive partitioning analysis method. Int J Radiat Oncol Biol Phys 2001; 51:426–34.

101. Kondziolka D, Patel A, Lunsford LD, et al. Stereotactic radiosurgery plus whole brain radiotherapy versus radiotherapy alone for patients with multiple brain metastases. Int J Radiat Oncol Biol Phys 1999;45:427–34.

102. Chougule PB, Burton-Williams M, Saris S, et al. Randomized treatment of brain metastases with gamma knife radiosurgery, whole brain radiotherapy or both [abstract]. Int J Radiat Oncol Biol Phys. 2000;48:114.

103. Andrews DW, Scott CB, Sperduto PW, et al. Whole brain radiation therapy with or without stereotactic radiosurgery boost for patients with one to three brain metastases: phase III results of the RTOG 9508 randomised trial. Lancet 2004;363:1665–72.

104. Aoyama H, Shirato H, Tago M, et al. Stereotactic radiosurgery plus whole-brain radiation therapy vs stereotactic radiosurgery alone for treatment of brain metastases: a randomized controlled trial. JAMA 2006;295:2483–91.

105. Sneed PK, Lamborn KR, Forstner JM, et al. Radiosurgery for brain metastases: is whole brain radiotherapy necessary? Int J Radiat Oncol Biol Phys 1999;43:549–58.

106. Ikushima H, Tokuuye K, Sumi M, et al. Fractionated stereotactic radiotherapy of brain metastases from renal cell carcinoma. Int J Radiat Oncol Biol Phys 2000;48:1389–93.

107. Loeffler JS, Siddon RL, Wen PY, et al. Stereotactic radiosurgery of the brain using a standard linear accelerator: a study of early and late effects. Radiother Oncol 1990; 17:311–21.

108. Werner-Wasik M, Rudoler S, Preston PE, et al. Immediate side effects of stereotactic radiotherapy and radiosurgery. Int J Radiat Oncol Biol Phys 1999;43:299–304.

109. Varlotto JM, Flickinger JC, Niranjan A, et al. Analysis of tumor control and toxicity in patients who have survived at least one year after radiosurgery for brain metastases. Int J Radiat Oncol Biol Phys 2003;57:452–64.

110. Urtasun RC, Band PR, Chapman JD, et al. Radiation plus metronidazole for glioblastoma. N Engl J Med 1977; 296:757.

111. Nelson DF, Schoenfeld D, Weinstein AS, et al. A randomized comparison of misonidazole sensitized radiotherapy plus BCNU and radiotherapy plus BCNU for treatment of malignant glioma after surgery;preliminary results of an RTOG study. Int J Radiat Oncol Biol Phys 1983;9:1143–51.

112. Nelson DF, Diener-West M, Weinstein AS, et al. A randomized comparison of misonidazole sensitized radiotherapy plus BCNU and radiotherapy plus BCNU for treatment of malignant glioma after surgery: final report of an RTOG study. Int J Radiat Oncol Biol Phys 1986;12:1793–800.

113. Overgaard J, Hansen HS, Overgaard M, et al. A randomized double-blind phase III study of nimorazole as a hypoxic radiosensitizer of primary radiotherapy in supraglottic larynx and pharynx carcinoma. Results of the Danish Head and Neck Cancer Study (DAHANCA) Protocol 5–85. Radiother Oncol 1998;46:135–46.

114. Rischin D, Peters L, Hicks R, et al. Phase I trial of concurrent tirapazamine, cisplatin, and radiotherapy in patients with advanced head and neck cancer. J Clin Oncol 2001;19:535–42.

115. Rischin D, Peters L, Fisher R, et al. Tirapazamine, Cisplatin, and Radiation versus Fluorouracil, Cisplatin, and Radiation in patients with locally advanced head and neck cancer: a randomized phase II trial of the trans-tasman radiation oncology group (TROG 98.02). J Clin Oncol 2005;23:79–87.

116. Urtasun RC, Kinsella TJ, Farnan N, et al. Survival improvement in anaplastic astrocytoma, combining external radiation with halogenated pyrimidines: final report of RTOG 86–12, Phase I–II study. Int J Radiat Oncol Biol Phys 1996;36:1163–7.

117. Prados MD, Seiferheld W, Sandler HM, et al. Phase III randomized study of radiotherapy plus procarbazine, lomustine, and vincristine with or without BUdR for treatment of anaplastic astrocytoma: final report of RTOG 9404. Int J Radiat Oncol Biol Phys 2004;58:1147–52.

118. Phillips TL, Scott CB, Leibel SA, et al. Results of a randomized comparison of radiotherapy and bromodeoxyuridine with radiotherapy alone for brain metastases: report of RTOG trial 89–05. Int J Radiat Oncol Biol Phys 1995;33:339–48.

119. Brada M, Ross G. Radiotherapy for primary and secondary brain tumors. Curr Opin Oncol 1995;7:214–9.

120. Viala J, Vanel D, Meingan P, et al. Phases IB and II multidose trial of gadolinium texaphyrin, a radiation sensitizer detectable at MR imaging: preliminary results in brain metastases. Radiology 1999;212:755–9.

121. Rosenthal DI, Nurenberg P, Becerra CR, et al. A phase I single-dose trial of gadolinium texaphyrin (Gd-Tex), a tumor selective radiation sensitizer detectable by magnetic resonance imaging. Clin Cancer Res 1999;5:739–45.

122. Magda D, Lepp C, Gerasimchuk N, et al. Redox cycling by motexafin gadolinium enhances cellular response to ionizing radiation by forming reactive oxygen species. Int J Radiat Oncol Biol Phys 2001;51:1025–36.

123. Meyers CA, Smith JA, Bezjak A, et al. Neurocognitive function and progression in patients with brain metastases treated with whole–brain radiation and motexafin gadolinium: results of a randomized phase III trial. J Clin Oncol 2004;22:157–65.

124. Greig N. Implications of the blood brain barrier and its manipulation. In: Neuwelt E, editor. Brain tumor and the blood tumor barrier. Vol 2. New York: Plenum;1989.

125. Franciosi V, Cocconi G, Michiara M, et al. Front-line chemotherapy with cisplatin and etoposide for patients with brain metastases from breast carcinoma, non small cell lung carcinoma, or malignant melanoma: a prospective study. Cancer 1999;85:1599–605.

126. Newlands ES, Blackledge GR, Slack JA, et al. Phase I trial of temozolomide (CCRG 81045: M&B 39831: NSC 362856). Br J Cancer 1992;65:287–91.

127. Stevens MF, Hickman JA, Langdon SP, et al. Antitumor activity and pharmacokinetics in mice of 8-carbamoyl-3-methyl-imidazo[5,1-d]-1,2,3,5-tetrazin-4(3H)-one (CCRG 81045; M & B 39831), a novel drug with potential as an alternative to dacarbazine. Cancer Res 1987;47:5846–52.

128. Stupp R, Dietrich PY, Ostermann Kraljevic S, et al. Promising survival for patients with newly diagnosed glioblastoma multiforme treated with concomitant radiation plus temozolomide followed by adjuvant temozolomide. J Clin Oncol 2002;20:1375–82.

129. Gilbert MR, Friedman HS, Kuttesch JF, et al. A phase II study of temozolomide in patients with newly diagnosed supratentorial malignant glioma before radiation therapy. Neuro-oncol 2002;4:261–7.

130. Christodoulou C, Bafaloukos D, Kosmidis P, et al. Phase II study of temozolomide in heavily pretreated cancer patients with brain metastases. Ann Oncol 2001;12:249–54.

131. Abrey LE, Olson JD, Raizer JJ, et al. A phase II trial of temozolomide for patients with recurrent or progressive brain metastases. J Neurooncol 2001;53:259–65.

132. Friedman H, Evans B, Reardon D. Phase II trial of temozolomide for patients with progressive brain metastases. Proc Am Soc Clin Oncol 2003;22:102.

133. Antonadou D, Paraskevaidis M, Sarris G, et al. Phase II randomized trial of temozolomide and concurrent radiotherapy in patients with brain metastases. J Clin Oncol 2002;20:3644–50.

134. Antonadou D, Coliarakis N, Paraskevaidis M. Whole brain radiotherapy alone or in combination with temozolomide for brain metastasis. a phase III study. Int J Radiat Oncol Biol Phys 2002;54(2 Suppl 1):93–94.

135. Verger E, Gil M, Yay R. Concomitant temozolomide (TMZ) and radiotherapy (RT) in patients with brain metastasis: randomized multicentric phase II study, a preliminary report. Proc Am Soc Clin Oncol 2002;21:78a.

136. Verger E, Gil M, Yaya R. Concomitant temozolomide (TMZ) and whole brain radiotherapy (WBRT) in patients with brain metastasis (BM): Randomized multicentric phase II study. Proc Am Soc Clin Oncol 2003;22:101.

137. Sunkara U, Walczak JR, Summerson L, et al. A phase II trial of temozolomide and IFN–alpha in patients with advanced renal cell carcinoma. J Interferon Cytokine Res 2004;24:37–41.

138. Park DK, Ryan CW, Dolan ME, et al. A phase II trial of oral temozolomide in patients with metastatic renal cell cancer. Cancer Chemother Pharmacol 2002;50:160–2.

139. Trinh QD, Cardinal E, Gallina A, et al. Sunitinib Relieves Renal Cell Carcinoma Spinal Cord Compression. Eur Urol. 2006 Nov 3;[Epub ahead of print]

140. Lipton A, Zheng M, Seaman J. Zoledronic acid delays the onset of skeletal-related events and progression of skeletal disease in patients with advanced renal cell carcinoma. Cancer. 2003;98:962–9.

141. Takahashi M, Rhodes DR, Furge KA, et al. Gene expression profiling of clear cell renal cell carcinoma: gene identification and prognostic classification. Proc Natl Acad Sci U S A 2001;98:9754–9.

142. Takahashi M, Sugimura J, Yang X, et al. Gene expression profiling of renal cell carcinoma and its implications in diagnosis, prognosis, and therapeutics. Adv Cancer Res 2003;89:157–81.

143. Tan MH, Rogers CG, Cooper JT, et al. Gene expression profiling of renal cell carcinoma. Clin Cancer Res 2004;10(18 Pt 2):6315S–21S.

144. Rogers CG, Tan MH, Teh BT. Gene expression profiling of renal cell carcinoma and clinical implications. Urology 2005;65:231–7.

# SUPPORTIVE CARE IN METASTATIC RENAL CELL CARCINOMA

## Palliative Care Considerations and Quality of Life Issues in Renal Cancer

**MELLAR P. DAVIS, MD, FCCP**

Renal cell carcinoma (RCC) accounts for 2 to 3% of all malignancies and is the third most common genitourinary cancer.[1] Over the last decade or 2 there has been a change in the stage and presentation of RCC. Incidental RCC is now found in 15 to 57% due to ultrasounds, computer tomography (CT) scans, and nuclear magnetic resonance imaging (MRI) done for other reasons.[2] Of the nearly 30,000 new diagnoses per year and 12,000 deaths in the United States, 2 of 3 will be men and over 60% will be due to a clear cell histologic subtype.[2] The median age of patients at diagnosis is 59 years.[3] This review will focus on the palliation of the clear cell subtype of RCC. Topics to be discussed are prognostic factors at presentation, symptoms and prognosis, symptoms associated with metastatic RCC, paraneoplastic syndromes, inflammatory cytokine symptoms, metastatic and cancer related complications and management, and individual systemic symptoms and management.

## PROGNOSIS AT PRESENTATION

The type of histology (clear cell, papillary medullary, and chromaphotae) is not as prognostic as Fuhrman grade, TMN Stage, and the Eastern Cooperative Oncology Group (ECOG) performance score (Table 1).[4] The rare sarcomatoid variant of RCC is highly aggressive, usually found within papillary or clear cell variants, and portends a poor outlook.[4] A large number of prognostic factors have been investigated at presentation (Table 2).

## SYMPTOMS AND PROGNOSIS

In all, 20 to 40% of patients present with local or systemic symptoms or signs. Of those symptomatic, 46% will complain of hematuria, 21% flank pain, 2 to 3% weight loss, and 1% fatigue, weakness, anemia, or bone pain.[5] The mean size of the

| Table 1. HISTOLOGIC SUBTYPES OF RENAL CELL CANCER | |
|---|---|
| Subtypes | Percentage of RCC |
| Clear cell | 70 to 80% |
| Papillary | 10 to 20% |
| Chromophobe (oncocytoma) | 5% |
| Collecting duct | < 5% |
| Sarcomatoid | < 5% |

RCC = renal cell carcinoma.

## Table 2. PROGNOSTIC FACTORS[4]

Tumor size
- Regional nodes
- Adrenal invasion
- Metastases
- Inferior vena cava tumor extending along the diaphragm

Tumor characteristic[4]
- Fuhrman grade
- Necrosis of tumor
- Microvascular invasion
- Sarcomatoid subtype
- Expression of hypoxia inducing factor (HiF$_x$)
- Vascular endothelial factor expression
- Mutations/overexpression TP53
- Low SMAC/Diablo expression
- Low P$_{27}$
- Low PTEN
- Low CAM expression
- Expression of IL$_6$

Patient characteristics
- Flank pain
- Hematuria
- Weight loss
- Anorexia
- Malaise

Laboratory characteristics
- High LDH
- Thrombocytosis
- Anemia

CAM = cellular adhesive molecule; IL = interleukin; LDH = lactate dehydrogenase; PTEN = ; SMAC = .

primary is usually larger in symptomatic patients than in patient with incidental RCC (3.7 vs 6.2 cm).[6] Tumor recurrence is more likely with symptomatic than asymptomatic presentations. Of those who do recur after nephrectomy, 72% will present with symptoms at the time of presentation.[7] Disease specific survival for asymptomatic presentations is 91% at 5 years but will be 69% at 5 years if patients present with symptoms.[8] Of those who die from RCC, 75% will present with symptoms at the time of diagnosis.[7] The risk of recurrence is greater in symptomatic presentations after controlling for tumor type, tumor grade, and ECOG performance score.[3]

Those who present with systemic symptoms fare worse than those who present with local symptoms.[7] The presentation with only one cachectic related symptom (malaise, weight loss of > 5% over 3 months, anorexia, albumin < 3.6 g %) in patients with limited disease (T$_1$) reduces disease specific survival by 15%.

## SYMPTOMS WITH METASTATIC RENAL CANCER

The symptoms of metastatic renal cell carcinoma (mRCC) are both highly prevalent and severe. The most prevalent symptoms are also the most severe. In a group of patients from the Cleveland Clinic Health Systems, 9 symptoms occurred in > 50% (pain, fatigue, weakness, anorexia, lack of energy, constipation, xerostomia, early satiety, and weight loss). More than 30% had depression, dyspnea, insomnia, and cough. The most prevalent symptoms are paraneoplastic (fatigue, weakness, anorexia, lack of energy, and weight loss) and probably relate to tumor cytokine production, particularly interleukin 6 (IL$_6$).[9]

## PARANEOPLASTIC SYNDROME

Renal cell cancer is the great masquerader of medicine due to its protean paraneoplastic manifestations.[9] Several of these syndromes are unique to RCC.

## NEPHROGENIC HEPATIC DYSFUNCTION

In 1961, Stauffer described nonmetastatic intrahepatic cholestasis in association with RCC.[9,10] Those with nephrogenic hepatic dysfunction present with increased serum alkaline phosphatase, gamma glutamine transaminase, gamma globulins platelets, and Westergren sedimentation rate. Reduced hepatic production of albumin and certain coagulation factors leads to edema and a prolonged prothrombin time. Patients will experience nausea and fatigue and will have hepatomegaly on physical examination. Some will have jaundice. The liver histology is nonspecific. Neutrophils, lymphocytes, and monocytes infiltrate the hepatic parenchyma with or without granulomas. Sinusoids will be dilated but not obstructed. Nephrectomy for localized tumor will

## Table 3. SYMPTOMS AT PRESENTATION AND RELATIVE RISK[4]

| Disease Status | Relative Risk |
| --- | --- |
| Disease free survival | 1.61 |
| Overall survival | 1.66 |
| Cancer specific survival | 1.9 |

reverse the syndrome. The syndrome may reappear with relapse. Failure to resolve the syndrome after nephrectomy is a poor prognosis. Clinicians who are unaware of the syndrome may assume that the signs and symptoms are due to metastatic disease and not pursue curative surgery.

## HYPERTENSION

Hypertension occurs in 40% of RCC and is twice the prevalence of the normal population.[9] It generally occurs with low grade histologies and is not associated with a poor prognosis. Elevated renin levels will be seen in 37%. The elevated serum renin may be caused either by proximal neoplastic tubular cells or in response to tumor compression and ischemia on the juxtaglomerular apparatus. Arteriovenous fistulas may occur within tumor leading to ischemia distal to the fistula, which occur more commonly in women.[9] Renin levels do not correlate with the degree of hypertension. Clinicians need to aggressively manage hypertension in order to avoid nephrosclerosis and renal failure.

## HYPERCALCEMIA

Hypercalcemia is reported with multiple malignancies, however, it is most common with RCC. In all, 13 to 20% will develop hypercalcemia during the course of disease, and 75% will have advanced stage cancer. Hypercalcemia does not correlate with tumor grade or survival and can be seen with limited stage disease. Etiologies are divided into metastatic and nonmetastatic. Fifty percent of those with hypercalcemia will have bone metastases. An elevated calcium in this situation is related to local release of prostaglandin ($PGE_2$) and may respond to hydration, bisphosphonates, radiation, and/or surgery.[9] Nonmetastatic hypercalcemia is related to tumor production of a PTH related protein ($PTH_{rp}$). $PTH_{rp}$ increases bone resorption, reduces renal calcium excretion, and inhibits 1,25 vitamin hydrolase, and thus 1,25-$(OH)_2$-vitamin $D_3$. As a result, serum PTH levels are low, calcium reabsorption from the gastrointestinal tract is low, and metabolic acidosis with an elevated serum chloride occurs from renal calcium wasting. Patients will experience lethargy, nausea, fatigue, confusion, and constipation, which mimics advanced cancer. The electrocardiographic changes include a prolonged PR interval and QT interval and bradyarrhythmias may supervene. Treatment is similar to hypercalcemia due to metastases and consists of hydration, bisphosphonates, and/or calcitonin. Those with limited disease may benefit from nephrectomy.

## POLYCYTHEMIA AND ANEMIA

Polycythemia is seen in 1 to 8% of patients with RCC. Erythropoietin is normally produced by peritubular interstitial cells. Production may be increased by local compression and ischemia or ectopically by tumor.[9] Ectopic production of erythropoietin occurs in as many as 66% of patients with RCC even though polycythemia is seen in only 1 to 8%. The presence of polycythemia with thrombocytosis (another paraneoplastic finding in RCC) may be mistaken for a chronic inflammatory disorder or myeloproliferative disorder. Anemia is much more common than polycythemia in RCC and appears to be related to tumor production of $IL_6$ and lactoferrin.[9]

## AMYLOID

Amyloidosis occurs in 3 to 8% of RCC. Amyloid is formed from SAA acute phase reactant proteins elaborated from the liver. β-Pleated sheets form in tissues and consist of AA proteins and amyloid P-protein. Cardiac involvement is rare and thus differs from amyloid secondary to a monoclonal protein or senile amyloid. Patients may present with fatigue, weakness, and weight loss and may have syncope that resembles cancer cachexia.[9] Rare paraneoplastic syndromes are listed in Table 4.

## INFLAMMATORY CYTOKINES AND RENAL CELL CANCER

$IL_6$ serum levels are increased in 70% of those with mRCC.[11] $IL_6$ levels increase with stage, tumor size, and grade and predict a poor prognosis.[12] Bone metastasis from mRCC highly express $IL_6$ and is associated with elevated levels of serum free $IL_6$ and

## Table 4. MISCELLANEOUS PARANEOPLASTIC SYMPTOMS ASSOCIATED WITH RENAL CANCER[9]

Galactorrhea and gynecomastia from elevated b HCG
Cushing syndrome from elevated ACTH
Hypoglycemia/hyperglycemia from ectopic production of insulin and glucagons
Motor neuron disease
Coagulopathies

ACTH = ; HCG = .

total IL₆.[12,13] Soluble $IL_6$ receptor binds to $IL_6$ and acts as a powerful agonist and reservoir for prolonged activity.[14] Fifty percent of renal cancers express $IL_6$.[15] Many of the paraneoplastic syndromes appear to be related to elevated serum $IL_6$, and these include anemia, nephrogenic hepatic dysfunction, anorexia, cachexia, hypercalcemia, thrombocytosis, and leukocytosis.[16–18] Increased $IL_6$ correlates strongly with serum C-reactive protein (CRP) levels.

$IL_6$ activates signal transducer and activator transcription 3 ($STAT_3$) via the Janus activating kinase (JAK), which phosphorylates tyrosine on $STAT_3$.[19] $IL_6$ is a intracrine stimulator of RCC proliferation through $STAT_3$.[19] Antibodies to $IL_6$ may block paraneoplastic manifestations of RCC but fail to stop $IL_6$ induced proliferation.[18,20] Either antisense oligonucleotides to the second exon of $IL_6$ or tyrosine kinase inhibitors to JAK block in vitro proliferation of RCC and induce apoptosis.[19] Mutations of the cell cycle regulating protein TP53 enhance $IL_6$ expression. TP53 normally suppresses $IL_6$ by interfering with specific transcription factor binding to the $IL_6$ promoter site.[19] Bisphosphonates inhibit osteoblastic production of $IL_6$, which may reduce hypercalcemia and decrease regional tumor proliferation.[17,21] Both dexamethasone and progesterone reduce $IL_6$ production, which ameliorates some of the paraneoplastic symptoms and signs associated with RCC.[15]

## METASTATIC PATTERN AND CANCER RELATED COMPLICATIONS AND MANAGEMENT

Renal cell cancer commonly spreads to bone, lung, liver, and brain. Recurrences occur in up to 50% postnephrectomy. Most recurrences occur within 12 to 18 months though disease free intervals can be greater than 10 years.[22] Renal cancer is one of the most frequent malignancies to present with isolated metastases. Aggressive surgical management that combines nephrectomy and metastectomy can lead to a prolonged disease free interval or cure. Spontaneous regressions (usually of metastatic lung lesions) can occur in 0.3 to 7% even after progression on immune therapy.[23,24]

Metastases to unusual sites are relatively common. These can occur years after nephrectomy and may be missed due to failure to recognize the association (Table 5).

## BONE AND SPINE METASTASES

The presence of bone metastases is usually associated with an elevated ECOG performance score and extraosseous metastases.[25,26] Alkaline phosphatase is elevated in half of patients but is a poor screening test. $IL_6$ increases alkaline phosphatase production from tumor and liver. Alkaline phosphatase is neither derived from bone metastases nor associated with hypercalcemia but is a paraneoplastic laboratory finding.[25] The sensitivity of bone scans in detecting metastatic bone lesions is controversial. Sensitivities range between 10 and 84%.[26] Bone scans will generally underestimate bone metastases because many metastases are osteolytic. Laboratory studies do not improve the sensitivity or diagnostic yield of bone scans.[26] At presentation, 17% will have bone metastases, 5% with $T_{1-2}$ NO primaries, and 35% with locally advanced cancer.[27] MRI and/or CT should be used to evaluate complaints of pain bone.

## Table 5. UNCOMMON METASTATIC SITES ASSOCIATED WITH RENAL CANCER

Endobronchial
Distal extremities
Gallbladder
Nasal structures
Paranasal sinuses
Pancreas
Orbit
Sublingual
Thyroid
Vagina

At postmortem examination, one-third to two-third will have bone metastases most commonly found in the pelvis followed by the spine.[28] Most of the patients with bone metastases (> 80%) will require radiation during the course of their cancer and a significant minority (40%) will need to undergo surgery for pain or pending fracture or spinal cord compression due to epidural extension of cancer.[25] Indications for surgery include isolated resectable bone metastases with resectable primary or as a recurrence; intractable mechanical bone pain; impending pathologic fracture; epidural extension of tumor with spinal cord compression; and vertebral fracture with bone fragment extending into the spinal canal with spinal cord compression. Renal cell cancers are highly vascular and will bleed profusely at the time of surgery. Preoperative embolization reduces the risk of intraoperative bleeding and facilitates surgical resection.[29,30] Median survival for those presenting with a single metastases treated surgically is 27 months, whereas the median survival of those with multiple bone metastases is 12 months.[31,32]

Renal cell cancer does symptomatically respond to radiation. Patients with mechanical (incident) pain are less likely to respond. Some claim that high biologic doses of radiation (TDF > 70) are required for best response, whereas others have not found a relationship between the biologic dose and response.[33,34] Single-fraction radiation (8Gy) will relieve bone pain but should not be used in cases of spinal cord compression.[35] Single-fraction radiation is ideally suited for those who show an expected survival and would benefit from a hospice transition.

Ablative procedures can be used to treat painful bony metastases that cannot be radiated or in situations where surgery is not an option. Injections of ethanol, radiofrequency heat ablation, or cryoablation can be done under conscious sedation and local anesthetics.[36] These ablative procedures also destroy trabecular, endosteal, and periosteal nerve endings, which may relieve pain. Cryoablation is better tolerated than radiofrequency ablation. Recent developments allow for the procedure to be done under CT scan guidance.[36] Ethanol ablation is technically not difficult and can relieve pain within 24 to 48 hours in part due to neurolysis. However, alcohol can extravasate through cortical fractures into vital structures or intraarticular areas.[37] Ablative procedures can destabilize bone or cause fractures. Osteoplasty, vertebroplasty, and kyphoplasty reduce bone or spine pain and stabilize fractures. In addition, the heat derived from polymethyl methacrylate cement will destroy cortical and endosteal nerve endings and reduce pain. Patients with epidural tumor extension and cord compression due to vertebral bone fragments are not candidates for vertebroplasty or kyphoplasty.[37] Kyphoplasty differs from vertebroplasty in that a balloon tamp creates a void in the vertebral body and restores the height of the vertebral body that allows low pressure prior to installation of cement. Both vertebroplasty and kyphoplasty require placing needles either unilateral or bilateral via the transpedicular route into the anterior vertebral body.[38] The polymethyl methacrylate is usually combined with some contrast material for visualization during the procedure, and cement is injected in a viscous state to avoid or minimize extraosseous extravasation. Three to four levels can be done under sedation and local anesthetics. The polymethyl methacrylate stiffens the vertebral body to prevent micromotion and incident pain and strengthens the bone on weight bearing.[38]

Complications to osteoplasty, vertebroplasty, and kyphoplasty include cement leak that is frequently asymptomatic but can lead to radicular pain or neurologic deficits. Infections can result from the procedure or the adjacent vertebral body collapse from kyphoplasty.[39] Contraindications to vertebroplasty and kyphoplasty are listed in Table 6.

| Table 6. CONTRAINDICATIONS TO VERTEBROPLASTY AND KYPHOPLASTY[39] |
| --- |
| **Absolute** |
| Asymptomatic fracture |
| Osteomyelitis, ascites, active systemic infection |
| Allergy to bone cement |
| Uncorrectable coagulopathy |
| **Relative contraindications** |
| Radicular pain |
| Tumor extension into vertebral canal or cord compression |
| Fracture or loss of integrity of posterior vertebral cortex |
| Fracture > 70% collapse |
| Spinal canal stenosis or retropulsion of bone fragment into the spinal canal |
| Diffuse metastases |
| Lack of surgical back up |

Bisphosphonates have been used to prevent bone complications resulting from mRCC. Zoledronate improves osteopenia, reduces risk of fracture, and improves pain related to the metastases.[40,41] Benefits from bisphosphonates may not only be due to interference with osteoclast activation induced by receptor activation for nuclear factor κB released from tumor and stroma but also by reduction in vascular endothelial growth factor levels and antiangiogenesis.[42] Complications from bisphosphonates include transient fever, 1 to 2 days postadministration, related to release of tumor necrosis factor-α (TNF) and IL₆.[43] In addition, osteonecrosis of the jaw is reported with long-term use. Osteonecrosis of the jaw presents with oral facial pain and facial swelling. Mandibular bone is usually exposed on physical examination. The risk of osteonecrosis of the jaw increases if dental procedures are performed while patients are on bisphosphonates. Once occurring, it is refractory to medical management.

## LUNG METASTASES

Lung metastases are associated with the highest prevalence of spontaneous regressions. Isolated metastases if resectable should be removed after nephrectomy if presenting synchronously with the primary. Endobronchial lesions are treated with external beam radiation, intralumenal brachytherapy, and/or laser photocoagulation.[44,45] Such an approach will successfully treat hemophysis and dyspnea in > 80%. Radiation for endobronchial procedures will relieve postobstructive pneumonia secondary to endobronchial metastases.[44] Metastatic renal cell cancer to the lung mimics stage IV nonsmall cell lung cancer but is managed differently. Lung cancer is usually treated with chemotherapy, which is ineffective in mRCC, whereas aggressive surgical resection should be done for both the primary and lung lesions for mRCC.[46]

## BRAIN METASTASES

Brain metastases occur in 5% with a median time from diagnosis to discovery of brain metastases of 18 months.[47,48] Brain metastases frequently present simultaneously with lung metastases and hence restaging is necessary once brain metastases are discovered before considering craniotomy. Patients with a limited number of metastases and a good performance score and no or limited cancer outside of the central nervous system should undergo surgical resection and radiation rather than whole brain radiation.[49,50] For patients with limited number of metastases but who are not surgical candidates due to location within the brain or for medical reasons, gamma knife radiation should be considered. Gamma knife radiation improves response over whole brain radiation (96 vs 30%) and extends survival (15 vs 2 months).[49,51,52] Whole brain radiation does not add gamma knife radiation for tumor control. Nearly half of intracranial metastases from mRCC are found to be hemorrhagic at autopsy, and intracranial hemorrhage is not an uncommon clinical event. Anticoagulation is a significant risk in patients with untreated intracranial metastases.[47,48] Gamma knife radiation and/or surgery may prevent this devastating complication even if not curative. Combined resection, brain and lung, may be considered in patients with resectable isolated metastases to both organs and a good performance score. A good prognosis is associated with resection of all metastases (brain and lung) supratentorial location, lack of neurological deficit, and primary arising from the left kidney.[50] Median survival from craniotomy is 12 months, and the majority of deaths are due to progressive systemic metastases outside of the central nervous system.[50] Long-term survivors have been reported who have had resections of brain metastases.[53]

## UNUSUAL METASTATIC SITES ASSOCIATED WITH RENAL CELL CANCER

Renal cell cancer is the most common primary to spread to the thyroid. Patients may present with a goiter years after nephrectomy, and those with a diagnosis of clear cell carcinoma of the thyroid should have mRCC excluded.[22] The presumed pathway of spread to the thyroid is by way of the paravertebral venous plexus of Bateson. RCC is also the most common cancer to spread to the nasal structures and paranasal sinuses. This may be the initial presenting site, and the most common symptom is epistaxis.[22] Renal cell cancer in a significant minority of patients can spread to the pancreas and mistaken for a secondary primary. Vaginal metastases usually arise from the left kidney primary, which invade the ovarian vein and uterovaginal venous plexus.[22] Renal cancers can invade the spermatic vein and may present as a varicocele. This also usually arises from the left kidney.

## PALLIATION BY NEPHRECTOMY AND ABLATIVE PROCEDURES

Debulking the renal primary may prevent tumor shedding, palliate local symptoms (pain and hematuria), and reverse paraneoplastic syndromes.[54] The presence of the primary site acts as an immunologic sink for the production of proinflammatory cytokines, which prevents responses to IL$_2$. Patients who benefit from nephrectomy are those who are ECOG 0 to 1, do not have brain metastases, have lung metastases only, and have greater than 75% of their primary tumor removed by nephrectomy or partial nephrectomy.[54] Unfortunately, only a minority of patients with mRCC are candidates for debulking nephrectomy due to either poor performance status or unresectable primaries. Nephrectomy plus interferon is reported to improve survival over interferon alone. Recent developments in targeted tyrosine kinase inhibitors (sunitinib and sorafenib) have demonstrated superiority over α interferons such that α interferon is no longer used and a trial of either tyrosine kinase inhibitor would be reasonable after debulking nephrectomy.[55,56]

Nephrectomy can be done by open procedure, laparoscopy, or robotic techniques with or without hand assistance methods. Laparoscopy is less morbid.[57] Renal sparing procedures in the rare individual with mRCC and without a large primary may also be an option.

Chronic pain syndromes can occur as a surgical complication of retroperitoneal laparoscopy. Trochar injuries have been reported to the ilioinguinal, iliogastric, and subcostal nerves.[57] Mechanical or cautery injuries during dissection may damage the same group of nerves. Treatment includes gabapentin, tricyclic antidepressants, and opioids. Pain may gradually improve over a period of months.[57]

Renal infarction is usually done prior to nephrectomy in order to reduce bleeding and facilitate resection. Epidural analgesia may be helpful in managing postinfarction pain prior to nephrectomy or may be continued in order to manage postoperative pain in addition to postinfarction pain.[58] Preemptive analgesia with morphine, clonidine, and ketamine prior to transperitoneal nephrectomy does not improve postoperative pain or reduce postoperative analgesic requirements.[59]

For those individuals who cannot undergo nephrectomy, percutaneous CT scanned guided cryoablation or radiofrequency ablation may be used to destroy small primaries or relieve symptoms from larger primaries.[60–62] For large tumors, preablation catheter embolization of the primary may enhance response by decreasing blood flow and perfusion, which would adversely affect ablative temperatures.[60] Large primaries may require several sessions. Symptoms and quality of life are reported to improve with ablative procedures.[62] Ablative procedures may also reduce symptoms due to retroperitoneal intraabdominal or pulmonary recurrences not amenable to surgery or radiation therapy.[62]

## MANAGEMENT OF INDIVIDUAL SYMPTOMS

### Introduction

Communication is the key to effective palliation. Effective palliation involves prevention and relief of suffering, optimizing quality of life, bolstering family and patient coping skills and strategies, and establish a plan of care consistent with the goals of care and trajectory of cancer.[63] Communication skills that are key to accomplishing these goals involve four domains: advanced care planning, empathetically communicating bad news, negotiating goals of care within the context of patient autonomy and prognosis, and withholding and withdrawing ineffective medical technologies.[63] The time spent in communication with patients and families will be a time well spent. The lack of communication leads to multiple calls, unrelieved symptoms, and psychologic distress, as well as reduced patient and family satisfaction. Principles of good communication are outlined in Table 7.

## Table 7. STRATEGIES FOR GOOD COMMUNICATION IN ADVANCED CANCER

Establish eye contact
Body position on level with the patient
Quiet atmosphere with family present
Attend to psychologic content of the conversation
Respond to the patients emotion with compassion and
  understanding
Summarize the main points
Ask if there are other questions or concerns not addressed

### Pain

Pain management has been guided by the World Health Organization 3 step ladder for analgesic use in cancer. This guideline has been validated and provides flexibility in choices depending upon analgesic availability.[64] For mild pains, nonopioid analgesics, such as acetaminophen or nonsteroidal anti-inflammatory drugs (NSAIDs), are the first drugs of choice prior to adding an opioid for more intensive pain. Patients who present with severe pain should be started with an opioid, which is titrated to a response. Morphine is generally accepted as the opioid of choice for cancer pain.[64,65] One concern physicians may involve the use of NSAIDs for those who have had a nephrectomy or renal reduction surgery. NSAIDs block prostaglandins that are necessary to maintain renal vascularity and blood flow. The fear of bleeding and renal failure is a theoretic concern. However, ketorolac has been used to manage acute postoperative nephrectomy pain without undue toxicity. Postoperative pain is better controlled with ketorolac and an opioid than with an opioid alone.[66] Hence, nephrectomy is not a contraindication to the use of NSAIDs though this drug class should be used with caution.

Pain patterns are variable (continuous, intermittent, or continuous with flares of pain), which dictate the opioid dosing strategy. For continuous opioids, around the clock is given either normal release morphine every 4 hours or sustained release morphine every 12 to 24 hours.[65] Initial doses of morphine are 5 mg every 4 hours for normal release and 15 mg every 12 hours for sustained release morphine. Patients do have a wide range of opioid requirements, hence the dose should be titrated to response.[67] If pain is uncontrolled, doses should be

increased 30 to 50% depending on the response in pain severity.[64] Recommendations for rescue dosing are 25 to 50% of the 4 hourly dose, the same as the 4 hourly dose, and 10% of the daily dose.[64,65,68,69] There is no maximum or ceiling dose with a pure mu opioid receptor agonist. Doses should be titrated until pain relief or dose limiting side effects occur (confusion, visual hallucinations, myoclonus, or nausea or vomiting). Patients who have acute severe pain should be treated with small frequent parenteral doses of morphine (1 to 2 mg every 1 to 2 minutes by parenteral injection) until response. The dose which is effective is the dose required every 3 to 4 hours for pain control.[70]

A minority of patients develop dose limiting side effects before achieving pain relief with morphine. Switching to a different opioid (hydromorphone, fentanyl, oxycodone, or methadone) will produce pain relief and resolve side effects in > 50%.[71,72] Switching to methadone is difficult and should be done only by those with experience.[67] Switching the route of administration particularly to epidural or intrathecal opioids in combination with local anesthetics and/or clonidine can relieve pain unresponsive to systemic opioids and nonopioids.[67] Guidelines to switch opioid route and convert to an alternative opioid are provided in Tables 20c–8 and 9.

Patients with neuropathic pain usually require higher opioid doses and either anticonvulsants or antidepressants to control pain.[73] Gabapentin, pregabalin, tricyclic antidepressant, or the 2 selective norepinephrine serotonin reuptake inhibitors duloxetine or venlafaxine are first line choices as adjuvants to opioids or as initial treatment.

## Table 8. OPIOID SWITCH

| Opioid | Dose |
| --- | --- |
| Morphine | 10 mg (oral) |
| Oxycodone | 10 mg (oral) |
| Hydromorphone | 2 mg (oral) |
| Fentanyl | 75 mcg (parenteral) |
| Methadone | linear ratio dependent upon morphine dose |
| | 1:4 < 09 mg morphine/24 h |
| | 1:8 > 90 mg < 300 mg/24 h |
| | 1:12 > 300 mg < 1,000 mg/24 h |

| Table 9. OPIOID ROUTE CONVERSION | | |
|---|---|---|
| | Oral | Parenteral |
| Morphine | 3 | 1 (steady state) |
| Oxycodone | 2 | 1 |
| Hydromorphone | 2 | 1 (steady state) |
| Methadone | 2 | 1 |

| Table 10. ANTICACHEXINS |
|---|
| Pentoxifylline |
| Melatonin |
| Cyclo-oxygenase inhibitors |
| Thalidomide |
| Anticytokine antibodies |
| NFκB inhibitors |
| Anti-inflammatory cytokines (interleukin$_{12}$, interleukin$_{15}$) |

## Cachexia

Cancer induces host proinflammatory cytokines (IL$_1$, IL$_6$, and TNF-$\alpha$) and is also a source of cytokine specific tumor specific cachexins. Both groups of cytokines reduce muscle synthesis by activation of NFκB, which reduces expression of MyoD.[74,75] Muscle catabolism is accelerated through activation of ubiquitin-mediated proteolysis. Cancer cachexia is also associated with elevated resting energy expenditures, accelerated lipolysis, decreased lipoprotein lipase, and continuous gluconeogenesis. There is a failure to convert from glucose to fat as the main source of energy resulting in ongoing somatic protein catabolism as a source of glucose. Appetite is inhibited through IL$_1$ effects on the hypothalamus. Markers of inflammation (elevated CRP and hypoalbuminemia) will be found on blood tests.[74] Clinically, patients will be anemic, have significant weight loss, have anorexia, may develop cognitive dysfunction, and will eventually become frail. Families will frequently mistake this for starvation. Initial management involves an explanation of the differences between starvation and the cancer cachexia process to families who mistakenly believe a loved one is dying from lack of calories.

Nutritional support will not reverse the catabolic effect of cancer and does not reduce morbidity or mortality. A subset of patients with secondary nutritional failure due to caloric deprivation from dysphagia, bowel obstruction, malabsorption, or short gut syndrome will benefit from nutritional support.[74] Appetite stimulants (megestrol acetate, cannabinoids, and corticosteroids) may be helpful for those who complain of anorexia. Ghercin an orexigenic hormone derived from the stomach, may also stimulate appetites. There are no standard anticachexins recommended to reverse the weight loss though some hold promise.[76,77] Classes of cachexins are listed in Table 10.

## Depression

Depression occurs in 30% of those with an advanced cancer and should not be considered a normal response to a serious illness.[63] Signs and symptoms of anorexia, weight loss, and reduced appetite cannot be taken as an indicator of depression in cancer. Patients who are depressed will experience a sense of worthlessness, guilt, and anhedonia and may complain of insomnia as a manifestation of their depression. The screening question "are you depressed?" may be helpful if there is a suspicion of depression. Treatment should consist of supportive psychotherapy and pharmacology.[78] Selective serotonin reuptake inhibitors have been used as first line because there are fewer side effects compared with tricyclic antidepressants. Sertraline, citralopram, and the selective norepinephrine serotonin reuptake inhibitors venlafaxine and duloxetine have fewer drug interactions than paroxetine and fluoxetine.[63] For those with a short expected survival, the psychostimulant methylphenidate may produce relief of depression within days where standard antidepressants take weeks.[79]

## Delirium

The incidence of delirium increases as death approaches. Forty percent of those admitted to a palliative unit will have delirium, and 80 to 90% will develop delirium within 2 weeks of death.[80,81] Delirium may be hyperactive and associated with paranoi, hypoactive and mistaken for depression, or mixed hyperactive and hypoactive. Delirium is associated with disturbances in consciousness (and thus differs from dementia), acute changes in cognition, and lack of the ability to concentrate. The course of delirium evolves over a short time (which also differs from dementia) and may wax and wane being frequently worse at night. The causes of delirium include medications (opioids, anticholinergics, psychotropics, and sedatives), infection, metabolic disturbances (hypercalcemia, hyponatremia), hypoxemia, pain, alcohol or nicotine withdrawal, or unknown causes.[80,82] Treatment involves reversing the underlying cause if known. Haloperidol is the gold standard for treatment of those with hyperalert delirium and paranoia. Doses should be high doses (5 mg bolus, 1 mg each hour until response, or 5 mg twice daily) in order to obtain a rapid response. Haloperidol can be given parenterally (intravenous or subcutaneous) in those unable to take oral medications.[81,83] Olanzapine or risperidone is an alternative medications for those with extrapyramidal reactions to haloperidol. In those with refractory agitation (terminal delirium), switching to chlorpromazine or adding lorazepam to haloperidol may control agitation.[83] Palliative sedation may be required in a few. Phenobarbital starting with 300 mg continuous subcutaneous or intravenous over 24 hours may be effective when usual measures fail to relieve terminal delirium. Doses may be titrated for sedation. The treatment of hypoalert delirium has been less well studied, however, the cautious use of a psychostimulant, such as methylphenidate, has been reported to improve delirium.[83,84]

## CONCLUSIONS

Renal cell cancer is an unpredictable and highly symptomatic cancer that requires a multidisciplinary approach to effectively reduce suffering. Oncologic care should be combined with palliative therapies in advanced disease.

## REFERENCES

1. Whang Y, Godley PA. Renal cell carcinoma. Current Opin in Oncol 2003; 15:213–6.
2. Lee B, Dantzer R, Langley KE, et al. A cytokine based neuroimmunologic mechanism of cancer related symptoms. Neuroimmunomodulation 2004; 11:279–92.
3. Kim H, Han KR, Zisman A, et al. Cachexia like symptoms predict a worse prognosis in localized T1 renal cell carcinoma. J Urol 2004; 171:1810–13.
4. Shuch B, Lam JS, Belldegrun A, Figlin R. Prognostic factors in renal cell carcinoma. Semin Oncol 2006; 33:563–75.
5. Schijns O, Kurt E, Wessels P, et al. Intermedullary spinal cord metastasis as a first manifestation of renal cell carcinoma: report of a case review of the literature. Clin Neurol Neurosurg 2000; 102:249–54.
6. Schlomer R, Figenshau R, Yan Y, et al. Pathological features of renal neoplasms classified by size and symptomatology. J Urol 2006; 176:1317–20.
7. Lee C, Katz J, Fearn PA, Russo P. Mode of presentation of renal cell carcinoma provides prognostic informaiton. Urologic Oncol 2002; 7:135–40.
8. Schips L, Lipsky J, Zigeuner R, et al. Impact of tumor associated symptoms on the prognosis of patients with renal cell carcinoma: a single center experience of 683 patients. Urology 2003; 62:1024–8.
9. Palapattu G, Kristo B, Rajfer J. Paraneoplastic syndromes in urologic malignancy: the many faces of renal cell carcinoma. Reviews in Urology 2002; 4:163–70.
10. Giannakos G, Papanicolaou X, Trafalis D, et al. Stauffer's syndrome variant associated with renal cell carcinoma. Int J Urol 2005; 12:757–59.
11. Negrier S, Perol D, Menetrier-Caux C, et al. Ravaud Douillard JY Interleukin-6, interleukin-10 and vascular endothelial growth factor in metastatic renal cell carcinoma: prognostic value of interleukin-6 from the Groupe Francais d'Immunotherapie. J Clin Oncol 2004; 22: 2371–8.
12. Yoshida N, Ikemoto S, Narita K, et al. Interleukin-6, tumor necrosis factor α and interleukin-1be patients with renal cell carcinoma. Br J Cancer 2002; 86:1396–400.
13. Kallio J, Tammela TL, Marttinen AT, Kellokumpu-Lehtinen PL. Soluble immunological parameters and early prognosis of renal cell cancer patients. J Exp Clin Cancer Res 2001; 20:523–8.
14. Yasukawa K, Saito T, Fukungaga T, et al. Purificaiton and characterization of soluble human IL-6 receptor expressed in CHO cells. J Biochem 1990; 108:673–76.
15. Takenawa J, Kaneko Y, Okumura K, et al. Inhibitory effect of dexamethasone and progesterone in vitro on proliferation of human renal cell carcinomas and effects on expression of interleukin-6 or interleukin-6 receptor. J Urol 1995; 153:858–62.
16. Blay J, Negrier S, Combaret V, et al. Serum level of interleukin-6 as a prognostic factor in metastatic renal cell carcinoma. Cancer Res 1992; 52:3317–22.
17. Paule B, Clerc D, Rudant C, et al. Enchanced expression of interleukin-6 in bone and serum of metastatic renal cell carcinoma. Hum Pathol 1998; 29:421–4.
18. Trika M, Corringha R, Klein B, Rossi JF. Targeted anti-interleukin-6 monoclonal antibody therapy for cancer: a review of the rationale and clinical evidence. Clin Canc Res 2003; 9:4653–65.
19. Angelo L, Talpaz M, Kurzrock R. Autocrine interleukin6 production in renal cell carcinoma: evidence for the involvement of p53. Cancer Res 2002; 62:932–40.
20. Alberti L, Thomachot MC, Bachelot T, et al. IL-6 as an intracrine growth factor for renal carcinoma cell lines. Int J Cancer 2004; 111:653–61.
21. Passeri G, Girasole G, Uliette V, et al. Bisphosphonates inhibit IL-6 production by human osteoblastic cells MG 63. J Bone Miner Res 1994:S320.

22.  Papac R, Poo-Hwu WJ. A paradigm of lanthanic disease. Am J Clin Oncol 1999; 22:223–31.

23.  Fakih M, Schiff D, Erich R, Logan TF. Intramedullary spinal cord metastasis in renal cell carcinoma: a series of six cases. Ann Oncol 2001; 12:1173–7.

24.  Giacosa R, Santi R, Vaglio A, et al. Late regressions of metastases from renal cancer after a period of disease progression continuing the same intermittent low dose immunotherapy regimen. Acta Biomed Ateneo Parmense 2004; 75:126–30.

25.  Lipton A, Colombo-Berra A, Bukowski RM, et al. Skeletal complications in patietns with bone metastases from renal cell carcinoma and therapeutic benefits of zoledronic acid. Clin Canc Res 2004; 10:6397s–403s.

26.  Staudenherz A, Steiner B, Puig S, et al. Is there a diagnostic role for bone scanning of patients with a high pretest probability for metastatic renal cell carcinoma. Clin Canc Res 1999; 85:153–5.

27.  Koga S, Tsuda S, Nishikido M, et al. The diagnostic value of bone scan in patients with renal cell carcinoma. J Urol 2001; 166:2126–8.

28.  Adiga G, Dutcher JP, Larkin M, et al. Characterization of bone metastases in patients with renal cell cancer. BJU Intl 2004; 93:1237–40.

29.  Stepanek E, Josph S, Campbell P, Porter M. Embolization of a limb metastasis in renal cell carcinoma as a palliative treatment of bone pain. Royal College of Radiologiss 1999:855–7.

30.  Munro N, Woodhams S, Nawrocki JD, et al. The role of transarterial embolization in the treatment of renal cell carcinoma. BJU Intl 2003; 92:240–4.

31.  Kollender Y, Bickels J, Price WM, et al. Metastatic renal cell carcinoma of bone: indications and technique of surgical intervention. J of Oncol 2000; 164:1505–8.

32.  Kierney P, van Heerden JA, Segura JW, Weaver AL. Surgeon's role in the management of solitary renal cell carcinoma metastases occurring subsequent to initial curative nephrectomy: an institutional review. Ann Surg Oncol 1994; 1:345–52.

33.  Onufrey V, Mohiuddin M. Radiation therapy in the treatment of metastatic renal cell carcinoma. Int J Radiation Oncol Biol Phys 1985; 11:2007–9.

34.  Wilson D, Hiller L, Gray L, et al. The effect of biological effective dose on time to symptom progression in metastatic renal cell carcinoma. Clin Oncol 2003; 15:400–7.

35.  Wu J, Wong RK, Lloyd NS, et al. Radiotherapy fractionation for the palliation of uncomplicated painful bone metastases - an evidence based practice guideline. BMC Cancer 2004; 4:71.

36.  Allaf M, Shayani S, Inagaki T, et al. Pain control requirements for percutaneous ablation of renal tumors: cryoablation versus radiofrequency ablation - initial observations. Radiology 2005; 237:366–70.

37.  Sabharwal T, Salter R, Adam A, Gangi A. Image guided therapies in orthopedic oncology. Orthop Clin N Am 2006; 37:105–12.

38.  Truumees E, Hilibrand A, Vaccaro A. Percutaneous vertebral augmentation. The Spine Journal 2004; 4:218–29.

39.  Gangi A, Sabharwal T, Irani F, et al. Quality assurance guidelines for percutaneous vertebroplasty. Cardiovasc Intervent Radiol 2006; 29:173–78.

40.  Michaelson M, Rosenthal DI, Smith MR. Long-term bisphosphonate treatment of bone metastases from renal cell carcinoma.

41.  Lipton A, Zheng M, Seaman J. Zoledronic acid delays the onset of skeletal related events and progression of skeletal disease in patients with advanced renal cell carcinoma. Cancer 2003; 98:962–69.

42.  Urch C. The pathophysiology of cancer induced bone pain: current understanding. Pall med 2004; 18:267–74.

43.  Dicuonzo G, Vincenzi B, Santini D, et al. Fever after zolendronic acid administration is due to increase in TNFα and IL-6. J Interferon Cytokine Res 2003; 23:649–54.

44.  Raju P, Roy T, McDonald RD, et al. IR-192 low dose rate endobronchial brachytherapy in the treatment of malignant airway obstruction. Int J Radiation Oncol Biol Phys 1993; 27:677–80.

45.  Hansen G, Sundset A. Transbronchial laser ablation of benign and malignant tumors. Minim Invasive Ther Allied Technol 2006; 15:4–8.

46.  Griniatsos J, Michail PO, Menenakos C, et al. Metastatic renal clear cell carcinoma mimicking stage IV lung cancer. Int Urol Nephrol 2003; 35:15–7.

47.  Harada Y, Nonomura N, Kondo M, et al. Clinical study of brain metastasis of renal cell carcinoma. Eur Urology 1999; 36:230–5.

48.  Yamanaka K, Gohji K, Hara I, et al. Clinical study of renal cell carcinoma with brain metastases. Int J of Urol 1998; 5:124–8.

49.  Maor M, Frias AE, Oswald MJ. Palliative radiotherapy for brain metastases in renal carcinoma. Clin Canc Res 1988; 62:1912–7.

50.  Wronski M, Arbit E, Russo P, Galicich GH. Surgical resection of brain metastases from renal cell carcinoma in 50 patients. J of Urol 1996; 47:187–93.

51.  Sheehan J, Sun MH, Kondziolka D, et al. Radiosurgery in patients with renal cell carcinoma metastasis to the brain: long term outcomes and prognostic factors influencing survival and local tumor control. J of Neurosurg 2003; 98:342–9.

52.  Hugeunin P, Kieser S, Glanzmann C, et al. Radiotherapy for metastatic carcinomas of the kidney or melanomas: an analysis using palliative end points. Int J Radiation Oncol Biol Phys 1998; 41:401–5.

53.  Hall W, Djalilian HR, Nussbaum ES, Cho KH. Long term survival with metastatic cancer to the brain. Med Oncol 2000; 17:279–86.

54.  Flanigan R. Debulking nephrectomy in metastatic renal cancer. Clin Canc Res 2004; 10:6335s–41s.

55.  Halbert R, Figlin R, Atkins M, et al. Treatment of patients with metastatic renal cell cancer. Cancer 2006; 107: 2375–83.

56.  Bankhead C. Three new drugs available to fight kidney cancer. J Natl Cancer Inst 2006; 98:1181.

57.  Oefelein M, Bayazit Y. Chronic pain syndrome after laparoscopic radical nephrectomy. J of Urol 2003; 170: 1939–40.

58.  Jordan G, Babcock NC, Mocnik JJ, Lynch DF. Pain control following renal infraction/ablation using continuous epidural combined anesthesia/analgesia. J Urol 1983; 130: 861–2.

59. Holthusen H, Backhaus P, Boeminghaus F, et al. Preemptive analgesia; no relevant advantage of preoperative compared with postoperative intravenous administration of morphine, ketamine, and clonidine in patients undergoing transperitoneal tumor nephrectomy. Reg Anesth Pain Med 2002; 27:249–53.

60. Gervais D, Arellano RS, Mueller PR. Percutaneous radiofrequency ablation of renal cell carcinoma. Eur Radiol 2005; 15:960–7.

61. Wagner A, Solomon SB, Li-Ming S. Treatment of renal tumors with radiofrequency ablation. J Endourology 2005; 19:643–53.

62. Zagoria R. Percutaneous image guided radiofrequency ablation. Radiol Clin N Am 2003; 41:1067–75.

63. Morrison L, Morris RS. Palliative Care and Pain Management. Med Clin N Am 2006; 90:983–1004.

64. Quigley C. The role of opioids in cancer pain. BMJ 2005; 331:825–29.

65. Hanks G, de Conno F, Cherny N, et al. Morphine and alternative opioids in cancer pain: the EAPC recommendations. Br J Cancer 2001; 94:587–93.

66. DiBiase S, Valicenti RK, Schultz D, et al. Palliative irradiation for focally symptomatic metastatic renal cell carcinoma: support for dose escalation based on a biological model. J of Urol 1997; 158:746–9.

67. Hanks G, Reid C. Contribution to variability in response to opioids. Support Care Cancer 2005; 13:145–52.

68. Portenoy R, Lesage P. Management of cancer pain. The Lancet 1999; 353:1695–1700.

69. Portenoy R, Payne D, Jacobsen P. Breakthrough pain: characteristics and impact in patients with cancer pain. Pain 1999; 81:129–34.

70. Davis M, Weissman D, Arnold R. Opioid dose titration for severe cancer pain: a systematic evidence based review. J Palliat Med 2004; 7:462–68.

71. Mercadante S. Opioid rotation for cancer pain. Cancer 1999; 86:1856–66.

72. Mercadante S, Bruera E. Opioid switching: a systematic and critical review. Cancer Treatment Reviews 2006; 32:304–15.

73. Davis M. What is new in neuropathic pain? Support Care Cancer 2006; 11.

74. Morley J, Thomas DR, Wilson MMG. Cachexia: pathophysiology and clinical relevance. Am J Clin Nutr 2006; 83:735–43.

75. Saini A, Nasser A, Stewart C. Waste management-cytokines, growth factors and cachexia. Cytokine & Growth Factor Reviews 2006; 17:475–86.

76. Boddaert M, Gerritsen WR, Pinedo H. On our way to targeted therapy for cachexia in cancer? Curr Opin Oncol 2006; 18:335–40.

77. Elamin E, Glass M, Camporesi E. Pharmacological approaches to ameliorating catabolic conditions. Curr Opin Clin Nutr Metab Care 2006; 9:449–54.

78. Williams S, Dale J. The effectiveness of treatment for depression/depressive symptoms in adults with cancer: a systematic review. Br J Cancer 2006; 94:372–90.

79. Sood A, Barton DL, Loprinzi CL. Use of methylphenidate in patients with cancer. Am J Hosp Palliat Care 2006; 23:35–40.

80. Lagman R, Davis MP, LeGrand SB, Walsh D. Common symptoms in advanced cancer. Surg Clin N Am 2005; 85:237–55.

81. Casarett D, Inouye SK. Diagnosis and management of delirium near the end of life. Ann Intern Med 2001; 135:32–40.

82. Caraceni A. Management in delirium. In: Grassil. Oxford: Oxford University Press; 2003. p. 131–57.

83. Stagno D, Gibson C, Breitbart W. The delirium subtypes: a review of prevalence, phenomenology, pathophysiology, and treatment response. Pall and Supportive Care 2004; 2:171–79.

84. Gagnon B, Low G, Schreier G. Methylphenidate hydrochloride improves cognitive function in patients with advanced cancer and hypoactive delirium: a prospective clinical study. J Psychiatr Neurosci 2005; 30:100–7.

# Index

Page numbers followed by f indicate figure. Page numbers followed by t indicate table.